REA's
Authoritative Guide to
MEDICAL
& DENTAL
SCHOOLS

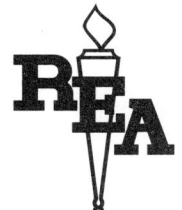 *Research & Education Association*

REA's Authoritative Guide to
MEDICAL & DENTAL SCHOOLS

Printed in the United States of America

Library of Congress Catalog Card Number 91-62039

International Standard Book Number 0-87891-874-4

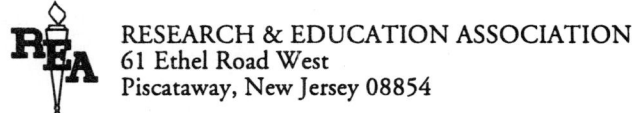 RESEARCH & EDUCATION ASSOCIATION
61 Ethel Road West
Piscataway, New Jersey 08854

PREFACE

This book was designed to help you, the prospective medical or dental school student, gain insight into the admissions process while learning about all types of medial and dental school programs. The guide contains profiles on every accredited medical, osteopathic, dental, chiropractic, and podiatric school in the United States and Canada, as well as information on how to apply to foreign medical schools.

At the beginning of each chapter you will find "At-a-Glance" statistical charts which allow you to easily and quickly compare facts on each school. The charts are then followed by detailed profiles of the schools which will help you narrow your decision in making your final selections of schools.

For greater insight into what to expect in the first year of medical or dental school, read the personal essays of two former students who share their unique experiences in a candid and forthright style. Tips on the admission process and what schools seek in reviewing applications can be discovered in the section written by our Pre-Med Advisor and Expert from Northern Kentucky University. Career options in various medical fields are also discussed in this section.

In addition, sections are provided on financial aid, the philosophy of osteopathic medicine, and careers in podiatry, and chiropractic medicine.

Applying to medical or dental school can be a difficult process, but with this book you will be able to make well-informed, educated choices about your professional health education.

ABOUT RESEARCH AND EDUCATION ASSOCIATION

Research and Education Association (REA) is an organization of educators, scientists, and engineers who specialize in various academic fields. REA was founded in 1959 for the purpose of disseminating the most recently developed scientific information to groups in industry, government, and universities. Since then, REA has become a successful and highly respected publisher of study aids, test preps, handbooks, and reference works.

Our Problem Solver series covers a wide range of topics in the sciences, social sciences, and mathematics. Each book is approximately 1000 pages and covers every type of problem in a step-by-step format. Our handbooks and references in math, science, and various technologies cover topics from a variety of fields that are current and of special interest.

Our Essentials series covers a variety of subjects including math, the physical and social sciences, statistics, business, accounting, computer sciences, economics, and history. Each book provides quick and easy access to critical information without the inconvenience of a large volume.

Our test prep series extensively prepares students and professionals for the Medical College Admission Test (MCAT), the Graduate Record Examinations (GRE), the Graduate Management Admission Test (GMAT), Fundamentals of Engineering Test (FE), Scholastic Aptitude Test (SAT), as well as the TOEFL and the Advanced Placement exams.

REA's publications and educational materials are highly regarded for their significant contribution to the quest for excellence that characterizes today's educational goals. We continually receive an unprecedented amount of praise from professionals, instructors, librarians, parents, and students for our books. Our authors are as diverse as the subjects and fields represented in the books we publish. They are well-known in their respective fields and serve on the faculties of prestigious universities throughout the United States.

ACKNOWLEDGMENTS

Special recognition is extended to the following persons:

Carl Fuchs, Director of Operations, for his overall guidance which has brought this publication to completion.

Rochelle L. Stern, Managing Editor, for coordinating the editorial staff throughout each phase of the project.

Judy Walters, Senior Editor, for her editorial contributions and management of the project.

Elizabeth Fili, Ellen Gong, and Susan Kennedy, for their editorial contributions.

Chris Martin, of the American Osteopathic Association, for additional help and suggestions.

Bruce Hanson, Graphic Design Manager, for the cover and interior book design.

Marty Perzan, for creating the database system and typesetting the manuscript.

TABLE OF CONTENTS

TABLE OF CONTENTS – ALPHABETICAL LISTING

U.S. Medical Schools

Canadian Medical Schools

Osteopathic Schools

Podiatric Schools

Chiropractic Schools

U.S. Dental Schools

Canadian Dental Schools

TABLE OF CONTENTS – BY STATE

U.S. Medical Schools

Canadian Medical Schools

Osteopathic Schools

Podiatric

Chiropractic

U.S. Dental Schools

Canadian Dental Schools

CHAPTER 1

Introduction

KEY TO THE CHARTS BEFORE EACH SCHOOL PROFILE

This key is designed to help you interpret the information given in the charts on each individual school. The categories are listed under each school and are as follows:

Accreditation refers to the institution accrediting the school. All U.S. medical schools in this book are accredited by the AAMC. All U.S. dental schools are accredited by the CDA. All other accreditations are on an individual basis, for example, by regional or other accrediting institutions.

Degrees offered refers to any degree a candidate may earn through the medical school. Joint programs consist of two degrees indicated by a slash: i.e., M.D./M.P.H.

 # Students Applied refers to the number of applicants who applied to that school for the school year 1991-1992. When 1991-1992 statistics were unavailable, data from the previous year has been used.

Enrollment refers to the number of matriculated students per class, except where the word "class" does not appear. In such cases, the figure represents the enrollment for the entire school.

UNIVERSITY OF CONNECTICUT SCHOOL OF MEDICINE

263 Farmington Avenue
Farmington, Connecticut 06030
(203) 679-2413

Accreditation	AAMC
Degrees Offered	M.D., M.S., Ph.D.
# Students Applied	1,596
Enrollment	Not Available
Mean GPA	3.48
% Men / % Women	53% / 47%
% Minorities	10%
Tuition	$5,550 In-State
	$12,300 Out-of-State
Application Fee	$50
Application Deadline	December 15

Mean G.P.A. refers to the mean grade point average for students accepted into the most recent freshman class.

Men/Women Ratio refers to the ratio of men to women matriculated in the most recent freshman class.

Minorities % refers to the percentage of minority students enrolled in the most recent freshman class based on the total enrollment of that class.

In-State Tuition is the tuition for permanent residents of the state in which the school is located.

Out-of-State Tuition is the tuition for students living in a state other than that in which the school is located. (Private schools have a set tuition rate for all students, regardless of residency.)

The **Application Fee** is the fee you must pay in order to process your application to that school.

The **Application Deadline** is the date by when the admissions department must receive your application.

FINANCING YOUR MEDICAL OR DENTAL EDUCATION

Deciding whether to apply to medical or dental school is not only about if you can get in, handle the work, and handle the pressure for four years. Another serious consideration to make is whether or not you can afford to go to medical school. Since few students (and their families) can afford to pay for a graduate health program without some sort of assistance, you will find that you are in good company as you wrestle with the question of how you will pay for your education. Medical and dental schools have high tuition costs, and with the cost of living, new medical books and tools, and the fact that students are discouraged from working to supplement their income during school, it is no wonder that financial aid is a major issue when contemplating medical or dental school.

As you'll see from the students who have described their experiences with medical and dental school, the key to practical financing appears to be in borrowing a minimum of money. While that may seem obvious, too many times students end up borrowing too much, with high repayments later. This leads to less money when you graduate, less money on which to live, and less money with which to begin your practice.

You can restrict your indebtedness by taking a number of positive steps. First of all, consider a public university. As a rule, public universities, which are always at least partially funded by the state, offer more competitive tuition rates. This means you will be paying less tuition for a quality education.

The best choice you can make with respect to your financial needs is to choose the medical school in your state. This will save you even more money. Although all state universities tend to be less expensive than private institutions, the medical school in your state will be even more economical for you. You will have to pay extra tuition to attend an out-of-state school. If you stick to in-state public schools, your tuition will be that much less.

You can also reduce your expenses by choosing a medical or dental school in a suburban area. Suburban areas, as a rule, are less expensive to live in than cities. When it comes time to find your living arrangements, you will discover that your dollar stretches a lot further in suburbia than in the cities. The same goes for food, car insurance, and the overall cost of living. Remember that the cost of medical school is not simply the tuition. When you take out loans, you will not only be financing your education, but also your life style.

There are many types of loans available to medical and dental students. First of all, there are five types of federal loan programs from which to choose. They are HPSL, Perkins, Stafford, HEAL, and SLS. Each has advantages and disadvantages. Where one student may find one loan perfect, another student may find the same loan inappropriate for his or her needs. Keep this in mind as you are introduced to each type of loan.

Health Professions Student Loans (HPSL)—These are need-based loans which can be attained through your school's financial aid office. You must be a U.S. citizen, U.S. national, or a U.S. permanent resident to apply. These loans will supply you with tuition plus $2,500 for living expenses. There is a 5 percent interest rate, but no interest accrues while you are in school, during deferment periods (internship, residency, up to three years of military duty, Public Health Service Corps, and Peace Corps, or two years of full-time approved educational activity). You have an automatic grace period of one year following graduation. There are no pre-payment penalties.

Perkins Loans—These are need-based loans which can be attained through your school's financial aid office. You must be a U.S. citizen, U.S. national, or U.S. permanent resident to be eligible. You can borrow up to $18,000 for your total schooling with these loans (includes undergraduate and graduate education). The rate of this loan is 5 percent, and no interest accrues while you are in school, during the nine-month grace period following graduation, or during deferments. (Deferments include up to three years active military duty, participation in the Public Health Service Corps, AC-TION/Peace Corps, temporary disability, two years of internship and residence training, up to six months of parental leave, or at least part-time student status.) There are no pre-payment penalties.

Stafford Loans—These are need-based loans which can be financed through a bank or state guarantee agency. You must be a U.S. citizen, U.S. national, or U.S. permanent resident in order to be eligible. The loan will supply you with $7,500 per year, with a total of no more than $54,750 for your entire schooling (includes undergraduate and graduate education). The rate of this loan is eight percent for the first four years of repayment, and 10 percent for each year thereafter. No interest accrues during school, the grace period (six months after graduation), or deferments. (Deferments include three years active military duty, service in the Public Health Service Corps, ACTION/Peace Corps, or the National Oceanic and Atmospheric Administration (NOAA), up to two years of internship/residency or unemployment, the care of a dependent, or part-time student status if the student has a Stafford or PLUS/SLS loan for that period.) There are no prepayment penalties.

Health Education Assistance Loans (HEAL)—These are need-based loans which can be financed through a bank or a state guarantee agency. You must be a U.S. citizen, U.S. national, or U.S. permanent resident in order to qualify. You can borrow up to $20,000 per year, with a total of $80,000. The interest rate can be variable or fixed on a 91-day Treasury Bill plus three percent. Interest does accrue during your schooling, the nine month grace period after graduation, and deferments. (Deferments include up to four years for internship and residency, three years for active military duty, Public Health Service Corps, ACTION/Peace Corps Service, and up to two years of a full-time educational activity.) There are no pre-payment penalties.

Supplemental Loans for Students (SLS)—These are not need-based loans and can be acquired through a bank or state guarantee agency. You must be a U.S. citizen, U.S. national, or U.S. permanent resident to qualify. You may borrow up to $4,000 a year with a total of no more than $20,000. The interest rate is variable. Interest accrues during school, and during deferments, which include up to three years active military duty, Public Health Service Corps, ACTION/Peace Corps, NOAA Corps service, temporary disability, care of a dependent, up to two years for internship and residency, up to six months for parental leave, or part-time student status if the student has a GSL, or PLUS/SLS loan for that period. There is no grace period after you graduate, and there is no prepayment penalty.

Federal loans are not the only way to secure finances for your medical or dental education. You can contact state agencies and nonprofit medical organizations (such as the American Heart Association, for example). Many of these organizations offer scholarships for medical and dental students. These scholarships may or may not be need-based, and are usually determined on some other qualification such as grades or specialty area of medicine/dentistry which the student wishes to pursue.

Additional scholarship sources can come from other nonprofit organizations such as womens' and minority groups and service organizations. These may or may not be need based, and are usually based on a qualification such as grades or specialty area of medicine/dentistry which the student wishes to pursue.

The Armed Services also offers financial assistance for men and women students who will pay back the money through service in one of the armed forces. This is not traditional financial aid where you borrow money which is paid back with interest. Instead, you give your time as a form of repayment.

Finally, be aware that you should always check with the financial aid office at your school. This is a good place to start your search for appropriate financial aid. Financial aid officers are trained to know where the money is and how to get it. A good financial aid officer will help you to find many sources of loans, scholarships, and other financial assistance as a combination package rather than focusing solely on one form of assistance. Your goal is to get the money you need with the least indebtedness possible.

CHAPTER 2

Medical Schools

TRENDS IN MEDICAL SCHOOL APPLICANTS

The number of medical school applicants is on the rise. The 1980s saw a decline in applications, but this appears to be reversing. For example, the number of students increased nine percent between 1989 and 1990. Since medicine has always been seen as a profession with financial and job security, the increase may be due to the recession the United States has been experiencing in the early part of the decade. Entering an advanced program such as medical school may avoid a job search during slower economic times while it also secures a good profession.

Not only are the number of applicants changing, the types of applicants desiring to become doctors are changing as well. For example, more women are entering medical school. In the school year 1970-71, there were 827 female applicants, as compared with a total of 5,584 female applicants in 1990-91. While the statistical average is 40.3 percent of female applicants, based on all U.S. medical schools, there could be as few as 17 percent or as many as 51 percent of women students at an individual school.

The number of minority applicants is also increasing. There were 591 Afro-American non-Hispanic female applicants in 1986-87, as compared to 701 in 1990-91. Between 1986 and 1990, the number of Asian/Pacific Islander men increased by over 600. During the same period, the number of Asian/Pacific Islander women increased by over 400. Minority applications appear to be on the rise.

The academic background of the applicants is also shifting. While most applicants are biology or chemistry majors, medical schools are now admitting more liberal arts majors. There is no reason why a liberal arts major cannot perform in a science-oriented environment, provided he or she has performed well in undergraduate science courses. This new trend is also evident in the revised Medical College Admissions Test (MCAT), which now includes an increased emphasis on liberal arts, in addition to the sciences.

Applicants are not the only people at medical school who have undergone a significant change. The educators have also been experiencing some changes. During the 1980s, medical educators suggested fundamental changes in the medical school curriculum. Medical educators now stress greater contact with patients, and less with textbooks. From 1980 to 1990, there was a 43 percent growth in clinical medical school faculty, which shows that there is a trend towards "hands-on" experience rather than textbook instruction.

Things are changing in the classroom as well as in the clinics. There is now more small-group teaching as compared to the typical "lecture-style" teaching of the past. More importantly, educators are concentrating on making textbook learning directly related to clinical experience by presenting real-life patient cases in the classroom. This encourages students to feel that what they learn in the classroom will have a visible effect on their patients. Textbook instruction has also been expanded to include an emphasis on social and ethical issues, making students more aware of the human side of being a physician.

Medical schools are becoming increasingly innovative in their instruction, also. New methods are giving students the chance to use what they have learned, rather than just answer objective questions. With methods such as multiple-station, "lab-practical" type exams, students can show their strengths and weaknesses through performance in actual situations.

There have also been significant trends in the financial aspects of attending medical school. The poor economy in the United States has reduced grants and contracts to only 25 percent of the total medical school revenue. Thirty years ago, these grants and contracts made up 50 percent of total revenue. Because of this forced reduction of revenue, tuition has increased greatly. In 1990-91, private school tuition increased by 33 percent. Tuition for an in-state public school student increased by 48 percent. Out-of-state tuition increased by 67 percent.

As you can see, medical education has undergone many changes since the 1980s. The number of women and minorities entering the field has increased. Patient-physician interaction has now become more valued than in the past. Medical education expenses have risen immensely, forcing tuition to increase.

You may want to take all these current medical profession trends into consideration when choosing your medical school. Choose the school that you feel can best help you meet your personal goals and objectives. This book will guide you with the first step in your medical career—your medical education.

COMMENTS FROM A PREMEDICAL ADVISOR

by Larry A. Giesmann, Ph.D.

What is a "Pre-med"?

Pre-medicine is a state of mind. It is not a curriculum, and it should not be an undergraduate major. Medical schools no longer favor or, in many cases, even accept, an undergraduate major identified as pre-med, and most undergraduate programs no longer offer this major. However, many undergraduate schools and most students have not yet accepted the reality that medical schools are now looking for applicants with a broad academic background that includes coursework in the natural sciences, social sciences, and the humanities. Specific course requirements (addressed later in this section) are few in number and allow consideration of applicants from a wide variety of disciplines.

The undergraduate or pre-professional years of preparation for a career in medicine should be a period of self discovery. During this time, a person considering medical school needs to determine if he or she possesses the attributes necessary to be successful in medical school and, by extension, to be content with the life of a physician.

A person who considers himself or herself to be a "pre-med" must enjoy being in school. This should be obvious to anyone who is in the pre-med state of mind, but for various reasons it is not. Far too many undergraduates have set acceptance into medical school as their goal. Once this goal is achieved, these individuals are often distressed to realize that they have four years of medical school and three to seven years of graduate medical education—a total of seven to 11 years of education—to complete before entering the practice that they envision. In fact, the educational process never ends. In addition to daily reading and formal continuing education programs, a practicing physician may have to prepare for and pass a certification exam periodically. Any change in specialty naturally requires additional education and examination.

An important part of the pre-med state of mind is understanding and being comfortable with delayed gratification. The current younger generation, and probably every previous younger generation, has been accused of being material-conscious, impatient, lazy, and generally not willing to work for their rewards. In the case of medical education, this may be true. Given the time commitment for formal education alone—four years of undergraduate school, four years of medical school, and three to seven years of graduate medical education—few people of any generation can be expected to accept such a challenge. The middle class life styles anticipated by many college students must be delayed by at least 10 years—well into residency training—for those who chose a career in medicine. The life style generally associated with a physician comes even later for some. During this time, former classmates and friends are well into family, career, and social success. Being content to delay gratification of one's personal wants in order to pursue career preparation is perhaps the most subtle of all the attributes of a successful pre-med student.

A part of the medical educational process that is least expected by undergraduates is the teaching role that physicians, residents, and even medical students must play. In fact, after a certain point in formal coursework, teaching may be the most effective way of learning. The location of the teaching varies—in seminars, at the bedside, in consultation, on patient rounds, in the classroom and laboratory—but the behavior continues throughout a physician's career. Some do it informally while others formalize the process and become teaching faculty at medical schools (usually in addition to their own practice), but all doctors teach. An undergraduate can easily discover whether he or she likes the teaching experience by serving as a tutor, working as an undergraduate laboratory teaching assistant (some colleges offer credit for this work), or simply by being active in group study.

Being a physician is difficult work, with long and/or unusual hours compared to many other professions. Most pre-med students understand this because of their knowledge of the medical profession. To be fully aware of the workload of a physician, however, one must spend some time in a health care environment. A pre-med has the responsibility of exploring the time commitment involved in medicine, and most admissions committees will expect to see evidence to this effect. Employment or volunteer experience in a hospital or other formal health care facility is generally the type of activity that best exposes students to the reality of a physician's professional life. While an internist may spend "only" 60 to 80 hours a week on the job, a surgeon may routinely work 80 to 100 hours. The actual numbers vary, of course, but one must understand the intensity and length of the typical physician's work schedule before making an intelligent decision about entering the profession.

A necessary practical consideration for most medical students is the willingness to assume large personal debt. For those members of the 1990 M.D. graduating class who had borrowed money to attend medical school, the average debt was about $46,000.[1] Indebtedness of $100,000 to $200,000 or more is possible for medical school graduates. While medical schools will tell applicants that no one is denied admission because of financial reasons, it is also true that a person aspiring to be a physician must be willing to commit future income to pay the expenses of medical school. While it is not necessary to become destitute, life style adjustments alluded to earlier must be willingly made. Becoming a pre-med means that the decision to invest in one's own future has also been accepted.

1. *AAMC 1992–93 Medical School Admissions Requirements.* 1991. Assoc. Amer. Med. Schools, Washington, D.C.

A final attribute valuable to a person desiring to become a physician is the ability to accept failure—the top student in high school may not be the best in his or her college class, the outstanding college graduate will probably not be at the top of the class in medical school, a resident may fail to fully comply with instructions of the attending physician. The physician's greatest failure is losing a patient. Even though it is the ultimate fate of every human, each physician must deal with the death of a patient in her or his own way, and reconcile doubts and decisions made in the course of treatment. The way that a pre-med student addresses failure in academic or personal affairs may be indicative of how comfortable life as a physician will be.

Why then, given this arduous and rigorous regimen, choose to become a physician? The practice of medicine is unique among professions. It presents the lifelong opportunity to practice a science in a social setting, to be intellectually challenged, and to be emotionally fulfilled. The real rewards of healing the human body or mind, assisting in the beginning of a new life, or improving the wellness of a patient are intangible but very powerful. No career is more satisfying than one which serves others, and a career in medicine serves most richly.

When to Choose a Specialty

Although it is important to think about what medical specialty or subspecialty one would like to practice, too many undergraduates enter the period of preparation for medical studies unduly concerned about this and other career considerations. Decisions about specialties, and the subsequent choice of an institution for the necessary graduate medical education, are probably best made while in medical school, not during undergraduate studies. Likewise, deciding which medical school to attend should be done during the latter part of one's undergraduate education, not while the student is in high school. While there are reasonable exceptions to this advice, as a general rule, one should take all available time to make decisions regarding career choice and training.

Undergraduate Curriculum

The first big decision a student must make is the choice of an undergraduate college. Most accredited schools have a pre-medical program of studies, and all of those will be glad to discuss their particular strengths. The prospective undergraduate student needs to examine a variety of factors: tuition and other costs, size of student body, geographic location, and academic reputation are just a few things that need to be considered. A visit to the campus and meetings with admissions personnel and a pre-medical advisor will help assess the "fit" between a student and an institution.

It is also very important to contact medical schools that regularly accept students from a given institution to find out how graduates of that institution perform in medical school relative to other students. Admissions officers and student affairs staff from medical schools probably have a better idea of the level of preparation received at undergraduate schools than anyone and will usually speak positively about the best places to obtain the necessary undergraduate education.

There are more than 120 medical colleges and schools in the United States. Most require a baccalaureate degree for entrance into their M.D. programs, although some will occasionally accept a student prior to completion of the B.S. or B.A. In addition, there are about two dozen schools that offer acceptance into a combined undergraduate/M.D. program to selected high school seniors.

Generally, the undergraduate curriculum is expected to include a year of biology, two years of chemistry (general and organic), and a year of physics. Competence in English and mathematics are also emphasized, although the requirement of specific courses, such as calculus, has gradually declined over the past decade. Increasingly, medical schools are favoring students with broad interests and coursework in nonscience content areas, to the extent that applicants with majors outside the biological and social sciences have equal or higher rates of acceptance.

The rigid pre-med course schedule of the past has been replaced with a flexible, cross-disciplinary approach that allows undergraduates to explore and experience courses in humanities, behavioral and social sciences, and the fine arts. Since undergraduate school usually presents the last occasion for physicians to study these subjects in any depth, someone considering medical school should take advantage of the opportunity. A broad-based curriculum has the additional advantage of presenting more options to the student who eventually chooses not to apply to medical school or is not accepted into a program of medical study. The curriculum is one of the best sources of information for a student's decisions about future directions, whether they involve career choices or simply which courses to take next term.

Most medical schools do not recommend that students take advanced-level science courses in subjects that are normally covered in medical school unless those courses are required for the undergraduate major. Enrolling in such courses with the exclusive purpose of improving chances for admission is unwise. On the other hand, successful completion of upper-division science courses demonstrates academic competence in difficult content areas. For someone with a poor early academic record or who has been out of school for some time, certain advanced science courses may be essential. Conversations with residents and current medical students reveal that upper-division undergraduate courses in biochemistry, animal or human physiology, histology, and embryology are especially valuable in dealing with the course content and methodologies encountered in the first two years of medical school; other undergraduate courses may be individually recommended. In any case, decisions regarding taking such courses should be made only after consulting your pre-med advisor and the admissions officers of the medical schools in which you are interested.

The Non-Traditional Student

Aggregate data for the 1990-91 medical school entering classes show that the mean age for accepted applicants was 23.8 years; six percent of that entering class was 32 years or older.[2] Although the acceptance rate for the 32 years-and-older group was lower than that for all applicants combined (39 percent vs. 58 percent), it is clear that chronological age alone is not an impediment to acceptance into medical school.

Non-traditional pre-med students have generally been out of school for a period of years, may be coming from careers other than the health professions, may have an early history of poor or inappropriate academic work, and may have commitments that effectively restrict their geographic mobility. For these reasons, it is essential that they consult an admissions officer at the medical school(s) they are most likely to attend. Since these students will almost certainly need to take additional coursework, probably at the undergraduate level, they should also talk to an undergraduate pre-med advisor. This person can help assess individual strengths and needs, an essential part of the strategy since each non-traditional student presents a unique experiential package.

A problem of special importance to non-traditional pre-med students is that of changes in life styles. Becoming a physician will forever change the way an individual deals with the rest of the world. Furthermore, the changes in life style that begin in medical school, and undergraduate preparation for medical school, are even more profound than those for traditional students who have just completed an uninterrupted high school and college education.

There are two principal reasons that a non-traditional student has more difficult adjustments to make in the process of becoming a physician. First is the fact that the individual is usually leaving a career in which he or she has already invested considerable time and money. Abandoning an existing career, or even admitting that the choice of that career was not appropriate, is often very difficult. In addition, colleagues or superiors may resent or be jealous of one's decision to strike out "at your age" in a new and potentially more rewarding profession. The reactions of these people and other possible consequences must be considered and dealt with if one is to make the career transition.

The second reason it is more difficult for a non-traditional student to make life style adjustments involves commitments to and responsibilities for other people. Marriage, parenthood, and care of parents or siblings are a few of the many types of obligations that must be reconciled with the demands that will be made by years of education and (probably) reduced income levels. One of the major concerns that admissions committees have regarding non-traditional students is, in fact, whether an applicant has carefully considered and made plans for dealing with personal and family obligations. One has to be quite certain that a spouse and/or other family members *fully* understand what attending medical school and becoming a physician entails and how that will affect their lives. While the final decision for a non-traditional student is still an individual one, it has far more implications for others than is the case for the traditional, single, undergraduate applicant.

Another concern of medical school admissions committees regarding non-traditional students *is* directly related to their age. Attending medical school and completing graduate medical education programs are strenuous activities. The non-traditional applicant needs to demonstrate the physical capacity to carry out these activities as well as the motivation and intellectual ability to compete with other superior students. For this reason, most medical schools want evidence of successful completion of upper-division undergraduate coursework prior to application as a measure of present ability. While the decision to return to school to test one's ability to compete at the appropriate level is a big one, an even more frightening one presents itself when it becomes apparent to the student that he or she can actually do the work! Again, the approach needs to be one of sequential problem solving; consider the possibilities and make decisions at the point they need to be made, not before.

Finally, not all undergraduate programs are designed to accommodate the needs of non-traditional pre-med students, although they are increasingly able and willing to do so. Often the college has a specific advisor who specializes in the needs of non-traditional students. This person probably has had considerable experience in advising and can answer questions directly, or suggest creative ways of solving problems. In any case, the question of whether one "could have gone to medical school" needs to be answered while the opportunity still exists.

The Application Process and Selection for Admission

Assuming one is still in the pre-med state of mind after considering the attributes necessary to become a physician, thoroughly investigating the rewards and demands of the profession, and taking enough of the required undergraduate coursework to confirm competitive academic ability, application to medical school should be the next major step.

One of the requirements for admission to medical school is the Medical College Admission Test, or MCAT (virtually all the schools in the United States and 13 in Canada require the MCAT). Information about the MCAT, including the application, can usually be obtained from undergraduate pre-med advisors. An applicant needs to be aware that the scores from the MCAT and their college grades are the two most important measures of potential to succeed in medical school (the others will be discussed later).

---

2. *Ibid.*

The MCAT is administered twice yearly, in April and September. The test has been extensively revised. The new version was first administered in April 1991. The new MCAT has four sections—Verbal Reasoning, Physical Sciences, a Writing Sample, and Biological Sciences (which includes Organic Chemistry). The writing sample is a subjective instrument and is scored accordingly on a low-to-high letter scale of J to T, respectively; scores for the other three sections are each reported on a low-to-high scale of 1 to 15, respectively. While it remains to be seen what constitutes a "good" score on the new version of the MCAT, scores of 8 to 9 and above on past tests have been viewed as acceptable by most medical schools. Each medical school has an independently developed policy regarding acceptance of "old" MCAT scores (some will accept only the new version).

Generally, it is not advisable to take the MCAT until completion, or expected completion, of the minimal coursework in biology, chemistry, and physics. For non-traditional students for whom time is more critical, it may be advisable to take the April MCAT while the student is still in the process of taking the basic science courses. The test can be retaken in September if the scores are not acceptable, and the student can remain in the same applicant pool.

Various MCAT preparation programs are available. These range from formal, structured on-site courses to self-guided test preparation books, such as REA's *MCAT Test Preparation* book. The advisability of such programs depends on one's academic background, test-taking skills, and time constraints. Consultation with an undergraduate pre-med advisor and discussions with other pre-med students experienced in preparing for the MCAT are invaluable aids in deciding this matter.

The application cycle for medical school admission begins in the academic year preceding matriculation and, according to guidelines issued by the Association of American Medical Colleges (AAMC), is generally completed by June 1 of the matriculating year. Specific dates and procedures can be obtained from the AAMC recommendations available from your advisor, a medical school admissions officer, or in various publications of the AAMC.

Special note should be made of the Early Decision Program (EDP), which was offered by 82 U.S. medical schools in 1990. Students who have acceptable MCAT scores and academic credentials, and who have a clear preference of one medical school over all others, should consider making EDP applications. The EDP application period is generally between June 1 and August 15, and application may be made to one school only under the terms of the program. A decision regarding acceptance will be given to the applicant by October 1, after which unsuccessful applicants may apply to any other medical school. Reapplication to the EDP-designated school is also permitted. If admission is offered under the EDP, the applicant must accept the offer. Violation of this stipulation or the one-school application rule jeopardizes a

student's chances of being enrolled in medical school until the next application cycle.

Application deadlines vary according to the medical school. For schools that participate in the American Medical School Admission Service (AMCAS), applications will be accepted no earlier than June 15. The last date for receiving applications to AMCAS-participating schools is determined by individual schools, but generally is between October 15 and December 15. All but 19 of the medical schools in the U.S. and Puerto Rico participate in AMCAS, and application may be made to any number of these schools through the service. Non-AMCAS schools have independent application materials and dates; be sure to contact these schools directly if you are interested in applying for admission.

Of all the selection criteria considered by medical school admission committees, MCAT scores and grade-point average (GPA) are typically the most heavily weighted. While individual schools differ, these two usually comprise half, or more, of the total assignable measures for a given applicant. GPAs from different undergraduate schools may be individually interpreted based on a given medical school's experience with graduates, or former students, from those institutions.

Other criteria used in selecting medical students include personal written statements, personal interviews, letters of evaluation, and, to a certain degree, the applicant's experience with the medical profession. While the form and content of the written statement may vary, it is always best to be straightforward in presenting oneself. The statement should include comments about reasons for wanting to be a physician, ways in which the applicant has prepared for medical school, and an indication why she or he is now ready to begin. The applicant should not point out perceived negative or weak areas of preparation but should be prepared to succinctly discuss or explain these areas if they are brought up during an interview. The written statement must be logically organized, well-written, and correct in syntax and grammar. Since this is the initial direct presentation by the prospective student, it should be the best possible effort.

Some undergraduate schools have pre-med review boards or committees, usually comprised of faculty who teach basic science courses and/or serve as pre-med advisors. If this is the case, a composite letter from the group is extremely important and sometimes essential because of individual medical school's admissions policies. Pre-med review boards may utilize an interview situation both to help assess an applicant's preparedness and to give the student experience in interviewing. These simulated interviews are invaluable preparation for the applicant's potential interview with admissions personnel and other medical school representatives. If a pre-med review committee or the undergraduate advisors do not routinely interview their applicants, they should be strongly encouraged to do so.

Letters of recommendation from other undergraduate faculty (i.e., not on a pre-med review board) or evaluators outside of academe should also be sought. These letters are very important and care must be taken in selecting the authors. They must be familiar with the applicant's intellectual and physical attributes, interpersonal skills, and rationale for wanting to become a physician. Candidates should provide resume or biographical information to their evaluators, and should make it clear when and where letters have to be sent. Letters from elected government officials or other politically influential people have no more impact than other letters and may even be viewed negatively unless the author is otherwise qualified to evaluate the applicant.

Most medical schools will ask applicants to identify the people who will be writing letters of evaluation. Until all of the letters, as well as other application material, are received, an application is *not* complete and will not be acted upon. A reminder to write a previously agreed upon letter does not offend an evaluator and is welcomed by most. Finally, the number of letters of evaluation should be reasonable—three at least, but no more than five or six. Admissions committee members don't like to read inordinate numbers of letters and may react negatively to the overall application as a consequence.

Throughout the application process, it is the applicant's responsibility to keep medical schools informed of any change in their status. Timely submission of academic transcript updates, secondary application materials, and other pertinent information not only shows a professional attitude on the part of the applicant but may also supply critical pieces of information needed by admissions committees in the latter stages of the process. Successful applicants may be offered admission to several medical schools. While it is understood that time may be needed to arrive at a final decision, the applicant should give prompt notification to all schools involved when that decision is made. Incidentally, pre-med advisors appreciate feedback, both short- and long-term, not only as a courtesy but also to help prepare future applicants.

Finally, applicants who have not been accepted need to ascertain ways to improve their applications for the next cycle. Admissions officers may be forced into a defensive posture by demands to explain an applicant's rejection, but will generally be quite helpful in pointing out areas of possible improvement in an applicant's file. Perseverance and action in addressing these areas will demonstrate the career commitment and dedication expected of a future physician.

—Larry A. Giesmann, Ph.D. is a pre-med advisor at Northern Kentucky University, in Highland Heights, Kentucky.

EXPERIENCES WITH MEDICAL SCHOOL

by Adam Isaacson, M.D., UMDNJ–Robert Wood Johnson Medical School

Medical school and the medical field demand a great deal of sacrifice, time, and commitment. There are many reasons for becoming a physician, and they vary for each person. I'd like to share with you some of my reasons for choosing medicine as a career.

I cannot say that I was born with a strong desire to help people, but I am happiest when I am around people, and I feel that I have an empathetic personality. For me, medicine is a profession which reflects my human nature and satisfies my own need to be around people.

I also took into consideration the fact that a medical career will provide both job and financial security, which are very important to me. The plethora of choices and opportunities that medicine has to offer gives me a sense of achieving "occupational freedom." This is extremely important. Other medically-related professions that I considered, such as podiatry, prosthetics and orthotics, chiropractic practice, and physical therapy, were more limited than that of a physician.

Having a professional title and being in a position of leadership within the community are also important considerations. As a physician, I will be well-regarded by my peers in the community as well as by my patients and family.

Lastly, I have found that personal experience also has a significant influence on one's desire to be a doctor. At age 13 I had successful spinal surgery, and since that time I have held a special admiration for doctors and medical science.

Becoming a physician means entering into an intimate relationship with human life and death. It means accepting the responsibility to continually learn and study new medical developments, and it means a commitment to tend to people's pain and suffering. Unfortunately, being a physician today also means being forced to practice an art under constant scrutiny and increasing regulation. Anyone entering the medical field should be aware of the litigation and politics which have changed, and will continue to change, the way doctors practice.

There is no question that medicine is emotionally, physically, and intellectually taxing, not to mention stressful and often, frustrating. But the rewards of medicine more than make up for the bad times, and make me glad that I chose this profession.

Once you have decided that you want to become a physician, you will have to choose a medical school. Initially, this may seem like an overwhelming decision. There are many important things to consider.

The suggestions of your college pre-med advisor and your college pre-med club will be most useful in helping you to formulate a strategy to pursue your goals. The standards and philosophies of each medical school are different and your advisor will be a guide to help tailor your curriculum to suit your career goals. He or she will also help you choose schools that are within your reach. Advisors are experts at putting things into perspective. Further, your advisor is also a good source of current information such as medical school brochures, MCAT study guides, and "how to apply" guides. Thus, knowing your advisor well and maintaining good rapport and close contact throughout your four years of undergraduate school is recommended.

The pre-med club at your school is an excellent way to learn about the medical field in general. My pre-med club invited guest speakers such as doctors from different fields, malpractice attorneys, and medical students so that the members could get an up-to-date overview of developments in the medical field. This is a great way to have your questions answered on the spot. Also, through other members of your club, you will get help with application strategies and trends in medical schools.

Now that you have your resources intact, there are other considerations to make when actually choosing the school.

Location is an important factor when choosing your medical school. Geographic location really has no bearing on your future, nor does it matter whether you are educated by a community or city program, but there are pros and cons you should think about when choosing a location. For instance, an inner-city school may have the benefit of exposing you to a large volume of patients with a broad scope of pathology in your clinical years, but the hospital environment may be impersonal and so busy that you may get less instruction. The opposite may exist in a community setting.

You might want to give strong consideration to the amount of recreation the school and/or the surrounding city has to offer. Medical school can be stressful at times, and you will need a way to blow off steam. If your school or the surrounding city has athletic or other non-medical activities for you to pursue, you will have a way to deal with the incredible stress and pressure you will feel.

Remaining close to home, if possible, is another consideration. When times get tough, having family nearby for support can mean a lot. Also, if you are unmarried and will be living alone, having parents nearby means getting those home-cooked care packages which you will need, particularly around exams when you have no time to shop or cook.

Cost is only as important as you make it. The education you will receive has no correlation with the price tag on it. (A higher-priced school does not necessarily guarantee you a better education.) Medical school can cost you as much as $40,000 a year and cost varies considerably between private and state schools. A goal should be to complete your studies while accumulating a minimum of loans and shelling out a minimum of your savings—unless your savings have already been earmarked for medical school. Then you will have a much easier time establishing your practice after residency is completed.

In any case, loans are easy to get as a medical school student. If you know that you will need to rely primarily on loans, check into the efficiency of the financial aid departments at the medical schools to which you are applying. If you have to deal with an inefficient, disorganized department, life can become quite difficult if loans are your primary source of income, and if there is a delay in getting your checks. This will make you feel more stress, and there will be enough stress just from attending medical school!

Yet another consideration when applying to medical school is the type of grading system the school uses. When I applied four years ago, grading systems varied, but the trend was toward a five point system. A five point system is typically broken down as: honors, high pass, pass, low pass, and fail. Although administrations claim that a five point system will further define the academic achievement of the student, I think it only increases stress and competition among students. The best advice I could give you is to be aware of the grading system, but don't make it a heavy consideration in your decision-making process.

The school's academic structure is something you should be more concerned with. Again, each school will have its own approach. In general, the first two years are devoted to the basic sciences and classroom-based introductory courses to clinical medicine, with some clinical (hands-on) exposure. An example of typical first-year courses include human histology, gross and developmental anatomy, biochemistry, medical physiology, cell biology, and neural science. The second year might include courses such as introduction to clinical medicine, introduction to clinical psychiatry, infectious diseases, pharmacology, pathology, and biostatistics/epidemiology. Some programs will give you more clinical exposure in the first two years than others.

Each school may arrange its courseload differently. For example, my school, UMDNJ-Robert Wood Johnson, takes a more traditional route by teaching complete subjects as separate units like undergraduate college. Other medical schools use the systems approach. This method coordinates subjects being taught to focus on the same major systems of the body simultaneously. For instance, when studying the respiratory system you will concentrate on the anatomy, histology, pathology, physiology, and clinical disease of that system simultaneously.

It is difficult for me to comment on which system is better, since I have been educated solely on the traditional system, but the systems approach may have the benefit of allowing more time to focus on all aspects of a system. On the other hand, the traditional system affords the opportunity to know exactly how your courses will be spread out. Usually an entire course is taught over one semester. Certain courses, such as physiology and pathology, encompass a large amount of material, and some schools will devote two semesters to them. Things like this can make your coursework more manageable.

You should also investigate course requirements, and which departments will teach them. Medical school curricula are usually a conglomeration of courses run by separate, relatively autonomous departments each with their own minimum passing grade cut-offs, assignments, small group, and laboratory requirements. You will need to know how time-consuming and worthwhile the department's requirements are for each school in which you are interested. To do this, you can ask students their opinion of course requirements. Be critical of what will be expected of you and what you can expect from the school.

Current students are the best way to get an accurate picture of the schools. I strongly recommend making an effort to speak or correspond with students. Medical schools usually have a body of students on the admissions committee who are available to speak with you.

As important as the structure of the curriculum is, so are the people who organize and teach the courses. Professors and administrators, for obvious reasons, are the people who determine how easy or difficult life in medical school will be.

Your first and second year courses will most often be taught lecture-style, usually by Ph.D.s who are experts in their field. Your hope should be that these professors will present the material in an organized, concise, understandable, and interesting manner, while highlighting facts and concepts pertinent to the impending exam. This may or may not happen.

As a medical student, you are looking for a professor who provides handouts highlighting the relevant concept which coincides with the format of the lecture. You also want someone who will point out what you should concentrate on when studying for an exam. Your goal will be to weed out the most important information so that your study time will be as productive as possible.

You need to find a school where there is a good student-faculty relationship, a supportive administration, and a "student-friendly" environment.

Exams will be your main concern during the first two years of medical school, since this will be primarily how your grades are determined. Each department works as an individual autonomous unit, and each department determines its own number of required exams, percent weight of each exam, exam format, exam content, and when to give the exams. The department professors, as mentioned above, control the amount and content of the study material to be covered. All of these factors contribute to the fairness of the exams.

In the best of situations, questions are formulated anew by each professor and are representative of the lecture material, without overemphasis on any one particular topic. What often happens is the opposite. While you will review for an exam on four particular topics, for example, you may only be actually tested on one of those topics. This actually happened to me during my second year. The Psychiatry Department gave an exam composed completely of questions taken from a single review book. This turned out to be extremely unfair, not only because the questions were poorly representative of the lecture material, but also because some of the students had been using that particular book to study from, while the majority had not.

How exams and assignments are planned is also a hot topic among medical school students. If several exams or laboratory and group projects are planned for the same week, it becomes very difficult to make time to study efficiently for anything.

The method of weighting exams is also an important factor in determining your final grade. It is ideal to have three to four exams of equal weight, and a non-cumulative final exam which is weighted equally with other exams you took throughout the semester. This gives you the opportunity to err somewhat on one exam without failing the course. The point here is that medical students are forced to learn voluminous amounts of material in short periods of time, and a system which favors cumulative finals that are worth a large part of your grade creates unnecessary stress and academic obstacles. Be sure to ask students about exam weighting, and be wary of schools which appear to favor grade determination on cumulative final exams.

In general, a "student unfriendly" school with an unsupportive administration ignores conflicts that complicate students' lives. On the other hand, a "student friendly" system polices lecturers, fairly spaces exams, regulates exam weighting, and is willing to make compromises to accommodate reasonable requests from students. Obviously, no system is perfect. Even in programs where students are unhappy, you will find exceptional, dedicated professors and administrators who care about the success of their students. But you should be aware that bad professors and "student unfriendly" environments exist so that, if possible, you can avoid those environments.

Finally, after you have composed that awesome application, been impressive on your interviews, visited schools, asked the right questions, and been accepted somewhere, you can begin to prepare yourself for medical school.

I felt fear and happiness simultaneously on the day I received my medical school acceptance. I felt wonderful about accomplishing what I considered impossible, but scared about the immense intellectual challenge I knew was ahead. From day one I had doubts about the commitment I was about to make.

The first two years of medical school can best be described as the fastest emotional roller-coaster ride you have ever been on. There are constant ups and downs which you live through, but never fully adjust to.

By the end of my first week, I felt helpless and totally out of my league. (Keep in mind that as I write this, I am one week away from graduation). I had only three courses (Anatomy, Biochemistry, and Histology) but each course covered nearly a college semester's worth of material by the first exam. That was distressing, to say the least.

Volume is the main challenge of medical school particularly in the first two years. While the material on the whole is not intellectually challenging, the amount of material you must cover verges on the impossible. I remember that by the end of anatomy, (a one semester course) in addition to 1400 pages of textbook, I accumulated a two foot tall pile of lecture notes and handouts. As bad as this may sound, there are ways to minimize the workload.

First of all, discipline is the key. Discipline in medical school means accepting that in order to survive, you will have to give up part of your recreational, social, and family life temporarily, and concentrate almost solely on your studies. This is one of the hardest adjustments I had to make, and definitely one of the down-slopes on that emotional roller-coaster. For instance, during my third year clinical rotations, my first nephew was born, and because I was so swamped with work, I didn't see him for the first time until two months later. I also had to cut a five-day-a-week workout to three days a week, and studied through practically every weekend. At times, I would get depressed about not seeing my family for long stretches and not being able to go on weekend escapes like the 9-5 world could. But I lived through the difficult times, and I feel that it was worth it.

There are those students, like my roommate, who have such a natural grasp of medical school that they can party right up until the week before the exam and still end up with the highest grades in the class. There is no question in my mind that if you are a fast reader and have a strong memory, medical school will be more manageable and you will have more time to play. As long as you are willing to put the time in and work very hard, though, you will make it through.

After you get organized, I also suggest that you look into Note Service, which is a student-run organization offered at many schools. This service gets every lecture summarized in detail by designated students (called scribes) who choose to be responsible for preparing a detailed summary of lectures for those in the service. There is usually a fee to join which is used to pay the scribes. Receiving Note Service allows you to go to lectures and concentrate because somebody else is taking the notes for you. Likewise, if you become a "scribe" you will make some extra money and digest the material fully the first time around during the lecture.

Naturally, digesting the pertinent material to pass the exam is the most important objective of the first year medical school student. The difficult part is finding the best way to get the key information and then to memorize it. Professors usually stress that the required textbook is the only pertinent source of information. Don't always assume this to be true; you will ultimately discover the best way to handle the material for yourself. People in my class have had equal success and failure when using different types of information and different methods of study.

I found that of all the study sources using simplified study guides and review of old exams were by far the most effective method. Study guides highlight the facts. When choosing guides, I suggest that you look for ones which are intended for National Board preparation. This way, you will be studying simultaneously for your current exam and for the National Board of Medical Examiners test without feeling the pain of studying for two exams.

Another highly regarded resource among students is old departmental exams, if they are available. Old exams are in themselves a list highlighting the concepts the department wants you to know. Occasionally, you will find that this is the only source you have, other times you will decide that this is the best available source, even though there are others available.

As you have probably figured out by now, the reality of the first two years of medical school is exams. In the first two years, you are constantly fighting to keep up with the flood of material and you constantly carry the stress of an impending exam. The worst part is that as quickly as you finish one exam, there is always another close behind. There is never enough time to feel adequately prepared for the exam. Being faced with this situation (for many of us for the first time!) challenges your emotions, and it is difficult to adjust to. One minute you will feel calm and in control because you have fully grasped one chapter, and the next minute you might feel intense despair and fear because there are still 20 chapters to go.

Your outlook on grades may also change when you begin medical school. To get into medical school, you had to be a high achiever. You are probably going to or already have graduated in the top one percent of your class. You are used to high grades, which I view as the high yield return on the investment of long hours of study. In medical school, your grades may suddenly plummet, and you are suddenly "just average" when you have never been "average" before. I achieved grades in the high sixties and low seventies on exams. Many times this was after I would put 15 hours a day into studying. Sometimes I even failed. This led me to thoughts of dropping out, and poor grades have led other students to consider dropping out also.

The bright spot is that most departments curve exam scores. Curved grades are every medical school student's saving grace, however, they are also the cause of great competition. Competition is an integral part of medical school no matter which school you attend. This is because most of the people in the class were competitive types when they entered medical school. I think the degree of competition may vary from school to school depending on the way the students are treated and the way the curriculum is structured. Many medical students have previously earned Ph.D.s. Others have had

careers as doctors of podiatry, physical therapists, and nurses. There are also foreign medical doctors who are trying to become American medical graduates, and there are honor students directly out of college. All of these people are highly motivated and are strongly determined to achieve their goal. They will compete heavily to do so.

The competition becomes apparent early on in your medical school career. For instance, by the second week I found that all the students did (including me) was compare how much material we had each learned so far, particularly near exam time. I also noticed that people would never hesitate to mention over and over again how much material they already reviewed, especially if they sensed that you were behind. Students would also discover or learn some great study secrets from upper classmates, and then not share them with anyone until the exam was over. Another stunt was for students to carry around piles of highlighted notes so that the class could observe how far ahead they were.

There are others who will hoard important books in the library. They will steal teaching models from anatomy lab. They will damage required audio-visual teaching aids. The only way to avoid these types of problems is to go to a school with a well-stocked medical library, and complete audio and visual materials.

There are many other forms of competition as well. Students have been known to give misleading information in Note Service with the hope that it will lower the mean exam average. Notes stolen from mail boxes and the stealing of personal notebooks also occur. Perhaps the worst situation I ever experienced was when there would be group discussions where the participants would be graded. Some classmates would deliberately make other students look bad by making degrading comments in response to answers given during the discussion period.

Every medical student carries the same fears, doubts, and anxieties about being able to handle medical school. Unfortunately, some choose to allay their fears in a cruel way. I have known some of these types of people, but I have also become friendly with students who are exceptionally caring and supportive people who respect your goals as well as their own.

A final topic I would like to address is failure. It is true that once you are in medical school, it is hard to fail out. This is true to a large extent because most departments will make the failing cut-off grade extremely low. But if you do fail a course, or courses, there is a lot of academic support provided. For example, each department gives a make-up exam over the summer, and they will even give you a short make-up course as a third chance to complete the course if you fail the first make-up. The prerequisite to move into the next year is to pass all your courses, and unfortunately, every year there are people who are held back because of repeated failure. Some schools also require passing Part 1 of the National Board Exam in order to move into your third year clinical rotations. Normally, you will be allowed three attempts at this test before dismissal. For academic support, schools do have skilled professional help available to assist anyone with academic difficulties. Be sure to investigate each school's policy for academic dismissal and what kind of support services they have in case you need them.

I chose not to discuss the third and fourth years because they are so different from the first two. The third and fourth years, in my opinion, are better years because what you have learned in the classroom begins to make sense. It is in the third year that you start to get a feel for the world of medicine and the fourth year is when you begin to feel like a physician.

I hope I have provided you with better insight to help you make a decision about becoming a doctor and about medical school. I hope I have made clear to you the commitment that medicine demands. Also, realize that your academic and clinical performance is far more important than the name of the institution from which you graduate. It is crucial that you choose an environment that will make you the happiest, and which provides maximum opportunities with minimum distractions.

—Dr. Isaacson is a May, 1991 graduate of UMDNJ-Robert Wood Johnson Medical School. He is currently serving an internship in internal medicine at Morristown Memorial Hospital. He plans to pursue a residency in rehabilitation medicine at Columbia University Hospital, New York City, in 1992.

THE MEDICAL COLLEGE ADMISSION TEST (MCAT)

Applying for medical school requires a thorough understanding of the preparation and administration of the Medical College Achievement Test (MCAT). Understanding when to take the test, what specifically to study, and how your score will be weighed is essential to making your application process easier and complete.

What is the MCAT?

The Association of American Medical Colleges (AAMC) designed the MCAT to evaluate the student's basic scientific knowledge as well as problem solving, critical thinking, and writing skills. It is designed to test a broad range of skills that you, as a potential physician, will need.

The MCAT vs. Academics (GPA)

Almost all American medical schools require the MCAT as criterion for admission. Every medical school will have its own formula for evaluating your application but, *as a general rule, MCAT scores are as equally important as your overall GPA.* A high MCAT score will give you an edge on getting into the highly competitive medical schools.

When to register for the MCAT

The MCAT is administered by the AAMC twice a year; once in the spring and once in the fall. It is advised that you take the MCAT in the spring prior to the year you plan to begin your studies. If you are currently an undergraduate, this means you would take the MCAT in the spring of your junior year. Spring test dates are more preferable because your test results will be ready for early processing of your medical school application. If your spring results are poor, you have the opportunity to retake the test in the fall and still complete your application that academic year.

MCAT registration materials for both the spring and fall administrations are available each February. You should contact your academic advisor or write to:

MCAT registration
The American College Testing Program
P.O. Box 414
Iowa City, Iowa 52243

Studying for the MCAT

You will want to study for the MCAT so that you may obtain the best possible score. It is important not only to know the scientific and other material presented, but also how the material will be presented. If you become familiar with the layout of the exam, how the questions will look and how much time you will have for each section, you will feel much more at ease on the day of the test, and ultimately improve your score.

REA publishes an MCAT Test Preparation Book which offers six full-length practice tests. Our practice tests will prepare you for the degree of difficulty and types of questions you will encounter on the actual exam. Each section offers detailed explanations of why the "right" answers are correct, and how you can avoid getting trapped by "trick" questions. Using our test prep book will allow you to further your understanding of the test material as well as to make accurate, confident choices on all test sections of the MCAT.

Format of the MCAT Test Sections

The MCAT is composed of four basic sections, each containing brief, informative passages. Following the passages are multiple-choice questions which are designed to test your knowledge of a particular subject.

Verbal Reasoning

The verbal reasoning section will require you to read passages of 500-600 words and answer interpretive, applicative, and inferential questions. The questions will not be based on detailed facts, but will include the following:

- Understanding the theme of a passage
- Determining and evaluating certain points of an argument
- Drawing inferences from facts and reaching conclusions

Medical knowledge is not needed to answer these questions. The passages will be drawn from many disciplines, such as the social sciences, the humanities, and philosophy. No one academic background will have an advantage.

Physical Sciences

Several informative mini-passages are included in the physical sciences section. You will be required to interpret and analyze information to:

- Understand and apply basic concepts
- Balance simple chemical equations
- Solve general physics problems

All questions asked will be on the first-year college level. You will not need advanced knowledge to answer these questions.

The Writing Sample

You will be asked to analyze a short statement or quote. You are then allotted time to write a logical, concise essay. Prior knowledge of medicine is not necessary, as topics on medicine will not be assigned. Two essays will be given and you will be expected to:

- Review and understand the topic statement or quote

- Formulate a clear position

- Support your position eloquently and effectively

- Incorporate correct grammar and word usage

Biological Sciences

Several informative mini-passages are included in the Biological Sciences section. You will be required to interpret, analyze, and apply the information to:

- Understand and apply basic concepts

- Balance simple chemical equations

- Solve general biology and organic chemistry problems

All questions will be at the level of first-year college material. You will not need advanced knowledge to answer these questions.

U.S. MEDICAL SCHOOLS AT A GLANCE

School	Accreditation	Degrees Offered	# Students Applied	Enrollment
University of Alabama School of Medicine	LCME	M.D., M.D./Ph.D., M.S., M.S./M.D.	1,055	165 / class
Albany Medical College	AAMC	M.D., M.D./Ph.D.	4,412	125 / class
Albert Einstein College of Medicine of Yeshiva University	LCME, AAMC	M.D., M.D./Ph.D.	4,045	200 / class
University of Arizona College of Medicine	AAMC	M.D., M.D./Ph.D.	255	88 / class
University of Arkansas College of Medicine	AAMC	M.D., M.S./Ph.D.	438	140 / class
Baylor College of Medicine	LCME, SACS	M.D., M.D./Ph.D.	1,588	164 / class
Boston University School of Medicine	LCME	M.D., B.A./M.D., M.D./M.A., M.D./Ph.D., M.D./M.P.H., M.D./DSc	5,340	135 / class
Bowman Gray School of Medicine of Wake Forest University	LCME	M.D., M.S.	3,135	108 / class
Brown University Program in Medicine	AAMC	B.A./M.D., B.S./M.D., M.M.S., M.S./M.D., M.D./Ph.D.	1,029	73 / class
University of California, Davis School of Medicine	AAMC	M.D., M.D./Ph.D.	2,956	93 / class
University of California, Irvine College of Medicine	AAMC	M.D., M.S., Ph.D.	3,266	92 / class
University of California, Los Angeles UCLA School of Medicine	LCME	M.D., M.D./Ph.D., M.D./M.P.H.	3,828	145 / class
University of California, San Diego School of Medicine	LCME	M.D., M.S., M.D./Ph.D.	4,000	122 / class
University of California, San Francisco School of Medicine	LCME	M.D., M.D./Ph.D., D.D.S./M.D., M.D./M.A., M.D./M.S., M.S./Ph.D., M.D./M.P.H.	3,705	153 / class
Case Western Reserve University School of Medicine	LCME	M.D., Ph.D.	4,527	138 / class
Universidad Central del Caribe School of Medicine	LCME	M.D.	572	61 / class
University of Chicago Pritzker School of Medicine	LCME	M.D., M.D./Ph.D., M.D./M.B.A., M.D./J.D.	3,797	113 / class
University of Cincinnati College of Medicine	LCME, AMA	M.D., M.D./Ph.D.	2,780	650
University of Colorado School of Medicine	AAMC	M.D., M.D./Ph.D., B.S., M.S.	986	131 / class

* Not Available   ** Not Applicable   C/S – Contact School   I/S – In-State   O/S – Out-of-State

Mean GPA	% Male / % Female	% Minorities	In-State Tuition	Out-of-State Tuition	Application Fee	Application Deadline
3.41	67% / 33%	13%	$4,098	$13,246	$25	November 1
3.2	57% / 43%	*	$18,900	**	$50	December 1
3.4	54% / 46%	*	$18,960	**	$60	November 1
3.52	59% / 41%	*	$6,192	**	C/S	November 1
3.5	64% / 36%	10%	$5,720	$11,440	$10	November 15
3.6	60% / 40%	*	$5,463	C/S	$30	November 1
3.23	59% / 41%	11%	$22,300	**	C/S	November 15
3.3	67% / 33%	*	$14,200	**	$40	November 1
*	50% / 50%	18%	$15,871	**	C/S	January 1
3.5	56% / 44%	22.5%	None	$6,416	$40	November 1
3.5	*	*	None	$6,416	$40	November 1
3.64	50% / 50%	33%	None	$5,916	$40	November 1
3.54	64% / 36%	*	None	$7,992	$40	November 1
3.69	58% / 42%	23%	None	$6,417	$40	November 1
3.4 / 3.5	55% / 45%	26%	$17,100	**	$30	November 1
3.10	67% / 33%	*	$15,000	$22,000	$50	December 15
3.58	65% / 35%	33%	$16,170	**	$45	December 15
3.42	61% / 39%	*	$7,650	$13,407	$25	November 15
3.5	59% / 41%	11.5%	$8,228	$34,132	$40	November 15

* Not Available   ** Not Applicable   C/S – Contact School   I/S – In-State   O/S – Out-of-State

School	Accreditation	Degrees Offered	# Students Applied	Enrollment
Columbia University College of Physicians and Surgeons	AAMC	M.D., M.D./Ph.D., M.D./M.P.H.	2,100	148 / class
University of Connecticut School of Medicine	AAMC	M.D., M.S., Ph.D.	1,596	*
Cornell University Medical College	AAMC	M.D., M.D./Ph.D.	4,000	101 / class
Creighton University School of Medicine	AAMC	M.D.	3,913	110 / class
Dartmouth Medical School	LCME	M.D., M.D./Ph.D.	4,189	87 / class
Duke University School of Medicine	AMCA	M.D., M.D./Ph.D., M.D./M.A., M.D./A.M., M.D./M.P.H., M.D./J.D.	4,545	105 / class
East Carolina University School of Medicine	LCME	M.D.	1,161	72 / class
East Tennessee State University James H. Quillen College of Medicine	LCME	M.D., M.S., Ph.D.	916	60 / class
Eastern Virginia Medical School of The Medical College of Hampton Roads	LCME	M.D.	2,831	97 / class
Emory University School of Medicine	AAMC	M.D., M.D./Ph.D., M.D./M.P.H.	3,060	112 / class
University of Florida College of Medicine	AAMC	M.D., B.S./M.D., M.D./Ph.D.	1,634	85 / class
George Washington University School of Medicine and Health Sciences	AAMC	M.D., Ph.D., M.D./Ph.D. and M.D./M.P.H.	5,687	150 / class
Georgetown University School of Medicine	LCME	M.D., M.D./Ph.D.	5,062	196 / class
Hahnemann University School of Medicine	LCME, MSACS	M.D./Ph.D./B.A.	5,051	690
Harvard Medical School	LCME	M.D., Ph.D., M.A.	*	*
University of Hawaii John A. Burns School of Medicine	LCME	M.D., Ph.D.	693	56 / class
University of Health Sciences Chicago Medical School	LCME	M.D., M.S., Ph.D.	4,807	149 / class
Howard University College of Medicine	AMA, MSASSC	M.D., B.S./M.D., M.S., Ph.D.	3,034	100 / class
University of Illinois College of Medicine	AAMC, LCME	M.D., Ph.D., M.D./Ph.D.	3,136	300 / class
Indiana University School of Medicine	LCME	M.D., M.D./Ph.D., M.D./M.S.	1,657	265 / class

* Not Available   ** Not Applicable   C/S – Contact School   I/S – In-State   O/S – Out-of-State

Mean GPA	% Male / % Female	% Minorities	In-State Tuition	Out-of-State Tuition	Application Fee	Application Deadline
3.5	61% / 39%	*	$17,892	**	$50	October 15
3.48	53% / 47%	10%	$5,550	$12,300	$50	December 15
3.5	50% / 50%	15%	$19,200	**	$50	October 15
3.0	67% / 33%	*	$15,900	**	$40	December 1
*	59% / 41%	9%	$20,650	**	$55	November 1
3.5	70% / 30%	9%	$14,200	**	$55	October 15
3.2	50% / 50%	19%	$1,344	$11,848	$25	November 15
3.27	63% / 37%	18%	$6,560	$10,410	$15	December 1
3.32	55% / 45%	10%	$10,000	$16,500	$50	December 1
3.5	66% / 34%	18%	$14,400	**	$50	October 15
3.67	60% / 40%	15%	$6,258	$15,301	$15	December 1
3.3	54% / 46%	*	$23,600	**	$45	December 1
3.3	76% / 24%	7%	$22,500	**	$55	November 15
*	60% / 40%	14%	$18,070	**	$50	October 15
*	*	*	$18,030	**	$60	October 15
3.3	*	*	$4,830	$14,490	None	December 1
3.2	70% / 30%	*	$24,300	**	$55	December 15
*	50% / 50%	80%	$9,450	**	$25	December 15
3.0	*	*	$7,136	$20,696	$20	December 1
3.56	62% / 38%	20%	$6,000	$13,560	$20	December 15

* Not Available   ** Not Applicable   C/S – Contact School   I/S – In-State   O/S – Out-of-State

School	Accreditation	Degrees Offered	# Students Applied	Enrollment
University of Iowa College of Medicine	LCME	M.D., M.D./Ph.D.	1,089	700
Jefferson Medical College of Thomas Jefferson University	MSACS, AMA, CAHEA, ADACDA	M.D., M.D./Ph.D., B.S./M.D., M.S./M.D.	4,675	223 / class
Johns Hopkins University School of Medicine	AMCA	M.D., M.D./Ph.D., M.D./M.P.H., Ph.D., M.A.	3,200	120 / class
University of Kansas School of Medicine	AAU	M.D., M.A., M.S., Ph.D.	1,115	178 / class
University of Kentucky College of Medicine	AAMC	M.D., M.D./M.S., M.D./Ph.D.	808	95 / class
Loma Linda University School of Medicine	AAMC, CME	M.D., M.D./Ph.D., M.S.	2,200	129 / class
Louisiana State University School of Medicine in New Orleans	LCME	M.D., M.D./Ph.D.	751	175 / class
Louisiana State University School of Medicine in Shreveport	AAMC	M.D., M.D./Ph.D.	508	100 / class
University of Louisville School of Medicine	AAMC, LCME	M.D.	809	125 / class
Loyola University of Chicago Stritch School of Medicine	AAMC	M.D., M.S., Ph.D.	4,116	130 / class
Marshall University School of Medicine	AAMC	M.D.	592	48 / class
University of Maryland School of Medicine	AAMC, LCME	M.D., M.D./Ph.D., M.D./M.S.	2,405	141 / class
University of Massachusetts Medical School	LCME	M.D., M.S., Ph.D., M.D./Ph.D.	651	100 / class
Mayo Medical School	AMCAS	M.D., M.D./D.M.S.	1,400	40 / class
Medical College of Georgia School of Medicine	AAMC, AMA	M.D.	860	180 / class
Medical College of Ohio	LCME	M.D.	1,907	135 / class
Medical College of Pennsylvania	LCME	M.D., M.D./Ph.D., M.D./M.S., M.D./M.B.A.	3,400	113 / class
Medical College of Wisconsin	LCME	M.D., M.D./Ph.D., M.S./M.D.	2,700	187 / class
Medical University of South Carolina College of Medicine	LCME	M.D., Ph.D.	1,447	129 / class
University of Medicine and Dentistry of N.J. New Jersey Medical School	LCME	M.D.	1,893	170 / class

* Not Available   ** Not Applicable   C/S – Contact School   I/S – In-State   O/S – Out-of-State

Mean GPA	% Male / % Female	% Minorities	In-State Tuition	Out-of-State Tuition	Application Fee	Application Deadline
3.5	*	*	$5,924	$15,350	$20	December 1
3.4	70% / 30%	10%	$18,200	**	$60	November 15
*	60% / 40%	*	$17,500	**	$60	November 15
3.5	35% / 65%	*	$5,770	$11,916	$15 Out-of-State	November 1
3.44	70% / 30%	5%	$5,030	$17,179	None	November 1
3.5	*	*	$15,990	**	$35	December 1
3.34	63% / 37%	*	$4,776	$12,576	$30	November 15
3.4	67% / 33%	*	$4,776	$12,576	$30	November 15
3.45	58% / 42%	*	$4,928	$17,078	$15	November 1
3.36	64% / 36%	*	$13,800	$17,650	$35	November 15
3.3	65% / 35%	*	$5,047	$9,017	$20	November 15
3.5	55% / 45%	*	$7,240	$14,652	$25	November 15
3.5	48% / 52%	5%	$6,500	**	$18	December 15
3.57	54% / 46%	*	$8,200	$17,650	$40	November 15
*	*	*	$3,942	$11,826	None	November 1
3.35	64% / 36%	14%	$7,749	$10,536	$30	December 1
3.40	*	20%	$15,590	**	$55	December 1
3.53	60% / 40%	33%	$7,674	$17,500	$45	December 1
*	*	*	$4,140	$8,820	$25	December 1
3.35	56% / 44%	22%	$10,457	$13,723	$25	December 15

* Not Available   ** Not Applicable   C/S – Contact School   I/S – In-State   O/S – Out-of-State

School	Accreditation	Degrees Offered	# Students Applied	Enrollment
University of Medicine and Dentistry of N.J. Robert Wood Johnson Medical School	LCME	M.D., M.D./Ph.D.	1,955	*
Meharry Medical College School of Medicine	AMA, AAMC	M.D., Ph.D., M.S.	2,143	80 / class
Mercer University School of Medicine	LCME	M.D.	585	42 / class
University of Miami School of Medicine	LCME	M.D., M.D./Ph.D.	685	128 / class
Michigan State University College of Human Medicine	LCME	M.D.	1,958	109 / class
University of Michigan Medical School	LCME	M.D., M.D./Ph.D.	3,279	170 / class
University of Minnesota—Duluth School of Medicine	LCME	M.D.	479	49 / class
University of Minnesota Medical School—Minneapolis	LCME	M.D., M.D./Ph.D.	1,409	180 / class
University of Mississippi School of Medicine	AMA, AAMC	M.D.	462	100 / class
University of Missouri—Columbia School of Medicine	LCME	M.D., M.D./M.S., M.D./Ph.D.	789	110 / class
University of Missouri—Kansas City School of Medicine	LCME	M.D., B.A.	455	102 / class
Morehouse School of Medicine	LCME, SACS, AAMC	M.D.	1,250	33 / class
Mount Sinai School of Medicine of the City University of New York	LCME	M.D., M.D./Ph.D.	2,323	115 / class
University of Nebraska College of Medicine	LCME	M.D., M.D./Ph.D.	925	126 / class
University of Nevada School of Medicine	LCME	M.D., M.D./Ph.D.	419	48 / class
University of New Mexico School of Medicine	LCME	M.D., M.D./Ph.D.	570	73 / class
New York Medical College	LCME	M.D., M.D./Ph.D.	3,409	190 / class
New York University School of Medicine	LCME	M.D., M.D./Ph.D.	2,327	156 / class
University of North Carolina at Chapel Hill School of Medicine	LCME	M.D., M.D./Ph.D., M.D./M.P.H.	2,286	160 / class
University of North Dakota School of Medicine	LCME, AAMC	M.D., M.D./Ph.D.	124	57 / class

* Not Available   ** Not Applicable   C/S – Contact School   I/S – In-State   O/S – Out-of-State

Mean GPA	% Male / % Female	% Minorities	In-State Tuition	Out-of-State Tuition	Application Fee	Application Deadline
3.29	61% / 39%	*	$10,547	$13,723	$25	December 15
*	52% / 48%	86%	$13,300	**	$25	December 15
*	50% / 50%	1%	$12,960	**	$25	December 1
*	*	*	$18,050	**	$50	December 1
3.46	49% / 51%	23%	$7,823	$16,823	$25	December 1
3.5	*	*	$10,000	$18,902	$10	November 15
3.4	80% / 20%	10%	$2,502 / per quarter	$5,005 / per quarter	None	November 15
3.44	54% / 46%	*	$2,379 / per quarter	$4,647 / per quarter	None	November 15
3.6	*	*	$6,000	$12,000	None	December 1
3.4	49% / 51%	6%	$7,130	$11,165	None	November 15
*	45% / 55%	*	$10,990	$14,960	$25 I/S $50 O/S	December 1
*	48% / 52%	97%	$12,700	**	$40	December 1
3.4	53% / 47%	39%	$16,000	**	$50	November 1
3.53	65% / 35%	*	$7,028	$12,640	None	November 15
3.4	75% / 25%	*	$5,566	$13,189	$35	November 1
3.4	57.5% / 42.5%	16.5%	$3,032	$8,468	$10	November 15
3.14	62% / 38%	*	$22,400	**	$50	December 1
3.5	62% / 38%	*	$19,325	**	$65	December 15
*	*	*	$1,344	$12,132	$35	November 15
3.49	60% / 40%	*	$7,800	$22,015	$25	November 1

* Not Available ** Not Applicable C/S – Contact School I/S – In-State O/S – Out-of-State

School	Accreditation	Degrees Offered	# Students Applied	Enrollment
Northeastern Ohio Universities College of Medicine	LCME, AAMC, AMA	B.S./M.D., M.D., M.D./Ph.D.	400	400
Northwestern University Medical School	LCME	M.D., B.A./M.D., B.S./M.D., M.D./Ph.D., M.D./M.M.	4,492	168 / class
Ohio State University College of Medicine	LCME	M.D., M.S., Ph.D.	2,279	210 / class
University of Oklahoma College of Medicine	LCME	M.D., M.D./Ph.D.	875	158 / class
Oregon Health Sciences University School of Medicine	LCME, AAMC	M.D., Ph.D.	802	94 / class
University of Pennsylvania School of Medicine	LCME	M.D., Ph.D., M.S.	4,721	154 / class
Pennsylvania State University College of Medicine	LCME, AAMC	M.D.	2,408	112 / class
University of Pittsburgh School of Medicine	LCME	M.D., Ph.D.	2,920	138 / class
Ponce School of Medicine	AMA	M.D., Ph.D	409	40 / class
University of Puerto Rico School of Medicine	LCME	M.D., M.S., Ph.D.	313	93 / class
University of Rochester School of Medicine and Dentistry	AAMC	M.D., Ph.D., M.S.	1,812	96 / class
Rush Medical College of Rush University	LCME	M.D., M.D./Ph.D	2,528	119 / class
Saint Louis University School of Medicine	LCME	M.D., M.D./Ph.D.	1,547	148 / class
University of South Alabama College of Medicine	AAMC, AMA, SACSS	M.D., M.D./Ph.D.	777	64 / class
University of South Carolina School of Medicine	LCME	M.D., M.D./Ph.D.	1,133	72 / class
University of South Dakota School of Medicine	LCME	M.D., M.S., Ph.D.	383	46 / class
University of South Florida College of Medicine	LCME	M.D.	565	96 / class
University of Southern California School of Medicine	LCME	M.D., M.D./Ph.D.	3,000	136 / class
Southern Illinois University School of Medicine	LCME	M.D., M.D./J.D.	872	74 / class
Stanford University School of Medicine	LCME	M.D., M.D./Ph.D., M.S./Ph.D.	4,189	86 / class

* Not Available   ** Not Applicable   C/S – Contact School   I/S – In-State   O/S – Out-of-State

Mean GPA	% Male / % Female	% Minorities	In-State Tuition	Out-of-State Tuition	Application Fee	Application Deadline
*	50% / 50%	*	$6,840	$12,840	$20	December 15
3.51	62% / 38%	*	$19,965	**	$50	November 15
3.0	48% 52%	*	$5,994	$18,147	$20	November 15
3.4	67% / 33%	22%	$5,370	$12,840	$10 I/S $15 O/S	November 1
3.5	55% / 45%	11%	$5,166	$11,958	$40	November 15
3.6	*	11%	$18,334	**	$55	November 1
3.53	66% / 34%	19%	$13,544	$19,442	$40	November 15
*	*	*	$14,500	$19,960	$50	November 15
3.15	65% / 35%	*	$14,000	$21,000	$50	December 15
3.54	51% / 49%	*	$2,500	C/S	$15	December 1
3.52	51% / 49%	10%	$17,300	**	$50	November 1
*	76% / 24%	*	$17,520	**	$35	November 15
3.49	78% / 22%	*	$18,700	**	$50	December 15
3.1	60% / 40%	*	$5,280	$10,560	$25	November 15
3.33	64% / 36%	12%	$4,800	$11,000	$20	December 1
3.39	57% / 43%	*	$6,670	$13,780	$15	November 15
3.5	66% / 34%	24%	$6,264	$15,307	$75	December 1
3.42	54% / 46%	22%	$20,600	**	$50	November 1
3.28	61% / 39%	19%	$7,892	$22,164	None	November 15
3.6	60% / 40%	20%	$17,925	**	$55	November 1

* Not Available   ** Not Applicable   C/S – Contact School   I/S – In-State   O/S – Out-of-State

School	Accreditation	Degrees Offered	# Students Applied	Enrollment
State University of New York Health Sciences Center at Brooklyn College of Medicine	LCME	M.D., M.D./Ph.D.	2,596	203 / class
State University of New York at Buffalo School of Medicine and Biomedical Sciences	LCME	M.D., M.D./Ph.D.	2,217	135 / class
State University of New York at Stony Brook Health Sciences Center School of Medicine	LCME	M.D., M.D./Ph.D.	2,755	100 / class
State University of New York at Syracuse Health Science Center College of Medicine	LCME	M.D., M.D./Ph.D., M.D./M.B.A.	2,652	150 / class
Temple University School of Medicine	LCME	M.D., M.D./Ph.D.	3,951	180 / class
University of Tennessee, Memphis College of Medicine	LCME	M.D.	602	138 / class
Texas A&M University College of Medicine	LCME	M.D., M.D./Ph.D.	904	48 / class
University of Texas Medical School at Galveston	SACS	M.D., M.D./Ph.D.	2,072	196 / class
University of Texas Medical School at Houston	LCME	M.D., M.D./Ph.D., M.D./M.P.H.	2,111	189 / class
University of Texas Medical School at San Antonio	LCME	M.D.	2,052	202 / class
University of Texas Southwestern Medical School at Dallas Southwestern Med. Sch.	LCME	M.D., M.D./Ph.D.	2,094	194 / class
Texas Tech University, Health Sciences Center School of Medicine	LCME	M.D., M.S./M.D., M.D./Ph.D.	902	100 / class
Tufts University School of Medicine	LCME	M.D., M.D./Ph.D., M.D./M.P.H.	5,038	152 / class
Tulane University School of Medicine	AAMC	M.D., M.D./M.P.H., M.D./M.S., M.D./Ph.D.	4,343	148 / class
Uniformed Services University of the Health Sciences F. Edward Hébert School of Medicine	LCME	M.D.	2,624	162 / class
University of Utah School of Medicine	LCME	M.D., M.S., Ph.D.	532	100 / class
Vanderbilt University School of Medicine	LCME	M.D., M.D./Ph.D.	3,215	97 / class
University of Vermont College of Medicine	LCME	M.D., M.D./Ph.D.	2,728	93 / class
University of Virginia School of Medicine	LCME	M.D., M.D./Ph.D.	2,750	139 / class

* Not Available   ** Not Applicable   C/S – Contact School   I/S – In-State   O/S – Out-of-State

Mean GPA	% Male / % Female	% Minorities	In-State Tuition	Out-of-State Tuition	Application Fee	Application Deadline
3.36	*	*	$5,850	$13,250	$50	December 15
3.51	59% / 41%	*	$5,850	$13,250	$50	December 1
*	*	*	$5,850	$13,250	$50	December 15
*	64% / 36%	*	$5,850	$13,250	$50	December 1
3.25	52% / 48%	12%	$14,212	$18,964	$40	December 1
3.4	*	*	$7,004	$11,224	$25	November 15
3.41	62% / 38%	*	$5,463	$21,852	$35	November 1
3.3	64% / 36%	30%	$5,463	$21,852	$35	October 15
3.41	60% / 40%	*	$5,463	$21,852	$35	October 15
3.38	60% / 40%	*	$5,463	$21,852	$35	October 15
3.56	69% / 31%	*	$5,463	$21,852	$35	October 15
3.2	79% / 21%	25%	$5,463	$21,852	$35	November 1
3.0	50% / 50%	*	$22,980	**	$55	November 1
*	*	*	$23,000	**	$55	December 15
3.45	78% / 22%	*	No Tuition	**	C/S	November 1
3.6	*	*	$4,896	$10,953	$25	October 15
3.6	61% / 39%	*	$14,580	**	$50	November 1
3.3	52% / 48%	*	$10,150	$21,700	$50	October 31
3.53	56% / 44%	*	$6,928	$14,728	$50	November 15

* Not Available   ** Not Applicable   C/S – Contact School   I/S – In-State   O/S – Out-of-State

School	Accreditation	Degrees Offered	# Students Applied	Enrollment
Virginia Commonwealth University Medical College of Virginia School of Medicine	LCME	M.D., M.S./M.D., M.D./Ph.D., M.P.H.	2,688	168 / class
University of Washington School of Medicine	LCME	M.D., M.D./Ph.D.	512	165 / class
Washington University School of Medicine	LCME	M.D., M.A./M.D., M.D./Ph.D.	3,544	121 / class
Wayne State University School of Medicine	LCME	M.D., Ph.D., M.S., M.D./Ph.D.	1,954	264 / class
West Virginia University School of Medicine	LCME	M.D., M.D./Ph.D.	1,276	83 / class
University of Wisconsin Medical School	LCME	M.D., M.D./Ph.D	1,255	143 / class
Wright State University School of Medicine	LCME	M.D.	1,304	91 / class
Yale University School of Medicine	LCME	M.D., M.D./Ph.D., M.D./M.P.H., M.D./J.D., M.D./M.Div.	2,219	*

* Not Available   ** Not Applicable   C/S – Contact School   I/S – In-State   O/S – Out-of-State

Mean GPA	% Male / % Female	% Minorities	In-State Tuition	Out-of-State Tuition	Application Fee	Application Deadline
3.21	70% / 30%	*	$6,600	$14,500	$50	December 1
3.53	59% / 41%	5%	$4,926	$12,513	$25	November 1
3.66	73% / 27%	*	$14,900	**	$45	November 15
3.35	70% / 30%	21%	$7,286	$14,517	$25	November 1
3.47	62% / 38%	*	$5,455	$9,865	$30	November 1
*	62% / 38%	*	$9,700	$14,200	$20	November 1
3.3	48% 52%	*	$7,035	$9,960	$25	November 15
*	68% / 32%	*	$16,950	**	$50	November 1

* Not Available   ** Not Applicable   C/S – Contact School   I/S – In-State   O/S – Out-of-State

UNIVERSITY OF ALABAMA SCHOOL OF MEDICINE

Box 100 - UAB Station
Birmingham, Alabama 35294
(205) 934-1111

Accreditation	LCME
Degrees Offered	M.D., M.D./Ph.D., M.S., M.S./M.D.
# Students Applied	1,055
Enrollment	165 / class
Mean GPA	3.41
% Men / % Women	67% / 33%
% Minorities	13%
Tuition	$4,098 In-State
	$13,246 Out-of-State
Application Fee	$25
Application Deadline	November 1

The University

The University of Alabama at Birmingham was accredited as an independent educational institution in 1970. The UAB Medical Center was established in Birmingham in 1945. The medical center encompasses six health schools and a hospital complex. The UAB schools of medicine are located in Birmingham, Huntsville, and Tuscaloosa. The medical educational program provides training in all facets of medicine, including medical education, research, and patient care. The first two basic science years of the predoctoral program are taught on the main campus in Birmingham. The last two clinical years are divided among the main campus and two branch campuses at Huntsville and Tuscaloosa.

The goals and priorities of the medical school are: care of the patient as the primary value; education of the student to be an expert on human biology; and promotion of the continuing education of the graduate, recognizing the physician as scholar.

Admissions

Completion of the MCAT and three years of college are required for admission. The admissions committee places more importance on the quality of the applicant's undergraduate work than on the subject matter taken. Other factors considered by the admissions committee include personality, character, and motivation; medical-related experience; and U.S. resi-

dency (legal residents of Alabama and citizens of the United States are given preference). UAB's nondiscrimination policy states that no applicant may be denied admission on the basis of race, color, religion, sex, national origin, or veteran status. An early decision plan is available to eligible applicants.

Undergraduate Preparation

The applicant's undergraduate coursework must include English composition and literature; two semesters of general chemistry with lab; two semesters of organic chemistry with lab; two semesters of general biology with lab; two semesters of general physics with lab; and two semesters of college mathematics.

Student Body

Characteristics of the 1990 entering class included a mean GPA of 3.41, six M.D./Ph.D. students, and 62 percent who majored in some type of science. Fifty-seven colleges and universities were represented.

Placement Records

The office of medical student affairs is responsible for assisting students in career placement and handling all aspects of the National Resident Matching Program.

Costs

Yearly tuition for in-state students based on a usual academic year of three terms is $4,098. The tuition for out-of-state students is $13,246. There are varying fees for students on the three campuses, including student activity fees, microscope fees, building fees, and other minimal fees.

Financial Aid

Numerous scholarships, fellowships, and loans are available to School of Medicine students, administered through the office of student financial aid for health professions.

Minority Programs

Scholarships and fellowships are available specifically for minority students, including National Medical Fellowships, and Martin Luther King, Jr. Fellowships for minority veterans.

Student Organizations

The Student Government Association is composed of representatives of each class. National honor societies include Omicron Delta Kappa and Alpha Omega Alpha. The Caduceus Club is an organization available to alumni and others for a membership fee of $200 per year.

Curriculum

The School of Medicine offers preclinical and clinical M.D. education as well as post-M.D. education in a wide variety of specialties and subspecialities. During the first two years of the program, the student will concentrate on the basic medical sciences, particularly as they relate to human biology and pathology. The third year and part of the fourth year consist of required rotation through clinical science disciplines. Students participate in the care of patients, both in the hospital and in ambulatory settings, under faculty supervision.

Facilities

The medical center consists of six health schools: Dentistry, Medicine, Nursing, Optometry, Health-Related Professions, and Public Health; and the University of Alabama Hospital. Facilities at Birmingham include approximately 40 research centers and clinics in fields such as Alzheimer's Disease and AIDS, epilepsy, lung health, and sleep/wake disorders. The Lister Hill Library, located in Birmingham, houses more than 240,000 volumes of monographs and bound journals and includes subscriptions to 3,000 of the world's leading biomedical journals.

Facilities at Tuscaloosa include the Capstone Medical Center, DCH Regional Medical Center, Veterans Administration Medical Center, AMI West Alabama Hospital, and Bryce State Hospital/Partlow State School and Hospital. The Health Sciences Library at Tuscaloosa serves all health professionals in the west Alabama area, housing a monograph collection of approximately 10,000 volumes and a reference collection of 425 volumes. The library subscribes to about 475 journals. The MEDLINE database is available, as well as a campus-wide on-line catalog, AMELIA.

Facilities at Huntsville include the Clinical Science Center-School of Primary Medical Care, UAH medical clinics, and a library with 8,825 monographs and 11,300 bound journals.

Grading Procedures

Grades in courses on academic segments consist of A, B, C, D, and F for most required elements of the program. Pass (P) or fail (F) are given for single elective experiences and for some experiences too short or otherwise unsuitable for letter grades.

Special Programs

UAB offers six- or seven-year M.D./Ph.D. opportunities, including a program that allows the student to pursue a doctorate in the biomedical sciences. The school also offers an M.S./M.D. program as well as specialized master's degrees in public health, dentistry, nursing, physical therapy, clinical nutrition, and other fields.

The EMSAP (Early Medical School Acceptance Program) is available to high school seniors who wish to pursue medicine as a career. These students should have at least a 3.5 GPA, an ACT score of 30, or an SAT of 1,300 or higher.

Application Procedures

Applicants must take the MCAT and have the results sent to the admissions committee. It is recommended that the MCAT be taken in the spring of the year in which the student will file an application. Transcripts and applications are processed through AMCAS. Applications to UAB School of Medicine should be filed with AMCAS between June 15 and November 1. Early application is encouraged. There is an application fee of $25.

Contact

Office of Medical Student Services/Admissions
University of Alabama School of Medicine
Box 100 - UAB Station
Birmingham, Alabama 35294
(205) 934-2330

ALBANY MEDICAL COLLEGE

47 New Scotland Avenue
Albany, New York 12208
(518) 445-3125

Accreditation	AAMC
Degrees Offered	M.D., M.D./Ph.D.
# Students Applied	4,412
Enrollment	125 / class
Mean GPA	3.2
% Men / % Women	57% / 43%
% Minorities	Not Available
Tuition	$18,900
Application Fee	$50
Application Deadline	December 1

The University

The Albany Medical College is a private medical school with a 150 year tradition of instructing students in the medical arts, as well as the practical science of medicine. Located in the capital city of New York, the college of medicine offers students a strong academic base as well as many opportunities for extracurricular cultural activity within the city itself. New York City, Boston, and Montreal are easily accessible by car or train.

Admissions

The Medical College, in selecting candidates for admission, looks for students with the potential to become competent and compassionate physicians who will continue to learn throughout their lives. A minimum of three years undergraduate study is required in order to be considered for admission to the Albany Medical College. Applicants who have undergraduate experience from a college or university in the U.S. or Canada will be given preference.

Undergraduate Preparation

Specific courses required for admission include one year each of general biology or zoology, organic chemistry, inorganic chemistry, and general physics. Proficiency in oral and written English is also required. The MCAT must be taken no later than the fall one year prior to intended medical school matriculation.

Student Body

Most students come from New York State although others may be admitted.

Costs

Tuition for the 1990-91 academic year was $18,900. Additional expenses for an unmarried student, including living costs, are estimated to total another $10,000.

Financial Aid

Albany Medical College offers eligible students assistance in the form of scholarships, loans, financial counseling and help in securing employment. It is possible to finance the complete cost of medical education through various loan programs. Full and partial merit scholarships are available for qualified applicants with outstanding academic records. Interested students may apply for an Armed Services Health Professions Scholarship which covers the entire cost of medical education and includes a stipend.

Minority Programs

The Assistant Dean for Minority Affairs reviews the applications of all minority applicants and is actively involved in the admissions process. The minority affairs office implements programs to ensure the admission, matriculation, retention, and graduation of qualified students from minority backgrounds and offers a variety of academic support services to students throughout the course of their four years of medical study. All accepted and alternate minority students are invited to attend a six-week summer pre-matriculation program at no cost.

Student Organizations

A variety of extracurricular groups and activities are available to medical students at Albany. There is an active student government, student newspaper, crew, choir, outing, and rugby clubs, squash and tennis courts as well as numerous informal cultural, social, and scientific groups.

Curriculum

The curriculum at the Albany Medical College integrates the teaching of basic sciences with clinical instruction. The first two years concentrate on the basic sciences but there are also associated patient presentations, and all teaching is done from a clinical perspective. In the third year, students devote most of their academic time to clerkships which rotate through each of the major clinical areas and gradually take on clinical responsibilities. Fourth year medical students are allowed, with the help of faculty advisers, to devise an individualized course of study which best suits their personal career goals and particular academic interests. A large variety of electives are available at Albany Medical Center Hospital, other affiliated hospitals and medical centers, and at other institutions in the United States and abroad.

Facilities

The Albany Medical Center is a 674-bed complex that serves as the main teaching hospital for the medical college. Directly adjacent to the main academic buildings, this facility is the only academic health sciences center in a 24-county region of northeastern New York and western New England,

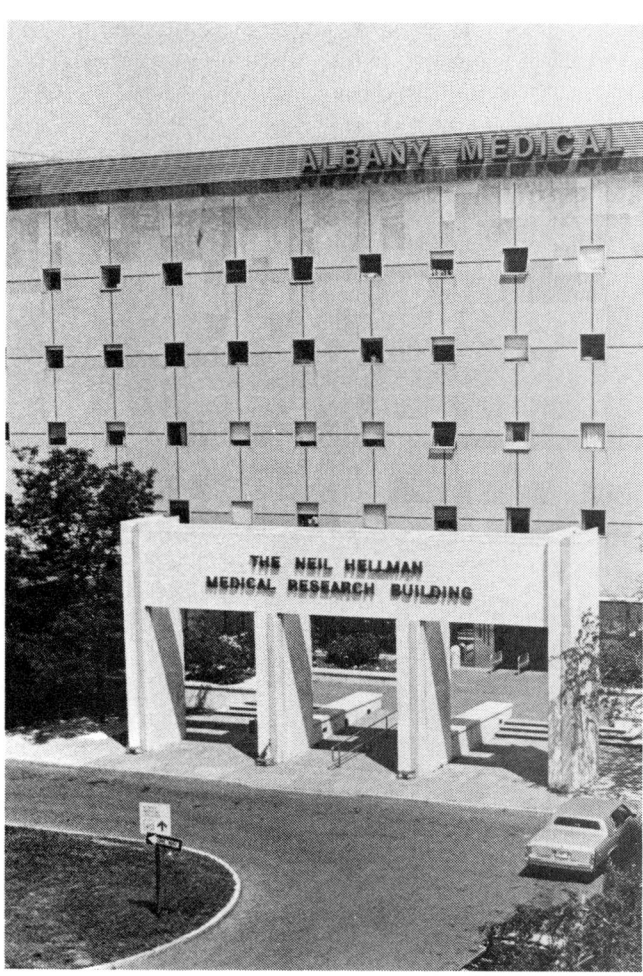

providing services for more than two million residents. Other affiliated institutions include the Albany Veteran's Administration Medical Center, a 750-bed facility, and the Capital District Psychiatric Center. A new seven-story addition to the Medical Center is underway as well. Scheduled to be completed by the spring of 1992, this $156 million facility will add a new ambulatory care facility, a new emergency department, and new surgery suites to the existing complex.

Special Programs

A six year combined M.D./Ph.D. degree program is available for students interested in pursuing careers in research and academic medicine. It is also possible to earn the M.D. degree with Distinction in Research by participating in research projects during the normal four-year period of medical studies.

Application Procedures

Applicants must submit an application to the Albany Medical College through the centralized service of the AMCAS. Supporting materials required include transcripts, MCAT results, and letters of recommendation. Candidates with records that demonstrate academic ability, interest in learning, concern for helping others, motivation for the difficult work of medical studies, emotional maturity, and a range of academic and non-academic interests are then selected to participate in on-campus personal interviews. The application deadline is December 1 of the year prior to desired entrance to medical school.

Contact

Office of Admissions A-3
Albany Medical College
Albany, New York 12208
(518) 445-5521

ALBERT EINSTEIN COLLEGE OF MEDICINE OF YESHIVA UNIVERSITY

1300 Morris Park Avenue
Bronx, New York 10461
(212) 430-2801

Accreditation	LCME, AAMC
Degrees Offered	M.D., M.D./Ph.D.
# Students Applied	4,045
Enrollment	200 / class
Mean GPA	3.4
% Men / % Women	54% / 46%
% Minorities	Not Available
Tuition	$18,960
Application Fee	$60
Application Deadline	November 1

The University

Albert Einstein College of Medicine, a constituent college of Yeshiva University, was founded in 1955 and has developed into one of the nation's foremost centers for medical education, research, and clinical care. The college is situated on a 17-acre campus in the Westchester Heights section of the Bronx, New York, 30 minutes from midtown Manhattan. The college is located in an area with six medical schools, nearly a dozen universities, and the largest complex of hospitals in the nation.

New York City offers an array of excellent libraries and the facilities of the New York Academy of Medicine and the New York Academy of Sciences.

The college has two postgraduate divisions, the Sue Golding Graduate Division of Medical Sciences and the Belfer Institute for Advanced Biomedical Studies.

Admissions

MCAT scores, undergraduate grades, recommendations, and the student's personal essay are all important elements in the admissions process. Interviews are only granted to those under serious consideration for admission.

The goal of the admissions committee of the college is to select a diverse and talented group of students who show the promise of becoming respected and distinguished members of the medical community in all areas including teaching, research, clinical practice, and administration. The committee seeks demonstrated academic excellence but also considers the personal qualities of applicants. Serious consideration is also given to applicants who have participated in extracurricular activities, service orientation, or have a research background, and previous experience in clinical health care settings.

Undergraduate Preparation

A firm foundation in the biological and physical sciences and mathematics is mandatory. Minimum premedical requirements include one formal year of laboratory work in biology, general chemistry, organic chemistry, and physics. One year of formal coursework in mathematics (including statistics and probability) and in English are required. Basic computer literacy is recommended.

Student Body

Among the class of 1994, students range in age from 19 to 41. Forty-six percent are women, as compared to 38 percent in the national pool. Sixty-three undergraduate colleges are represented. Eighteen students among the class are considered of minority status.

U.S. students come primarily from the northeast, although the south and midwest are also represented. Almost two dozen foreign countries are represented in the student body.

Placement Records

The college assists students in obtaining residency positions through the National Residency Matching Program. Members of the class of 1990 were assigned residencies in hospitals primarily in the northeast states—New York, New Jersey, Connecticut, Massachusetts.

Costs

For 1990-91, the tuition was $18,960. Other fees, including laboratory fees, housing costs, books, supplies, and instruments totaled about $4,000.

Financial Aid

Qualified students may be eligible for a maximum of $5,000 per academic year from the Einstein Scholarship Fund and the Einstein College Loan Fund. Health Professional Student Loans are available to U.S. citizens and permanent residents. More information on financial assistance can be obtained by contacting the student finance office at the college.

Minority Programs

The College of Medicine maintains an office of minority student affairs (OMSA). OMSA provides counseling and tutoring to underrepresented minority students, especially in the basic biomedical science courses during the first two years of study. OMSA also plans and administers programs designed to recruit minority and disadvantaged students.

Student Organizations

In addition to the Student Council, the college hosts chapters of the American Medical Students Association and the American Medical Women's Association. Chapters of the Stu-

dent National Medical Association and the Boricua Health Organization organize activities designed especially for minority students.

Faculty

The college's full-time faculty of more than 1,000 teachers delivers health care and conducts studies in every major medical specialty and area of biomedical research. Several faculty members have been elected to the National Academy of Sciences, and two faculty members have been awarded the National Medal of Science in recent years.

Curriculum

The goals of the student are: to understand the scientific bases of disease; to develop the ability to recognize disease states and determine the need for medical care; to learn how to evaluate information critically; to learn to value the integrity of patients and relate to them with sensitivity and compassion; to acquire the knowledge, skills, and attitudes required for prevention of disease and health maintenance; and to develop skills for self-evaluation and a commitment to lifelong continuing education.

The preclinical curriculum stresses biological sciences taught in a traditional setting, but also offers instruction in clinical skills. During the clinical curriculum, students learn to apply their knowledge and to treat patients. The clinical curriculum begins in the third year, when the student embarks on a 46-week sequence of clerkships in the hospitals affiliated with the college. The fourth-year curriculum features a subinternship and a choice of electives.

Facilities

The college's physical complex has comprehensive facilities for teaching, research, and clinical experience. These include the Leo Forchheimer Medical Science Building, the Ullmann Research Center for Health Sciences, and the Irwin S. & Sylvia Chanin Institute for Cancer Research, one of the largest cancer research centers in the East affiliated with a medical school.

Students pursue their clinical experience in one of a large number of college-affiliated community-based hospitals, including Bronx Municipal Hospital Center, Montefiore Medical Center, the Bronx Psychiatric Center, and the Bronx-Lebanon Hospital Center.

The D. Samuel Gottesman Library houses 160,000 monographs and bound journals, and has 2,300 current periodical subscriptions, archival materials, audiovisual media, and computer software. The MEDLINE database is available as well as other bibliographic and information databases.

Grading Procedures

Grading in preclerkship courses are honors, pass, and fail. Grades in clinical courses are honors, high pass, pass, low pass, and fail.

Special Programs

The Einstein Medical Scientist Training Program is a six- or seven-year course of study that leads to a combined M.D./Ph.D. degree. One of the oldest programs of its kind in the country, the MSTP is designed to train students for a career in biomedical research and teaching. MSTP trainees study the basic science that is taught to M.D. students in their core curriculum and also pursue advanced coursework in several specific areas of medicine.

Application Procedures

The College of Medicine will only accept applications processed through the AMCAS. Applications must be received by AMCAS by November 1 of the year preceding anticipated matriculation. Applicants must also submit letters of recommendation and a $60 application fee. The composite evaluation of a premedical advisory committee is preferred, although letters of recommendation from two members of the undergraduate faculty will be considered instead.

Students being seriously considered for admission may be called for a personal interview.

Contact

Albert Einstein College of Medicine of Yeshiva University
Jack and Pearl Resnick Campus
Office of Admissions
1300 Morris Park Avenue
Bronx, New York 10461
(212) 430-2106

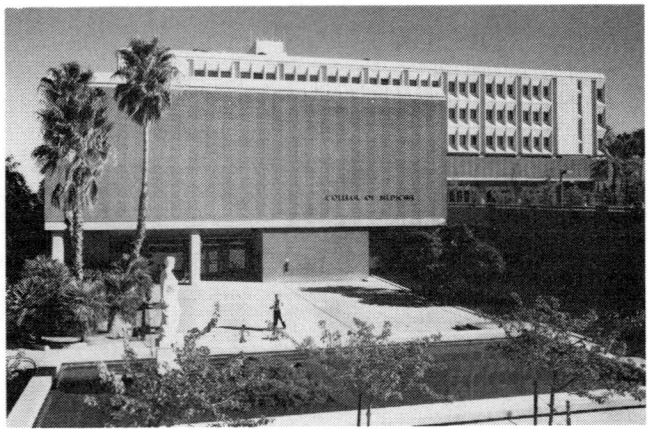

UNIVERSITY OF ARIZONA COLLEGE OF MEDICINE

Tucson, Arizona 85724
(602) 621-2211

Accreditation	AAMC
Degrees Offered	M.D., M.D./Ph.D.
# Students Applied	255
Enrollment	88 / class
Mean GPA	3.52
% Men / % Women	59% / 41%
% Minorities	Not Available
Tuition	$6,192
Application Fee	Contact School
Application Deadline	November 1

The University

The University of Arizona was established in 1885 as a land-grant institution, 27 years before Arizona was admitted to the Union. It is one of three public institutions of higher learning in Arizona. Today, the university is a major southwestern institution comprising 10 colleges, four faculties, eight schools, 119 academic committees or departments, and 52 research and special service units. The university enrolls over 36,000 students and offers nearly 400 fields of study.

Established in the mid-1960s, the College of Medicine graduated its first class in 1971. The mission of the college is: to educate physicians and other biomedical scientists; to make nationally and internationally recognized contributions to both basic and clinical biomedical research; and to provide models of excellence in patient care.

The university is located near downtown Tucson, a rapidly growing metropolitan area of more than 650,000 residents.

Admissions

The College of Medicine accepts students from Arizona (including Native Americans living on reservations contiguous with the state of Arizona); and, if they are highly qualified, students from Alaska, Montana, and Wyoming are considered (these students must provide evidence of full and uninterrupted funding from their state of origin). The college will not consider students from any other state.

Admission is based on academic record, MCAT scores, personal statement, college preprofessional committee evaluations (or letters of recommendation), and results of personal interviews. Course load, breadth of undergraduate education, work experience, extracurricular pursuits, and other factors also influence the admissions decision.

Undergraduate Preparation

The college encourages interested students of all majors to apply; however, the following minimum requirements must be met by the end of the spring semester prior to matriculation: completion of at least three full years of study (90 semester hours or 135 quarter hours); and completion of two full semesters or equivalent in general chemistry; organic chemistry; physics; general biology or zoology; and English. In addition, applicants are urged to take the MCAT in the spring of the year of application and to have their premedical requirements completed at the time of application.

Student Body

Students hold an average GPA of about 3.52 and average MCAT score in the sciences, math, and reading of about 9.3 (the average score in biology is 9.8).

Placement Records

The faculty assists students in applying for and successfully competing for residency programs in Arizona and throughout the United States.

The class of 1990 residency appointments were made primarily in the southwest, but many graduates took posts in the midwest and the east, including Ohio, Iowa, New York, and Pennsylvania.

Costs

Tuition and fees total approximately $6,192 for the first and second years (charges for the third and fourth years can be obtained from the medical financial aid office). Books and supplies are estimated to cost about $1,300, and room and board are estimated to cost between $5,600 and $6,700.

Financial Aid

With some exceptions, most assistance is granted solely on the basis of need and according to the availability of funds.

Loans from outside the university include Stafford Loans, Health Education Assistance Loans, and Supplemental Loans for Students. Applications can be obtained from the college's student financial aid office.

Minority Programs

The College of Medicine has an active program dedicated to the recruitment, admission, education, and graduation of an increasing number of students from minority ethnic groups.

Student Organizations

The various committees in which students may participate include the American Holistic Medical Association, the American Medical Student Association, the American Medical Women's Association, the Christian Medical Society, Commitment to Underserved People, and the Student Committee on Medical Education.

Curriculum

The curriculum comprises three years of required studies and one year of elective rotations. Half of the program focuses on the basic sciences critical to modern medical understanding and practice; the other half introduces the student to patient contact and clinical science instruction.

Methods of instruction include lectures, small group instruction, independent study, clinical clerkships, practicums in physical diagnosis, computer-based instruction, and a variety of other learning modes.

The first part of the curriculum deals with biologic, cultural, psychosocial, economic, and sociologic concepts and data. Emphasis is placed on problem solving and developing an awareness of the milieu in which medicine is practiced. The third year is devoted to clinical clerkships and the fourth year is composed solely of elective rotations.

Facilities

The Arizona Health Sciences Center is a complex of buildings located just north of the main campus. The center comprises the Basic Sciences Building, the Clinical Sciences Building, outpatient clinics, the University Medical Center, the Arizona Cancer Center, and Life Sciences North. Other facilities include the Family Practice Center, biomedical research laboratories, and a radiology research building.

University Medical Center, a private 300-bed hospital, is the primary setting used for the education of medical students. It houses the only lithotripsy unit in Tucson, a magentic resonance imaging facility, and other modern diagnostic and therapeutic apparatus. Other clinical buildings include Tucson Veterans Administration Medical Center, Tucson Medical Center, Kino Community Hospital, and Crippled Children's Clinic. Clerkships are also conducted at hospitals in Phoenix.

The library maintains a collection of 165,000 volumes and 3,400 media programs, and subscribes to 3,500 journals and serial publications. Most services of the library are computer enhanced.

Grading Procedures

The College of Medicine employs an honors/pass/fail grading system along with narrative evaluation of student performance for each course or clerkship. Class members are not ranked, but the honors and awards committee reviews all written evaluations in order to identify outstanding student performance.

Special Programs

The college offers a program that leads to the M.D./Ph.D. degree. Completion of both degrees normally takes six to seven years. Those interested must be accepted into the College of Medicine and the Graduate College of the university.

Application Procedures

Candidates must apply directly to AMCAS. The deadline for applications is November 1. Those selected through prescreening will be sent additional materials from the college and invited for a personal interview.

Contact

University of Arizona College of Medicine
Admissions Office
Tucson, Arizona 85724
(602) 626-6214/6215

UNIVERSITY OF ARKANSAS COLLEGE OF MEDICINE

4301 West Markham Street - Slot 551
Little Rock, Arkansas 72205
(501) 569-3000

Accreditation	AAMC
Degrees Offered	M.D., M.S., Ph.D.
# Students Applied	438
Enrollment	140/class
Mean GPA	3.5
% Men / % Women	64% / 36%
% Minorities	10%
Tuition	$5,720 In-State
	$11,440 Out-of-State
Application Fee	$10
Application Deadline	November 15

The University

The University of Arkansas for Medical Sciences (UAMS) was established in 1879 as the medical department of the Arkansas Industrial University. In 1975, the medical center was renamed the University of Arkansas for Medical Sciences and designated as one of the five campuses within the University of Arkansas system. Today, the university is a comprehensive health center for teaching, service, and research. UAMS comprises five colleges—Medicine, Nursing, Pharmacy, Health-Related Professions, and the Graduate School.

UAMS operates as a referral center for physicians through-out the state with patients who have special problems and is the only biomedical research facility in the state.

Admissions

A broad undergraduate education of at least 90 semester hours is a prerequisite to admission, and a bachelor's degree from an accredited school is strongly recommended. Undergraduate transcripts and MCAT scores are considered in the admissions process, along with recommendations from the applicant's premedical advisory committee and a personal interview for in-state applicants. Certain personal attributes are sought in the applicant, including compassion, integrity, stamina, dedication to human service, and a sustained ability to learn.

State law permits the admissions committee to accept a limited number of nonresident applicants provided no qualified resident applicant is displaced. Nonresident applicants with less than a 3.5 GPA will not be considered.

Undergraduate Preparation

A broad cultural background is highly valued in the applicant. While no specific courses are required of the undergraduate, a recommended course of undergraduate study includes general biology or zoology and botany; a full year of general chemistry, organic chemistry, or physical chemistry; physics and mathematics; behavioral science courses, such as anthropology and sociology; and humanities courses that include English composition and speech.

Student Body

For the 1990 entering class, 280 resident applicants applied and 150 were admitted. The average GPA was 3.5. MCAT scores averaged between 7.9 and 8.9. Of the class, about 36 percent were female, 64 percent were male, and these included 10 percent minority students. Eighty-four percent of undergraduate majors were in the science disciplines. About one quarter of the class obtained all or part of their undergraduate education outside Arkansas.

Placement Records

All internships, residencies, and fellowships offered by UAMS are accredited by the Accreditation Council for Graduate Medical Education. Most transitional intern and first-year residency positions are appointed through the National Resident Matching Program.

Costs

Tuition for 1990-91 was $5,720 per year for Arkansas residents and $11,440 for nonresidents. Diagnostic equipment was $670 for the first academic year. Books are estimated to cost $450 per year. Various other living expenses, including room, board, and transportation, bring the estimated total of first-year expenses to $15,554.

Financial Aid

Types of aid available include federal loans (Stafford Loans and Supplemental Loans to Students), institutional loans, service-connected loans/scholarships, institutional scholarships, and a wide variety of other kinds of scholarships.

Students accepted for admission must be U.S. citizens or permanent residents of the United States to qualify for financial aid. Eligibility for aid is determined by the Graduate and Professional School Financial Aid Service (GAPSFAS) needs analysis. Students must also have a financial aid transcript (FAT) sent to the university from each school previously attended.

Financial aid packets are mailed to students following acceptance of admission. The suggested date for filing the GAPSFAS is March 31. Applicants should submit the university's application for student financial assistance by April 30.

Faculty

Medical students are taught by a full-time faculty of approximately 400 members augmented by a voluntary faculty of more than 800 practicing physicians throughout Arkansas. In addition, about 450 interns, residents, and fellows are in specialty postdoctoral training and participate in medical student instruction.

Curriculum

Lectures, laboratory periods, conferences, and tests are conducted in such a way as to encourage the student to develop initiative, self-reliance, intellectual curiosity, and independence. Students are encouraged to participate, where possible, in the research carried out by members of the staff.

Basic medical courses, such as gross anatomy, microanatomy, medical biochemistry, and neuroscience are taken in the first year. Clinical clerkships begin in the third year in areas such as surgery and obstetrics/gynecology. The senior program is mostly elective. Participation in research can be part of the senior electives.

Facilities

The medical complex is located in the west-central section of Little Rock near the War Memorial Stadium. Facilities include the 400-bed University Hospital of Arkansas and Clinics; a nine-story building for biomedical sciences; the T.H. Barton Institute for Medical Research; the Child Study Center; a nine-story education building; the Isaac Folsom Clinic; and the Arkansas Cancer Research Center.

Throughout the 1970s, six area health education centers were developed in selected Arkansas cities as outreach training sites for predoctoral, postdoctoral, and continuing physician education programs.

Grading Procedures

UAMS uses a letter grading system—A, B, C, D, and F. Elective courses are graded as P (pass) or F (fail).

Special Programs

Special degree programs include graduate work leading to the Master of Science degree in any of the following fields: anatomy, biochemistry and molecular biology, interdisciplinary toxicology, microbiology and immunology, pathology, physiology and biophysics, and pharmacology. Programs are also offered that lead to the Ph.D. in anatomy, biochemistry and molecular biology, interdisciplinary toxicology, microbiology and immunology, pharmacology and physiology, and biophysics.

Application Procedures

The standard AMCAS application form and transcripts must be received by AMCAS by November 15 for the class entering the following fall. A $10 fee will be requested by the university admissions office.

Students should take the MCAT by the fall of the year preceding the year of desired admission. College transcripts should be sent directly to the university office of admissions. Recommendations should be mailed directly to the office of admissions. In-state applicants may be called for an interview.

Contact

University of Arkansas
College of Medicine
Office of Student Admissions
4301 West Markham Street
Little Rock, Arkansas 72205
(501) 686-5354

BAYLOR COLLEGE OF MEDICINE

One Baylor Plaza
Houston, Texas 77030
(713) 799-4951

Accreditation	LCME, SACS
Degrees Offered	M.D., M.D./Ph.D.
# Students Applied	1,588
Enrollment	164
Mean GPA	3.6
% Men / % Women	60% / 40%
% Minorities	Not Available
Tuition	$5,463 In-State
	Contact School for Out-of-State
Application Fee	$30
Application Deadline	November 1

The University

Baylor College of Medicine is an independent medical school affiliated with the Texas Medical Center, a group of 13 hospitals and other health care facilities in metropolitan Houston. Founded in 1900 as part of the University of Dallas, the college was later named for its affiliation with Baylor University in Waco. Baylor College of Medicine moved to Houston in 1943 and in 1969 became independent of Baylor University. Besides the extensive educational and research opportunities available to students through the Texas Medical Center, the city of Houston, centrally located only 50 miles from the Texas Gulf Coast beaches, offers extensive cultural and recreational diversions.

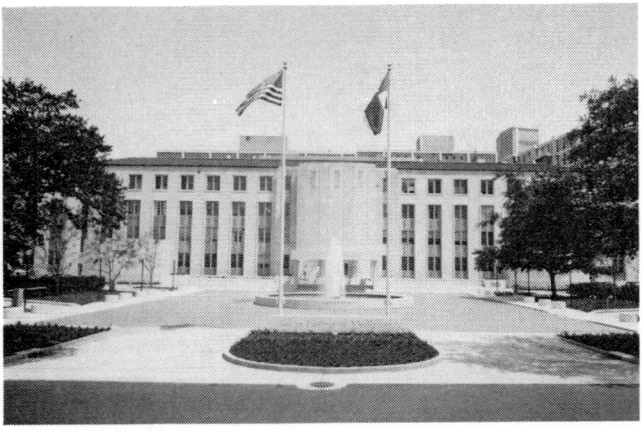

Admissions

Baylor generally requires applicants to have an undergraduate GPA of at least 3.0, with the average GPA of successful applicants at 3.6. Average MCAT scores are in the 10 range.

Undergraduate Preparation

Required undergraduate coursework consists of one year each of general chemistry, organic chemistry, general biology, and physics (all with lab), as well as one year of English composition or literature. Baylor does not require an applicant to have a science major, but students must demonstrate the ability to successfully handle scientific concepts. A minimum of 90 semester hours is required, but the completion of a baccalaureate degree prior to enrollment is preferred. Pass/fail grades in undergraduate science courses are not recommended.

Student Body

Members of the entering class of 1989 represented 71 undergraduate colleges, 29 undergraduate majors, and approximately 25 states. Sixty-four percent were men, 36 percent were women.

Costs

As the result of an agreement between Baylor and the state, legal Texas residents attending Baylor College of Medicine are charged tuition comparable to the cost of state-supported medical colleges in Texas. In-state tuition is $5,463. Tuition for non-Texans is comparable to that charged by other private U.S. medical schools; a specific breakdown is available upon request. Fees total $700 per year, with books adding another $1,000. Baylor estimates total living expenses at $10,781 annually.

Financial Aid

Federal need-based loans are available to students who qualify and other privately financed loans may be available. Since only limited scholarship aid is available from the school, Baylor advises that the student explore outside organizations for further funds. The financial aid office helps students locate these sources of assistance. The deadline for financial aid applications is March 15.

Minority Programs

The Baylor Association of Minority Medical Students is a student organization that works to recruit and retain underrepresented minority students and faculty to the College of Medicine. The organization also acts as a support group and is open to any interested person.

Student Organizations

Extracurricular opportunities for students at Baylor are extensive. Organizations on campus include the American Medical Student Association, American Medical Women's Association, Day with a Doctor, the Family Practice Club, and the Texas Medical Association chapter of the American Medical Association. Alpha Omega Alpha, the national medical honor fraternity, has a chapter on campus as well. Also available are the student newspaper, yearbook, intramural athletic league, and several academic and social support groups.

Faculty

Baylor has 1,505 full-time faculty members, 131 part-time faculty members, and approximately 1,700 voluntary faculty.

Curriculum

Generally, requirements for the M.D. degree are 150 weeks of academic work distributed to include 54 weeks in basic science courses, 68 weeks in required clinical science clerkships, and 28 weeks (56 credits) in elective courses or clerkships. Baylor allows students flexibility in designing their schedules to allow opportunities for advanced completion of the basic science requirements as well as the ability to slow the pace of medical education if academic difficulty is encountered.

Facilities

Baylor's affiliation with the Texas Medical Center affords students access to many educational facilities. The Houston Academy of Medicine-Texas Medical Center Library is one of the nation's largest medical libraries with 83,500 books, 134,800 journal volumes, 4,155 audiovisual materials, and 3,000 current journals. Baylor is also a major biomedical research center with opportunities available to students at the DeBakey Heart Center, the nation's only Children's Nutrition Research Center, and a national center for the study and control of influenza.

Grading Procedures

Grades at Baylor are based on a combination of objective exams and written evaluations of student performance. In preclinical courses, grades are designated as honors, pass, marginal pass, or fail. In the clinical curriculum an additional grade of high pass is used to designate exceptional performance in most areas. Baylor does not require students to take Part I or Part II of the National Boards, but subject National Boards are required.

Special Programs

An M.D./Ph.D. program is available for students interested in the biomedical sciences. A Ph.D. program in Biomedical Engineering is also offered in conjunction with Rice University. A Medical Scientist Training Program (MSTP) is available through a grant from the National Institutes of Health. The purpose of the MSTP is to integrate medical and graduate education and offer training in basic medical sciences, clinical medicine, and biomedical research.

Application Procedures

Applicants to Baylor College of Medicine should submit an application to the office of admissions no later than November 1 of the year before desired medical school entrance. The deadline for early decision candidates is August 1. All applications must be accompanied by transcripts of undergraduate work, a letter of evaluation from the chair of the premedical advisory committee at the undergraduate college, and a $30 application fee. MCAT scores are also required; the test should be taken in April of the year before desired enrollment. All applicants offered places in the entering class will be invited to personal, on-campus interviews.

Contact

Office of Admissions
Baylor College of Medicine
One Baylor Plaza
Houston, Texas 77030
(713) 798-4841

BOSTON UNIVERSITY SCHOOL OF MEDICINE

80 East Concord Street
Boston, Massachusetts 02118
(617) 638-5300

Accreditation	LCME
Degrees Offered	M.D., B.A./M.D., M.D./M.A., M.D./Ph.D., M.D./M.P.H., M.D./DSc.
# Students Applied	5,340
Enrollment	135 / class
Mean GPA	3.23
% Men / % Women	59% / 41%
% Minorities	11%
Tuition	$22,300
Application Fee	Contact School
Application Deadline	November 15

The University

Boston University is an independent, coeducational, nonsectarian institution with an enrollment of about 19,100 full-time students and a faculty of over 2,500. The university traces its heritage back to 1839 and was incorporated by the

Commonwealth of Massachusetts in 1869. Today, the university system comprises 15 schools and colleges. Most of the university's schools and colleges are situated on the Charles River near downtown Boston.

The School of Medicine was established in 1873 when Boston University merged with the New England Female Medical College, which had been founded in 1848 as the first medical school for women in the world. The School of Medicine is situated in the South End of Boston between Boston City Hospital and University Hospital.

Admissions

Applicants must hold a bachelor's degree from an approved college of arts and sciences or engineering. Factors considered by the admissions committee include academic record, college recommendations, involvement in college and community activities, personality, and maturity of character. Applicants should take the MCAT in the spring of the year of application.

Students of the 1987 entering class had a mean GPA of 3.23 and an average MCAT score of about 9.0 in each subtest.

Undergraduate Preparation

The following courses are prerequisites to enrollment in the School of Medicine: one year of English composition or literature; one year of humanities; one year each (with lab) of general chemistry, organic chemistry, physics, and biology.

Students should have a broad education in the humanities, behavioral sciences, and social sciences. A knowledge of quantitation in chemistry is recommended, and a course in calculus is recommended but not required.

Costs

For 1988-89, tuition was $22,300 per year for the four-year M.D. program. The first two years of the six-year program (B.A./M.D.) are $12,800 plus fees of $175 per year and $210 per credit for summer courses. Fees for medical insurance, which is required, varies by plan. There are other service charges, including National Board of Medical Examiners fees.

Financial Aid

Loans and grants are offered to student applicants after need is determined. Applications are based on income, assets, family size, and other relevant information. Low-interest deferred loans are the main source of financial aid at the School of Medicine. Grant funds make up about one-tenth of the direct assistance offered by the school.

There are numerous scholarships and loan funds. Also available are Guaranteed Student Loans, Health Education Assistance Loans, Supplemental Loans for Students, and the federally-funded college work-study assistance programs. There is also a wide variety of awards, prizes, and fellowships.

Minority Programs

The School of Medicine has an office of minority affairs that offers programs and resources to attract students from groups underrepresented in the physician population.

Student Organizations

Student organizations include Alpha Omega Alpha; the American Medical Student Association; American Medical Women's Association; Gay and Lesbian Students of BUSM; the Maimonides Society (a national organization for Jewish medical students); Physicians for Social Responsibility; and the Primary Care Society.

Curriculum

The first-year curriculum focuses on the study of human biology. Courses cover the traditional disciplines that lead to an understanding of normal structure and function. In addition to gross anatomy, physiology, introduction to physical diagnosis, and biochemistry, courses are offered in the psychological and sociological aspects of health, illness, and the medical system.

Second-year courses include microbiology, pharmacology, biology of disease, and physical diagnosis and history taking.

The third year is the principal clerkship year. The fourth year consists of 32 weeks of elective time, four weeks of home medical service or community diagnosis, and a basic sciences in clinical medicine seminar.

The Boston University School of Medicine is known for the outstanding relationships that develop between students and members of the faculty.

Facilities

Facilities include the 14-story instructional building, the Housman Research Building, and the Silvio O. Conte Medical Research Center. Clinical facilities include University Hospital, the Centers for Advancement in Health and Medicine, Boston City Hospital, and the Veterans' Administration Medical Center.

The combined Boston University libraries contain more than 1.6 million volumes in paper, 2.4 million in microfilm, 29,000 current journals, and access to hundreds of bibliographic databases.

The Alumni Medical Library houses about 99,000 volumes and regularly receives approximately 1,600 current periodicals and serial publications. The Mugar Memorial Library provides central library service to all students of the university. The Boston City Hospital Medical Library is also open to BU's medical school students.

Grading Procedures

Student evaluation is conducted on an honors-pass basis. Departments or course instructors employ methods of examining and evaluating students that are most appropriate to their course content.

Special Programs

The MMEDIC (Modular Medical Integrated Curriculum) program is a combined eight-year program designed to integrate the liberal arts and the basic medical sciences. Qualified seniors in secondary schools may apply for admission to the six-year Program of Liberal Arts and Medical Education, which leads to the B.A. and M.D. degrees. The M.D./Ph.D. program is open to highly-qualified individuals who are strongly motivated toward an education and a career in both medicine and research. The university also offers a combined M.D./M.P.H. (Master of Public Health) program, the coursework for which is generally completed in four to five years.

Application Procedures

Candidates for admission to the four-year M.D. program should register with AMCAS. Applicants are urged to take the MCAT in the spring of the year of application.

Candidates can apply between July 1 and November 15, but early application is strongly recommended.

Contact

Admissions Office
Building L, Room 124
Boston University
School of Medicine
80 East Concord Street
Boston, Massachusetts 02118
(617) 638-4630

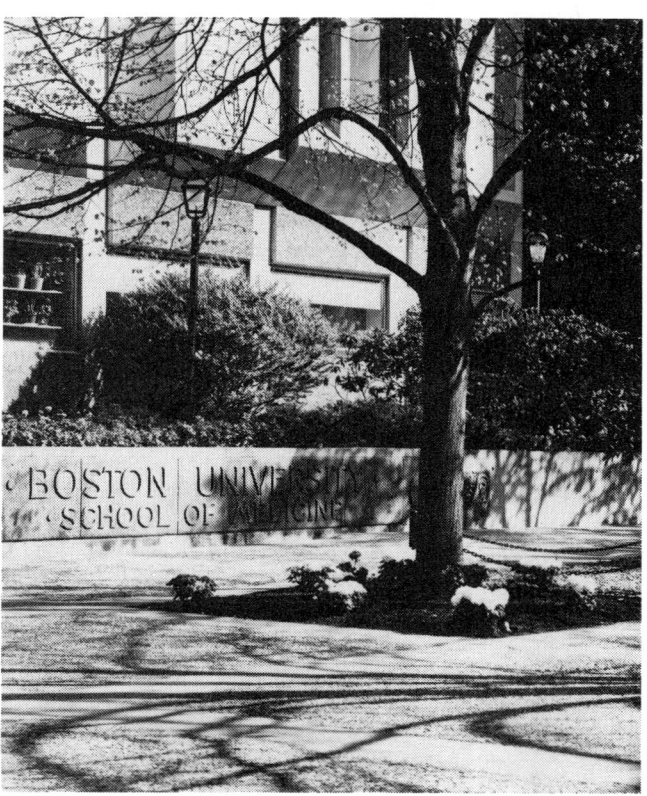

BOWMAN GRAY SCHOOL OF MEDICINE OF WAKE FOREST UNIVERSITY

300 South Hawthorne Road
Winston-Salem, North Carolina 27103
(919) 748-4424

Accreditation	LCME
Degrees Offered	M.D., M.S.
# Students Applied	3,135
Enrollment	108 / class
Mean GPA	3.3
% Men / % Women	67% / 33%
% Minorities	Not Available
Tuition	$14,200
Application Fee	$40
Application Deadline	November 1

The University

The Wake Forest Institute was founded in 1834. In 1956, the school moved from Wake County to Winston-Salem; in 1967 it became a university. The Wake Forest Medical School, established in 1902, later renamed itself after Bowman Gray, the benefactor who made the move from Wake County possible. The Bowman Gray School of Medicine became the second four-year medical school in North Carolina.

The campus is located within walking distance of Winston-Salem's Hanes Park and is only a 10-minute drive from the Forsyth County's Tanglewood Park where students and faculty can enjoy PGA championship golf courses, tennis courts, swimming pools, and horseback trails. Winston-Salem has a population of approximately 153,000. The middle class neighborhood around the school contributes to a pleasant academic environment.

Admissions

Every applicant is required to take the Medical College Admissions Test (MCAT). It is advisable to take the exam in the spring of the year applying. Scores of the test can be no older than three years. North Carolina residents have admissions preference.

Undergraduate Preparation

Although a minimum of 90 undergraduate semester hours are required of all applicants, it is strongly desired that the student satisfactorily complete the graduate degree prior to enrollment. Almost every medical student holds a baccalaureate before matriculation in the medical school. Minimum preparation consists of eight semester hours each in general biology, general chemistry, organic chemistry, and physics. In addition, students are encouraged to study the humanities and to develop a diverse background of interests.

Student Body

Approximately 60 percent of the student body is made up of North Carolina residents. The 108 students of the most recent entering class represent more than 100 undergraduate colleges and universities. The admissions committee makes efforts to keep the student body as diverse as possible.

Placement Records

In several departments (such as anesthesia) residents score at or above the 90th percentile on in-training examinations. Over 92 percent of the eligible residents pass full National Board Examinations.

Costs

The Bowman Gray School of Medicine reported for the 1990-91 year a tuition of $13,000. It is expected that textbooks and supplies will run about $1,000. For the nine-month school year, a minimum of $8,500 should be reserved for room and board.

Financial Aid

Qualified applicants are awarded loans or scholarships on the basis of established criteria. Financial assistance needs are reviewed on the day of the interview when students have the opportunity to talk privately with a financial officer. Students are advised to contact the financial aid office for questions and information.

Faculty

Many of the BGSM faculty have held national professional offices. The school employs 541 full-time faculty and 498 part-time teachers in the basic and clinical sciences.

Curriculum

The School of Medicine provides two approaches to learning. One is a traditional formal lecture and laboratory approach, and the other is a more advanced problem-based, multidisciplinary format known as Parallel Curriculum, which emphasizes self-directed learning in tutorial groups of six students led by faculty members. Interested students apply to this curriculum through an additional application. Students are exposed to most of the multidisciplinary departments, including cardiology, endocrinology and metabolism, gastroenterology, oncology, infectious disease, and internal medicine.

Facilities

The School of Medicine provides 24-hour quiet study areas, small meeting rooms, and first-year lecture halls. An extensive library contains more than 110,000 volumes, including 2,300 journals of all aspects of medical science. The computerized bibliographic services of the National Library of Medicine can be accessed through MEDLINE and TOXLINE. BGSM has affiliations with several medical centers including the Reynolds Health Center, and hospitals in Hickory, Salisbury, and Boone. The school also participates in the teaching program of the Northwest Area Health Education Center (AHEC). A Student Life and Fitness Center contains aerobic and fitness areas as well as saunas and showers and Next Generation Nautilus equipment.

Grading Procedures

All students must pass Parts I and II of the NBME in order to graduate.

Special Programs

Students of the Bowman Gray School of Medicine have access to several special programs, awards, and unique study opportunities. For example, up to seven Academic Merit Awards covering complete tuition are made annually to exceptional North Carolina freshmen. The Medical Student Scholars Program allows students interested in an academic medicine career to do independent research with a faculty advisor. The school also has the only Comparative Medicine Clinical Research Program in the United States.

Application Procedures

The School of Medicine participates in the American Medical College Application Service (AMCAS). Applications should be made through AMCAS from July 1 to the November 1 deadline. A supplemental application form will be sent by December 15. Letters of recommendation should be written by the applicant's premedical advisory committee members or supervisor. Bowman Gray will ask about 12 percent of the applicants to come in for interviews. Accepted applicants are asked to respond within two weeks. At the time of response, a holding place fee must be submitted.

Contact

Office of Medical School Admissions
The Bowman Gray School of Medicine of Wake Forest
  University
300 South Hawthorne Road
Winston-Salem, North Carolina 27103
(919) 748-4264

BROWN UNIVERSITY PROGRAM IN MEDICINE

Box G-A212
Providence, Rhode Island 02912
(401) 863-3330

Accreditation	AAMC
Degrees Offered	B.A./M.D., B.S./M.D., M.M.S., M.S./M.D., M.D./Ph.D.
# Students Applied	1,029
Enrollment	73 / class
Mean GPA	Not Available
% Men / % Women	50% / 50%
% Minorities	18%
Tuition	$15,871
Application Fee	Contact School
Application Deadline	January 1

The University

Brown University, a private Ivy League college, was founded in 1764 as the third college in New England and the seventh in the nation. The college is situated on a 133-acre campus in Providence, Rhode Island's capital city.

Although Brown offered a medical program in the early 1800s, the more recent history of medical education at Brown University started in 1963. The Program in Liberal Medical Education (PLME) as it is known today admitted its first class in 1985. The PLME is an eight-year program that combines a strong liberal arts foundation with a professional education. This flexible approach allows each student to develop an individualized course of study.

Admissions

For the PLME, Brown seeks highly qualified and motivated students committed to medicine who wish to pursue an area of academic interest to an advanced level of scholarship within the framework of a broad liberal education. Students must take the SAT and three Achievement Examinations. In 1989, students admitted to the PLME averaged scores of 650 on the verbal and 720 on the math sections of the SAT (these are somewhat higher than the scores for the overall Brown applicant pool).

Personal qualities—motivation, maturity, character, and intellectual breadth—also substantially influence the decision process.

Undergraduate Preparation

In the four undergraduate years of the PLME program, a variety of courses in the natural, social, and behavioral sciences and mathematics are recommended. During these four years, students have flexibility in choosing a major, which may be in the sciences, humanities, social sciences, or behavioral sciences. Students can also choose from several interdisciplinary concentrations, such as biomedical ethics or international relations.

Student Body

For the university as a whole, the following statistics apply: about half of the approximately 5,500 undergraduate students are men and half are women; 1,350 are from New England and 3,650 are from outside New England. There are 290 students enrolled in the PLME.

Costs

For 1990-91 undergraduate tuition and fees (first four years of the PLME) total $15,871. Room and board costs $4,980, and books and personal expenses are estimated to cost $1,500.

Tuition for the last four years of the PLME is somewhat higher than the tuition mentioned above; these costs are determined on a year-to-year basis.

Financial Aid

University-wide, nearly 2,000 undergraduates each year receive a total of almost $26 million in assistance. Usually assistance is awarded in a package consisting of loans, campus jobs, and scholarships. The financial aid office makes awards on the basis of need.

Loans are the most common form of financial aid for PLME students, particularly in the last two years of the eight-year program.

Assistance during the last four years of the PLME is administered by the Office of Medical Admissions and Financial Aid, 97 Waterman Street, Providence, RI 02912

Minority Programs

The university's Associate Dean of Biology and Medicine for Minority Affairs serves as an advocate for minority students and provides academic and personal counseling as well as numerous other services for minority students pursuing a medical education. The Daniel Hale Williams Student Medical Society offers academic support to undergraduate minority students enrolled in the PLME.

Student Organizations

Brown students are involved in over 200 organizations involving political, athletic, service, social, dramatic, recreational, and ethnic interests, as well as a wide-ranging program in intercollegiate, intramural, and recreational sports for men and women.

PLME students may be particularly interested in groups such as the Center for Public Service, the Center for Environmental Studies, or the Brown Community Outreach Program.

Faculty

The university-wide student/faculty ratio is 9:1; the school employs 540 full-time faculty members and 120 visiting and adjunct professors. The PLME also offers an excellent student/faculty ratio.

Curriculum

The eight-year PLME allows flexibility in planning an individualized course of study. The program fosters competency in the preclinical sciences and advanced scholarship, as well as an appreciation for the social context of medicine. The continuum concept allows students to continue study in their undergraduate concentration to an advanced level and to engage in creative, original work.

There are no premedical curriculum requirements; however, students must demonstrate competence in the natural, behavioral, and social sciences during the preclinical phase of study. Students must complete a program of clinical instruction of at least 12 months. Students may choose from a number of electives during the clinical phase.

Facilities

The Biomedical Center includes the Center for Gerontology and Health Care Research and the Multidisciplinary Teaching Laboratory. Other research centers operating in conjunction with the university include the Center for Alcohol and Addiction Studies, the Cancer Research Center, and the International Health Institute.

Eight community-based teaching hospitals in the greater Providence area offer affiliated residency programs. Among these are the Emma Pendleton Bradley Hospital, Memorial Hospital, the Miriam Hospital, Rhode Island Hospital, and the Women & Infants Hospital of Rhode Island.

The Sciences Library, one of a network of university libraries, offers MEDLINE, the bibliographical retrieval system.

Special Programs

Special degree programs in the medical field include the M.M.S.; the M.S. in community health, gerontology, and chronic disease epidemiology; and the combined M.D./Ph.D. program.

A physician visitation program offers PLME students a chance to spend a day observing physicians in their daily routine in a clinical setting. Other special extracurricular opportunities include a foreign studies fellowship and a summer research assistantship program.

Application Procedures

Each applicant is considered first as an applicant to the university college and second as an applicant to the PLME. Interested students should request the application for Brown "The College" and check the box marked "PLME." The ad-

missions office reviews all candidates and notifies them in the same way as other Brown applicants.

Admission to the PLME is considered extremely competitive. The number of PLME applicants is anticipated to greatly exceed the 60 spots available each year.

The application deadline is January 1 for April notification.

Contact

Brown University
Admission Office
Box 1876
45 Prospect Street
Providence, Rhode Island 02912
(401) 863-2378

UNIVERSITY OF CALIFORNIA, DAVIS, SCHOOL OF MEDICINE

Davis, California 95616
(916) 752-1360

Accreditation	AAMC
Degrees Offered	M.D., M.D./Ph.D.
# Students Applied	2,956
Enrollment	93 / class
Mean GPA	3.5
% Men / % Women	56% / 44%
% Minorities	22.5%
Tuition	None – In-State
	$6,416 Out-of-State
Application Fee	$40
Application Deadline	November 1

Admissions

The school seeks students who have both the academic potential and personal characteristics necessary for the study of medicine. The admissions committee considers the applicant's scholastic record; MCAT results; reports from teachers, advisors, and interviewers regarding intellectual capacity, motivation, emotional stability, and personal dedication; and the applicant's awareness of the scientific, organizational, social, and economic problems facing modern medicine. Experience in the health sciences and a service- or community-oriented background are also important.

Preference is given to California residents and to applicants who are either United States citizens or permanent residents.

Undergraduate Preparation

Applicants must have completed at least three years of study at an accredited college or university in the United States or Canada. A minimum of 90 semester hours or 135 quarter units of college-level work is required. The following are mandatory undergraduate prerequisites for admission: one year of English; one year of biology (with lab); one year of general chemistry (with lab); one year of organic chemistry; one year of physics; and coursework in math that satisfies the prerequisites for integral calculus. Coursework in biochemistry, genetics, and embryology is helpful.

Student Body

Profiles of the school's classes have consistently shown a highly diverse student body in age, ethnic identification, and background. Recent surveys have consistently ranked UC Davis' medical school among the top 10 schools nationwide in the number of ethnic minority admissions.

Costs

First-year medical students who are legal California residents pay no tuition costs. Currently, the total four-year academic fee for state residents is $8,902. Books and other instructional materials are estimated to cost $2,090 for the first year of study; these costs tend to diminish in the second through fourth years. On-campus room and board is estimated to cost $5,120 for the 1990-91 academic year. (Student family housing and off-campus housing are also available.)

Financial Aid

A wide variety of financial assistance is available. All entering students are automatically considered for university-awarded scholarships, fellowships, and endowment monies. Some forms are restrictive; others are open to all students.

Types of assistance include Regents Scholarships (based on exceptional academic performance and promise); UC Davis School of Medicine opportunity grants (four are awarded each year to outstanding first-year minority students); University of California grants; university student loans; Health Professionals Student Loans; and Guaranteed Student Loans.

Minority Programs

The university offers a Health Resources Development Program that specifically addresses the needs of minority and disadvantaged students. Services provided by this federally funded project include a National Boards preparation program, tutorial assistance, peer group counseling and tutoring, and various issues seminars.

Student Organizations

Student organizations include the American Medical Student Association and the Student National Medical Association. Each class has a representative to the Organization of Student Representatives of the Association of American Medical Colleges.

Alpha Omega Alpha honor society members are chosen from third- and fourth-year classes on the basis of scholarship, personal integrity, and potential leadership qualities.

Faculty

The School of Medicine has a full-time faculty of approximately 370; 1,300 volunteer clinical faculty also offer students individual attention in a clinical setting. The faculty are involved in more than 300 ongoing research projects.

The UC Davis School of Medicine ranks 14th among American and Canadian schools whose faculty are principal investigators for the National Institutes of Health.

Curriculum

The curriculum leading to the M.D. degree is normally a four-year course of study that provides comprehensive training for the practice of medicine. Core courses emphasize primary care; electives provide a basis for specialization. Although the first two years stress the basic sciences as a foundation of medicine, the student is introduced to patient care during the very first quarter of study.

The first and second years include the study of anatomy, physiology, biochemistry, systemic pathology, the reproductive system, pharmacology, microbiology, the behavioral aspects of medicine, and a physical diagnosis practicum. The third year consists of required clinical clerkships in surgery, medicine, maternal and child health, and psychiatry. The fourth year consists of flexible clerkships, including 16 weeks of clinical electives. Also included is a two-week course in medical ethics, jurisprudence, and economics.

To complete the M.D. program, students must successfully complete 255 credits of coursework and clerkships.

Facilities

Teaching, research, and administrative facilities are located on the UC Davis campus. The majority of the school's clinical space is located at the UC Davis Medical Center in Sacramento, 19 miles east of campus. The medical center is one of northern California's busiest hospitals, serving as a referral center for a regional area of over four million residents. The medical center has 480 beds, 100 specialty clinics, and eight specialized intensive care units. A new Career Center is scheduled for completion in 1991.

Grading Procedures

All work is assessed using the letter grading system, A, B, C, D, F, I (incomplete), Y (provisional), or IP (in progress).

Special Programs

The university offers postgraduate specialty training and a joint program leading to a degree in medicine and an academic doctorate in a basic science related to medicine. The course of study for the M.D./Ph.D. usually lasts six years.

Application Procedures

The School of Medicine participates in AMCAS. Applications are available after April 1. One application and only one set of transcripts need to be submitted. Two letters of recommendation and an application fee of $40 should be sent on request to the Chairperson of the Admissions Committee at UC Davis. Interviews are held at the medical school and at the UC Davis Medical Center in Sacramento.

Applications are accepted between June 15 and November 1. Early application is encouraged.

Contact

Office of Student Affairs
University of California, Davis
Davis, California 95616
(916) 752-3170

UNIVERSITY OF CALIFORNIA, IRVINE, COLLEGE OF MEDICINE

E112 Medical Sciences Building
Irvine, California 92717
(714) 634-6545

Accreditation	AAMC
Degrees Offered	M.D., M.S., Ph.D.
# Students Applied	3,266
Enrollment	92 / class
Mean GPA	3.5
% Men / % Women	Not Available
% Minorities	Not Available
Tuition	None In-State
	$6,416 Out-of-State
Application Fee	$40
Application Deadline	November 1

The University

Located on a park-like campus adjacent to the main university grounds in Irvine, the College of Medicine offers students the opportunity to study in the year-round relaxing, mild climate of southern California. Academically, one of the College of Medicine's greatest strengths is basic sciences research; medical students have many opportunities to participate in this ongoing work.

Admissions

Applicants are selected on the basis of their intellectual and emotional potential to provide comprehensive and continuing medical care, their ability to guide patients and cope with disease, their commitment to remain sensitive to individual needs, and their dedication to strive for the advancement of the art, science, and practice of medicine long after obtaining a medical degree. As part of the University of California system, the College of Medicine gives admissions preference to residents of California. Also, the College of Medicine participates in the Western Interstate Commission for Higher Education. Under this program, qualified residents of certain states without medical schools (Alaska, Idaho, Montana, and Wyoming) are considered along with California residents and are charged academic fees at the in-state rate.

Undergradute Preparation

The College of Medicine advises premedical students to take advantage of the intellectual maturation afforded by a well-rounded liberal arts education. Specific required courses include one year of general chemistry, one year of organic chemistry, one year of physics, one and one-half years of biology or zoology, and study of college-level calculus. Genetics, vertebrate embryology, and physical chemistry are recommended but not required. The MCAT is required and scores must be from within the previous three years.

Costs

For the 1990-91 academic year, fees for California residents came to $694.50 per quarter, totalling $2,083.50 annually. There is no tuition for California residents. For out-of-state students, tuition and fees were $2,666.50 per quarter, totalling $7,999.50 annually.

Student Organizations

Extracurricular organizations for medical students at the College of Medicine include Women in Medicine, the Student National Medical Association, the Chicano Medical Student Association, the American Indian Medical Student Association, and Asians in Medicine.

Faculty

The College of Medicine currently has more than 450 full-time and 1,800 volunteer faculty members.

Curriculum

The first two years consist of basic science and preclinical instruction scheduled on a modified quarter system. Each quarter spans nine to 15 weeks, including eight to 14 weeks of teaching with one week for final or midcourse exams. Basic science subjects include gross anatomy and embryology, biochemistry, histology, neuroanatomy, physiology, microbiology, behavioral sciences, and nutrition. Preclinical subjects include pathology, clinical pathology, behavioral sciences II, preventive medicine, examination of the patient, mechanisms of disease, and introductory courses to the clinical clerkships. The second two years of medical study are spent in clinical rotations and are scheduled according to 10-week quintiles. Clerkships include medicine, pediatrics, obstetrics and gynecology, surgery, anesthesiology, opthalmology, psychiatry, physical medicine and rehabilitation, neurosciences, primary care, and radiological sciences. There are also many opportunities for students to participate in elective clinical and research experiences.

Facilities

The UCI Medical Center is the main teaching hospital for the College of Medicine and is the only designated Level I trauma center in Orange County, houses the county's only burn center, and offers the only 24-hour poison center in a five-county area. Other research and learning facilities include a cardiac transplantation program, an air pollution effects lab, a geriatric assessment center, a diabetes research program, an Alzheimer's disease research center, a sleep disorders center, a brain imaging center, the cancer surveillance program of Orange County, in infant special care unit, the Center for Reproductive Health/Fertility program, and the Beckman Laser Institute.

Grading Procedures

The College of Medicine assigns letter grades on an A through E basis.

Special Programs

Currently more than 100 medical students are pursuing biomedical graduate degrees in a program offered in conjunction with the university's School of Biological Sciences. Also, the Medical Scientist Training Program offers highly qualified students the chance to simultaneously complete their M.D. and Ph.D. degrees.

Application Procedures

Students must first submit a preliminary application through AMCAS between June 15 and November 1 of the year before desired admission to medical school. After an initial screening of MCAT and grades, selected applicants will be asked to submit additional materials including letters of recommendation, two photographs, and a nonrefundable application fee of $40. From this group of applicants, interviews will be granted and final admissions decisions made.

Contact

Office of Admissions
University of California - Irvine
College of Medicine
E112 Medical Sciences Building
Irvine, California 92717
(714) 856-5388

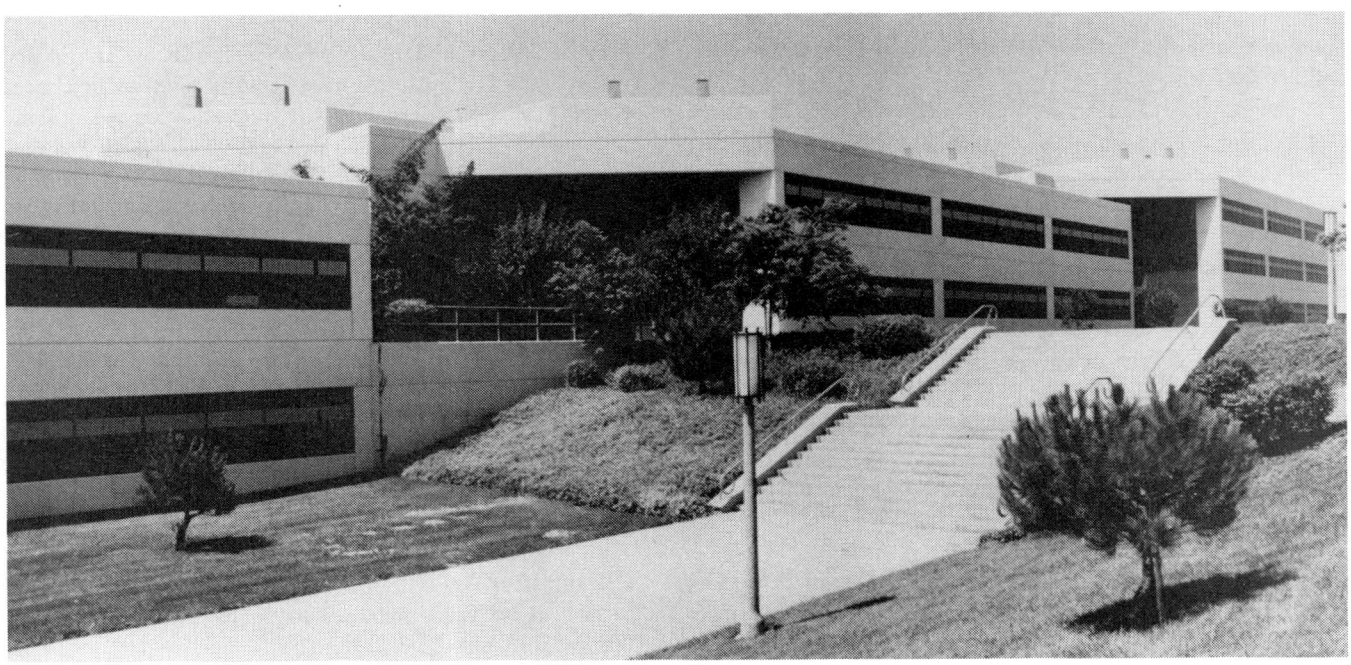

UNIVERSITY OF CALIFORNIA, LOS ANGELES, UCLA SCHOOL OF MEDICINE

Los Angeles, California 90024-1720
(213) 825-4321

Accreditation	LCME
Degrees Offered	M.D., M.D./Ph.D., M.D./M.P.H.
# Students Applied	3,828
Enrollment	145 / class
Mean GPA	3.64
% Men / % Women	50% / 50%
% Minorities	33%
Tuition	None In-State
	$5,916 Out-of-State
Application Fee	$40
Application Deadline	November 1

The University

The UCLA School of Medicine, established in 1946, was the first University of California medical school in southern California. The School of Medicine has evolved into an internationally recognized leader in education and research. Through its 17 departments of instruction, the school prepares undergraduate and graduate students for careers in all branches of medicine.

The growth of Los Angeles into a major metropolitan center has affected the growth of the School of Medicine and the Medical Center. A vast network of teaching hospitals offer a wide range of educational opportunities for students.

Admissions

A bachelor's degree is ordinarily required for admission, but students who have completed three full academic years at an accredited college or university may, in certain cases, be accepted. The MCAT is required. Preference is given to students who present evidence of broad training and high achievement in college, have an interest in biomedical research, and show an ability to communicate effectively.

Undergraduate Preparation

The following undergraduate courses are required for admission: one year of English, including composition; one year of physics with laboratory; two years of chemistry, including inorganic chemistry, quantitative analysis, and organic chemistry; two years of biology, including one year of upper division courses; and one year of mathematics, including algebra. Introductory calculus is highly recommended. In addition, courses in biochemistry and Spanish are also highly recommended.

Courses with subject matter overlapping those taught in the School of Medicine (e.g., human anatomy) are not recommended. Knowledge of practical computer applications is very desirable.

Costs

There is no tuition cost for residents, but academic fees total $2,128.50 per year; for nonresidents, $5,916.00. Senior medical student fees include an additional $382.50 for the required summer period.

Books, supplies, and equipment are estimated to cost $1,800 the first year, $1,400 the second year, $630 the third year, and $770 the fourth year. Average room and board expenses are $7,100 the first and third years. $7,900 the second year, and $9,500 the fourth year. Personal expenses vary greatly, but generally range from $2,000 to $2,600 per year.

On-campus housing is available but competitive. Off-campus housing is in great demand in the Los Angeles area, and arrangements should be made as soon as possible. An automobile is required for transportation to affiliated hospitals in the third and fourth years and for some students in the second year.

Financial Aid

Financial assistance is available through the office of financial aid at the UCLA School of Medicine. A limited number of Regents scholarships are available for outstanding students. California State Graduate Fellowships are awarded on a competitive basis for undergraduates in their senior year and first-year medical students who have demonstrated financial need. National Medical Fellowships, Inc., provides financial assistance to minority medical students for the first two years. Also available are Stafford Student Loans, Health Education Assistance Loans, and Perkins Loans. Many other awards, scholarships, and loans are available from several private, state, and federal offices. Applicants for admission receive financial aid application forms only after they have been accepted for admission.

Student Organizations

Student organizations include the Association of American Medical Colleges, Organization of Student Representatives, The American Medical Student Association, Alpha Omega Alpha, and Phi Delta Epsilon. All students belong to the UCLA Medical Student's Association.

Curriculum

Many courses are presented cooperatively by faculty in several departments and disciplines.

The first year consists of courses in introductory basic sciences, social medicine, medical ethics, and interdisciplinary clinical correlates, which presents clinical correlations relevant to subjects being taught.

The second year includes advanced basic science courses, clinical fundamentals, genetics, clinical correlates, and pathophysiology of disease.

The third and fourth years, covering 94 weeks, include 50 weeks of required clerkships and 28 weeks of electives. Electives consist of three types: in-depth electives emphasizing clinical skills; advanced clinical clerkships, which allow students to build on the basic information and skills learned during required rotations; and subinternship and subinternship/in-patient courses, where students function as interns, assuming more responsibility.

Facilities

The School of Medicine is located in the Center for Health Science, a large building complex that includes the Brain Research Institute, the UCLA Medical Center, the Neuropsychiatric Institute and Hospital, and the Louise Darling Biomedical Library, which contains over 471,000 volumes and regularly receives over 6,000 current serial titles.

The School of Medicine is also affiliated with Los Angeles County Harbor-UCLA Medical Center, a 700-bed hospital staffed exclusively by full-time members of the UCLA faculty.

Grading Procedures

Promotion from one grade to the next is determined by a promotion committee, which is made up of faculty members. Part I of the National Board of Medical Examiners (NBME) exam must be taken upon completion of the second medical school year, and Part II at the beginning of the senior year.

Special Programs

The Medical Scientist Training Program (MSTP), available for exceptional students, is a concurrent degree program (M.D./Ph.D.) that may be earned in seven years.

The M.D./M.P.H. degree may be earned through elective choices by students who wish to earn a Master's of Public Health degree while attending medical school.

The Dred/UCLA Undergraduate Medical Program accepts up to 24 students per year. This education and research program is of special interest to students who wish to serve in disadvantaged communities.

In the UCR/UCLA Biomedical Sciences Program, undergraduates follow a three-year premedical program at the University of California, Riverside Campus. Following the completion of the third year, up to 24 students are admitted to the UCLA School of Medicine. These students continue with two years of basic medical sciences study at Riverside and the Harbor-UCLA Medical Center. Students complete the last two years at the UCLA School of Medicine.

Application Procedures

Preliminary applications are processed by the American Medical College Application Service (AMCAS). Completed applications are accepted between June 15 and November 1, a year before the August of planned enrollment. Applicants are encouraged to take the MCAT in the spring, rather than the fall, of the year preceding admission. The admissions committee will not consider applications received after the deadline. If the candidate is accepted for an interview, a processing fee of $40 is required. Students not admitted upon the first application may apply a second time the following year, but a third application is discouraged. Interviews are required. A few transfer students who have completed two years in a medical school program equivalent to the UCLA School of Medicine's will be considered for the third-year class. These students must also have successfully completed Part I of the National Board medical exam.

Contact

Office of Admissions
UCLA School of Medicine
Los Angeles, California 90024-1720
(213) 825-6081

UNIVERSITY OF CALIFORNIA, SAN DIEGO, SCHOOL OF MEDICINE

9500 Gilman Drive
La Jolla, California 92093
(619) 534-4431

Accreditation	LCME
Degrees Offered	M.D., M.S., M.D./Ph.D.
# Students Applied	4,000
Enrollment	122 / class
Mean GPA	3.54
% Men / % Women	64% / 36%
% Minorities	Not Available
Tuition	None In-State
	$7,992 Out-of-State
Application Fee	$40
Application Deadline	November 1

The University

An institution of learning with a four-year study program for men and women, the University of California, San Diego was originally envisioned as a leading research and education center for all of the natural sciences. The School of Medicine carries the wisdom of the university's 77-year history to its major affiliate programs, including the Basic Science Building, the Veterans Administration Medical Center, the Salk Institute, Research Laboratories, and Clinical Teaching Facilities. LaJolla, considered the "Jewel By The Sea," is surrounded by such beautiful attractions as Del Mar, Solana Beach, and Encinitas. Attractions such as the Del Mar Race Track, Rancho Santa Fe, and the San Diego Zoo are in close view. In addition, southern California contains several museums, theaters, art galleries, botanical gardens, parks, and boardwalks.

Admissions

Early application is strongly advised. Scores from the Medical College Admissions Test (MCAT) are required. Students are urged to take the MCAT in the spring of the year applying. The admissions committee seeks students with excellent scholastic portfolios.

Undergraduate Preparation

The School of Medicine seeks applicants with four years of undergraduate study. However, the minimum requirement is three years of academic attendance at an approved college of arts and sciences. Students must have successfully completed one year of biology, one year of physics, two years of chemistry (including organic), and one year of mathematics. Preference is given to California residents.

Placement Records

Most students find residency within California and the major affiliated medical centers. The options for medical students and residency are open due to the fact that California issues Physicians and Surgeons Certificates that are unrestrictive.

Costs

For the 1991 academic year the academic fees were $2,076 for in-state students, and tuition and fees were $7,992 for out-of-state admittants. The off-campus rent, utilities, and food costs range about $670/month. Total expenses and fees for nonresidents reach upwards of $16,000/year. Residents can approximate a total annual expense of $10,000.

Financial Aid

Financial aid is available through loans, grants, and scholarships, including the Stafford Loan, the Alumni Medical Student Loan, Armed Forces Health Professions Scholarship Program, and Regent Scholarships. For detailed information students are asked to inquire at the student financial services office of the School of Medicine.

Minority Programs

Minority students are encouraged to apply. A Special Admissions Subcommittee makes efforts to consider the social and financial barriers of applicants. Minority students can participate in the summer program which offers additional training and help.

Student Organizations

The UCSD General Catalog offers listings of campus organizations and student facilities.

Faculty

The School of Medicine has a large faculty comprised of hundreds of full-time M.D. professors. In addition, there are over a thousand part-time and volunteer instructors from Ph.D.s to R.N.s.

Curriculum

During the first year, the curriculum is academic, encompassing anatomy, psychiatry, biochemistry, and physiology. The second-year student selects one of seven areas of concentrated study. These areas, or pathways, are designed to expand from and build upon the core curriculum. Beginning in the third year, both required and elective clerkships are scheduled. During the final month of the fourth year, a course on the mechanisms of disease and advanced cardiac life support is given.

Facilities

The UCSD Medical Center serves as a full-fledged hospital and teaching facility for a 9,000 square mile area. The Salk Institute has a worldwide reputation as a research center mingling the likes of Jonas Salk, Francis Crick, and Roger Guillemin. The Biomedical Library houses over 100,000 volumes and works in close association with other San Diego and Los Angeles medical/scientific libraries. In addition, the clinical resources for the School of Medicine includes the Veterans Administration Medical Center, the Naval Hospital of San Diego, the Children's Hospital and Health Center, the Green Hospital of Scripps Clinic, and the U.S. Public Health Service Outpatient Clinic.

Grading Procedures

The School of Medicine utilizes an honors/pass/fail system of grading. Students cannot be ranked nor can the school provide information regarding class standing.

Special Programs

During an intense Medical Scientist Training Program students can earn the combined M.D./Ph.D. degrees in six to seven years. There are opportunities for research in prominent fields of discovery including the Dr. Theodore Friedmann research team at the UCSD Center for Molecular Genetics.

Application Procedures

Official transcripts and AMCAS applications are due no later than November 1. There is a $40 application fee. Part of the screening process includes letters of recommendation and personal interviews. Decisions by the Admissions Committee are communicated during the fall quarter. After notification students have two weeks to respond to the Office of Admissions. All new students are required to complete a Health History Form and physical examination.

Contact

Admissions Office
UCSD School of Medicine M-021
LaJolla, California 92093
(619) 534-3880

UNIVERSITY OF CALIFORNIA, SAN FRANCISCO, SCHOOL OF MEDICINE

Room S224
San Francisco, California 94143-0410
(415) 476-2342

Accreditation	LCME
Degrees Offered	M.D., M.D./Ph.D., D.D.S./ M.D., M.D./M.A., M.D./M.S., M.S./Ph.D., M.D./M.P.H.
# Students Applied	3,705
Enrollment	153 / class
Mean GPA	3.69
% Men / % Women	58% / 42%
% Minorities	23%
Tuition	None In-State
	$6,417 Out-of-State
Application Fee	$40
Application Deadline	November 1

The University

The University of California, San Francisco is the only one of the nine campuses of the University of California that is devoted solely to the health sciences. Dating back to 1873, the university is today a state-supported institution that com-

prises four professional schools: Dentistry, Medicine, Nursing, and Pharmacy; a graduate program in basic and behavioral sciences; two health policy institutes; plus a medical center with three hospitals. The programs at the university encompass teaching, research, patient care, and public service.

Admissions

A primary objective of the School of Medicine is to select students who share its educational objectives, who reflect the diversity of the applicant pool (age, sex, race, culture, etc.), and whose past achievements as well as personal qualities are outstanding. All applicants must take the MCAT. Academic performance as well as the difficulty of the course of study are also weighed in the admissions process. In general, applicants who have achieved a 3.0 GPA or better are more favorably considered.

Undergraduate Preparation

The School of Medicine requires completion of three years (90 semester units or 135 quarter units) of acceptable college credit. These must include: one year of general chemistry (with lab); two quarters of organic chemistry; one year of physics (with lab); and one year of biology (with lab). Mathematics, upper-division biology, and humanities courses are also recommended. California residents are given priority in the admissions process.

Student Body

The average age of the entering student for the first-year class of 1989 was 23. Forty-two percent were women. Forty-eight percent were nonwhite, and 23 percent were minorities. The average first-year student of that year had an overall GPA of 3.69, a science GPA of 3.72, and MCAT scores of 12 on biology, chemistry, physics, and science.

Placement Records

The student and career placement office provides counseling and assistance with placement in on- and off-campus jobs to enrolled students, spouses, and alumni.

Appointments to residencies are handled through the National Resident Matching Plan. Professional postdoctoral programs for residents are provided at facilities in Fresno, Salinas, San Francisco, and Sonoma. The resident program offers curricula in 16 disciplines. Records indicate that 100 percent of the graduates of the class of 1989 who were seeking employment found employment upon graduation.

Costs

Tuition per quarter for legal nonresidents is $1,972. There is an educational fee for all students of $300. Registration is $214 per quarter. Most other fees are minimal.

The cost of textbooks, instruments, and other supplies is estimated to cost $1,750 for the first year; these costs tend to decrease for the succeeding three years.

Financial Aid

Financial assistance is available in the form of loans, scholarships, grants, and work-study programs, including National Health Service Corps Scholarships, Exceptional Financial Need Scholarships, federal loans, medical student loans, Stafford Loans, and Supplemental Loans for Students. Veterans benefits may also be available. Funds are awarded only to students who demonstrate need. Students should apply for financial aid as soon as they have been accepted for admission.

Minority Programs

In the last 15 years, UCSF has had one of the highest minority enrollments of Continental U.S. medical schools. In the last three years, the school has offered a total of 145 places to minority applicants and 103 of these students have enrolled in the medical school.

Student Organizations

UCSF has several student organizations, including the Associated Students of the University of California, San Francisco, Associated Students of the School of Medicine, the Student-Faculty Liaison Committee, and the Alumni-Faculty Association.

Curriculum

A core curriculum in the basic sciences is prescribed for the first two years of study. During the second year, the student selects a major pathway for concentrated study from the following choices: behavioral specialist, family medicine, general, medical scientist, medicine, social and administrative specialist, and surgery. About one-quarter of the curriculum is devoted to elective courses and clerkships that are arranged to meet pathway requirements.

Starting in the third year, required and elective clerkships are scheduled for full-time study in two-to-eight week blocks, rather than by quarter.

The course of study also includes the economic, ethical, and legal issues, social and cultural factors, and governmental policies that affect the practice of medicine.

During the final month of the fourth year, students are required to take a course in the mechanisms of disease and advanced cardiac life support.

Facilities

The campus hospitals are Moffit/Long (including the Children's Medical Center); and Langley Porter Psychiatric Hospital. There is also a large ambulatory care program. Clinical instruction also takes place at a host of other major medical care facilities throughout the area.

Ten research facilities are affiliated with the campus, including the Cancer Research Institute, the Institute for Health Policy Studies, Laboratory of Radiobiology and Environmental Health, and the Cardiovascular Research Institute.

The UCSF medical library is considered to be one of the most preeminent of its kinds. The collection contains more than 680,000 volumes, including more than 200,000 foreign medical dissertations and nearly 10,000 journal titles. There are special collections and an Oriental Medicine Collection. The library has the MELVYL online catalog. MEDLINE is also accessible.

Grading Procedures

Grades are P (pass) and E (provisional nonpassing). Grade E is assigned as an initial nonpassing provisional grade; it will be converted to a passing grade when the requirements for the course are met satisfactorily.

Special Programs

Special programs include: the Medical Scientist Training Program; M.D. with thesis program; D.D.S./M.D. Oral and Maxillofacial Program; M.D./M.S.; and M.S./Ph.D. There is also a joint degree that leads to the M.D./Master of Public Health degree.

Application Procedures

The School of Medicine processes applications through AMCAS. Applications are available from AMCAS in April and must be submitted no later than November 1 of the year preceding expected enrollment. AMCAS must receive official transcripts from undergraduate colleges or universities. Applicants for the fall semester must take the MCAT in the fall of the previous year to be eligible.

Applicants who pass a preliminary review are asked to submit a minimum of three letters of recommendation.

There is a $40 application fee.

Contact

University of California, San Francisco
School of Medicine
Office of Admissions
San Francisco, California 94143-0410
(415) 476-2342

CASE WESTERN RESERVE UNIVERSITY SCHOOL OF MEDICINE

2119 Abington Road
Cleveland, Ohio 44106
(216) 368-2820

Accreditation	LCME
Degrees Offered	M.D., Ph.D.
# Students Applied	4,527
Enrollment	138 / class
Mean GPA	3.4
% Men / % Women	55% / 45%
% Minorities	26%
Tuition	$17,100
Application Fee	$30
Application Deadline	November 1

The University

Case Western Reserve University, founded in 1826 as Western Reserve College, was formed in 1967 when Western Reserve University merged with Case Institute of Technology. The university has a total enrollment of approximately 8,500 students. The School of Medicine, added to the school in 1843, is the largest biomedical research institution in the state of Ohio. Located in University Circle, a neighborhood only four miles from downtown Cleveland (which is home to several other institutions of higher learning), the university offers students both the comfortable environment of an academic community and the resources and cultural diversity of a large, metropolitan city.

Admissions

Admission to the School of Medicine is based primarily on overall undergraduate academic achievement. Most successful applicants rank in the top third of their classes; however, the general potential and ability displayed by a student in non-academic areas is also considered. An undergraduate degree in a science is not necessary because the School of Medicine emphasizes the importance of a broad, general college education. Completion of a B.A. or B.S. degree prior to enrollment is preferred. Consideration is also given to students who have been out of college for several years, as well as to older applicants with non-traditional backgrounds who wish to change career direction and study medicine. Because the university receives financial support from the state of Ohio, 60 percent of students must be state residents. All applicants must submit MCAT scores.

Undergraduate Preparation

A solid foundation in the sciences is necessary for an understanding of modern biochemical knowledge. It is expected that applicants will have taken undergraduate coursework that includes one year each of biology, general chemistry, organic chemistry, and basic physics. Applicants must also demonstrate a proficiency in writing, generally by taking at least a freshman course in expository writing. Aside from these specific requirements, applicants are encouraged to develop their course of study around their particular area of academic interest, rather than limit their studies to subjects in the natural sciences.

Student Body

Students at the School of Medicine come from diverse backgrounds. Forty-five percent of the students are women, 55 percent are men, and 26 percent are from minority backgrounds. Members of the class of 1992 represent 74 different undergraduate institutions and 18 states. Fifty-nine percent of students were between the ages of 20 and 23 when they enrolled in the School of Medicine while the mean age of all medical students is 24.3.

Placement Records

In the class of 1990, 68 percent of the students gained their first choice of residency program, while 91 percent got one of their top three selections. Seventeen different speciality choices were represented.

Costs

Tuition costs (including all fees) for the 1990-91 academic year was $17,100. Annual living expenses, including cost of housing, food, and incidentals in the Cleveland area, are estimated at $9,200.

Financial Aid

Approximately 75 percent of the students at the School of Medicine receive some form of financial aid. Students are expected to obtain about $10,000 of their financial support from outside sources, such as Guaranteed Student Loans, family resources, and personal savings. Once this amount has been obtained, the medical school generally offers loans and scholarships to students with further need.

Curriculum

The curriculum at the School at Medicine has three main components in which all students participate: the Core Academic Program, the Flexible Program, and the Patient-Based Program. The Core Academic Program prepares students in the fundamental medical sciences using a multidisciplinary, team-teaching approach that facilitates clinical understanding. The Flexible Program portion of the curriculum allows students to take preclinical or clinical electives, conduct research, participate in apprenticeships, and concentrate in one particular area of medical study. In the Patient-Based Program, students are gradually introduced to clinical responsibility during the first two years of medical school. When clerkships begin in the third and fourth years, students have had experience working directly with patients and are contributing members of the ward team.

Facilities

The medical school has centers for arthritis, bioarchitectonics, biomedical ethics, environmental health sciences, international health, neurosciences, genetics, geriatrics, health systems management, and cancer research. A new $60 million biomedical research building is scheduled to be completed in 1992. The School of Medicine is also affiliated with five hospitals in the Cleveland area: University Hospitals of Cleveland, MetroHealth Medical Center, The Veterans Affairs Cleveland Medical Center, the Mt. Sinai Medical Center, and St. Luke's Hospital.

Grading Procedures

Students are evaluated on a pass/fail basis.

Special Programs

The School of Medicine offers a Medical Scientist Training Program (MSTP) for highly-qualified students who wish to pursue the M.D. and Ph.D. degrees simultaneously. This program generally takes six to seven years to complete; financial assistance, includes both stipend and tuition support.

Application Procedures

Interested students must first apply through AMCAS; selected applicants are sent final applications from CWRU. After further consideration, strong candidates for admission are invited to on-campus interviews. Applicants are notified of admissions decisions no later than May 1.

Contact

Case Western Reserve University
School of Medicine
Associate Dean for Admissions and Student Affairs
2119 Abington Road
Cleveland, Ohio 44106
(216) 368-3450

UNIVERSIDAD CENTRAL DEL CARIBE SCHOOL OF MEDICINE

Bayamón, Puerto Rico 00621-6032
(809) 798-3001

Accreditation	LCME
Degrees Offered	M.D.
# Students Applied	572
Enrollment	61 / class
Mean GPA	3.10
% Men / % Women	67% / 33%
% Minorities	Not Available
Tuition	$15,000 In-State
	$22,000 Out-of-State
Application Fee	$50
Application Deadline	December 15

The University

The School of Medicine at the Universidad Central del Caribe was established in 1976. It is a private, non-profit institution. The school is located on 56 acres in the city of Bayamón, Puerto Rico.

Admissions

The admissions committee evaluates an applicant's undergraduate academic record, GPA (general and science scores), MCAT scores, letters of recommendation, and personal interview.

Undergraduate Preparation

At least three years of college (90 semester hours) are required for admission. Completion of a Bachelor's degree is preferred. Required courses include eight semester hours each of general biology or zoology, general chemistry, organic chemistry, and general physics (all with lab). At least six semester hours of college mathematics, English and Spanish are also required. A broad background in the humanities, arts, and behavioral sciences is encouraged. Proficiency in both English and Spanish is required.

Student Body

One-third of the students accepted to the 1990-91 entering class were women. Approximately 90 percent of students accepted to this class had completed their baccalaureate degrees. The mean GPA was 3.10.

Costs

Estimated tuition costs amount to $15,000 per year for residents and $22,000 for nonresidents. Student fees amount to $97.

Financial Aid

Financial aid is available from federal and commonwealth scholarship and loan programs. The Office of the Dean for Student Affairs offers financial aid counseling.

Curriculum

The school concentrates on training students toward orientation of primary health care, with emphasis on community health and family medicine. The first two years of study include basic science courses, presented with clinical correlations. The second year consists of basic sciences and Introduction to Clinical Medicine. The third year consists of required clinical clerkships in internal medicine, pediatrics and obstetrics-gynecology. A clinical clerkship in community and family medicine is offered in an ambulatory care facility. The fourth year includes clerkships in psychiatry and surgery, and 16 weeks of electives.

Facilities

The school's teaching hospital is the Dr. Ramon Ruiz Arnau University Hospital. Adjacent to the hospital is a new building which houses the basic sciences teaching facilities, administration offices, and library.

Grading Procedures

A letter grading and pass/fail system is used. Electives are graded on an honors/pass/fail basis.

Application Procedures

The School of Medicine participates in AMCAS. Applications should be filed between June 15 and December 15 of the year prior to anticipated entry. The school participates in the early decision plan. Candidates for the EDP should apply from June 15 to August 1 of the year prior to entry. The MCAT should be taken in the spring of the year before planned enrollment. There is an application fee of $50. Interviews are required and are arranged by the office of admissions. Rejected applicants may reapply for admission.

Contact

Office of Admissions
Universidad Central del Caribe
School of Medicine
Ramon Ruiz Arnau University Hospital
Call Box 60-327
Bayamón, Puerto Rico 00621-6032
(809) 740-4265

UNIVERSITY OF CHICAGO PRITZKER SCHOOL OF MEDICINE

5841 S. Maryland Avenue - Box 69
Chicago, Illinois 60637
(312) 702-6500

Accreditation	LCME
Degrees Offered	M.D., M.D./Ph.D., M.D./ M.B.A., M.D./J.D.
# Students Applied	3,797
Enrollment	113 / class
Mean GPA	3.58
% Men / % Women	65% / 35%
% Minorities	33%
Tuition	$16,170
Application Fee	$45
Application Deadline	December 15

The University

The University of Chicago is located in Hyde Park, approximately seven miles from downtown Chicago. This town of about 45,000 people offers much culture, including the Museum of Science & Industry, Oriental Institute Museum, and DuSable Museum of African-American History, as well as the Chicago Symphony Orchestra. The campus also provides a large indoor athletic facility, art galleries, and a number of student theater groups. Lake Michigan is just a short walk from campus. The School of Medicine was founded in 1927 and offers many opportunities for interdisciplinary study, as the Pritzker School of Medicine is part of the Division of Biological Sciences of the University of Chicago.

Admissions

In order to apply, students must take the MCAT and have completed a minimum of three years of college, although a baccalaureate degree is preferable. Students entering in the 1990 class had a science GPA average of 3.9 and a nonscience GPA average of 3.5.

Undergraduate Preparation

To apply, students must have one year each of biology, physics, inorganic chemistry, and organic chemistry, all with lab. Social science, humanities, English composition, and mathematics courses are recommended but not required. The admissions committee looks for applicants with a broad education and a strong record of extracurricular activities and interests.

Student Body

Approximately 40 percent of the entering class comes from Illinois. In 1990, a total of 113 students were enrolled, including 73 men, 40 women, 35 Asians, 2 Blacks, and 75 Caucasians. They come from diverse geographic, cultural, and academic backgrounds.

Placement Records

Upon graduation, most Pritzker students enter a residency through the National Resident Matching Program. Over the past four years, 56 percent of the students have been matched to their first choice and 83 percent to one of their first three choices.

Costs

Total estimated costs for 1990-91 including tuition and most other expenses are $28,460 for the first and second year and $38,575 for the third and fourth year.

Financial Aid

Students may receive financial aid in the form of scholarships and low interest loans. Approximately 60 percent of all Pritzker students receive some form of financial aid.

Minority Programs

Minority students are encouraged to apply. The University of Chicago offers a summer program for MCAT preparation, study skills, and test taking skills development as well as local outreach programs with high school and college students.

Student Organizations

Among the organizations for medical students are the American Medical Students Association, the American Medical Women's Association, the American Medical Association-Medical Student Section, and the Organization of Student Representatives.

Faculty

The School of Medicine employs approximately 780 full-time faculty members.

Curriculum

First year courses consist of anatomy, biochemistry, cell and organ physiology, neurobiology, immunobiology and medical genetics, medical ethics, and an elective. Second year courses include pharmacology, clinical pathophysiology, microbiology, cell and general pathology, human development and psychopathology, medical statistics, nutrition, and an elective. The third year consists of five major clinical clerkships, including internal medicine, surgery, pediatrics, psychiatry, obstetrics and gynecology. The fourth year consists of elective courses as well as subinternships, ambulatory experiences, and away rotations in other countries.

Facilities

By 1993, the School of Medicine will have a new Biological Sciences Learning Center. Clinical teaching is done in the University Hospitals and two other major off-site community-based hospitals. There are also many research laboratories as well as a new institute for molecular medicine. The Crerar Library has over 996,000 volumes and 7,000 periodicals, making it one of the largest science holdings in the U.S.

Grading Procedures

Most courses in the first two years are graded on a pass/fail basis. Clinical clerkships are graded in terms of honors, high pass, pass, low pass, and fail. However, only pass or fail is recorded on the student's transcript.

Special Programs

Students who desire both clinical and laboratory research experience may apply simultaneously for admission into the School of Medicine and the Medical Scientist Training Program. The School of Medicine also allows students to pursue joint M.D./Ph.D, M.D./M.B.A., and M.D./J.D. degrees.

Application Procedures

Application must be made through the American Medical College Application Service (AMCAS). MCAT scores are required and should be preferably from the year prior to intended matriculation. Applications will be accepted between June 15 and December 15. Interviews will be requested after review of other application materials.

Contact

The Pritzker School of Medicine
Office of the Dean of Students
Billings Hospital, G-115A
5841 South Maryland Avenue
Chicago, Illinois 60637
(312) 702-1939

UNIVERSITY OF CINCINNATI COLLEGE OF MEDICINE

231 Bethesda Avenue
Cincinnati, Ohio 45267-0552
(513) 558-7338

Accreditation	LCME, AMA
Degrees Offered	M.D., M.D./Ph.D.
# Students Applied	2,780
Enrollment	650
Mean GPA	3.42
% Men / % Women	61% / 39%
% Minorities	Not Available
Tuition	$7,650 In-State
	$13,407 Out-of-State
Application Fee	$25
Application Deadline	November 15

The University

Founded in 1819, the University of Cincinnati College of Medicine is the oldest medical college west of the Allegheny Mountains. The college is housed in the Medical Sciences Building which is part of the Cincinnati Medical Center. The Medical Center also comprises the colleges of nursing and pharmacy.

Admissions

The admissions committee seeks students with diverse backgrounds, interests, and talents. Personal characteristics and learning skills are as important as demonstrated academic performance. Academic record, MCAT performance, and AMCAS applications are evaluated for admissions. The admissions committee also weighs the student's motivation, integrity, leadership skills, interpersonal skills, and intellectual qualities. Applicants who are being seriously considered are called for interviews. Ohio residents are given preference in the admissions process.

Undergraduate Preparation

A bachelor's degree is preferred but not required for admission. Students must have completed 90 semester hours at an accredited four-year college or university. Both science majors and nonscience majors are considered for admission. Minimum prerequisite courses are: basic chemistry (10 semester hours); organic chemistry (six semester hours); biology (eight semester hours); physics (eight semester hours); and English (six semester hours). Both CLEP and AP credits may be applied toward these requirements.

Costs

Tuition and fees for Ohio residents totaled $7,650 for the entering class of 1989-90. Nonresidents paid $13,407. Apartments near the college rent for about $250/month.

Financial Aid

More than 67 percent of students receive some form of financial aid. Both need- and merit-based awards are available, and most students have access to low-cost loans. Work-study opportunities are also available. Students are encouraged to apply for assistance before May 31. Financial aid information will be mailed to accepted students after January 1.

Student Organizations

Academic organizations include the American Medical Association and the Ohio State Medical Association, as well as the American Medical Student Association and the Medical Students Association. Other academic groups include the Urban Health Project and Women in Medicine. Social organizations include the Bridge Club, the Christian Medical Fellowship, the Medical Cycling Enthusiasts, and the Note-O'chords music group.

Curriculum

The College of Medicine has a strong basic sciences program for the first two years that focuses on preparing students to handle a dynamic and rapidly expanding body of medical knowledge. Clinical experience is introduced early in the curriculum, with Introduction to Clinical Practice I and II in the first and second years, respectively. Students can participate in clinical application in a number of fields, including internal medicine, pediatrics, environmental health, psychiatry, and neurology. Legal and ethical issues of medicine are also taught in these years. The third year features a series of eight-week clerkships in a variety of areas, including some elective areas. The fourth year allows students to develop their individual interests further and to continue to obtain clinical experience.

Facilities

The University of Cincinnati Medical Center includes the medical, pharmacy, and nursing colleges, two research institutes, and a 766-bed university hospital. There are five other associated teaching hospitals that are easily accessible to students. They represent over 3,500 beds and include the Veterans' Administration Medical Center, Children's Hospital Medical Center, and Christ Hospital.

Grading Procedures

Evaluation of students is by an honors/pass/fail grading system in the first and second years. An honors/high pass/

pass/fail system is used in the third and fourth years.

Special Programs

The College of Medicine offers an M.D./Ph.D. program designed to prepare physician-scientists for academic careers in medical research. In addition to applying to the College of Medicine, applicants to the M.D./Ph.D. program must apply to the Medical Science Scholars Program.

Application Procedures

All applicants are required to take the MCAT, in the year prior to the intended matriculation date. Students must submit an AMCAS application as well as a University of Cincinnati College of Medicine application. Transcripts must be submitted to AMCAS by November 1. Candidates will receive a College of Medicine application packet, which contains forms for the student to document the completion of the premedical required courses and residency status.

There is also an early decision program (all AMCAS materials must be received by August 1). There is an application fee of $25.

Contact

Office of Admissions
University of Cincinnati College of Medicine
231 Bethseda Avenue
Cincinnati, Ohio 45267-0552
(513) 558-7314

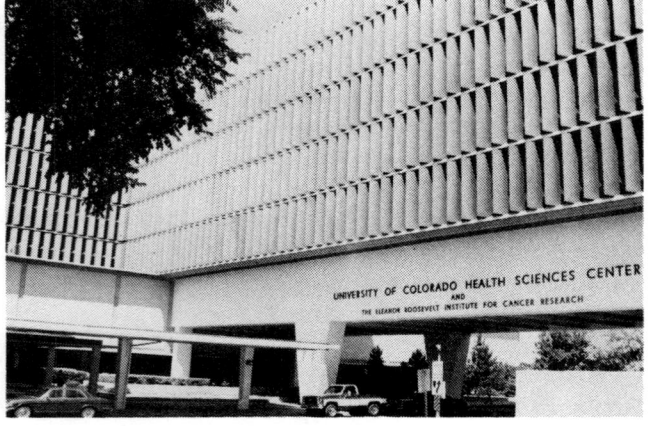

UNIVERSITY OF COLORADO SCHOOL OF MEDICINE

4200 East Ninth Avenue
Denver, Colorado 80262
(303) 270-7563

Accreditation	AAMC
Degrees Offered	M.D., M.D./Ph.D., B.S., M.S.
# Students Applied	986
Enrollment	131 / class
Mean GPA	3.5
% Men / % Women	59% / 41%
% Minorities	11.5%
Tuition	$8,228 In-State
	$34,132 Out-of-State
Application Fee	$40
Application Deadline	November 15

The University

The University of Colorado Graduate School and the Schools of Medicine, Nursing, and Dentistry comprise the University of Colorado Health Sciences Center. The center also houses two hospitals and eight affiliated institutes. Originally located on the Boulder campus, the medical school has been in Denver since 1911. Denver's proximity to the Rocky Mountains and its pleasant seasons allow for skiing, hiking, and other outdoor activities. This city of about 1.5 million residents also has many cultural and urban recreational facilities.

Admissions

Admission to the medical school is based on college grade point average, Medical College Admissions Test (MCAT) scores, recommendations from professors and others, and a required personal interview. Students in each entering class have a mean GPA of 3.5 and an average MCAT score of 9.5. About 12.5 percent of all applicants are accepted to fill a freshman class of 130 students. About 10 students each year are accepted through the early decision program.

Undergraduate Preparation

Undergraduate academic requirements include eight semester hours each of biology or zoology, general chemistry, organic chemistry, and physics, all with lab; six semester hours of college mathematics, six semester hours of English literature or equivalent; and three semesters hours of English composition or creative writing or equivalent. Calculus and a quantitative mathematically-oriented physics course are recommended with a view toward understanding rates of physiological change.

Student Body

The majority of students in each entering class are Colorado residents. Preference is also given to applicants from the WICHE states of Wyoming, Montana, and Alaska. The mean age of students is 26.

Costs

Entering students must pay a fee of $200 when they respond positively to the acceptance offer. This deposit is applied to the tuition of the last term at UCHSC. Another $300 deposit is due by August 1 and is applied to the first term. Disadvantaged students may have application fees and interview costs defrayed. Tuition is $8,228 for residents and $34,132 for nonresidents.

Financial Aid

Any degree candidate is eligible for financial aid, but full-time students are given preference. Foreign students desiring financial aid must be an immigrant with a permanent visa. Aid is offered based on financial need through part-time employment, long-term low-interest loans, and grants. Applications for financial aid are due by March 15 preceding the entrance date or 30 days after the letter of acceptance is sent to the student. Students must reapply for financial aid each year.

Minority Programs

The Center of Multicultural Enrichment (CME) recruits and provides services for students whose ethnic groups are underrepresented on the UCHSC campus. African-American, Asian, Hispanic, and Native American students benefit from CME efforts.

Faculty

The clinical courses are taught by about 1,000 community physicians in private practice.

There are 575 full-time and 1,200 volunteer instructors.

Grading Procedures

Courses are graded on an honors/pass/fail basis.

Special Programs

A combined M.D./Ph.D. program, as well as various allied health profession programs, is offered by the medical school. The Child Health Associate (CHA) program offers physician-assistant training to 16 to 20 students each year in the health care of infants, children, and adolescents. During October of the third and final year of the program, certification is earned by passing the National Certifying Examination for Physician Assistants. The Medical Scientist Training Program (MSTP) offers an M.D./Ph.D. degree by combining medical school and graduate school curricula in about a seven-year period. Students choose their Ph.D. program from among the offerings of six departments, which include biochemistry, biophysics, and genetics; cellular and structural biology; microbiology and immunology; pathology; and pharmacology. The B.S in medical technology is a one-year program designed to train 14 to 16 students for medical laboratory service. The B.S. may be earned from UC School of Medicine after completion of required undergraduate coursework in chemistry, biology, and mathematics. The B.S. may also be earned at the undergraduate institution by combining credits earned there with Medical Technology Program credits. The Master of Science in physical therapy may be earned in two years. The program is located in the medical school but the degree is awarded by the UC Graduate School.

Application Procedures

Applications must be filed through the American Medical College Application Service (AMCAS) by November 1 and by August 1 for early decision program (EDP) candidates. Nonresidents are urged to apply through EDP. EDP applicants are notified by October 1 and regular applicants are notified by March 15.

Contact

Office of Admissions and Records
University of Colorado Health Sciences Center
4200 East Ninth Avenue, Box A054
Denver, Colorado 80262
(303) 270-7676

COLUMBIA UNIVERSITY COLLEGE OF PHYSICIANS AND SURGEONS

630 West 168th Street
New York, New York 10032
(212) 305-3592

Accreditation	AAMC
Degrees Offered	M.D., M.D./Ph.D., M.D./ M.P.H.
# Students Applied	2,100
Enrollment	148 / class
Mean GPA	3.5
% Men / % Women	61% / 39%
% Minorities	Not Available
Tuition	$17,892
Application Fee	$50
Application Deadline	October 15

The University

Founded in 1754, Columbia University was originally known as King's College. The college organized its first medical faculty in 1767 and was the first learning institution in the North American colonies to graduate M.D.s. In 1912, the college was renamed Columbia University in the City of New York, and in 1928 the Columbia-Presbyterian Medical Center was established.

Admissions

In its search for students, the college looks nationally as well as locally. The college admits about 148 students from a very large applicant pool each year. A wide range of factors is considered in the admissions decision, including results of an interview, MCAT scores, and academic achievement. The college seeks independent, self-motivated students, and those who seek continuous self-education. Important personal qualities include maturity, leadership capabilities, and the ability to take responsibility.

Undergraduate Preparation

The necessary prerequisites for admission to the college are English, physics, biology, organic chemistry (including at least one semester of lab), and another one-year course in chemistry. The student's major is not important, but a well-rounded education and proven ability in the natural sciences is favored. All students must have completed at least three years of un-

dergraduate study, but the student who holds a baccalaureate degree is preferred in admissions.

The MCAT must have been taken within four years before the date of application; the latest time the MCAT should be taken is the fall before the date of anticipated enrollment.

Costs

1990-91 tuition is $17,892. Additional fees include a health service fee of $500 per year and a hospital insurance premium of $413 per year. Books, supplies, and microscope fees are estimated to cost about $1,300 per year.

Financial Aid

The college awards financial aid based on demonstrated need. A GAPSFAS form must be submitted for the Scholarship for Students of Exceptional Financial Need and the Financial Assistance for Disadvantaged Health Professions Students scholarship.

Students are encouraged to seek scholarship assistance from the state in which they live. Nongovernmental sources of assistance include the National Medical Fellowships, Inc., which awards funds to needy minorities. There are also numerous scholarships administered by the college's financial aid office.

Full-time students are eligible to receive loans, including Health Professions Student Loans, Perkins Loans, and Stafford Loans. There is also a dean's loan fund and there are other loan funds available through the university as supplements.

For more information, contact the Health Sciences Office of Student Financial Planning at (212) 305-4100.

Student Organizations

Student organizations include the P&S Club, founded by Nobel Peace Prize winner John R. Mott. All medical students are automatically members. The club has numerous committees and organizes a variety of extracurricular activities, including concerts, choral society, winetasters, athletics, and community youth work.

The Alpha Omega Alpha honor society was founded at the college in 1907. Select students are appointed to membership in this national honor society in their senior year.

Curriculum

The first year emphasizes the basic sciences, but also includes clinics designed to highlight the application of the sciences to the physician's practice. First-year students are introduced to the health care system in society and its effects on both patient and physician. The second year brings the basic sciences closer to the clinical experience, as second-year students begin their clinical education in the second semester of this year.

The third year is the major clinical year, consisting of clerkship rotations in all the clinical disciplines (these include dermatology, neurology, anesthesiology, psychiatry, surgery, and pediatrics). Students learn history-taking and participate in the physical examination of patients as they learn to develop professional relationships with patients.

In the fourth year, students can choose from a variety of basic science electives, clinical electives, and research programs. All fourth-year students must take a one-month elective in ambulatory care. Students are encouraged to choose electives in a broad range of fields and to participate in research.

Facilities

The campus spans about 20 acres and includes the main 17-story structure that adjoins Presbyterian Hospital. Other major facilities include the William Black Medical Research Building and the Julius and Armand Hammer Health Sciences Center, which houses teaching, research, and library facilities.

The college comprises the divisions of the University Faculty of Medicine (the College of Physicians and Surgeons, the School of Nursing, the School of Public Health); the University School of Dental and Oral Surgery; the Presbyterian Hospital and its subdivisions; the New York State Psychiatric Institute; and the Washington Heights Health and Teaching Center.

The Augustus C. Long Health Sciences Library houses nearly 450,000 volumes and is one of the largest medical center libraries in the nation. The library regularly receives over 4,000 periodicals. Students have access to computer literature searching and a microcomputer library and classroom.

Grading Procedures

The college uses an honors-pass-fail grading system. In addition, faculty members write a narrative description of student performance in the preclinical courses, major clinical clerkships, and elective courses.

Special Programs

The college has an M.D./Ph.D. program, which is cooperatively sponsored by the college and by the Graduate School of Arts and Sciences. Motivated students who are strong in the sciences and committed to biomedical research can select one of the basic sciences for which the graduate school has a Ph.D. program.

The college and the School of Public Health offer a dual M.D./M.P.H. degree program. Candidates must be accepted into the college before making application to the School of Public Health. The degree prepares students for careers in public health or in research or practice.

Other special programs include the Integrated M.D./Oral and Maxillofacial Surgery Program.

Application Procedures

Students must file a special application available through the Admissions Office of the Faculty of Medicine. Students are encouraged to file the application early. The filing deadline is October 15. Students must submit a nonrefundable $50 application fee along with undergraduate transcripts, MCAT scores, and letters of recommendation. A personal interview may be required.

Contact

Columbia University
College of Physicians and Surgeons
Admissions Office
630 West 168th Street
New York, New York 10032
(212) 305-3595

UNIVERSITY OF CONNECTICUT SCHOOL OF MEDICINE

263 Farmington Avenue
Farmington, Connecticut 06030
(203) 679-2413

Accreditation	AAMC
Degrees Offered	M.D., M.S., Ph.D.
# Students Applied	1,596
Enrollment	Not Available
Mean GPA	3.48
% Men / % Women	53% / 47%
% Minorities	10%
Tuition	$5,550 In-State
	$12,300 Out-of-State
Application Fee	$50
Application Deadline	December 15

The University

The University of Connecticut is a state-supported institution with an educational tradition dating back to 1881; in 1939, its name officially became the University of Connecticut. The School of Medicine graduated its 19th class in May 1990.

Admissions

The admissions committee considers closely the GPA and the MCAT scores of applicants. In addition, the committee considers evidence of academic achievement beyond the regular coursework, motivation, ability, character, evidence of intellectual growth, and extracurricular activities. Applicants must demonstrate skill in areas such as communication and observation. Preference for both first-year and transfer applicants is given to Connecticut residents.

Undergraduate Preparation

The School of Medicine believes that a broad liberal arts education is the best background for those entering medical school, and that applicants should have proficiency in the English language and in mathematics. Applicants should hold a bachelor's degree or its equivalent and must complete the following undergraduate courses or their equivalents: general chemistry, organic chemistry, physics, biology or zoology, and English (courses in composition and literature are recommended). Students should have taken the introductory courses required of those majoring in the subjects listed above rather than nonmajor "survey" type courses.

Student Body

Ninety percent of the 1990 entering class are Connecticut residents. The average age is about 23 years at the time of application. Slightly less than half are female, and 10 percent are underrepresented minorities. The average MCAT score is 58. Forty-four undergraduate schools are represented in the student body. About one-quarter are nonscience majors.

Costs

Connecticut residents pay $5,550 for tuition; non-residents pay $12,300. Annual fees are $2,250. Books, equipment, and other supplies are estimated to cost $850 per year, and living expenses average $9,500 for the single student.

Financial Aid

Financial need is determined by standard needs analysis through GAPSFAS. The most commonly used noninstitutional programs are Stafford Loans, Supplemental Loans for Students, and Health Education Assistance Loans. There are numerous other grants, scholarships, and loans for which students may be eligible, including Health Professions Student Loans; Perkins Loans; Robert Wood Johnson Fund Loans; and the Health Professions Exceptional Financial Need Scholarships.

Minority Programs

The university maintains an Office of Minority Student Affairs. The School of Medicine provides educational opportunities and financial assistance to students from educationally disadvantaged groups who are underrepresented in American medicine. Special programs include both tutorial and counseling help for these students.

Student Organizations

Students may be elected to the Medical Council and several student committees. Other student organizations include the Organization of Student Representatives, the Student National Medical Association, the Family Medicine Interest Group, and the Medical-Dental Student Government.

Faculty

The faculty is large and represents a wide variety of disciplines, including a department of Nuclear Medicine and a department of Psychiatry.

Curriculum

The first two years expose students to the fundamental knowledge and skills necessary to all physicians. The curriculum features a blend of departmental and interdisciplinary courses, each designed and taught by a faculty team. In an effort to integrate basic science with clinical experience, the school provides an introductory clinical medicine course that runs throughout the first two years, in which the student learns to establish the vital physician-patient relationship. In the third and fourth years, the student applies the knowledge gained in the first half of the academic curriculum. The last two years are characterized by intensive clinical work. The third year is a full-time clinical year. Required clerkships include medicine, surgery, obstetrics and gynecology, and psychiatry. There are also 150 elective clerkships from which students can choose. Third- and fourth-year clerkships take place in a wide variety of community hospital settings.

Facilities

The School of Medicine comprises a 232-bed University Hospital staffed and equipped for teaching purposes, medical outpatient teaching clinics, extensive medical research facilities, multi-discipline laboratories, the Lyman Maynard Stowe Library, and a host of allied and affiliated community-based hospitals. Most of the university-sponsored residencies and fellowships take place in a health consortium of eight hospitals in the Greater Hartford area.

Grading Procedures

The basic sciences program uses a pass/fail system of grading. There is no class ranking. Clinical clerkships and elective activities are judged by the faculty to be either "satisfactory" or "unsatisfactory."

Special Programs

The university offers a combined M.D./Ph.D. program. Those interested must apply to the School of Medicine through AMCAS. A detailed description is available from the graduate office or the medical student affairs office.

Application Procedures

Applicants must submit a standardized application directly to AMCAS. The application deadline for submitting applications to AMCAS for first-year entry is December 15. The deadline for submission of all supplementary materials (recommendations, personal statements, etc.) is December 31. For early notification, the application deadline is August 1. Note: All applicants are required to take the MCAT exam no later than the fall of the year preceding their expected date of matriculation.

Contact

University of Connecticut School of Medicine
Admissions Office
263 Farmington Avenue
Farmington, Connecticut 06030
(203) 679-2152

CORNELL UNIVERSITY MEDICAL COLLEGE

445 East 69th Street
New York, New York 10021
(212) 746-5454

Accreditation	AAMC
Degrees Offered	M.D., M.D./Ph.D.
# Students Applied	4,000
Enrollment	101 / class
Mean GPA	3.5
% Men / % Women	50% / 50%
% Minorities	15%
Tuition	$19,200
Application Fee	$50
Application Deadline	October 15

The University

The Cornell University Medical College is located on the Upper East Side of New York City in close proximity to six other nationally renowned medical facilities, including the Memorial Sloan-Kettering Cancer Center. Founded in 1898, the Medical College sends many graduates on to prominent positions in academic medicine and, because of its location, is able to provide students with unique clinical and research opportunities.

Admissions

The average MCAT score of successful applicants to Cornell is 10.9, while the cumulative undergraduate GPA of accepted students averages 3.5. However, these are not the only criteria used by the college to evaluate candidates for admission. Other factors given serious consideration are extracurricular activities, independent investigation of the field of medicine and the applicant's overall suitability and motivation for medicine as a career. While a B.A. degree is not necessary for admission to the Medical College, a minimum of three years of undergraduate study must be completed. A science major is not required.

Undergraduate Preparation

In accordance with the regulations of New York State, the Medical College requires the completion of at least six semester hours each of English, physics, biology or zoology, general chemistry, and organic chemistry. However, the college advises students to consider these requirements the minimum and to pursue further study in these subjects as individual academic interests suggest. The MCAT is also required.

Student Body

Approximately 50 percent of the students at the Medical College are female. Fifteen percent of the student body are members of minority groups. Students come from 47 different undergraduate institutions in 22 states and three foreign countries. The average age of entering medical students at Cornell is 22.

Placement Records

Recent graduates have accepted positions at facilities including the New York Hospital, Brigham and Women's Hospital, the Johns Hopkins Hospital, University of California Hospitals in San Francisco, Yale-New Haven Medical Center, Columbia-Presbyterian Medical Center, and UCLA Medical Center.

Costs

Tuition for the 1990-91 academic year was $19,200. Other expenses, including books, instruments, food, lodging, utilities, and personal expenses, are estimated to total another $7,900.

Financial Aid

The Medical College helps many students with economic needs finance their education. Accepted students apply for financial aid by completing an application with the graduate and professional school financial aid service. Once need is determined, Cornell tries to balance financial aid between loans and grants. Assistance is also given to help students find summer employment prior to beginning their first year of medical training.

Minority Programs

Cornell conducts a research fellowship program for about 20 minority premedical students. The Medical College makes a nationwide effort to enroll qualified minority students.

Faculty

The Medical College has over 1,500 faculty members, many of whom also hold staff positions at nearby New York City hospitals. Cornell emphasizes individualized academic attention, and therefore classes are usually small. Elective courses often have only seven or eight students each, and students interact closely with the faculty.

Curriculum

The first year emphasizes basic medical sciences, the second year brings in more specialized aspects of basic medical sciences and introductory clinical work, the third year fully integrates the student into the clinical environment, and in the fourth year continues clinical experiences while allowing for electives. Recently the college has implemented curricular changes. Some specific changes include an increased amount of time for electives in the first and second years, an increase in the amount of class time that must be devoted to small group teaching, and the expansion of the third year to allow students to have more clinical experience before making career decisions.

Facilities

The New York Hospital, with 1,460 beds, is the main teaching facility for the Medical College. Cornell is also affiliated with a number of other hospitals in the New York City area.

Grading Procedures

Performance is graded by an honors/pass/fail system supplemented by faculty evaluations.

Special Programs

Joint M.D./Ph.D. programs are offered in conjunction with both Rockefeller University and Memorial-Sloan Kettering Cancer Center. Also, the Medical College participates in the National Institutes of Health Medical Scientist Training Program. Students accepted into this program receive full tuition and stipend support to cover living expenses for the entire six year period.

Application Procedures

Students must submit an application to the AMCAS by October 15 of the year prior to desired entrance into medical school. Once the Medical College receives this information from the AMCAS, students will receive a supplemental Cornell application to complete. This must be submitted by November 1, accompanied by a $50 application fee. Also required is one letter of recommendation from the undergraduate premedical advisory committee or, if no such committee exists, two letters from faculty members familiar with the student. MCAT scores are also required and Cornell recommends that students submit only scores from the "new" version of the standardized test. Strong candidates for admission will be invited to the Medical College for personal interviews, and all applicants will be advised of their admissions status by March 1.

Contact

Committee on Admissions
Cornell University Medical College
445 East 69th Street
New York, New York 10021
(212) 746-1067

CREIGHTON UNIVERSITY SCHOOL OF MEDICINE

California at 24th Street
Omaha, Nebraska 68178
(402) 280-2600

Accreditation	AAMC
Degrees Offered	M.D.
# Students Applied	3,913
Enrollment	110 / class
Mean GPA	3.0
% Men / % Women	67% / 33%
% Minorities	Not Available
Tuition	$15,900
Application Fee	$40
Application Deadline	December 1

The University

The Creighton University School of Medicine opened in 1892 and currently has an enrollment of 440. Creighton is the smallest university in the four major health sciences.

Admissions

The MCAT and at least 90 semester hours of accredited college work are mandatory. Preference is given to applicants who hold baccalaureate degrees. Up to 27 hours of credits are accepted under CLEP and/or advanced placement programs. Candidates are not restricted by state of residence, but preference is given to students who live in mid-western states and to students from states that do not have medical schools. Preference is also given to applicants who have done their undergraduate work at Creighton.

Undergraduate Preparation

Creighton encourages applicants to take the MCAT in the

spring of the year before entry into medical school. MCAT scores from before 1987 will not be considered. Students must meet all requirements the June before entry. At least 90 semester hours of credit are mandatory in the following areas: English, six hours; general biology, physics and inorganic chemistry, eight hours each; and organic chemistry, 8-10 hours, all including lab.

Student Body

The mean age of the 1989 entering class was 24. Their cumulative GPA was 3.3. Thirty-three percent of the class were women, and 90 percent had their undergraduate degree in science.

Costs

Tuition for 1990-91 was $15,900. Fees come to $254. Room and board is estimated at $9,670, and books and supplies total $940.

Financial Aid

Approximately 72 percent of students receive some form of financial aid during their years of study. Eligibility requirements include U.S. citizenship or eligible nonresidents, good academic standing, maintenance of at least half-time status, and completion of the Financial Aid Form (FAF). Eleven scholarship funds support student financing. Nebraska residents may apply for two different loan funds. About 20 long- and short-term loans are available.

Minority Programs

Financial aid in the form of grants and long-term loans is available to minority students on the basis of proven need.

Curriculum

During the first year and a half, students learn traditional preclinical sciences along with courses in behavioral science, public health, and epidemiology. A half-year of programs follows in clinical medicine and physical diagnosis. The third year consists of required clerkships lasting 50 weeks. The fourth year, which is entirely elective, offers courses in preclinical and clinical disciplines. Some portion of this year may be spent off-campus.

Facilities

The Medical Center has a new $75 million teaching hospital, and a $5 million Bio-Information Center. Integrated into the hospital design is the Omaha Health Professions Center. A library is conveniently located on the health science campus. The Boys Town National Institute for Communication Disorders in Children is a special facility for study and research. Some instruction is also done at Children's Memorial, Omaha Veteran's Administration, and Archbishop Bergan Mercy Hospitals. Clinical services are also available at other local area hospitals.

Special Programs

Other than the M.D., Creighton offers programs in nursing, pharmacy, and dentistry.

Application Procedures

Students must apply through AMCAS between June 1 and December 1 of the year before desired entry. The fee is $40, but Creighton will waive the fee if AMCAS has waived its costs. Students should also submit academic recommendations, a recent photo (2" x 2"), and supplementary personal information. After written notice of acceptance, students must reply in writing within 14 days. Prior to March 1, students must pay a $100 enrollment fee. After March 1, deposits are not refundable. Applications for advanced standing are considered.

Contact

Medical School Admissions Office
Creighton University
California at 24th Street
Omaha, Nebraska 68718
(402) 280-2798

DARTMOUTH MEDICAL SCHOOL

Hanover, New Hampshire 03756
(603) 646-7480

Accreditation	LCME
Degrees Offered	M.D., M.D./Ph.D.
# Students Applied	4,189
Enrollment	87 / class
Mean GPA	Not Available
% Men / % Women	59% / 41%
% Minorities	9%
Tuition	$20,650
Application Fee	$55
Application Deadline	November 1

The University

Dartmouth Medical School was founded in 1797, and it is the fourth oldest medical school in the United States. The Medical School is fully accredited by the LCME. The college is located on a 250-acre wooded site in Hanover, New Hampshire. Hanover is located in the heart of one of America's winter wonderlands and offers opportunities for year-round outdoor sporting activities. Boston, one of America's premier cultural and historic centers, is within driving distance.

Admissions

Out of the 4,189 applications Dartmouth receives for its first-year medical programs, only 84 are selected. Dartmouth has two first-year programs, one at Dartmouth proper and one in conjunction with Brown University in Providence, Rhode Island. Approximately 500 students are selected for interviews each year. Students in the Brown-Dartmouth Program in medical education complete their first two years at Dartmouth and then transfer to Brown at the beginning of the third year. For detailed information inquire at the office of admissions.

Undergraduate Preparation

Requirements include one year each of general chemistry, organic chemistry, biology, and physics. A half-year of calculus is required. Applicants must have facility in written and oral English. All candidates must take the MCAT and have completed the equivalent of at least three years of college at a United States college or university. Nonscience majors who have demonstrated competence in science are encouraged to apply.

Student Body

Sixty-four new students are enrolled each year to the Dartmouth M.D. program, and the Brown-Dartmouth program admits 20 students. The whole student body consists of 300. On the average, 25 states are represented in the incoming class. Nine percent of the student body are minorities.

Placement Records

For the class of 1991, 57 graduates received residency appointments. Virtually all medical graduates go on to three years or more of residency training following medical school. Eighty-five percent of the class of 1991 received one of their top three choices, 54 percent received their first choice.

Costs

Tuition for 1990-91 was $20,650. Living expenses are estimated at $6,650. During the first year, students pay $140 for microscope use. Books cost approximately $190, and incidental living expenses come to about $1,850 for first year students. Limited housing is available for students in a college-owned community of apartments and townhouses just south of Hanover.

Financial Aid

Dartmouth supports students who show documented financial need through GAPSFAS analysis and additional financial information. Financial awards are made beginning April

15. During 1990-91, more than 77 percent of the students received financial aid. About 42 percent received loans and scholarship aid, and 35 percent received loans only. The base loan was $17,000. Federal loan programs available include some six other loan funds.

Minority Programs

The Afro-American Society and the Native American Council support minority students on the Dartmouth College campus.

Student Organizations

Physicians for Social Responsibility has a chapter on campus. Other organizations include The Christian Medical and Dental Society, DMS Social Issues in Medicine, The American Medical Student Association, Family Medicine Interest Group, and Women in Medicine.

Curriculum

The first two years focus on the function of the human organism in its physical and psychosocial contexts and cover the basic sciences. The third year entails required clerkships, about 45 percent of which are in the outpatient setting. The fourth year is given over to electives, and three required courses in health, society, and the physician; clinical pharmacology and therapeutics; and advanced cardiac life support. In the Brown-Dartmouth Program, the requirements for clerkships and electives vary slightly from those of Dartmouth Medical College.

Facilities

The Dartmouth-Hitchcock Medical Center, completed in 1991, is the heart of the college. In the 1990s, preclinical instruction will be relocated to the new campus, 2.5 miles from the present site. A new Conference and Education Building is scheduled for completion in the mid-1990s. Dartmouth is also affiliated with the Veterans Administration Hospital in White River Junction and the Community Health Center. Other facilities include the Dartmouth-Hitchcock Mental Health Center, the Norris Cotton Cancer Center, the Dartmouth-Hitchcock Hemophilia Center, and a number of local hospitals and clinics. The Dana Biomedical Library at the Hitchcock Center houses over 185,000 volumes and 3,200 journals.

Special Programs

Datrmouth offers the M.D./Ph.D. and programs in physiology, pharmacology and toxicology, biochemistry and bioengineering. Graduate Medical Education is carried on at a number of centers. Graduates may study at the Maine-Dartmouth Family Practice Residency based in central Maine.

Application Procedures

Applications must be obtained and processed through

AMCAS. The nonrefundable application fee is $55. Applicants will need a composite recommendation from their school's premedical committee; otherwise, two individual letters of recommendation are required. Regular applications are reviewed September through April. Interviews follow for accepted candidates. The early decision plan is available, and interested applicants must file by August 1.

Contact

Office of Admissions
Dartmouth Medical School
Hanover, New Hampshire 03756
(603) 646-7505

DUKE UNIVERSITY SCHOOL OF MEDICINE

Durham, North Carolina 27706
(919) 684-3403

Accreditation	AMCA
Degrees Offered	M.D., M.D./Ph.D., M.D./ M.A., M.D./A.M., M.D./ M.P.H., M.D./J.D.
# Students Applied	4,545
Enrollment	105 / class
Mean GPA	3.5
% Men / % Women	70% / 30%
% Minorities	9%
Tuition	$14,200
Application Fee	$55
Application Deadline	October 15

The University

In 1930, James Buchanan Duke established the School of Medicine, the School of Nursing, and the hospital central to Duke University. The Private Diagnostic Clinic, organized in 1932, provides care to private patients with moderate incomes. The modern Duke Hospital North, with 1,048 beds, opened in 1980. The Medical Center is located on 140 acres on Duke's West Campus. Duke is a leader in contemporary medicine, maintaining standards of high quality patient care, dedication to educational programs, national and international

distinction in research, and service to the region. Durham (pop. 100,000) is in the Piedmont region of North Carolina, close to the sea and coast.

Admissions

The MCAT is required of all applicants, and students should take the test in April of the year they plan to apply. The earliest Notification of Acceptance is November 1 for students entering the following August. A personal interview is conducted. Candidates are admitted based on merit. Students with Ph.D. degrees may apply for a three-year program for the M.D. degree.

Undergraduate Preparation

Duke requires a minimum of 90 hours of approved undergraduate credit for admissions including one year each of the following: college English (composition), inorganic chemistry, organic chemistry, physics, biology or zoology, and calculus. Students must complete all science requirements not more than seven years prior to entrance.

Student Body

The University has an enrollment of 10,826 students from all 50 states and from many foreign countries.

Costs

Officials estimate $22,000 per year for student expenses. Tuition is $14,200. Rental rates for townhouse apartments, utilities not included, are $2,525. Other apartments range from $2,535 to $3,913 for singles. Deposits are required with all applications.

Financial Aid

Fifty-four scholarships awarded for merit are available, ranging from $5,000 to full four-year tuition and other costs based solely on academic excellence. Seven scholarships are available annually to academically excellent freshmen minority students who are North Carolina residents. Need-based full-tuition scholarships from the Armed Forces Scholarships programs are available; loans, from both inside and outside the university, are also available.

Student Organizations

Alpha Omega Alpha Honorary Medical Fraternity has a chapter on campus. All medical students are members of the Davison Society, which conducts medical student group activities and social events. The Engel Society promotes intellectual and social interaction between students and faculty. The Duke University Medical Alumni Association sponsors several social functions each year.

Faculty

The faculty are from all medical fields and disciplines.

Curriculum

The Medical School curriculum is designed to give students solid academic as well as clinical knowledge. The first-year student will study basic scientific principles, working toward a second-year program of clinical sciences. The third and fourth years allow the student to design his own programs, with the aid of a faculty advisor. The program may involve research, as well as the opportunity to evaluate the research of others. Clinical courses in the third and fourth years enhance the scientific curriculum of the first two years.

Facilities

The Medical Center Library/Communications Center consists of 239,000 volumes, 2,650 journals, and houses the Trent Collection in the history of medicine. The Veterans Administration Medical Center and Sea Level Hospital and Extended Care Facility all have representatives who serve as advisors to students. Lenos Baker Children's Hospital and Durham County General Hospital also participate in training experiences.

Grading Procedures

Grading consists of "passing" a course or "passing with honors." Students not meeting course requirements get an "incomplete." Failures cannot be erased from the record; however, students may repeat a course. To advance a year, the student must be awarded Satisfactory Progress.

Special Programs

Duke offers the M.D./Ph.D. (six to seven years). The Medical Historian Program offers an M.D./Ph.D. (six years) or an M.D./M.A. (four to five years). The M.D./A.M. program (maximum five years) offers multidisciplinary education with complete medical science and clinical training, as well as training in health services. The M.D./J.D. program offers combined medical and legal education. Also offered is the M.D./M.P.H. program.

Application Procedures

Applicants must obtain application forms from their undergraduate premedical advisor through the AMCAS. AMCAS receives applications any time after June 15 until October 15. The supplemental application deadline is December 15. Interviews may be required. The application fee is $55, and a $50 deposit is required within three weeks of acceptance.

Contact

Office of Admissions
Medical Center
Duke University
Durham, North Carolina 27706
(919) 684-2985

EAST CAROLINA UNIVERSITY SCHOOL OF MEDICINE

Greenville, North Carolina 27858-4354
(919) 551-2201

Accreditation	LCME
Degrees Offered	M.D.
# Students Applied	1,161
Enrollment	72 / class
Mean GPA	3.2
% Men / % Women	50% / 50%
% Minorities	19%
Tuition	$1,344 In-State
	$11,848 Out-of-State
Application Fee	$25
Application Deadline	November 15

The University

The East Carolina University School of Medicine opened in 1977. The school's facilities are located on the 100-acre Health Sciences Center campus in Greenville.

Admissions

The school seeks competent students of diverse personalities and backgrounds. Factors considered in the selection process cover aspects of the social, personal, and intellectual development of the individual applicant. MCAT scores, academic performance, letters of recommendation, and the results of personal interviews are all important factors in considering students for admission. Preference is given to qualified residents of North Carolina.

Undergraduate Preparation

A minimum of three years of undergraduate preparation is required. Required coursework includes one year of biology or zoology (with lab), one year of inorganic chemistry (with lab), one year of organic chemistry (with lab), one year of physics (with lab), and one year of English. Additional courses in the social sciences and humanities and a second year of English are recommended.

Student Body

The 1989 entering class totaled 72 students; only two of these were from out of state. The mean GPA of the class was 3.2. Thirty-five were women and 13 were minorities. All students in the class held bachelor's degrees at the time of enrollment.

Costs

Tuition of the 1989-90 first-year class was $1,344 for state residents and $11,848 for nonresidents. Student fees were $458 per year.

Financial Aid

Financial aid awards are based on need as determined by confidential information supplied by the applicant. Both loans and scholarships are available. Sixty-five percent of the student body receives some type of financial aid.

Minority Programs

The school's Center for Student Opportunities offers a wide range of services to assist and guide minority students, and minority representation on the school's admissions committee is substantial. The school encourages members of minority groups, especially those who reside in North Carolina, to apply for admission.

Curriculum

The first year includes the study of anatomy, biochemistry, physiology, microbiology/immunology, genetics, and the psychosocial basis of medical practice. Courses in primary care and philosophy and medicine are also included, as well as clinical lectures. The second year features courses that are directed toward clinical medicine, including pharmacology, pathology, clinical pathophysiology, psychiatry, human sexuality, physical diagnosis, and family medicine. The third year consists of six required clerkships of eight weeks each, and the fourth year is composed of 36 weeks of clerkships and both clinical and basic science electives. The fourth year offers the opportunity for the student to select an individualized curriculum, in consultation with faculty advisors.

Facilities

Facilities include the Brody Medical Sciences Building for preclinical instruction; the Pitt County Memorial Hospital, a 566-bed institution where clinical instruction is carried out;
the Child Development Evaluation Clinic; the Mental Health Center; an alcoholic rehabilitation center; the Intensive/Intermediate Care Neonatal Unit; and the new Biotechnology Building.

Grading Procedures

Student performance is evaluated by letter grade, and promotion to the next year is recommended to the dean by the promotions committee of the respective year.

Application Procedures

The school participates in AMCAS. The earliest date for filing the AMCAS application is June 15, and the deadline for receipt of the application is November 15. MCAT scores previous to 1988 will not be considered. Students will be notified of acceptance after October 15. Applicants for early decision must submit applications between June 15 and August 1.

Students enrolling in the first-year class must make a $100 advance tuition deposit when accepting an offer of admission.

Contact

Associate Dean, Office of Admissions
East Carolina University
School of Medicine
Greenville, North Carolina 27858-4354
(919) 551-2202

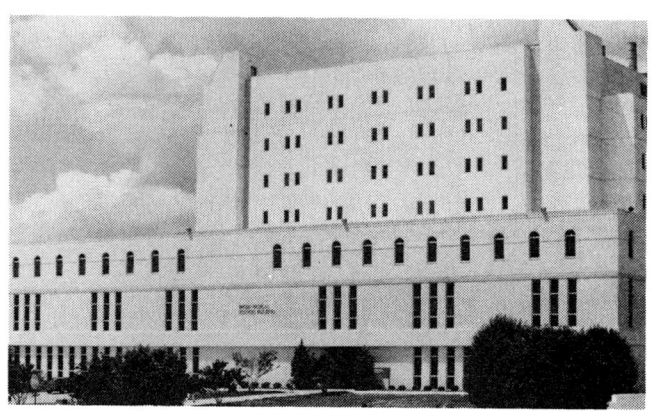

EAST TENNESSEE STATE UNIVERSITY JAMES H. QUILLEN COLLEGE OF MEDICINE

Johnson City, Tennessee 37614-0002
(615) 929-6315

Accreditation	LCME
Degrees Offered	M.D., M.S., Ph.D.
# Students Applied	916
Enrollment	60 / class
Mean GPA	3.27
% Men / % Women	63% / 37%
% Minorities	18%
Tuition	$6,560 In-State
	$10,410 Out-of-State
Application Fee	$15
Application Deadline	December 1

The University

Located on the main campus of East Tennessee State University, James H. Quillen College of Medicine is one of the newest fully accredited medical schools in the United States. Established in the 1970s, the college is a community-based medical school whose goal is to provide more physicians and premium medical care to northeast Tennessee and the surrounding region.

The college is situated in the tri-cities area—Johnson City, Bristol, and Kingsport. The area is rich in American cultural heritage and offers the scenic beauty of the Appalachian Mountains, Appalachian Trail, and the Blue Ridge Parkway.

Northeast Tennessee is a rapidly developing region and ranks nationwide as the 80th largest Standard Metropolitan Statistical Area.

Admissions

Admission is competitive and is based on a range of factors, including demonstrated academic achievement, MCAT scores, letters of recommendation, pertinent extracurricular research and work experience, evidence of nonacademic accomplishment, and demonstrated motivation to study and practice medicine. Important personal characteristics include maturity, integrity, and willingness and ability to assume responsibility.

Preference in admission is given to residents of Tennessee.

The college also gives preference to veterans of U.S. military service and to applicants who have received at least a bachelor's degree from an accredited institution.

Undergraduate Preparation

Completion of a minimum of 90 semester hours of undergraduate courses at an accredited institution is required for admission. These courses must include eight semester hours each of general chemistry, organic chemistry, physics, and biology; nine semester hours of communications skills; and 49 semester hours of electives.

Majors in the sciences or humanities are equally acceptable. Competence in communication skills, the humanities, and other nonscience areas is viewed favorably in the admissions process.

Candidates for admission must have taken the MCAT within the two years prior to applying in order to be considered for admission. It is recommended that applicants complete the MCAT in the spring of the year in which they will file their application.

Student Body

Total student enrollment is approximately 234, with an entering class of 60. The makeup of the student body is approximately 63 percent men and 37 percent women. Minorities comprise approximately 18 percent. Three percent are from out of state. The mean age is 25 years.

The MCAT average is 7.97. The average undergraduate GPA is 3.27.

Placement Records

About 81 percent of Quillen College graduates receive one of their three choices of residency appointments. Graduates are placed in residency positions in all areas of the country.

Costs

Tuition and fees for state residents in 1990 totaled $6,560. Nonresidents paid $10,410. Books and supplies for the 1990 first-year class cost about $600. Health insurance costs $244, on-campus room and board costs at least $4,300, and other required expenses amount to $250. The microscope rental fee is $125.

Financial Aid

The amount of aid awarded to students is limited to each student's determined need, program limitations, and the availability of funds. Complete financial aid packets are distributed upon the student's acceptance to the college.

Faculty

The college faculty numbers 155 full-time and 454 part-time and volunteer members. The total faculty (paid and volunteer)-to-student ratio is 1:.44.

Curriculum

The college provides a community-based program with an emphasis on the education of primary care physicians. The first two years of the program are devoted to the study of the basic medical sciences. Clinical application is introduced during these years, providing early exposure to patient care. The third and fourth years provide extensive clinical experience and allow students flexibility in choosing their area of interest.

Facilities

Instructional facilities are located on the main campus of the university and on the grounds of the U.S. Veterans Affairs Medical Center in Mountain Home, Tennessee. On campus, several modern buildings provide spacious teaching, research, and laboratory space. The newest building was added in 1983.

The college operates a range of clinics in the tri-cities area and a state-of-the-art rural family practice clinic in Mountain City. The five affiliated hospitals are Bristol Memorial Hospital, Holston Valley Medical Center, Johnson City Medical Center Hospital, the VA Hospital, and Woodridge Psychiatric Hospital. They represent a total of over 2,000 beds. The newest addition to the clinical facilities are a neonatal unit, children's hospital, and a level I trauma center. All are located within a 30-minute drive of the college. The medical library houses over 60,000 books and journals.

Application Procedures

The college participates in AMCAS. Applications must be filed with AMCAS between June 15 and December 1 of the year prior to intended enrollment. The college will request supplemental information from the applicant along with an application fee. Well-qualified applicants may be invited to participate in a personal on-campus interview.

The college also participates in the AMCAS early decision program. The application period for early decision is June 15 to August 1 of the year prior to the year of intended enrollment.

Contact

East Tennessee State University
James H. Quillen College of Medicine
Office of Student Affairs
P.O. Box 19900A
Johnson City, Tennessee 37614-0002
(615) 929-6219

EASTERN VIRGINIA MEDICAL SCHOOL OF THE MEDICAL COLLEGE OF HAMPTON ROADS

700 Olney Road
Norfolk, Virginia 23507
(804) 446-5812

Accreditation	LCME
Degrees Offered	M.D.
# Students Applied	2,831
Enrollment	97 / class
Mean GPA	3.32
% Men / % Women	55% / 45%
% Minorities	10%
Tuition	$10,000 In-State
	$16,500 Out-of-State
Application Fee	$50
Application Deadline	December 1

The University

Eastern Virginia Medical School (EVMS) was created to serve the Hampton Roads area and eastern Virginia with health care and health care education. A community-centered institution, EVMS focuses on educating primary care physicians, and students are exposed to community-based health care facilities. The school also promotes medical research.

Admissions

The school examines a wide range of factors in the admissions decision, as it seeks to graduate concerned and competent physicians. The mean GPA and MCAT scores are evaluated, as well as a variety of factors relating to the candidate's familiarity with the medical field, level of maturity, overall character, and integrity. Factors such as community involvement and volunteer work in a medical setting are important. While preference is given to residents of Virginia, there has recently been a rise in the number of nonresidents admitted to EVMS.

Undergraduate Preparation

Applicants must have at least 100 college semester hours from an accredited college or university to be considered for admission. Required courses include one year of biology, two years of chemistry (including organic chemistry), and one year of physics. A grade of "C" or above is required for each preprofessional course. In recent years, the enrolling classes at

EVMS have had an average overall GPA of 3.32, and a score of 9 in each area of the MCAT. The MCAT must have been taken within two years prior to the time of application.

Student Body

EVMS admitted 97 new students in 1990-91. Seventy-six were residents of Virginia. In recent years, nonresidents have comprised 33 to 40 percent of enrolling classes.

Costs

For the 1990-91 first-year class, tuition was $10,000 for residents and $16,500 for nonresidents. Yearly fees, which include health insurance, are $1,386.

Financial Aid

Most types of financial assistance available are based on need as determined by the GAPSFAS form. The main forms of financial aid are scholarships, grants, and loans, as well as the college work-study program. While many types of assistance are obtained from the state or federal sources, there are also scholarships and low-interest loans available from EVMS.

Minority Programs

The school actively encourages minorities to apply, and has an Assistant Dean for Minority Affairs and minority counseling. Scholarships designed for black students are available. EVMS also has faculty liaison committees and student groups that support minority students.

Faculty

In addition to its full-time faculty, EVMS has about 800 volunteer faculty who are practicing community-based physicians.

Curriculum

The first two years consist of basic science courses, introduction to clinical skills, and courses related to ethics in the practice of medicine. Students have the opportunity to learn in a small group setting for problem-solving and for the stimulation of independent thinking. The third year introduces students to clinical clerkships in internal medicine, family medicine, obstetrics/gynecology, pediatrics, psychiatry, and surgery. The fourth year is a combination of rotations in various surgical specialties and in substance abuse treatment, along with individually chosen electives.

Facilities

Students obtain their clinical training in one of twenty-nine hospitals located in communities throughout eastern Virginia.

Grading Procedures

Students are evaluated using the grades of honors, high pass, pass, or fail.

Application Procedures

The school participates in AMCAS. Candidates for admission should file the AMCAS application between June 15 and December 1 of the year prior to the year of intended enrollment. The dates of application for early decision are June 15 to August 1. There is an application fee of $50. Applicants are notified of acceptance after October 15 (early decision applicants are notified by October 1). There is a $200 deposit required for holding the applicant's place in the class; the deposit is applied toward tuition.

Contact

Eastern Virginia Medical School
Office of Admissions
700 Olney Road
Norfolk, Virginia 23507
(804) 446-5812

EMORY UNIVERSITY SCHOOL OF MEDICINE

Atlanta, Georgia 30322
(404) 727-5660

Accreditation	AAMC
Degrees Offered	M.D., M.D./Ph.D., M.D./M.P.H.
# Students Applied	3,060
Enrollment	112 / class
Mean GPA	3.5
% Men / % Women	66% / 34%
% Minorities	18%
Tuition	$14,400
Application Fee	$50
Application Deadline	October 15

The University

The Emory University School of Medicine, founded in 1915, is located on 620 acres in the Druid Hills section of Atlanta and in the Emory medical facilities in downtown Atlanta. Emory is a privately controlled university affiliated with the Methodist Church, awarding over 2,000 degrees annually. The campus acres are heavily wooded, six miles northeast of downtown Atlanta, and offer a pleasant, bucolic setting in which to work.

Admissions

A GPA of 3.3 or higher is expected, with a cumulative mean of 3.5. Students must take the MCAT. Applications must be filed through AMCAS. Some applicants will be invited for an interview. Early acceptance is available to students from Emory College and Oxford College of Emory University.

Undergraduate Preparation

Applicants must take the MCAT in the spring before the fall of the academic year for which they applied and have a minimum of three years of college. Students must complete at least 90 semester or 135 quarter hours in arts and sciences at an accredited institution before enrollment. CLEP credit is accepted if no more than 25 percent of the total. Specific minimum requirements include biology, inorganic chemistry (with lab), organic chemistry (with lab), physics, English, and humanities. Majors in the sciences or nonsciences are equally acceptable, but nonscience majors must be competent in basic mathematics. Completion of the bachelor's degree is mandatory if listed on the AMCAS application.

Student Body

Students from the Southeast receive some preference. Of the entering class of 1989, 35 percent were women, 24 percent were minorities.

Costs

Tuition and fees are approximately $14,400. A student activity fee of $100 is payable each year. There is a $20 fee for athletic programs. Housing is available on- and off-campus. Rental rates range upwards to $400 per month.

Financial Aid

Awarded based on need, about 200 scholarships given annually range from $500 to $7,200. Georgia residents are eligible for awards from the State Medical Education Board of Georgia. Six first-year students receive fellowships. One full-tuition and some half-tuition scholarships are available. Veterans benefits, special Dean's Scholars Awards for minorities, and loans are available.

Minority Programs

The School of Medicine provides significant financial aid to qualified minority students in the form of Dean's Scholar Awards, need-based grants and/or loans.

Student Organizations

Honor societies include Alpha Psi Omega, Alpha Omega Alpha, Phi Beta Kappa, Sigma Xi, and Omicron Delta Kappa. The Black Student Alliance promotes black culture, ideas, and goals. The Emory Medical Women's Association offers a network of support among women students, residents, faculty, and staff.

Faculty

The medical faculty consists of 1,700 members from all fields of medicine and research. The student/faculty ratio is about 10:1.

Curriculum

The first two years are devoted to classroom study of the basics of medicine. During the second year, the student is introduced to clinical medicine. The third and fourth years are entirely clinical, but allow the student 16 weeks at the end of the senior year for elective opportunities which may be spent in clinical areas, basic science subjects, or on research work. Opportunities for study abroad are available.

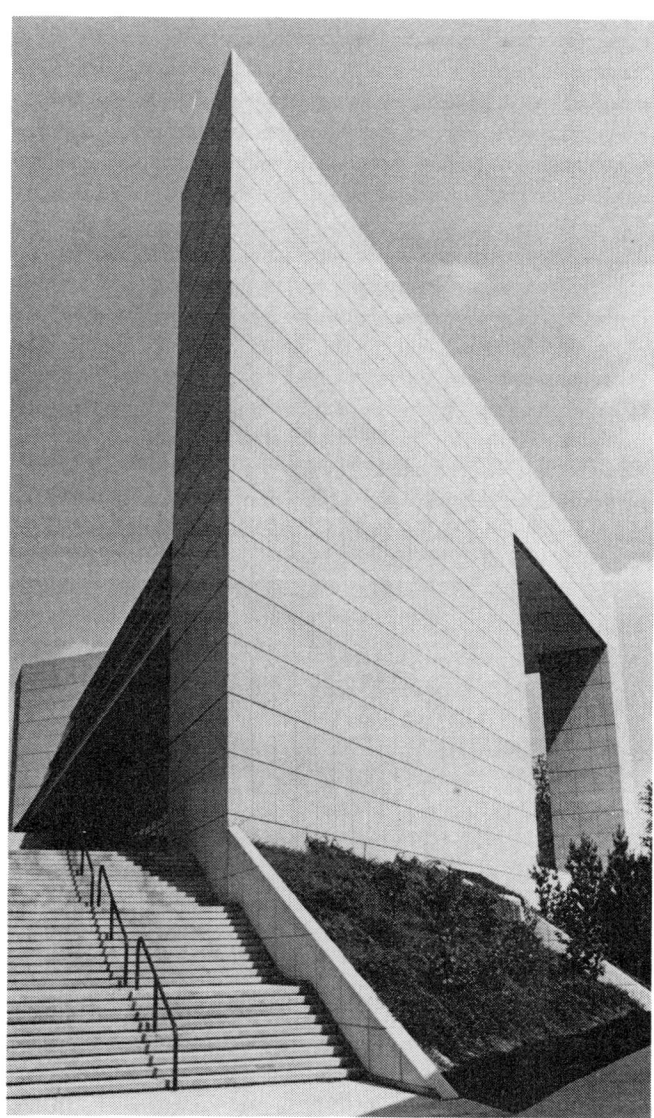

Facilities

The Emory campus has eight specialized libraries. The Health Sciences Library consists of more than 190,000 volumes. The Clifton Corridor consists of about 250 acres of facilities and the world's largest volunteer health organization. The O. Wayne Rollins Research Center offers 25,000 square feet of space for research. The Yerkes Regional Primate Research Center is located nearby.

Grading Procedures

Emory uses letter grades A through F, except for senior electives which are graded satisfactory/unsatisfactory. Student evaluations are not part of the grading system.

Special Programs

Emory offers a six-year joint M.D./Ph.D. program, a five-year M.D./M.P.H., and the Master of Medical Science, Master of Physical Therapy, Bachelor of Medical Science, and Associate in Medical Science. Certificate programs are available in Hospital Pharmacy Technology and Ultrasonography. Residencies and fellowship training are available at the Emory University affiliated hospitals. Summer fellowships, continuing education courses, and a special program at the Georgia Institute of Technology are available.

Application Procedures

Applicants must apply through the American Medical College Application Service. AMCAS accepts applications up to October 15; Emory must receive Supplemental Application forms and recommendation letters by December 1. Medical Scientist Training Program Applications must be received at Emory by December 1. Applicants should submit recommendations from a premedical advisor or three letters of recommendation to be received no later than December 1. Two of the letters should be from faculty who can assess the applicant's academic qualifications (one from the natural sciences).

Contact

Medical School Admissions
Room 303, Woodruff Health Sciences Center
Administration Building
Emory University
Atlanta, Georgia 30322
(404) 727-5660

Include your full name and Social Security number on all correspondence.

UNIVERSITY OF FLORIDA COLLEGE OF MEDICINE

J. Hillis Miller Health Center
Gainesville, Florida 32610
(904) 392-3701

Accreditation	AAMC
Degrees Offered	M.D., B.S./M.D., M.D./Ph.D.
# Students Applied	1,634
Enrollment	85 / class
Mean GPA	3.67
% Men / % Women	60% / 40%
% Minorities	15%
Tuition	$6,258 In-State
	$15,301 Out-of-State
Application Fee	$15
Application Deadline	December 1

The University

The University of Florida College of Medicine admitted the first class of students in September 1956. Located in north central Florida, the college is engaged in intramural and extramural programs with local medical centers and cities. The college occupies the southeast corner of the 2,000-acre campus of the University of Florida. Full national accreditation was first achieved in 1960 and again in 1976; in 1983 the college was accredited by the LCME. Residency programs are accredited individually by each respective specialty of the Accreditation Council on Graduate Medical Education, and all 21 programs are approved. Set in sunny Florida, the college is within striking distance of Orlando (Seaworld and Disneyworld), Ocala National Forest, and other cultural and resort centers of the state.

Admissions

Applicants must take the MCAT before the application deadline. Florida residents are given preference; however, a limited number of exceptionally qualified nonresidents are accepted each year. The College of Medicine does not discriminate on the basis of race, sex, creed, or national origin.

Undergraduate Preparation

Applicants should complete the bachelor's degree at an accredited university or college by matriculation. Students should have eight semester hours each (including laboratories) in biology, general and organic chemistry, and physics. Some college-level calculus and statistics courses are strongly recommended. The remainder of undergraduate work should be distributed among the humanities.

Student Body

Most students are Florida residents; a few are from out of state. Through an active recruitment program, the College of Medicine is developing a broader ethnic mixture in the student body. The whole student body consists of about 570 students, and the classes of 1990-1993 range from 86 to 120 full-time students. About 140 other graduate students study on campus. A few students take continuing education courses.

Costs

The fee structure changes from year to year. Tuition and fees are listed in the Bulletin of the Graduate School. Textbooks and instruments for the first year run from $700 to $900. The minimal annual cost for a single Florida resident for the year is about $8,000 plus tuition. Students may obtain fee information after July 1 by contacting Student Financial Services, Room 100, THE HUB, Gainesville, Florida 32610.

Financial Aid

Aid is available to students who show either financial need or academic excellence. About 18 scholarships and 47 scholastic awards are awarded. The College of Medicine also offers about a dozen different loan programs based solely on need. For more information write to the Office for Student Financial Affairs, 111 Anderson Hall, University of Florida, College of Medicine, Gainesville, Florida 32610.

Student Organizations

Alpha Omega Alpha medical honor society has a chapter on campus. The Student Government Organization on campus advocates student interest and needs.

Faculty

The most current catalog lists about 1,050 full-time and volunteer faculty at the college. Of these, 157 are graduate faculty, suggesting a student/teacher ratio of about 3:1.

Curriculum

The four years of study are divided into three blocks. During the preclinical coursework (two years), students study the core of basic science and general clinical information. Next, the required clinical clerkships (one year) include anesthesiology, community health, medicine, neurology, obstetrics and gynecology, pediatrics, psychiatry, and surgery. The postclerkship electives and required courses (one year) include four weeks each of required rotations in surgery and medicine, and four weeks of advanced pharmacology. The remainder of the fourth year is for electives.

Facilities

In addition to the research laboratories and animal facilities in the university Health Science Center and The Veterans Administration Medical Center, animal research facilities exist at the Health Science Center Animal Research Farm. A new 240,000-square-foot biomedical research building houses additional laboratories. Other facilities include the Chandler A. Stetson Medical Sciences Building; the Communicore Building (housing a main library of over 215,000 books and periodicals); the Academic Research Building; the Colleges of Dentistry, Health-Related Professions, Medicine, Nursing, Pharmacy, and Veterinary Medicine; Shands Hospital; and the Gainesville Veterans Administration Center. MEDLINE computer retrieval system is available to support teaching and research.

Grading Procedures

The College of Medicine uses letter grades A through F or pass-fail. Passing grades are A through C. The D grade connotes unsatisfactory performance, and remediation is required. In addition to all coursework, students must have a GPA of 2.0 or better and must have completed all remedial work with a C or higher. Parts I and II of the National Board Examination must be taken before graduation is possible.

Special Programs

The College of Medicine offers degrees in the basic medical sciences, residency programs in various specialties, and numerous fellowship programs of clinical or scientific orientation. Degrees offered include the M.S., Ph.D., and the M.D./Ph.D. program.

The seven-year Junior Honors Medical Program combines the B.S./M.D. degrees for undergraduates who have demonstrated superior academic and personal qualities in their first two years of college. Students should apply during their sophomore year of college; specific prerequisites are listed in the College of Medicine catalog.

Application Procedures

Students must apply through AMCAS. Return the completed form with a preprofessional committee evaluation or letters of recommendation. The fee is $15, and the deadline is December 1. Requests for an interview may follow. Students must send a letter of intent to the college within two weeks of acceptance.

Contact

Office of Student Admissions and Affairs
College of Medicine
Box J-216, J. Hillis Miller Health Center
University of Florida
Gainesville, Florida 32610-0216
(904) 392-3071

GEORGE WASHINGTON UNIVERSITY SCHOOL OF MEDICINE AND HEALTH SCIENCES

Walter G. Ross Hall
2300 Eye Street, N.W.
Washington, D.C. 20037
(202) 994-3727

Accreditation	AAMC
Degrees Offered	M.D., Ph.D., M.D./Ph.D., M.D./M.P.H.
# Students Applied	5,687
Enrollment	150 / class
Mean GPA	3.3
% Men / % Women	54% / 46%
% Minorities	Not Available
Tuition	$23,600
Application Fee	$45
Application Deadline	December 1

The University

Established in 1825, the George Washington University School of Medicine is the eleventh oldest medical school in the country. During the Civil War, the school was occupied by union soldiers, totally destroyed, and later rebuilt at its present site along Pennsylvania Avenue. Only a few blocks from the White House, the School of Medicine is in the heart of Washington, D.C. Nearby places of interest include historic Georgetown, the State Department, and the World Health Organization, as well as the Kennedy Center for the Performing Arts.

Admissions

When considering applicants for admission, the School of Medicine looks for students with a broad base of knowledge. A science major is not required and, in fact, the school encourages candidates with a background in the arts, humanities, and social sciences to apply. It is most important to the admissions committee that a student show scholarly interest and significant achievement in the chosen area of concentration as well as in the basic medical sciences. Although the School of Medicine is a private institution, "special consideration" is granted to students applying from the Washington, D.C. area as well as those applicants who attended George Washington University as undergraduates. The mean GPA for a recent

entering class was 3.3. The same class had a mean MCAT score of above 9.

Undergraduate Preparation

A minimum of 90 semester hours at an accredited U.S. or Canadian college are required prior to matriculation. Specific requirements include eight semester hours each (including two semester hours of lab work) of biology or zoology, general chemistry, organic chemistry, and physics. Six hours of English are also required for admission.

Student Body

Of the total medical school enrollment of approximately 600, the student body is about evenly split between men and women (the class of '93 comprises 68 women and 84 men). Students come from all over the country and represent a cross section of academic backgrounds. The age range of the class entering in September 1989 was from 20 to 51; the average age was 25.

Placement Records

In 1990, the School of Medicine reports, 85 percent of fourth-year students got one of their first three choices of training programs in the National Residency Matching Program, and 55 percent got their first choice. Salaries for these post-graduate positions ranged from $19,000 to $26,000.

Costs

Tuition for the 1990-91 academic year was $23,600. This figure includes all charges except for living expenses, which can vary widely depending on the housing arrangements made by individual students in the Washington area. Average monthly rent last year for the class of 1993 was $460.

Financial Aid

Approximately 78 percent of the medical students at George Washington receive some form of financial aid. The School of Medicine itself has limited resources and available funds are reserved for the neediest students, approximately 25 percent of financial aid recipients. Alternative sources of assistance include various federally funded loan programs, as well as scholarships and grants from outside organizations.

Faculty

There are over 1,600 faculty members at the School of Medicine. Seventy basic science faculty and 500 clinical faculty have full-time appointments, while the remaining clinical staff members are voluntary. Many faculty members maintain active practices in the Washington area and some serve on the staffs of the National Institutes of Health and other federal medical facilities.

Curriculum

The first year's studies are devoted to basic medical subjects, while the second year begins to prepare the student to function in the clinical environment. The third and fourth years consist of a continuum of clinical clerkships designed to provide experience and background for postgraduate training. Part I of the National Board Examination is required after the second year. The School of Medicine emphasizes cooperative effort rather than competition, and students on planning committees participate actively in evaluating and restructuring the curriculum.

Facilities

The main clinical setting for the School of Medicine is the George Washington University Hospital, a 511-bed, acute-care facility located across the street from the primary school academic buildings. The seven-story Ross Hall contains over ten acres of floor space, and is where basic and introductory clinical sciences are taught. One floor is devoted to sophisticated audiovisual support services. In the adjoining health sciences library are three computer-based reference systems, an audiovisual center, and a vast collection of books and periodicals. The school is also affiliated with more specialized institutions throughout the Washington area.

Grading Procedures

Students are evaluated using grades of honors, pass, conditional, or fail. The conditional grade is equivalent to an incomplete grade and can be changed, without having to repeat the course completely, if a student participates in a departmentally tailored academic program. All remedial work to remedy grades of conditional and fail is done during the summer at no additional cost to the student.

Special Programs

A variety of M.D./Ph.D. options are available in more than 50 research fields and usually take six years to complete. Interested students must apply and be accepted to both the School of Medicine and the Graduate School. A joint M.D./M.P.H. (Master of Public Health) program is offered and may be completed in four years in conjunction with M.D. studies. Also, the School of Medicine awards summer research fellowships that allow students to spend up to three months working on special projects at a number of health care centers affiliated with the university.

Application Procedures

The School of Medicine participates in the centralized application program of the AMCAS. Students must submit an application to AMCAS by December 1 of the year prior to desired admission and a supplemental George Washington application form is then due by January 15. MCAT scores are required; no results more than three years old will be accepted for evaluation. Also, letters of recommendation are required from the premedical advisory committee to the undergraduate college or from a student's professors. Approximately 20 percent

of the most promising candidates will be invited to the School of Medicine for personal interviews.

Contact

Office of Admissions
The George Washington University
School of Medicine and Health Sciences
Walter G. Ross Hall
2300 Eye Street, N.W.
Washington, D.C. 20037
(202) 994-3506

GEORGETOWN UNIVERSITY SCHOOL OF MEDICINE

3900 Reservoir Road, N.W.
Washington, D.C. 20007
(202) 687-4600

Accreditation	LCME
Degrees Offered	M.D., M.D./Ph.D.
# Students Applied	5,062
Enrollment	196 / class
Mean GPA	3.3
% Men / % Women	76% / 24%
% Minorities	7%
Tuition	$22,500
Application Fee	$55
Application Deadline	November 15

The University

Located in the Georgetown section of Washington, D.C., the university was founded in 1789 and is the oldest Catholic, Jesuit institution of higher learning in the United States. The campus is located on the banks of the Potomac River and covers 106 acres. Aside from the activities to be found at the university itself, students also have the almost limitless cultural and recreational opportunities of the nation's capital at their disposal.

Admissions

Students are selected to Georgetown on the basis of undergraduate academic achievement, character, maturity, and motivation. MCAT scores are also required. Strong candidates for admission are invited to campus for personal interviews before final evaluation of applications.

Undergraduate Preparation

One year each of inorganic chemistry, organic chemistry, biology, and physics, all with laboratory, as well as one year of mathematics and English, are required for admission to the School of Medicine. While not required, Georgetown also recommends courses in computer science, cellular physiology, genetics, embryology, biostatistics, quantitative analysis, and physical chemistry.

Student Body

Applicants who enrolled in 1989 had a mean GPA of 3.3. Sixty-one percent had degrees in the biological sciences, 14 percent in the physical sciences, 10 percent in social sciences, 15 percent in various humanities and other majors. Thirty-four percent were women, 11 percent were minorities.

Costs

Tuition for the academic year 1990-91 was $22,500. Included in this fee are all laboratory, university, registration, yearbook, graduation, and recreational complex charges. Living expenses were not included.

Financial Aid

The School of Medicine provides all interviewed applicants with financial aid information and application forms. Scholarships, grants, and private Georgetown loans are available on a limited basis depending on need. Students are also advised to seek aid from federally funded loan programs, as well as independent organizations. The Office of Financial Aid provides a list of such sources for applicants to use. Medical students are also encouraged to work part-time jobs, which are available through the university.

Minority Programs

The Georgetown Experimental Medical Studies Program is a one-year prematriculation program for qualified minority students.

Student Organizations

A variety of extracurricular activities are available to Georgetown medical students, including the Saint George Society, the American Medical Student Association, the Student National Medical Association, and the American Medical Women's Association. Alpha Omega Alpha, the medical honor society, has a chapter on campus. Students also elect representatives to the School of Medicine Student Council, which sponsors occasional social events and publishes a monthly newspaper.

Curriculum

The first and second years of instruction in the M.D. program consist of departmental courses providing the student with scientific knowledge basic to the practice of medicine, a series of interdepartmental courses on the introduction to the patient and a series of elective courses. The third year contains 48 weeks of instructional time, which the students spend in various clinical clerkships. The fourth year consists of more in-depth clerkships where the student gets experience in the clinical management of patients and more elective courses.

Facilities

The School of Medicine operates in conjunction with the Georgetown University Hospital, a 535-bed teaching facility that offers clinical programs in all specialties and subspecialties. The Lombardi Cancer Research Center, completed in 1982, is also on campus providing medical care for cancer patients while also allowing opportunity for multidisciplinary cancer research and treatment activities. The Research Resources Facility employs animal models to study the causes of human diseases. The collection at the John Vinton Dahlgren Memorial Library includes 42,000 books, 93,000 bound journals, 1,750 current journal subscriptions and over 3,700 audiovisual/computer programs.

Grading Procedures

The grading system consists of honors, high pass, pass, and fail.

Special Programs

Through the Office of International Programs, Georgetown allows fourth-year medical students to fulfill part of the 20-week elective requirement by traveling to Third World countries and gaining practical medical experience. Opportunities are available in the Bahamas, the Dominican Republic, and Southeast Asia. An M.D./Ph.D. program is also offered in combination with several academic departments.

Application Procedures

Applicants must submit an AMCAS application as well as a secondary Georgetown form. A letter of recommendation is required from the premedical advisory committee at the applicant's undergraduate college. If no such committee exists, then two faculty recommendations are required. Also, the MCAT must be taken and scores submitted to Georgetown no later than the fall prior to desired entrance. A $55 application fee is required. The deadline for regular applicants is November 15, while early decision candidates are required to have their applications complete by August 1.

Contact

Office of Admissions
School of Medicine
Georgetown University
Washington, D.C. 20007
(202) 687-1154

HAHNEMANN UNIVERSITY SCHOOL OF MEDICINE

Mail Stop 442 — Broad & Vine
Philadelphia, Pennsylvania 19102-1192
(215) 448-4401

Accreditation	LCME, MSACS
Degrees Offered	M.D./Ph.D./B.A.
# Students Applied	5,051
Enrollment	690
Mean GPA	Not Available
% Men / % Women	60% / 40%
% Minorities	14%
Tuition	$18,070
Application Fee	$50
Application Deadline	October 15

The University

Hahnemann University is a private, not-for-profit institution founded in 1848. Located in attractive center-city Philadelphia, Hahnemann University includes the School of Medicine, the Graduate School, the School of Health Sciences and Humanities, and Hahnemann University Hospital. The campus includes 10 buildings containing modern state-of-the-art facilities for health care service, teaching, and research. Hahnemann is chartered by the Commonwealth of Pennsylvania to award doctorate, master, baccalaureate, and associate degrees.

Hahnemann is located in the center-city area of Philadelphia, providing students with access to museums, theaters, restaurants, and major athletic events. Philadelphia is within a few hours drive to the New Jersey shore and Pennsylvania's Pocono mountain resorts.

Admissions

All applicants must take the Medical College Admission Test (MCAT) within four calendar years of matriculation. Applicants must have completed a minimum of 90 semester hours or the equivalent in a course of study leading to the baccalaureate degree.

Undergraduate Preparation

A major in science is not required. A background in the sciences as well as in the humanities and social sciences is needed. The minimum requirements for admission are eight semester hours in general biology, general or inorganic chemistry, organic chemistry, and general physics. Also, six semester hours in English composition and literature, social sciences, and humanities are required.

Student Body

Characteristics of students in the 1989 entering class were: average science GPA, 3.21; average total GPA, 3.11; mean MCAT scores, 5.5 or better in each subtest. Forty percent were from Pennsylvania, 40 percent were women, 14 percent were minorities.

Placement Records

Postgraduates are accepted into numerous hospitals across the country.

Costs

The estimated expenses for a first-year student are as follows: tuition $18,070, living expenses (estimated) $9,350, activity fee $50, books and instruments $1,350.

Financial Aid

The University offers monthly payment plans through Academic Management Services (AMS) and Tuition Management Systems (TMS). University aid is awarded to students based on financial need. Scholarships are awarded based on need and/or academic performance. Students who wish to be considered for aid must file the PHEAA (Pennsylvania Higher Education Assistance Agency) State Grant and Federal Aid Application no later than May 31 prior to the academic year for which funds are needed. More complete information regarding financial aid programs is available from the student financial aid office.

Minority Programs

The Resource System is a program for minority medical students and provides the following special services: pre-appli-

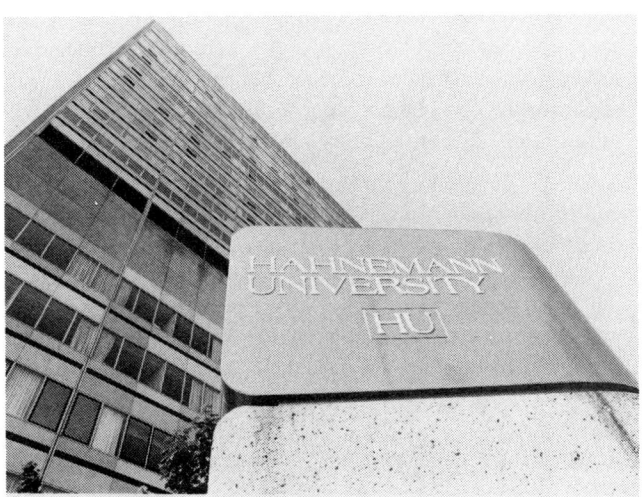

cation and application services including recruiting, counseling, and support for prospective applicants. The Summer Academic Enrichment Program is an eight-week summer program required for all minority students accepted to the School of Medicine. Student Resource Services provides tutoring and counseling, and students may be offered the flexible curriculum for a five-year course of study, which expands the first year of medical school into two years.

Student Organizations

The Medical Student Institute is one of the most active student organizations at Hahnemann. It consists of five executive officers and six members from each medical school class, two yearbook editors, and the medical student representatives on Hahnemann's standing committees.

Faculty

The faculty and staff of the University total more than 6,000. The faculty/student ratio is approximately 3:1.

Curriculum

The first two years of instruction emphasize the basic sciences. In the first year, the disciplines of gross and microscopic anatomy, neuroscience, biochemistry, human behavior, microbiology and immunology and physiology and biophysics are taught. During the second year pathology and laboratory medicine, molecular and human genetics, pharmacology, psychopathology, and clinical medicine are taught. In the third year, the curriculum provides a broad base of clinical experience through intensive clinical clerkship training in each of the major divisions of medical practice. In the fourth year, hands-on responsibility of patient care is provided.

Facilities

The Lucy F. Cooke Room houses Hahnemann's archives and special collections in the history of medicine and homeopathy. The Hahnemann library houses over 85,000 publications and contains individual study carrels and group study rooms. The Audiovisual Learning Laboratory and the Microcomputer Learning Laboratory give access to a collection of slides, videocassettes, microcomputer equipment, and software applications. The Hahnemann on-line catalog (HAL) provides information about the library's books and other holdings.

Grading Procedures

All courses in the School of Medicine are graded on an honors—satisfactory—marginal satisfactory—unsatisfactory basis. Departmental honors and distinction are awarded at graduation.

Special Programs

The School of Medicine and the Graduate School offer a program for students to pursue both the M.D. and Ph.D. degrees. In-depth experience in clinical medicine and basic science are required. Application to the M.D./Ph.D. program is accepted only after successful completion of one year of medical education. A 30-month program leading to the degree of Doctor of Medicine is offered to dental surgeons who have completed a residency in oral and maxillofacial surgery prior to entrance. For entering college students, Hahnemann University is affiliated with an accelerated seven-year B.A./M.D. program at Boston University for Pennsylvania residents only, a seven-year B.A./M.D. program at Gannon University, and a standard eight-year B.A./M.D. program at Rosemont College.

Application Procedures

The MCAT must be taken within four calendar years of matriculation. Applications are accepted by AMCAS between June 15 and October 15. Applications, fees, letter(s) of recommendation, and the Supplemental Information Form must be received by the Hahnemann University Admissions Office no later than January 31. Letters of recommendation should be sent directly to the admissions office. A composite letter of recommendation submitted by the applicant's pre-medical advisor is preferred. If this service is not available, three recommendation letters are required. Two of these letters must be from faculty members in the applicant's biology, chemistry, physics, or mathematics courses. A third letter must be by a faculty member in the department of the student's major.

Contact

Admissions Office
Hahnemann University School of Medicine
Mail Stop 442
Broad & Vine
Philadelphia, Pennsylvania 19102-1192
(215) 448-7600

HARVARD MEDICAL SCHOOL

25 Shattuck Street
Boston, Massachusetts 02115
(617) 432-1501

Accreditation	LCME
Degrees Offered	M.D., Ph.D., M.A.
# Students Applied	Not Available
Enrollment	Not Available
Mean GPA	Not Available
% Men / % Women	Not Available
% Minorities	Not Available
Tuition	$18,030
Application Fee	$60
Application Deadline	October 15

The University

The Harvard Medical School was established in 1782. Since 1906, the school has been located in the Longwood Avenue Quadrangle. The Medical School still occupies its original buildings, although each has undergone extensive interior renovation to accommodate the needs of modern medical teaching and research facilities. In addition, the Medical Education Center was opened adjacent to the Medical School in 1987.

Admissions

Although no minimal specific GPA or MCAT score is required for admission to the Medical School, academic excellence is expected. Applicants must demonstrate that their intellectual and personal credentials are of such quality as to predict success in the study and practice of medicine.

Undergraduate Preparation

Students are encouraged to pursue work in honors courses and independent research wherever possible during their undergraduate years. Applicants are also advised to follow a "balanced and liberal" curriculum, not limiting their studies to topics in the biological or physical sciences. Specific, required undergraduate coursework includes: one year of biology with lab, two years of chemistry (organic and inorganic) with lab, one year of physics, one year of calculus, and one year of expository writing. At least 16 hours of courses in literature, language, the arts, humanities, and the social sciences are also recommended.

Costs

Tuition for the academic year 1990-91 was $18,030. A health insurance fee of $1,105 per year is also required. Microscopes are available for rental at a rate of $270 for the academic year. The average cost of living for a first year medical student at Harvard, including tuition, health service, health insurance, room, board, books, transportation, laundry, and incidentals, is estimated at approximately $31,200 for the 10-month academic year.

Financial Aid

Applicants are admitted to the Medical School without regard to their ability to pay. Once accepted, the student is encouraged to file a financial aid form with the Graduate and Professional School Financial Aid Service. The individual student must take primary responsibility for financing the cost of a medical education at Harvard; however, the Financial Aid Office attempts to help students with financial need find access to resources. Job opportunities for students are posted in the Student Employment Office and the Harvard University Personnel Office helps students' spouses find employment within the university.

Student Organizations

Students admitted to the Medical School are randomly assigned to one of four academic societies. These groups offer students a chance to interact with faculty and administrators in an informal setting. The societies also give students personal counseling, general support, and help in planning the overall academic program at Harvard.

Curriculum

The first year consists of required basic science courses. The second year continues this core curriculum as well as including time for electives. In the third and fourth years, students devote most of their time to the core clinical clerkships as well as advanced research or independent study, and a wide variety of electives.

Recent changes in the Medical School curriculum have resulted in the implementation of new approaches to learning. Presently, interdisciplinary courses, small group tutorials, and independent study are the primary methods of instruction.

Special Programs

The Harvard Medical School offers a Health Sciences and Technology (HST) program in conjunction with the nearby Massachusetts Institute of Technology. This special curricular program is designed for students with a strong interest and background in areas of quantitative science, including biology, chemistry, physics, engineering, and mathematics. The program enrolls 30 students each year. Participants are simultaneously enrolled at the Harvard Medical School and at MIT and are taught in courses outside of the main medical school teaching structure. A thesis is required for the M.D. degree in the HST program. Harvard also offers medical students a variety of opportunities to pursue either a Master's or a Ph.D. degree while concurrently enrolled in the M.D. program.

Application Procedures

Applications to the Medical School must be postmarked no later than October 15 and be accompanied by a $60 application fee. Supporting materials, including premedical advisory committee recommendations, individual letters of recommendation, transcripts, and MCAT scores, must be received by the admissions office before November 15. The MCAT should be taken in the spring or no later than the fall prior to desired entrance into medical school. MCATs more than five years old must be retaken. In January, highly qualified applicants will be selected for on-campus or regional personal interviews, and final admissions decisions will be made at that time. All applicants will be notified of their admissions status during the last week of February.

Contact

Harvard Medical School
Office of Admissions
25 Shattuck Street
Boston, Massachusetts 02115
(617) 432-1550

UNIVERSITY OF HAWAII JOHN A. BURNS SCHOOL OF MEDICINE

1960 East-West Road
Honolulu, Hawaii 96822
(808) 956-8287

Accreditation	LCME
Degrees Offered	M.D., Ph.D.
# Students Applied	693
Enrollment	56 / class
Mean GPA	3.3
% Men / % Women	Not Available
% Minorities	Not Available
Tuition	$4,830 In-State
	$14,490 Out-of-State
Application Fee	None
Application Deadline	December 1

The University

The University of Hawaii at Manoa is located in Honolulu and has a total student body of approximately 21,000. The John A. Burns School of Medicine was founded in 1965 as a two-year medical education program and expanded in 1973, graduating its first class of 62 physicians two years later.

Admissions

Candidates for admission to the School of Medicine are selected on the basis of their undergraduate academic work, MCAT scores, as well as an applicant's potential to contribute to the health profession in the Pacific and succeed as a humanistic physician. Preference is given to residents of Hawaii and applicants with ties to the American Pacific Basin.

Undergraduate Preparation

While only 90 semester hours, and not a bachelor's degree, are required for admission to the School of Medicine, most successful applicants will have completed their undergraduate work before they enroll. Specific required courses include eight hours of biology, eight hours of physics, four hours of general chemistry, and eight hours of organic chemistry, all with lab. A science major is not required, and the School of Medicine recommends that students expand their studies to include work in the humanities. Applicants must also take the MCAT with the preferred date being either April or September of the year prior to desired medical school admission.

Student Body

Because of its location students at the University of Hawaii come from diverse, multicultural backgrounds, including Caucasian, Chinese, Korean, Japanese, Hawaiian, Filipino, Samoan, Micronesian, and Charmorran.

Placement Records

Of the 978 students who have graduated from the M.D. program since 1975, approximately 260 are currently in various residency training programs and 767 have completed their residencies. Four percent of these students are in various branches of the armed services and one percent hold full-time academic positions.

Costs

For Hawaii residents, tuition is $4,830 annually, while out-of-state students are charged $14,490 per year. Other fees include a $25 Campus Center fee and a $13 Board of Publications charge. Living expenses vary depending on a student's accommodations. Many students are local residents and commute to and from the medical school. Out-of-state students can find apartments close to campus but at a somewhat higher cost than elsewhere due to Hawaii's high cost of living.

Financial Aid

Financial aid is available on the basis of need and comes mostly in the form of federally administered student loans. The Office of Financial Aid has limited scholarship and loan funds available. Applicants are encouraged to seek assistance from outside organizations; such aid is available particularly to students of Hawaiian, Samoan, and Filipino backgrounds. Also, the governments of American Samoa, Guam, the Federated States of Micronesia, the Commonwealth of the Northern Marianas, the Republic of Belau, and the Republic of the Marshall Islands offer scholarships at the University of Hawaii for their residents.

Curriculum

The curriculum at the School of Medicine is problem-based and aims to familarize students with clinical concepts and responsibilities immediately upon entrance to medical school. In the first two years of the M.D. program, students learn the basic medical sciences in a sequence of small-group tutorials and are introduced to the practice of clinical medicine through electives. Part I of the National Board Examination is required at the end of the second year. In the third year, students participate in a series of clinical clerkships in the areas of surgery, obstetrics and gynecology, pediatrics, psychiatry, and internal medicine. The fourth year is then devoted to further clerkships and electives, as well as an eight-week preceptorship in which students spend time with primary care physicians from various areas of Hawaii, Samoa, and Micronesia. The goal of this approach is to encourage students to enter primary care fields and spend at least part of their medical careers in the underserved areas of Hawaii and the Pacific.

Facilities

The School of Medicine is affiliated with 13 hospitals and health care facilities in the Hawaiian Islands that offer students a broad variety of research and clinical opportunity. The university has two libraries devoted to the collection of medical material. The Hamilton Library, with 70,000 books and bound journals and 2,500 journal subscriptions, consists of texts on both the basic medical sciences and clinical topics, while the Hawaii Medical Library offers another 73,000 books and bound journals and 1,400 journal subscriptions, which focus primarily on clinical subjects.

Grading Procedures

In the first two years of the M.D. program, while students are primarily studying the basic medical sciences, grades are on a satisfactory/unsatisfactory basis. In the third and fourth years, when the emphasis shifts to the study of clinical problems, grades are on a credit/no credit/honors basis and are supplemented with written evaluations of a student's clinical skills.

Special Programs

It is possible for a student at the School of Medicine to work toward the M.D. degree while simultaneously studying for a Ph.D. Interested applicants must apply both to the medical school and the university's Graduate Division, and admissions decisions are made on an individual, case-by-case basis. The university also offers a program that grants early admission notification to undergraduate students at the Manoa campus. Once accepted into this program students complete their undergraduate work, choosing their own curriculum in a Liberal Studies major.

Application Procedures

Candidates for admission to the School of Medicine must file an application with the AMCAS, a copy of which will be forwarded to the University of Hawaii. Students are also required to submit letters of recommendation and MCAT scores. Applicants who reach a secondary screening level will be invited to on-campus interviews. The application deadline is December 1 for regular decision candidates and August 1 for early decision.

Contact

Assistant Dean for Admissions
University of Hawaii
John A. Burns School of Medicine
1960 East-West Road, Biomed T-101
Honolulu, Hawaii 96822
(808) 956-8300

UNIVERSITY OF HEALTH SCIENCES/ CHICAGO MEDICAL SCHOOL

3333 Green Bay Road
North Chicago, Illinois 60064
(708) 578-3000

Accreditation	LCME
Degrees Offered	M.D., M.S., Ph.D.
# Students Applied	4,807
Enrollment	149 / class
Mean GPA	3.2
% Men / % Women	70% / 30%
% Minorities	Not Available
Tuition	$24,300
Application Fee	$55
Application Deadline	December 15

The University

The University of Health Sciences is a private institution of higher education chartered by the state of Illinois and founded in 1912. The School of Medicine is the main component of the university and also embodies the School of Graduate and Postdoctoral Studies, which grants advanced degrees in the basic sciences and clinical psychology, and the School of Health Related Professions, which grants baccalaureate and master's degrees in physical therapy and medical technology.

Admissions

Students are selected on the basis of various criteria, including scholarship, character, motivation, and educational background. Potential for the study and practice of medicine is evaluated on the basis of academic achievement, MCAT scores, personal evaluations by preprofessional advisory committee or individual instructors, and a personal interview, if requested by the student admissions committee.

Undergraduate Preparation

A minimum of three years of undergraduate study must be completed in order for an applicant to be considered for admission into the Chicago Medical School and most applicants have completed their B.A. degree upon enrollment. No specific undergraduate major is necessary although one year each, with lab, of biology/zoology, inorganic chemistry (including quantitative and qualitative analysis), organic chemistry, and physics are required. Applicants are encouraged to take courses in mathematics, such as calculus and statistics, as well as courses in social sciences, English, and fine arts.

Student Body

Thirty percent of the students at the Medical School are women, while seventy percent are men. The majority of students are from out of state and range in age from 19 to 36 at the time of enrollment, with the average entering age being 23.

Costs

For the 1989-90 academic year, tuition was $24,300 and living expenses were estimated at $8,800. Books and supplies, including microscope rental, totaled another $2,650.

Financial Aid

The university has some limited funds available to supplement student resources and governmentally administered financial aid programs. Awards are based on an analysis of a student's financial need as determined by the GAPSFAS. Approximately 75 percent of students receive some form of financial aid, whether it be university administered or from an outside source. The average award of university administered funds is $2,000 for full need medical students.

Curriculum

The four-year curriculum at the Chicago Medical School consists of 13 terms. Six terms are devoted to basic science, the first three primarily to the study of the structure and function of the human body and the second three to the study of disease, processes, therapy, and prevention. During this time, students also study principles of basic life support in emergency situations, become certified in cardiopulmonary resuscitation and are trained in physical diagnosis, medical interviewing, and history-writing. The final seven terms are divided between 48 weeks of junior clinical rotations and 36 weeks of senior clinical electives, electives, or basic science courses. Required junior clerkships include medicine, surgery, obstetrics and gynecology, psychiatry, and pediatrics. Parts I and II of the National Board Exam are required for graduation.

Facilities

Affiliated facilities offering clinical training at various levels to students at the Medical School include Cook County Hospital, Mt. Sinai Hospital, North Chicago Veterans Administration Hospital, Jackson Park Hospital, and Great Lakes Naval Medical Center.

Application Procedures

In addition to the centralized AMCAS application form, all applicants are required to submit supplemental materials to the Medical School, including three letters of recommendation from professors or one single evaluation from the premedical advisory committee. At this point, all applications are screened and selected candidates (approximately 10 percent of all applicants) will be invited for personal interviews and then notified of final admissions decisions.

Contact

University of Health Sciences
Chicago Medical School
Office of Admissions
3333 Green Bay Road
North Chicago, Illinois 60064
(708) 578-3206/3207

HOWARD UNIVERSITY COLLEGE OF MEDICINE

520 W. Street, N.W.
Washington, D.C. 20059
(202) 806-6100

Accreditation	AAMC, AMA, MSASSC
Degrees Offered	M.D., B.S./M.D., M.S., Ph.D.
# Students Applied	3,034
Enrollment	100 / class
Mean GPA	Not Available
% Men / % Women	50% / 50%
% Minorities	80%
Tuition	$9,450
Application Fee	$25
Application Deadline	December 15

The University

A traditionally black university, founded in 1868 and located in Washington, D.C., Howard University enrolls over 12,000 students from all over the world. With over 4,000 living alumni, the College of Medicine has educated a substantial percentage of the nation's minority physicians. With the university providing the educational opportunities, students can supplement their medical education by using the resources offered by the nearby Walter Reed Army Medical Center and the National Institutes of Health. Cosmopolitan Washington also offers many diversions to occupy students' free time.

Admissions

Admission to Howard is not based on academic achievement alone. The College of Medicine also evaluates the individual applicant's intellectual, personal, and social traits. Successful candidates are selected on the basis of these qualities as well as their potential to practice in communities needing physician services.

Undergraduate Preparation

All applicants to the College of Medicine must have completed a minimum of 62 semester hours of undergraduate work including eight hours each of biology, general chemistry, organic chemistry, and physics, as well as six hours each of mathematics and English. Although not required for admission, Howard also recommends coursework in biochemistry, cell biology, and embryology. The MCAT is also required.

Student Body

Traditionally, the students of Howard University College of Medicine have been predominantly black. Black students compose 70-80 percent of the student population each year. More than 20 states, as well as several African and Caribbean nations are represented. Approximately 20 percent of the students in most entering classes have attended Howard as undergraduates. Fifty percent of the student body are men, while 50 percent are women.

Costs

Tuition for the academic year 1990-91 was $9,450 while other fees totalled $848. Housing costs are not included in the tuition and vary depending on the accommodation selected by the student.

Financial Aid

Approximately 85 percent of the students in the College of Medicine receive some form of financial assistance. Financial aid at Howard is based on a combination of need and academic merit and includes scholarships, loans, and summer research fellowships. Applicants for financial aid are required to submit the financial aid form to the College Scholarship Service.

Faculty

Traditionally, Howard University has had the largest gathering of black scholars of any institution in the United States.

Curriculum

The first year consists of required courses, including gross and developmental anatomy, histology, biochemistry, microbiology, physiology, and psychiatry. The second year consists of further required courses in basic medical subjects and electives. The third and fourth years require students to participate in a variety of clerkships and examinations in clinical subjects. Twenty weeks of the fourth year are reserved as elective time to provide students the opportunity for additional clinical and research opportunities. Parts I and II of the National Board Examination are required.

Facilities

The Howard University Hospital, completed in 1975, is a 500-bed teaching hospital utilizing the latest technical advances to provide patient care. Facilities include computerized tomography, magnetic resonance imaging, and a completely integrated intraoperative radiation therapy suite, the first such facility in the world.

Grading Procedures

Grades are recorded on the transcript as H (honors), S (satisfactory), or U (unsatisfactory).

Special Programs

An extended medical curriculum is available and allows the student to use three years to complete what is normally the first two years of the M.D. program. An M.D./Ph.D. program is also offered.

Application Procedures

Howard College of Medicine participates in the American Medical College Application Service. The deadline for filing this application is December 15 of the year preceding desired entrance to medical school. Applicants must also submit two letters of recommendation from a health professions committee at the undergraduate college or from two science instructors. A personal interview may also be required. The application fee is $25.

Contact

Admissions Office
College of Medicine
Howard University
520 W. Street, N.W.
Washington, D.C. 20059
(202) 636-6270

UNIVERSITY OF ILLINOIS COLLEGE OF MEDICINE

Box 12149
Chicago, Illinois 60612
(312) 996-3500

Accreditation	LCME
Degrees Offered	M.D., Ph.D., M.D./Ph.D.
# Students Applied	3,136
Enrollment	300 / class
Mean GPA	3.0
% Men / % Women	Not Available
% Minorities	Not Available
Tuition	$7,136 In-State
	$20,696 Out-of-State
Application Fee	$20
Application Deadline	December 1

The University

The University of Illinois was chartered in 1867 as a land grant institution. Currently, the College of Medicine educates over 1,300 medical students a year at four campuses across the state in Chicago, Urbana-Champaign, Peoria, and Rockford.

The University of Illinois College of Medicine at Chicago is located in the heart of the West Side Medical Center District, approximately two miles west of downtown Chicago. The college is convenient to public transportation. The cultural resources of the city are easily accessible.

Admissions

As part of a state university the College of Medicine gives admissions preference to Illinois state residents, although nonresidents usually account for approximately 10 percent of each entering class. The college selects applicants who demonstrate qualities of academic achievement, good communications skills, emotional stability, maturity, integrity, diversity of interests, leadership, and motivation. The committee considers academic accomplishments, including achievement in advanced projects, as well as work and extracurricular experience.

Undergraduate Preparation

Specific requirements for admission include coursework in biology, chemistry, physics, and behavioral sciences, as well as college mathematics including calculus. Any undergraduate major is acceptable, but a B.A. degree is required. An applicant's undergraduate GPA as well as MCAT scores are considered.

Student Body

The majority of students (approximately 90 percent) are Illinois state residents. Percentages of men, women, and minority students vary from campus to campus.

Costs

The College of Medicine in Urbana-Champaign follows the semester system. On this campus, in-state tuition and fees are $3,005 per semester and $8,090 for out-of-state students. The College of Medicine campuses in Chicago, Peoria, and Rockford all follow the quarter system. At these campuses tuition and fees total $2,045 per quarter for Illinois residents and $5,435 per quarter for non-residents. Living expenses vary from campus to campus depending on the type of housing a student selects.

Financial Aid

The University Office of Financial Aid administers all state and federal aid programs and offers limited grant and scholarship support to students on the basis of need. Applicants requesting financial aid must complete the Family Financial Statement (FFS) supplied by the American College Testing program. The financial aid office also operates a short-term emergency loan service from which students can borrow up to $200 to meet unexpected expenses.

Minority Programs

The College of Medicine administers an Urban Health Program that is dedicated to the recruitment, retention, and graduation of minority medical students. Currently 280 students from all of the four campus sites participate. As part of the program, students are offered a Summer Prematriculation Program, academic support, and career counseling services throughout their four years of education. The college is one of the leading educators of minority physicians among public institutions in the country.

Student Organizations

Student activities and organizations at the College of Medicine vary from campus to campus. However, each campus offers several professional and preprofessional societies as well as chapters of Alpha Omega Alpha, the national medical honor society. The Chicago campus has a centralized recreation center as well as a full-time day care center.

Faculty

There are over 4,000 teaching faculty at the four campuses of the College of Medicine.

Curriculum

All students must spend the first year at either Chicago or Urban-Champaign studying basic medical subjects and completing a generalized medical curriculum. Chicago-based students continue at the campus for the entire four years while students at Urbana-Champaign may elect to remain or continue their training in either Peoria or Rockford. Clinical emphases and specialties vary from campus to campus.

Facilities

The Library of the Health Sciences at Chicago is the primary medical reference facility for the University of Illinois and also serves several Chicago-based health care centers. The library's holdings include over 6,700 current periodicals, more than 525,000 bound periodical volumes, books, government documents and 161,000 audiovisual items. Each campus division of the College of Medicine is affiliated with many different hospitals and community health care facilities in their geographical region of the state of Illinois.

Grading Procedures

The specifics of grading vary from campus to campus. Generally, however, some combination of objective examinations and written evaluations are used. National Board Examinations are required.

Special Programs

The College of Medicine offers an M.D./Ph.D. program as well as Medical Scientist Training Program fellowships, which allow students to work towards the two degrees simultaneously over a course of six to seven years. Participating departments include Anatomy, Biological Chemistry, Genetics, Microbiology and Immunology, Pathology, Pharmacology, and Physiology.

The College of Medicine cooperates with a joint committee of the Illinois State Medical Society and the Illinois Agricultural Association in a program designed to increase the number of practitioners in rural areas of Illinois. The Medical Student Loan Fund Program's board annually recommends a number of rural candidates for admission.

Application Procedures

Applications must be submitted to AMCAS no later than December 1 of the year prior to desired enrollment. The University may then request the applicant to submit a Supplemental Application form, for which a $20 fee is required. MCAT scores are required and the test must be taken by the fall of the year prior to entrance. Also, a minimum of three letters of recommendation from an applicant's professors, or a single letter from a preprofessional committee, is required. Certain candidates will be invited for personal interviews.

Contact

(for admission to all campuses)
Office of Medical College Admissions (M/C 783)
The University of Illinois at Chicago
Box 12149
Chicago, Illinois 60612
(312) 996-5635

INDIANA UNIVERSITY SCHOOL OF MEDICINE

1120 South Drive
Indianapolis, Indiana 46202-5113
(317) 274-8157

Accreditation	LCME
Degrees Offered	M.D., M.D./Ph.D., M.D./M.S.
# Students Applied	1,657
Enrollment	265 / class
Mean GPA	3.56
% Men / % Women	62% / 38%
% Minorities	20%
Tuition	$6,000 In-State
	$13,560 Out-of-State
Application Fee	$20
Application Deadline	December 15

The University

The Indiana University School of Medicine, located on the Bloomington campus, awarded the Doctor of Medicine (M.D.) degree to its first class of 25 in 1907. In 1908, all medical schools in the state were united with Indiana University. In that same year, upon mandate of the General Assembly of Indiana, Indiana University assumed responsibility for medical education in the state of Indiana. A School of Medicine faculty committee in 1965 recommended a comprehensive plan for medical education throughout the state, and in 1971, the assembly authorized legislation that led to the completion of the Indiana Statewide Medical Education (ISME) system. Henceforth, the Indiana University School of Medicine has been responsible for the selection, admission, and assignment of students; for curricular development; and for evaluation and accreditation of the ISME system.

Admissions

Preference is given to residents, although a significant number of well-qualified nonresidents are accepted each year. The applications of nonresidents who have significant ties to the state of Indiana may be given greater consideration. Applicants who are Indiana residents should have a GPA above 3.0. Nonresidents should have outstanding MCAT scores and a GPA equal to that of the previous year's entering class. Applicants are evaluated on the basis of scholarship, character, personality, references, MCAT scores, and the personal interview. The admissions committee gives greater weight to the quality of work than to the amount of credit hours of work completed. A student who has withdrawn from or been dismissed from another medical school is usually not eligible for admission to the first-year class.

Undergraduate Preparation

Applicants must have completed a minimum of 90 credit hours (excluding physical education and ROTC courses). It is strongly recommended that the applicant complete a bachelor's degree in a college or university accredited by one of the regional accrediting agencies. Any major is acceptable. Students with educational backgrounds in areas outside the usual liberal arts and sciences curriculum (education, business, engineering, pharmacy, etc.) will be evaluated based on a minimum of 90 credit hours of college-level arts and sciences. Applicants must complete at least eight to ten credit hours (or one academic year) of the following science courses (including lecture and laboratory): general chemistry, organic chemistry, physics, and the biological sciences. Applicants are also expected to have a significant number of courses in the humanities and social sciences, and be competent in speaking and writing the English language.

Costs

Tuition fees for resident students amount to $6,000 per year. Tuition for nonresident students amounts to $13,560 per year. The health service fee is included in these rates.

Financial Aid

Financial assistance application materials will be sent to all prospective medical students who have been accepted for the fall first-year class. The financial aid form (FAF) is used to determine the student's eligibility for financial assistance. Students are encouraged to investigate other sources of aid that may be available through bank trusts, church endowments, fraternal, and professional organizations. Emergency student loan funds are available.

Student Organizations

There is a branch of the Alpha Omega Alpha honor society on campus.

Faculty

The faculty consists of both volunteer physicians in private practice and geographic full-time clinicians and investigators.

Curriculum

At this time, students may take their first two years of medical school courses on one of the nine Centers of Medical Education. The last two years of clinical instruction take place at the School of Medicine at Indianapolis. The curriculum allows some integration across disciplines in the basic medical sciences, promotes interdisciplinary teaching in the second year, and introduces a twelve-month "core" clinical third year and a fourth year reserved exclusively for electives. As a functioning part of the medical team, the student is introduced to patient care through an intensive and multidepartmental introduction to medicine course.

During the clinical years, students make use of the full calendar year and are integrated into the medical care program of the hospitals. The clinical clerk is a full member of a medical team, serving with increasing responsibility in all aspects of a patient's problem. Night and weekend calls are served on essentially the same schedule as that of the house staff. Extensive and varied elective programs are available for fourth-year students. Student research is supported through a fellowship program.

Facilities

The Medical Center campus is located approximately one mile from the center of Indianapolis. The basic sciences are taught in the medical science building, which also houses the medical library. Additional instructional facilities are located at the Centers for Medical Education, at the University of Notre Dame, Purdue University, Ball State University, Indiana State University, the University of Evansville, and Indiana University Northwest. The medical sciences program is housed in Myers Hall on the Bloomington campus.

Clinical instruction takes place in Indianapolis. Indiana University hospitals have 692 beds. The Wishard Memorial Hospital, a 618-bed institution, offers clinical teaching facilities to the three upper classes. Clinical clerkships are offered at various hospitals and community hospitals throughout the state. The total number of beds on the Medical Center campus exceeds 2,000.

The Indiana University School of Medicine Library serves the schools of medicine and nursing. It contains approximately 160,000 volumes and subscribes to 1,800 journals. Books and journal articles not available in the library may be requested through interlibrary loan. Computerized literature services are available.

Grading Procedures

In order to graduate, students must have achieved a passing score on the National Board of Medical Examiners Comprehensive Examination, Parts I and II.

Special Programs

The School of Medicine and the Graduate School offer selected students an opportunity to pursue the M.S. or Ph.D. degrees, concurrently or sequentially, with the M.D. Applicants must be approved by both the School of Medicine and the Graduate School.

Application Procedures

The School of Medicine participates in the American Medical College Application Service (AMCAS). The application form is available between May 1 and December 1 of each year. The completed application form must be received by AMCAS by December 15 of the year preceding planned enrollment. The school participates in the early decision plan (EDP). EDP applications must be received by August 1. The MCAT is required and should be taken in the spring of the year preceding the submission of their application. Ordinarily, acceptance will not be granted in the absence of the student's score on this test. Students must ensure that their schools send an official transcript of record to the AMCAS at the time of application. An application fee of $20 is required. Interviews with selected applicants will be arranged by the admissions committee.

Transfer applicants who are Indiana residents enrolled in another U.S. or foreign medical school, or nonresidents who are enrolled in the U.S., will be considered for admission to the second- and third-year classes only. Nonresidents enrolled in foreign medical schools and students in other professional or graduate schools will not be considered for transfer.

Contact

Admissions Office
Fesler Hall 213
1120 South Drive
Indianapolis, Indiana 46202-5113
(317) 274-3772

UNIVERSITY OF IOWA COLLEGE OF MEDICINE

Iowa City, Iowa 52242
(319) 335-3500

Accreditation	LCME
Degrees Offered	M.D., M.D./Ph.D.
# Students Applied	1,089
Enrollment	700
Mean GPA	3.5
% Men / % Women	Not Available
% Minorities	Not Available
Tuition	$5,924 In-State
	$15,350 Out-of-State
Application Fee	$20
Application Deadline	December 1

The University

Formed in 1850, the College of Medicine has grown into an important center for medical research and patient care. The College of Medicine is part of the University of Iowa, a 900-acre campus located in Iowa City, whose population is 54,000, including Iowa University students. Two new campus buildings are designed specifically for studies in human biology and research into the design and construction of lasers.

Admissions

Applicants must have earned a minimum grade of 2.5 and have taken the Medical College Admission Test to be considered for admission. Average MCAT scores of classes admitted in recent years have been near 9.5 (on a 15-point scale) for the sciences and 9.0 for Reading and Quantitative Skills Analysis. Applicants must have completed a baccalaureate degree, or three years of a curriculum qualifying them to receive a baccalaureate degree after completing the first year in medicine. Strong preference is given to residents, although nonresidents are considered.

Undergraduate Preparation

Prospective students must have earned at least 94 semester hours of credit, or the equivalent, including: a complete introductory course in physics, a complete introductory course in organic chemistry, ordinarily following a complete introductory course in general chemical principles, advanced college mathematics or college algebra and trigonometry, a complete intro-

ductory course in the principles of animal biology, or zoology and botany (not botany alone), and an advanced biology course. A major in one of the natural sciences is not required.

Student Body

The university places special importance to attracting minorities and women to the student body. Seventy percent of University students come from Iowa, 24.5 percent come from out of state, and the rest from foreign nations.

Placement Records

Nearly two-thirds of the seniors match with their first choice of residency sites, and 85 percent receive assignments from among their first three choices. Placement is done with help from the National Resident Matching Program.

Costs

Tuition and fees are $5,924 for residents and $15,350 for nonresidents. Housing costs vary between $160-$580 per month. Books and equipment are $1,000 for the first year, $1,453 for the second year, and roughly $600 for each of the third and fourth years.

Financial Aid

Financial assistance is provided on the basis of demonstrated need. Most aid is in the form of loans. Federally funded loans include the Health Professions Student Loan and the Stafford Student Loan Program (formerly the Guaranteed Student Loan Program). Eligibility for financial aid is based on information given on the College Scholarship Service's Financial Aid Form (FAF). This should be completed as soon as possible after January 1. A limited number of grants are awarded each year, ranging in value from $500 to $9,500. These grants are awarded in cases of exceptional need.

Minority Programs

The Educational Opportunities Program offers financial and academic assistance to disadvantaged students from minority groups underrepresented in American medicine.

Student Organizations

Student organizations include the Medical Student Council, the American Medical Student Association, Los Curanderos, Women in Medicine, Physicians for Social Responsibility, Alpha Omega Alpha, and the Iowa Family Practice Club.

Faculty

There are approximately 500 faculty members teaching 3,200 students, including 700 medical students. Most faculty members work full time, combining their practice and research with their work in teaching.

Curriculum

The first three semesters present a core of science study

basic to the study of medicine. The fourth semester is an intensive introduction to clinical medicine. The third year includes required clinical clerkships, where students work with physicians as they care for their patients. The fourth year is spent in selective study of areas ranging from advanced courses in specialty areas to community-based clerkships in primary care.

Facilities

The Health Center is an integral part of the University. At the University Hospital and Clinics medical students receive clinical training in the nation's largest (more than 900 beds) university-owned teaching hospital. The university also has facilities such as The Human Biology Research Facility, where interdisciplinary research is conducted. Facilities there include electron microscopy, mass spectrometry, computer-assisted image analysis, and DNA and radiobiology technology. Other facilities include the College of Pharmacy, which contains an FDA-approved pharmacy manufacturing facility. The Hardin Library holds approximately 213,000 volumes, 2,700 periodicals and has computer access to the National Library of Medicines collections and other data bases. At the Veterans Administration Medical Center medical students and physicians in residencies receive clinical training in this 327-bed hospital.

Grading Procedures

Promotion from one grade to the next is determined by the promotions committee, which consists of five faculty members and the associate dean. Scholastic performance is reported by using the honors/pass/fail system.

Special Programs

The Medical Scientist Training Program provides integrated graduate education and original research for the Ph.D. program combined with the clinical studies necessary for the M.D. degree. It is usually accomplished within six to seven years. Equal consideration is given to all applicants, regardless of state of residence.

There are also interdisciplinary programs available through the Center for Health Services Research, the Mental Health Clinical Research Center, the Cardiovascular Research Center, the Diabetes and Endocrinology Research Center, the Cancer Center, and the Alzheimer's Disease Research Center.

Application Procedures

Preliminary applications are processed by the American Medical College Application Service beginning June 15. The closing date for applications is December 1. Applications that are not completed by February 1 will not be reviewed. There is an application fee of $20. The MCAT must be taken no later than the fall preceding the year in which the applicant wishes to enroll. Personal interviews are occasionally requested by the admissions committee. Applicants who feel that an interview is necessary may request that an interview be arranged

by contacting the coordinator of admissions (requests should be made before January 1). Early decision is available.

Contact

Coordinator of Admissions
College of Medicine
HRBF
The University of Iowa
Iowa City, Iowa 52242
(319) 335-8052

JEFFERSON MEDICAL COLLEGE OF THOMAS JEFFERSON UNIVERSITY

1025 Walnut Street
Philadelphia, Pennsylvania 19107
(215) 928-6000

Accreditation	MSACS, AMA, CAHEA, ADACDA
Degrees Offered	M.D., M.D./Ph.D., B.S./M.D., M.S./M.D.
# Students Applied	4,675
Enrollment	223 / class
Mean GPA	3.4
% Men / % Women	70% / 30%
% Minorities	10%
Tuition	$18,200
Application Fee	$60
Application Deadline	November 15

The University

Dr. George McClellan and his colleagues founded Jefferson Medical College in 1824, two years before Thomas Jefferson's death. Jefferson soon became the largest private medical school in the country. The number of graduates now totals 25,056, of whom more than 8,500 are living. The Postgraduate College of Graduate Studies has granted 524 degrees. On July 1, 1969 Thomas Jefferson University was established. The Medical College is situated on a 13-acre urban campus. Located in historic Philadelphia, the college sits in the midst of history, architecture, and urban life. Independence Hall, the Liberty Bell, Penn's Landing, The Philadelphia Museum of Art, and a host of parks, restaurants, and shopping areas in the city make Jefferson an attractive locale serving many cultural and social needs. Thomas Jefferson University is fully accredited by the MSACS, CAHEA, AMA, ADACDA, the Pennsylvania State Board of Nurse Examiners, and the Commission on Accreditation in Education of the American Physical Therapy Association. Continuing medical education at Jefferson Medical College is accredited by the ACCME.

Admissions

All applicants must take the MCAT no more than four years before the year of their application. The admissions committee reviews the undergraduate college attended, the applicant's academic record, and letters of recommendation, and assesses the applicant's personal qualities, motivation, compassion, integrity, and commitment in nonacademic areas.

Undergraduate Preparation

Preference is given to candidates who have a bachelor's degree from an accredited university or college in the United States or Canada. However, some exceptional candidates are admitted with 90 semester hours completed. Minimum course requirements include one year each (with lab) of general biology, organic and inorganic chemistry, and general physics. Jefferson expects broad study in the natural and social sciences and in the humanities.

Student Body

Each year more than 1,200 students apply. The estimated number of students admitted to each new class is 223. The total enrollment for 1989-90 was 876. Of these, 452 were from Pennsylvania, 117 from New Jersey, 58 from Delaware, 48 from New York, and the rest from around the country and other nations.

Costs

A comprehensive fee of $18,200 per year for students entering in September 1990 (which doesn't change throughout the four years) covers tuition, student health services, Commons fee, 20 residency recommendations, and graduation expenses. A health insurance fee of $711 is required, unless the student is covered by other health insurance. A microscope, which typically costs about $700, is required for the first year. Books and supplies are estimated at $335; room and board, $7,800; transportation, $525; medical/dental, $400; and miscellaneous, $725.

Financial Aid

Where need is established (through GAPSFAS), students may apply for financial aid. About 62 scholarships are available along with some two-dozen loan funds. Nine loan programs assist the extremely economically disadvantaged and the handicapped. Some federal scholarships are available, including educational fellowships from the Office of Indian Education

Program. About a dozen outside sources of aid are available from local agencies.

Minority Programs

No specific minority programs exist; however, Jefferson Medical College encourages members of all minority groups to apply for entry to the Medical College. Some on-campus student organizations help provide support for minority concerns.

Student Organizations

Jefferson houses chapters of the Alpha Omega Alpha honor medical society, Kappa Beta Phi, and the Hobart Amory Hare Honor Medical Society. Among the regular social organizations and over 30 medical specialty groups are included the Ethical Society of Jefferson Medical College, American Medical Women's Association, the Jewish Medical Society, the Christian Medical Society, Family Physicians Society, Arsmedica, Physicians for Social Responsibility, and the Jefferson Medicolegal Society.

Faculty

The full-time university and hospital-based faculty at Jefferson totals 544; in addition, there are 38 part-time and nearly 5,000 volunteer faculty.

Curriculum

The curriculum for the M.D. covers four years. The first two years encompass a departmental and systems approach covering the basic sciences. The clinical program consists of two phases. Phase I covers 42 weeks of required clerkships. Phase II covers 42 weeks of required clerkships and electives.

Facilities

The Samuel Parson Scott Library-Administration Building on the urban campus contains 155,000 volumes and over 2,200 periodicals. Jefferson Alumni Hall houses all the preclinical departments and the Commons facility with a cafeteria, social, music, and reading lounges, swimming pool, and gymnasium. The Stein Research Center on campus is dedicated to specific activities in radiology, embryology, and cancer research. Over 20 local hospitals, clinics, and medical centers work in close affiliation with the Medical College for training and research.

Grading Procedures

Courses in the basic medical sciences are given numerical grades. Courses in the clinical curriculum for all Phase I and II required courses and all electives are graded as follows: high honors: 4; above expected competence: 3; expected competence: 2; marginal competence: 1; incomplete: I; failure: F. To complete the record, a numerical examination grade is assigned for clinical and elective courses, and a faculty member writes an evaluation of the student's performance in each course.

Special Programs

Jefferson offers the M.S. and Ph.D. at its College of Graduate Studies. Two combined M.D./Ph.D. programs are available to students enrolled in the Jefferson Medical College who wish to pursue a career in research. The College of Allied Health Sciences offers M.S., B.S., and certificate programs in dental hygiene, diagnostic imaging, laboratory science, nursing, and occupational therapy, physical therapy, and general studies.

Application Procedures

Students should apply through AMCAS between June 15 and November 15. Following this, applicants send all supplementary materials, including the applicant data card, the application fee ($60), MCAT scores, and the required letters of recommendation directly to the office of admissions. Jefferson prefers a recommendation from a preprofessional committee. Otherwise, letters (one each) from faculty members in biology, chemistry, physics, and the humanities should be sent. Deadline for letters is January 15. The earliest notification date is October 15. Applicants must respond within two weeks of notification and pay a $100 deposit fee to hold their places in class.

Contact

Associate Dean for Admissions
Jefferson Medical College
1025 Walnut Street
Philadelphia, Pennsylvania 19107
(215) 955-6983

JOHNS HOPKINS UNIVERSITY SCHOOL OF MEDICINE

720 Rutland Avenue
Baltimore, Maryland 21205
(301) 955-3182

Accreditation	AMCA
Degrees Offered	M.D., M.D./Ph.D., M.D./ M.P.H., Ph.D., M.A.
# Students Applied	3,200
Enrollment	120 / class
Mean GPA	Not Available
% Men / % Women	60% / 40%
% Minorities	Not Available
Tuition	$17,500
Application Fee	$60
Application Deadline	November 15

The University

The Quaker merchant and philanthropist Johns Hopkins bequeathed $7,000,000 to establish a university, hospital, and teaching center. The university was founded in 1876, and the School of Medicine, which opened in 1893, signaled the completion of Hopkins' dream. The main campus for the School of Medicine is in eastern Baltimore, about 20 minutes from the Homewood campus of the university.

Baltimore is an active and attractive city. The Johns Hopkins Medical Institutions are one mile from the Inner Harbor at the head of Chesapeake Bay. In July 1980, Harborplace opened, a renovation of the harbor complete with old world charm and modern attractions, which consists of two pavilions containing 135 shops and restaurants. The Maryland Science Center and the popular National Aquarium are also at the harbor and historic Annapolis and Washington are not more than an hour away.

Admissions

Although MCAT scores may be used, they are not required for acceptance. Applicants should submit the official scores of a single SAT, GRE, or ACT; however, the MCAT may be used as a substitute if any of these tests haven't been taken. If used, the MCAT should be taken no later than October before anticipated matriculation. All scores should be sent to the committee on admission.

Undergraduate Preparation

All applicants must be or must have been attending an institution on the "Accredited Institutions of Postsecondary Education" list. Hopkins requires one semester of calculus, one year each of college-level chemistry, organic chemistry, biology, and physics. The applicant must also have a minimum of 24 semester hours in the humanities, social sciences, and behavioral sciences. Candidates must be proficient in English and should have received a B.A. degree or its equivalent before matriculation.

Student Body

The student body is made up of students from 46 states and foreign countries.

Placement Records

Many Johns Hopkins students enter highly selective residency programs that are well suited to their career interests. Hopkins alumni go on to medical careers in hospitals, labs, and academic institutions around the world.

Costs

The tuition for medical students entering in September 1991 was $17,500. The tuition rate, which covers all normal charges, remains in effect until students in that class receive the M.D. degree. Additional fees include living expenses, health insurance, a $100 microscope rental fee, and a $380 matriculation fee. Students in residence pay an annual $25 fee. Visiting medical students registered for clinical or research electives pay a $250 registration fee per quarter or fraction thereof. Hospitalization insurance (currently $1,344 for single students) is mandatory. On-campus and off-campus housing is available.

Financial Aid

Financial aid for students in residence is awarded solely on the basis of need. Over 100 scholarships from memorial funds and organizations are available. Research fellowships vary from $500 to $1,250. A limited number of prizes and awards are offered for academic excellence. Students may appeal to more than 30 loan funds offered by the university.

Student Organizations

The Johns Hopkins Medical Student Society consists of all students actively seeking the M.D. degree. The Black Student Organization of the JHU School of Medicine acts as a liaison between The Johns Hopkins medical institutions and the neighboring Black community. The Johns Hopkins Graduate Student Association conducts seminars and schedules speakers, and the American Medical Student Association contributes to educational and social policy. Alpha Omega Alpha conducts seminars, lectureships, and visiting professorships. The International Club plans trips and social events during the year.

Faculty

The faculty comes from all disciplines, and the university is world renowned for its contributions to medicine and scientific research.

Curriculum

The curriculum for the M.D. comprises four academic years. With special approval, students may complete the curriculum in three years. Basic requirements for graduation include (1) two consecutive semesters as a full-time resident student; (2) fulfilled departmental requirements; (3) one foreign language; (4) a dissertation; and (5) an oral examination. There is a separate M.D./Ph.D. program. Individual department requirements vary.

The first year of medical study focuses mainly on normal human structure and function. Second-year students study causes and effects of disease, and also learn about pharmacology and elements of patient exams. Thereafter, students follow an educational program adapted to one's particular interests, in various clinical clerkships.

Facilities

The Johns Hopkins Hospital offers unparalleled opportunity for research and study. The Johns Hopkins Medical Institutions include the School of Hygiene and Public Health, and the School of Nursing. The Welch Medical Library contains more than 300,000 bound volumes. The Johns Hopkins Hospital offers a complex of "minihospitals" for reference and research. The Francis Scott Key Medical Center treats the chronically ill. A number of local hospitals support research activities.

Grading Procedures

Letter grades are given in required courses and clerkships; students in elective courses are graded honor-pass-fail. Students may get an incomplete but must pass every course to remain in good standing. No more than one D is allowed during each academic year.

Special Programs

Johns Hopkins offers the M.D., the M.D./Ph.D., the M.D./M.P.H., the Ph.D., and M.A. Graduate degree programs are offered in biochemistry, cellular and molecular biology, neuroscience, molecular biophysics, biomedical engineering, human genetics and molecular biology, and other graduate programs.

For undergraduate juniors and seniors of accredited U.S. colleges who demonstrate a commitment to medicine, the Johns Hopkins FlexMed program assures admission, upon graduation, to the School of Medicine. Upon acceptance, FlexMed applicants are treated as Johns Hopkins students for program planning and advising.

Application Procedures

The deadline for applying is November 15. Submit supporting credentials by January 1 of the following year. Notification occurs between November 15 and March 31. Other requirements include (1) an official transcript, (2) either MCAT scores or official scores of the SAT, GRE, or ACT, and (3) a letter from the applicant's premedical advisor or college premedical committee. Two letters from senior faculty members in science departments who taught the applicant may be substituted if the applicant's college has neither a premed advisor nor a committee. Send test scores to the committee on admission. The applicant will be notified when the admissions committee determines that a personal interview is necessary.

Contact

Office of Admissions
The Johns Hopkins University School of Medicine
720 Rutland Avenue
Baltimore, Maryland 21205
(301) 955-3182

UNIVERSITY OF KANSAS SCHOOL OF MEDICINE

39th and Rainbow Boulevard
Kansas City, Kansas 66103
(913) 588-5287

Accreditation	AAU
Degrees Offered	M.D., M.A., M.S., Ph.D.
# Students Applied	1,115
Enrollment	178 / class
Mean GPA	3.5
% Men / % Women	35% / 65%
% Minorities	Not Available
Tuition	$5,770 In-State
	$11,916 Out-of-State
Application Fee	$15 for Out-of-State Applicants
Application Deadline	November 1

The University

As the first state university on the Great Plains, the University of Kansas opened in 1866 with 55 students and three faculty members. The School of Medicine opened in 1905 in Bell Memorial Hospital, a facility with only 35 beds. Today the university has over 28,000 students and the School of Medicine has approximately 700 students completing their medical training on two campuses, one in Kansas City and another in Wichita.

Admissions

Candidates for admission are evaluated on the basis of undergraduate academic achievement, MCAT scores, letters of recommendation, and impressions made during personal interviews. There is no established quota for admission of out-of-state students, but well-qualified Kansas applicants will be given first preference.

Undergraduate Preparation

A baccalaureate degree is required before enrolling in the School of Medicine. Specific coursework required for admission includes: one year each, with lab, of general chemistry, organic chemistry, biology and physics, one college mathematics course that includes integral and differential calculus or one course in computer science, one year of English, and electives from areas other than the natural sciences. All applicants should have a substantial academic background in the liberal arts.

Costs

Tuition for Kansas residents is $5,770 annually, while out-of-state resident pay $11,916 per year. Books and supplies are estimated to cost between $400 and $750 annually. Other fees include a $100 library fee and a $25 health-service fee. Students are also required to have a microscope for their own use during the basic science courses. A new microscope costs $725, while a used one may be obtained for $350.

Financial Aid

Financial assistance for medical school expenses is limited and is most frequently awarded through state- and federally funded student loan programs. Students who are admitted to the School of Medicine receive notification in January and must submit the Family Financial Statement to the American College Testing Service by May 1. Applicants will be notified of their financial aid awards by June. In-state students at the School of Medicine may also apply for aid through the Kansas Medical Scholarship Program. This program, authorized by the state legislature, offers scholarships to 35 students annually, covers tuition, and provides monthly stipends.

Student Organizations

Extracurricular organizations at the School of Medicine include the Medical Student Assembly, the Student National Medical Association, the American Medical Student Association, the American Medical Women's Organization, and the Christian Medical Society. During annual Research Days students have the opportunity to report on their original research. Rural Health Weekends familiarize students with the practice of medicine in community settings by placing them in doctor's offices and hospitals in Kansas.

Curriculum

All students at the School of Medicine spend the first two pre-clinical years at the Kansas City campus, where they complete required courses in basic medical sciences. For the third and fourth years of clinical training and clerkships, students have the option of staying in Kansas City or completing their studies at the campus in Wichita. Required and elective clerkship opportunities vary between these two sites and students choose the location which best fits their career goals.

Facilities

The Archie R. Dykes Library of the Health Sciences contains more than 170,000 books, journals, and other medical-related informational materials. The Clendening History of Medicine Library has one of the top five rare medical book collections in the nation and contains 21,000 first or early editions of almost all important works in medical literature. The School of Medicine also operates the KU Cancer Center, the Center on Aging, the Radiation Therapy Center, and the Center on Environmental and Occupational Health.

Grading Procedures

Students at the School of Medicine are evaluated with grades of superior, high satisfactory, satisfactory, low satisfactory, and unsatisfactory. In the third and fourth years of clinical clerkships, students take objective examinations and also receive written evaluations of their ability to diagnose medical problems, make recommendations for patient care, and interact with patients. A 4.0 grade-point system is used to determine class ranking.

Special Programs

Students are permitted to pursue the M.D. alone or simultaneously with a Master's degree or Ph.D. Interested students must also apply to the Graduate School.

Application Procedures

Students must submit applications to the School of Medicine no later than November 1 of the year prior to desired entrance. Applications must be supported by a report from the undergraduate premedical advisor or committee. Students in graduate school must submit a letter of recommendation from the major advisor and/or department chair. The MCAT is also required and must be taken no later than the fall of the year prior to admission. After evaluation of these materials, certain applicants will be invited to Kansas City for personal interviews.

Contact

Associate Dean of Admissions
University of Kansas School of Medicine
39th and Rainbow Boulevard
Kansas City, Kansas 66103
(913) 588-5245

UNIVERSITY OF KENTUCKY COLLEGE OF MEDICINE

Office of Education
MN 104 UK Medical Center
Lexington, Kentucky 40536-0084
(606) 233-6582

Accreditation	AAMC
Degrees Offered	M.D., M.D./M.S., M.D./Ph.D.
# Students Applied	808
Enrollment	95 / class
Mean GPA	3.44
% Men / % Women	70% / 30%
% Minorities	5%
Tuition	$5,030 In-State
	$17,179 Out-of-State
Application Fee	None
Application Deadline	November 1

The University

The Lexington campus of the University of Kentucky is the site of the University's College of Medicine. The College of Medicine, Colleges of Allied Health Professions, Dentistry, Nursing and Pharmacy, and the University of Kentucky Hospital make up the UK Medical Center, which was established in 1956.

Admissions

Ninety-five students are selected for admission to each entering class at the College of Medicine. As a condition of state support, 90 percent of all the students enrolled are Kentucky residents. Applicants are considered on the basis of MCAT scores, grades, coursework, dedication to the field of medicine, activities, accomplishments, and recommendations. Applicants should have obtained a bachelor's degree.

Undergraduate Preparation

Required coursework for admission to the University of Kentucky College of Medicine includes biology, chemistry, physics, and English. Coursework in mathematics, social sciences, and the humanities is also desirable, but not required.

Placement Records

Of the more than 2,000 alumni of the College of Medicine, more than 33 percent live in Kentucky. The remainder practice medicine elsewhere in the United States. The University of Kentucky Medical Center has provided postgraduate training to 2,500 residents.

Financial Aid

Approximately 80 percent of the medical students attending the University of Kentucky College of Medicine receive financial aid in some form.

Faculty

One hundred basic science and 300 clinical, full-time faculty members teach at the College of Medicine.

Curriculum

During the first two years of medical school, students study basic sciences including anatomy, biochemistry, behavioral science, and pathology. Students are also instructed in patient interviewing techniques and physical diagnosis. In the third year, students evaluate and manage the health care status of their patients. Fourth year studies combine required and elective clerkships including two experiences in other medical facilities, one at an Area Health Education Center where students work with physicians in underserved regions of Kentucky.

Facilities

Among the many facilities available to students at the College of Medicine are the Bone Marrow Transplant Program, the Center on Drug and Alcohol Abuse, the Critical Care Center, the Kentucky Heart Institute, the Lucille Parker Markey Cancer Center, the Magnetic Resonance Imaging and Spectroscopy Center, the Neonatal Intensive Care Unit, and the Sanders-Brown Center on Aging.

Special Programs

The College offers many programs allowing students to pursue their special interests. The Integrative Studies Program provides students an opportunity to consider complex medical issues. The Osler Program uses literature, philosophy, art, and history as a vehicle for studying medicine. In the Nurse Preceptor Program, second-year medical students accompany members of the nursing staff on their rounds. Extramural clerkships are available to fourth-year students who wish to study at other medical facilities in the U.S. and internationally. Students may participate in Summer Research Fellowships in basic science or clinical research. In the Post-Sophomore Fellowship Program in Pathology, eligible students are given a chance to take on the responsibilities of first-year pathology residents.

Application Procedures

Only students whose applications have been screened are interviewed in the fall or early spring.

Contact

Office of Education
MN 104 UK Medical Center
Lexington, Kentucky 40536-0084
Admissions: (606) 233-6161

LOMA LINDA UNIVERSITY SCHOOL OF MEDICINE

Loma Linda, California 92350
(714) 824-4481

Accreditation	AAMC, CME
Degrees Offered	M.D., M.D./Ph.D., M.S.
# Students Applied	2,200
Enrollment	129 / class
Mean GPA	3.5
% Men / % Women	Not Available
% Minorities	Not Available
Tuition	$15,990
Application Fee	$35
Application Deadline	December 1

The University

Founded in 1909, the School of Medicine is part of Loma Linda University, owned and operated by the Seventh-Day Adventist Church. Full accreditation is given by the AAMC and the Council on Medical Education of the American Medical Association. Located in sunny California, the School of Medicine is not far from Los Angeles or Hollywood, and the social and cultural amenities of these great western cities.

Admissions

Students must take the new MCAT. Students are selected based on a review of their complete college record, letters of recommendation, extracurricular activities, and a personal interview. The School of Medicine does not encourage transferring into the program they offer with advanced standing.

Undergraduate Preparation

Students are urged to complete a bachelor's degree at an accredited liberal arts college or technical institute before entering the School of Medicine. Some exceptional students may apply after 85 semester hours (128 quarter hours). The School of Medicine expects letter grades on transcripts. Students should have one year each of biology, general and organic chemistry, physics (all with lab), English composition and, as the college attended may require, religion. General study in the humanities and social sciences is also expected.

Student Body

Preference is given to members of the Seventh-Day Adventist Church; however, a few non-church members who have demonstrated a commitment to Christian principles are admitted. Total Loma Linda University enrollment is about 5,000 students.

Costs

The tuition is $15,990. Books, supplies, and living expenses are about $6,000 per student.

Curriculum

The first two years cover the study of the basic medical sciences and clinical applications, including introduction to human behavior and physical diagnosis. Students must pass Part I of the National Boards to progress to their junior year. Clinical training in major areas includes surgery, medicine, pediatrics, obstetrics-gynecology, and psychiatry. Electives are possible in clinical and research subjects in the fourth year.

Facilities

Instruction takes place primarily at Loma Linda University Medical Center, the Jerry L. Pettis Memorial Veterans Hospital, Riverside General Hospital, and the White Memorial Medical Center in Los Angeles. San Bernadino County General Hospital, Kaiser Foundation Hospital, and Glendale Adventist Medical Center are used for training and research.

Special Programs

The School of Medicine offers the M.D., and qualified students may earn the M.S. or Ph.D. simultaneously. Students must submit separate applications to the School of Medicine and to the Graduate School.

Application Procedures

Candidates must apply through AMCAS. Applications may be obtained between June 15 and December 1. Applicants who wish to enter the summer of a following year must apply between these dates. After evaluation, the admission committee may request a supplementary application with letters of recommendation. An interview may follow for selected candidates. Fees are required for each application and for supplementary applications.

Contact

Admissions Office
School of Medicine—Medical Center A-505

Loma Linda University
Loma Linda, California 92350
(714) 824-4467 or (714) 824-4468

LOUISIANA STATE UNIVERSITY SCHOOL OF MEDICINE IN NEW ORLEANS

1901 Perdido Street
New Orleans, Louisiana 70112-1593
(504) 568-6262

Accreditation	LCME
Degrees Offered	M.D., M.D./Ph.D.
# Students Applied	751
Enrollment	175
Mean GPA	3.34
% Men / % Women	63% / 37%
% Minorities	Not Available
Tuition	$4,776 In-State
	$12,576 Out-of-State
Application Fee	$30
Application Deadline	November 15

The University

The School of Medicine in New Orleans was established in 1931 by the Louisiana State Board of Supervisors and the governing board of the Charity Hospital of Louisiana at New Orleans. After World War II, the Residence Hall, Student Center, Medical Education Building, and the Lions-LSU Clinics Buildings were added.

The School of Medicine was constructed adjacent to Charity Hospital and is located on the edge of the city's central business district, in a metropolitan urban area of approximately 1.2 million people.

Admissions

Applicants are required to take the Medical College Admissions Test (MCAT). Scores must be received before the November 15 application deadline. State residents are given priority. Nonresidents who are transfer students are considered for enrollment, usually after completion of the first two years of medical school. For certain highly competitive curricula, nonresident applications will not be considered.

Undergraduate Preparation

Prospective students must have completed the following required courses (including necessary laboratory work): six credit hours of general chemistry and six credit hours of organic chemistry; eight credit hours of physics covering heat, light, sound mechanics, electricity, and magnetism; eight credit hours of biology, which should include general zoology, vertebrate embryology, comparative vertebrate anatomy, and microscopic anatomy; and nine credit hours of English.

Applicants who are enrolled in the coursework specified by their college for a baccalaureate degree or other advanced degree will be given preference over those who simply complete the subjects required for admission and the minimal credit hours required. Other helpful courses include mathematics, statistics, computer sciences, economics, history, foreign languages, philosophy, and social studies.

Placement Records

Approximately 60 percent of the graduates of the School of Medicine have remained in Louisiana.

Costs

Annual tuition for resident M.D. candidates is $4,776; for nonresidents, $12,576. First-year books and equipment are estimated to cost $2,795 (including microscope); second year, $1,795; third year, $2,395. Students must purchase group health insurance from the school or prove they are covered by another plan.

Financial Aid

Financial aid is given to students from a variety of different sources. Examples of available loans and grants include the Stafford/Guaranteed Student Loan, the Pell Grant, the Supplemental Educational Opportunity Grant, and the Health Education Assistance Loan. The supplemental loans for students are non-need based.

Financial aid, including grants, loans, scholarships, and part-time employment, is handled through the Office of Financial Aid and Insurance. Completed applications for fall enrollment should be received by March 17, or by June 1 for priority consideration.

Minority Programs

Applications from minority students are encouraged. The School of Medicine employs an Assistant Dean for Minority Affairs.

Student Organizations

Student organizations include the Student Council, Alpha Omega Alpha, and the Aesculapians.

Faculty

The faculty of the Medical Center comprises approximately 3,700 appointees, of which nearly 1,400 are involved in full-time teaching and research activities. They are augmented by more than 2,300 part-time faculty.

Curriculum

The first two years of study are devoted to the basic medical sciences and clinical medicine. The third year begins with eight days of ophthalmology, a day of radiology, followed by four consecutive 12-week blocks which include general surgery, otorhinolaryngology, obstetrics and gynecology, pediatrics, and psychiatry. The fourth year consists of nine four-week blocks providing clerkships in ambulatory care, general medicine, neural sciences, and an acting internship.

Facilities

The Louisiana State Medical Center is a statewide teaching, research, and health care facility. The LSU Medical Center conducts a broad spectrum of teaching programs for medical students and residents at the adjacent Charity Hospital of Louisiana. Most students at the School of Medicine obtain their clinical education at Charity Hospital. The 555-bed hospital is state owned, and has a history and tradition of providing medical care to the indigent of Louisiana.

The Library of the Medical Center serves the six professional schools with approximately 258,000 volumes and a periodical title list in excess of 3,400. Through a cooperative program of interlibrary loan, the holdings of any LSUMC facility, regional biomedical library, or the National Library of Medicine is available to faculty and students.

Grading Procedures

Official final grades are recorded as honors, high pass, pass, fail, and withdrawal. Part I of the National Board of Medical Examiners (NBME) examination must be taken and passed after satisfactory completion of the second year of medical school. Students entering the fourth year of study will be required to take Part II of the NBME and achieve a passing score prior to graduation.

Special Programs

A combined M.D./Ph.D. program is available for highly-qualified students.

Application Procedures

The School of Medicine participates in the American Medical College Applications Service (AMCAS). Preliminary materials and instructions for application will be furnished by AMCAS. Transcripts, personal letters of recommendation, biographies, and other related material should not be sent to the admissions office until the applicant has received instructions from the school and a secondary application has been filed. All official recommendations must be in the admissions office by December 1. Interviews are mandatory and are arranged by invitation only.

The earliest date for filing an application is July 1 for

admission in the fall of the following year. Applications must be filed after July 1 and on or before November 15 for admission in the fall of the following year. The application fee is $30. First offers of acceptance are mailed on October 15.

Contact

Office of Student Admissions
Louisiana State University
School of Medicine in New Orleans
1901 Perdido Street
New Orleans, Louisiana 70112-1593
(504) 568-6262

LOUISIANA STATE UNIVERSITY SCHOOL OF MEDICINE IN SHREVEPORT

1501 Kings Highway
Shreveport, Louisiana 71130-3932
(318) 797-5000

Accreditation	AAMC
Degrees Offered	M.D., M.D./Ph.D.
# Students Applied	508
Enrollment	100 / class
Mean GPA	3.4
% Men / % Women	67% / 33%
% Minorities	Not Available
Tuition	$4,776 In-State
	$12,576 Out-of-State
Application Fee	$30
Application Deadline	November 15

The University

The School of Medicine in Shreveport was established in 1966. Permanent medical school facilities include a comprehensive care teaching facility, basic and clinical science buildings. These facilities are adjacent to the Louisiana State University Hospital (650 beds), the school's principal teaching hospital.

Admissions

Applicants are required to have attended at least three full academic years at an approved college and must have completed at least 90 semester hours before registration at the School of Medicine. A baccalaureate degree (B.A. or B.S.) is preferred. The MCAT is required. The School of Medicine admits only Louisiana residents.

Undergraduate Preparation

Completion of the following courses (including necessary laboratory work) is required: six credit hours each of inorganic and organic chemistry, eight credit hours each of biology and physics, and six credit hours of English.

Acceptable grades in all acceptable college courses must have been received before registration. Students are encouraged to pursue broad educational interests.

Costs

Annual tuition for a resident is $4,776. A nonresident pays $12,576. In addition, first-year students will need approximately $1,400 for the purchase of books, equipment, and supplies.

Financial Aid

Financial aid is given to students from a variety of different sources. Examples of available loans and grants include the Stafford Student Loan, the Pell Grant, the Supplemental Educational Opportunity Grant, and the Health Education Assistance Loan. The supplemental loans for students are non-need based.

Financial aid, including grants, loans, scholarships, and part-time employment is handled through the Office of Financial Aid and Insurance. Completed applications for fall enrollment should be received by March 17.

Outside employment is not encouraged, because of the exacting curriculum requirements.

Minority Programs

Applications from minority students are encouraged. The School of Medicine employs a Special Coordinator of Minority Affairs.

Student Organizations

Student organizations include the Student Executive Council and Alpha Omega Alpha.

Curriculum

The school believes that early patient contact should be presented from the beginning, to avoid an abrupt transition from study of the basic sciences to the clinical responsibilities of later years. The first-year curriculum includes introductory basic science courses, plus introductory courses in comprehensive care and a course entitled "Perspectives in Medicine I." Live clinics are given weekly. During the second year, advanced basic sciences are offered as well as a major course in clinical diagnosis, which introduces the students to the clinical works of the third and fourth years. During the second year, the student begins to work with patients. The third and fourth years consist of supervised patient care. Forty-four percent of the fourth-year curriculum is elective.

Facilities

The 650-bed Louisiana State University Hospital (formerly the Confederate Memorial Medical Center) is the primary teaching facility. Teaching and research are also conducted at the affiliated 450-bed Veterans Administration Medical Center and other regional hospitals. The Library of the Medical Center serves the six professional schools with approximately 258,000 volumes and a periodical title list in excess of 3,400. Through a cooperative program of interlibrary loans, the holdings of any LSUMC facility, regional biomedical library, and the National Library of Medicine can be made available to faculty and students.

Grading Procedures

All required courses have a letter grading system. Comprehensive care and all electives are graded on a pass/fail basis. Promotion from one grade to the next is determined by the promotion committee.

Special Programs

The School of Medicine offers a combined M.D./Ph.D.; interested students should note this on their secondary application so the appropriate department can provide you with further information.

Application Procedures

The School of Medicine participates in the American Medical College Application Service (AMCAS). All applicants are automatically sent a secondary application when the medical school receives a verified preliminary application from AMCAS. The secondary application is brief and asks for certain supplemental information and a passport-type photograph. A nonrefundable $30 fee must accompany the secondary application. Copies of an admission information brochure describing the application and selection processes may be obtained directly from the Office of Admissions at the School of Medicine in Shreveport at any time.

All candidates being seriously considered for acceptance will be interviewed by members of the faculty.

Contact

Office of Student Admissions
Louisiana State University
School of Medicine in Shreveport
1501 Kings Highway
Shreveport, Louisiana 71130-3932
(318) 674-5190

UNIVERSITY OF LOUISVILLE SCHOOL OF MEDICINE

Louisville, Kentucky 40292
(502) 588-5184

Accreditation	AAMC, LCME
Degrees Offered	M.D.
# Students Applied	809
Enrollment	125 / class
Mean GPA	3.45
% Men / % Women	58% / 42%
% Minorities	Not Available
Tuition	$4,928 In-State
	$17,078 Out-of-State
Application Fee	$15
Application Deadline	November 1

The University

The School of Medicine was originally affiliated with the Louisville Medical Institute when it was founded in 1833. In 1846 the school changed affiliations to the University of Louisville, which is part of the state university system. The school is part of the Health Sciences Center, which also comprises the School of Dentistry, the Health Sciences Instructional Building, and the Health Sciences Library and Commons Building. There is also a teaching hospital affiliated with the medical school.

Admissions

Candidates for admission are evaluated on an individual basis. The school examines college transcripts, MCAT scores, and recommendations of the preprofessional committee. The college also considers the applicant's involvement in community activities, personality, and level of motivation. The school gives preference to residents of Kentucky and to those who will have completed the baccalaureate degree prior to matriculation.

Undergraduate Preparation

Applicants must have completed at least three years (90 semester hours) of undergraduate coursework. Two semesters of each of the following preprofessional college subjects are required: general biology (with lab); general or inorganic chemistry (with lab); organic chemistry (with lab); general physics (with lab); college math (or one semester of calculus); and English. All candidates for admission must take the MCAT.

Student Body

The 1990 entering class was comprised of 125 students; 58 percent men and 42 percent women. The mean GPA was 3.45. Virtually all entrants held bachelor's degrees. Six members of the class were from out of state.

Costs

Yearly tuition (resident) for the 1990-91 first-year class was $4,928. Tuition for nonresidents was $17,078.

Financial Aid

About 90 percent of the school's students receive some form of financial assistance during the course of the program. Scholarships are awarded on the basis of both demonstrated financial need and academic and professional potential.

Minority Programs

The school gives special consideration in the admission of minorities, especially qualified Black candidates from the region.

Curriculum

The core curriculum consists of the basic science and clinical subjects generally taught at all medical schools. During the first two years, students have the opportunity to take elective courses as well. The school has a very flexible elective program, which allows students to tailor their medical education to suit their individual goals. About half of the fourth year comprises clinical electives, in which the student works closely with a faculty member.

Facilities

In addition to University Hospital, the school is affiliated with four other hospitals. Together, there are about 1,000 beds that represent clinical teaching experience for students. The school also has comprehensive outpatient facilities.

Grading Procedures

In preclinical courses, pass/fail and percentage grades are used to evaluate student performance. In clinical core and clinical elective courses, students are graded on a pass/fail basis in addition to a subjective evaluation.

Application Procedures

The school participates in AMCAS. Applications must be filed with AMCAS between June 15 and November 1 of the year preceding the year of desired entry. The school will not accept MCAT scores that are older than 1989. There is an application fee, payable to the school, of $15. For the early decision plan, applications must be submitted to AMCAS between June 15 and August 1. Upon acceptance, students must submit a $100 deposit to hold their place in the class; the deposit is applied toward tuition.

Contact

University of Louisville
School of Medicine
Office of Admissions
Health Sciences Center
Louisville, Kentucky 40292
(502) 588-5193

LOYOLA UNIVERSITY OF CHICAGO STRITCH SCHOOL OF MEDICINE

2160 South First Avenue
Maywood, Illinois 60611
(708) 216-3229

Accreditation	AAMC
Degrees Offered	M.D., M.S., Ph.D.
# Students Applied	4,116
Enrollment	130 / class
Mean GPA	3.36
% Men / % Women	64% / 36%
% Minorities	Not Available
Tuition	$13,800 In-State
	$17,650 Out-of-State
Application Fee	$35
Application Deadline	November 15

The University

A four-year college for men and women, Loyola is an independent, urban school of Jesuit/Roman Catholic affiliation. The university has served for 120 years as an institution that stresses social, moral, and spiritual growth within the Judeo-Christian framework. Only blocks away from Lake Michigan and downtown Chicago, Loyola is surrounded by a multi-resource metropolis. Students and faculty have access to an array of facilities. These include opera houses, libraries, professional sports complexes, and Sears Tower, the world's tallest building. In addition, the Medical Center of Loyola works closely with several prominent hospital facilities in Chicago.

Admissions

Scores from the Medical College Admission Test (MCAT)

must be included with the application. It is advised to take the MCAT in the spring of the year applying. The results of the test must be no more than four years old.

Undergraduate Preparation

A bachelor's degree is required of all applicants. Specific undergraduate majors are not recommended; it is the intensity of the program rather than one's GPA that is stressed. A combination of liberal arts with sciences is preferred. In addition, four prerequisite courses for the medical school curriculum are one academic year each of general chemistry, organic chemistry, general biology, and general physics, all with labs.

Student Body

About half of the enrolled students come from Illinois.

Placement Records

Loyola's reputation includes an 85 percent occupancy rate for graduates at the Foster G. McGaw Hospital. Most postgraduates establish residency within Chicago.

Costs

Loyola-Stritch reported a 1989-90 annual tuition of $13,800 for in-state students. The out-of-state charge was $17,650. No on-campus housing is available; however, suburban housing can be found for an average cost of $500 per month. Additional living expenses, books, and supplies are expected to range around $4,300. Students must supply their own microscopes.

Financial Aid

Students are strongly advised to refer to the "Guidelines for Student Financial Aid" booklet available at the admissions interview. Eighty-five percent of Loyola-Stritch students receive financial aid offered through a variety of scholarships and loans, each bound by a set of restrictions. The requirements for each program are spelled out in the "Guidelines" packet.

Minority Programs

In an effort to enhance the diversity of the student body, members of minority groups are encouraged to apply. Tuition scholarships are offered to students with disadvantaged backgrounds. The restrictions are explained in the "Guidelines" packet.

Student Organizations

Members of the Medical Student Union (MSU) are actively involved in various committees on the Loyola campuses, including the Financial Aid Committee, the Basic Science and Clinical Curriculum Committee, and the Committee on Admissions. Stritch also has chapters of the American Medical Student Association, the American Medical Association, the American Medical Women's Association, Physicians for Social Responsibility, and Amnesty International.

Faculty

The professional staff of Loyola-Stritch comprises 450 basic and clinical scientists. Enrollment of medical students total 520; in addition, there are 400 resident physicians and postgraduate students in training programs, making a student/faculty ratio of about 2:1.

Curriculum

The first two years of coursework are designed to help students acquire complete knowledge of both normal body functions and disease mechanisms. The semesters run for 18 weeks. The required course/lab work consists of anatomy, biochemistry, physiology, neuroscience, microbiology, pharmacology, and physical diagnosis. In the third and fourth years students, under supervision, begin making diagnoses, recommending treatment, and commencing their clerkships.

Facilities

The Stritch School of Medicine is fortunate to have the major city of Chicago as a haven of resources. The school itself contains a Learning Resource Center designed to improve the diagnostic skills of students with videotapes and heart sound simulators. At the newly expanded Medical Center Library, 126,000 volumes are housed for student access. The library also subscribes to 2,000 periodicals and newspapers. Much of the clinical training is performed at the Hine's Veteran's Administration Hospital and the Foster G. McGaw Hospital.

Grading Procedures

A pass/fail system of grading is used, with the possibility of high pass and honors grades for exceptional work.

Special Programs

Research opportunities are available in areas such as heart transplantation, Interleukin 2, and infection in premature infants. A dual degree program is offered where students can earn their M.D./M.S. and Ph.D. at the same time. Also of interest is a clinical experience offered on the island of St. Lucia in the Caribbean. This clinical rotation gives students a greater appreciation of modern medicine by practicing medical science in a Third World country.

Application Procedures

All applicants must complete a standardized AMCAS application. The school's application schedule runs from June 15 to November 15. Applicants who pass the initial screening are sent the Stritch Supplemental Application. Included is a personal experience essay due no later than February 1. Following this, a Recommendation Inventory Form is sent for letters of support. Prospective students are invited for interviews to supplement their application.

Contact
> Associate Dean for Admissions
> Loyola University Medical Center
> 2160 South First Avenue, Room 1752
> Maywood, Illinois 60153
> (708) 216-3229

MARSHALL UNIVERSITY SCHOOL OF MEDICINE

1542 Spring Valley Drive
Huntington, West Virginia 25755
(304) 696-7000

Accreditation	AAMC
Degrees Offered	M.D.
# Students Applied	592
Enrollment	48 / class
Mean GPA	3.3
% Men / % Women	65% / 35%
% Minorities	Not Available
Tuition	$5,047 In-State
	$9,017 Out-of-State
Application Fee	$20
Application Deadline	November 15

The University

Marshall University was established in 1837. Today, the university has an enrollment of more than 12,000 students. The School of Medicine was created in 1978, under the Veteran's Administration Medical School Assistance and Health Training Act. Through its growing research program, the school hopes to improve rural health care, as well as study such areas as diabetes, hypertension, and an AIDS vaccine.

Huntington is the trade and cultural center for a large portion of West Virginia, Ohio, and Kentucky. It offers the combination of modern business and cultural activities with low crime rates, a relaxed lifestyle, and quick access to rural areas and recreational activities.

Admissions

Applicants should have a bachelor's degree from an accredited college or university, but exceptionally well-qualified candidates will be considered after three years of college education or its equivalent. All applicants must take the Medical College Admission Test (MCAT) no later than the fall of the year they apply. They must have taken the MCAT within three calendar years of the year they wish to enter. Preference is given to residents, although consideration is given to well-qualified nonresidents from states adjoining West Virginia, or to applicants with strong ties to West Virginia. Only U.S. citizens or those with permanent resident visas are considered.

Undergraduate Preparation

All applicants must have completed the following courses: eight semester hours each of zoology or biology, inorganic chemistry, advanced chemistry (must include at least one semester of organic chemistry), and physics, all with lab, six semester hours of social or behavioral sciences, and six semester hours of English composition and rhetoric.

Beyond these required courses, applicants are encouraged to pursue their own educational interests. The quality of an applicant's work is considered to be more important than the field studied.

Student Body

Most students are residents of West Virginia. Class size is small.

Placement Records

In the class of 1989, more than 75 percent of the graduates received their first-choice residencies and another 12 percent received their second choice.

Costs

Annual tuition and fees for residents come to $5,047; nonresidents are charged $9,017. The estimated cost of books is $600 per year.

Financial Aid

Marshall's financial aid office gives assistance to students in need. There are a variety of scholarships and loans available. For information, contact the office of financial assistance.

Student Organizations

Organizations on campus include a chapter of the American Medical Student Association, a Family Medicine Interest Group, and a chapter of Alpha Omega Alpha. Students and faculty from both the School of Medicine and the main campus participate in the activities of Sigma Xi, a national research honorary.

Curriculum

The first year includes basic medical sciences as well as courses in communication in medicine, human sexuality, introduction to medicine, and behavioral medicine. Second year courses include medical sciences and introduction to clinical medicine, as well as psychotherapy, genetics, and community medicine.

Third-year clerkships are taught at Marshall's three affiliated hospitals in Huntington. Students are rotated through six eight-week clerkships in obstetrics/gynecology, psychiatry, medicine, surgery, pediatrics, and family practice. The fourth year includes three four-week blocks of medicine, surgery, emergency medicine, and 26 weeks of electives. Four weeks of these electives must be taken in rural West Virginia and in ambulatory care (these two requirements may be combined in a single elective). No more than 12 weeks of electives may be spent outside Huntington without special permission.

Grading Procedures

A student is promoted to the next year after being recommended by the Academic Standards Committee, the Dean's Advisory Committee, and the Dean. A letter grading system is used. Students must pass Part I of the National Board of Medical Examiners (NBME) examination before being promoted to year three. To graduate, students must take Part II of the NBME exam.

Special Programs

The biomedical sciences graduate program offers a master of science degree; the doctor of philosophy may be pursued through arrangements with West Virginia University. More information about the graduate program may be found in MU's graduate catalog.

Application Procedures

Application should be made through the American Medical College Application Service (AMCAS). Applications for admission are accepted by AMCAS from June 15 to November 15 of the year prior to enrollment for the fall semester. Supplemental application materials are provided by the School of Medicine and must be completed by September 1 for early decision, and December 31 for regular admission. Interviews are arranged only by invitation of the admissions committee.

Contact

The Marshall University School of Medicine
Office of Admissions
1542 Spring Valley Drive
Huntington, West Virginia 25755
(304) 696-7312 or (800) 544-8514

UNIVERSITY OF MARYLAND SCHOOL OF MEDICINE

655 West Baltimore Street
Baltimore, Maryland 21201
(301) 328-7410

Accreditation	AAMC, LCME
Degrees Offered	M.D., M.D./Ph.D., M.D./M.S.
# Students Applied	2,405
Enrollment	141 / class
Mean GPA	3.5
% Men / % Women	55% / 45%
% Minorities	Not Available
Tuition	$7,240 In-State
	$14,652 Out-of-State
Application Fee	$25
Application Deadline	November 15

The University

The University of Maryland School of Medicine is the fifth oldest medical college in the United States. Its first class graduated in 1810, and in 1823 it became one of the first medical colleges to build its own hospital for clinical instruction. The university also established the first intramural residency for senior students. Other professional schools of the university include the schools of dentistry, nursing, and pharmacy. The school is located on the Baltimore City Campus, which is adjacent to the downtown Charles Center and Baltimore's Inner Harbor.

Admissions

Selection of students for admission is based on evaluation of academic achievement, MCAT scores, letters of recommendation, extracurricular involvement, and the results of interviews conducted by faculty members. The school rarely admits applicants who are not citizens and permanent residents of the United States and Canada. Preference is given to residents of Maryland.

Undergraduate Preparation

Students must have taken at least 90 semester hours of arts and sciences at an accredited college to be considered for admission. Preference is given to applicants who hold bachelor's degrees. The following courses must be completed prior to matriculation: eight semester hours of biology; eight semester hours of inorganic chemistry; six semester hours of organic chemistry; eight semester hours of physics; and six semester hours of English.

Student Body

There were 142 students enrolled in the 1989 first-year class. Twenty-four were from out of state and 118 were residents of Maryland. All of those enrolled held bachelor's degrees. The 1989 class had an average GPA of 3.5 and an MCAT average of 60. About 52 percent were science majors. Forty-five percent were women.

Costs

1989 tuition costs were $7,240 for residents and $14,652 for nonresidents. Student fees were $1,058 per year.

Financial Aid

Approximately 70 percent of the student body receives some type of financial assistance. The school offers both scholarships and loans to those students with demonstrated economic need. The amount of the award varies according to the student's need and the amount of funding available.

Minority Programs

The school has an assistant dean for minority affairs who actively participates in the search for qualified minority students. More information can be obtained by contacting Dr. Robert Harrell, Assistant Dean for Minority Affairs, Room M-006 at the School of Medicine.

Curriculum

The first two years of the four-year curriculum consist mainly of the study of the basic medical sciences with some elective experiences and some time for research and interdisciplinary study. The third year is devoted to basic clinical clerkships and the fourth year to advanced clinical work, both elective and required. Ambulatory care and some medical specialties are introduced at this time. During a large part of the fourth year, students may pursue elective experiences on the Baltimore campus or elsewhere.

Facilities

The University of Maryland Medical System and affiliated hospitals in and around Baltimore have more than 1,400 general hospital beds for teaching purposes.

Special Programs

The school offers the joint M.D./Ph.D. degree. The first two years of this program consist of medical school (preclinical study). Students then pursue two years of full-time graduate study in their Ph.D. field and two years of clinical clerkships. Elective time during the clinical years may be used to complete the Ph.D. research.

For the M.D./M.S. in preventive medicine, the student usually completes the M.S. portion during summers and elective periods.

Application Procedures

The school participates in AMCAS. All Maryland residents who apply will be permitted to submit an application directly to the school after the AMCAS application is received. Nonresident applicants are sent a second application only upon recommendation of the admissions committee. Interviews are arranged only for selected qualified applicants.

AMCAS application and materials must be submitted by November 15 of the year prior to intended year of matriculation; the school application must be submitted by December 1 accompanied by a $25 fee. The school has an early decision program.

Contact

University of Maryland School of Medicine
Committee on Admissions
Room 14-015
655 West Baltimore Street
Baltimore, Maryland 21201
(301) 328-7478

UNIVERSITY OF MASSACHUSETTS MEDICAL SCHOOL

55 Lake Avenue, North
Worcester, Massachusetts 01655
(508) 856-0011

Accreditation	LCME
Degrees Offered	M.D., M.S., Ph.D., M.D./Ph.D.
# Students Applied	651
Enrollment	100 / class
Mean GPA	3.5
% Men / % Women	48% / 52%
% Minorities	5%
Tuition	$6,500
Application Fee	$18
Application Deadline	December 15

The University

The University of Massachusetts, established in 1863, is a small, affordable learning institution with campuses in Amherst, Boston, and Worcester. The medical school, which accepted its first students in 1970, was specifically designed to train residents of the commonwealth and, in turn, furnish underserved sections of the state with quality health care professionals. The school receives substantial research funds and ranks first among 12 public medical schools in the Northeast. The University of Massachusetts teaching hospital hosts a regional trauma center as well as New England Life Flight, the first air ambulance in the area. The UMass Medical Center is nationally recognized for its work in diabetes research.

The city of Worcester boasts a population of 164,000 and is a bustling community rich with cultural events. There you will find business and industry as well as history. The school itself is situated on the beautiful banks of Lake Quinsigamond.

Admissions

The average MCAT score of UMass applicants is 10.3, the average GPA (for all majors) is 3.5. The University only accepts prospective students who reside in Massachusetts. (Requirements may differ from legal residency.)

Undergraduate Preparation

In preparing for a career in medicine, the university strongly encourages diversity of interests and an education that reflects that diversity. Students should be well rounded, able to communicate effectively, and should have completed the minimal preparation in biology, preferably a one-year course in general biology or zoology, one year each of inorganic and organic chemistry, a one-year course in general physics, and one year of college-level study in English literature or composition. Courses in the following areas are also useful: calculus, statistics, cell biology, embryology, genetics, comparative anatomy, biochemistry, psychology, sociology, economics, and ethics.

Student Body

UMass Medical School admits only students who are certified legal residents of Massachusetts. The average age of the UMass student is 25; however, many fall into the 26 to 45 range, providing a wealth of backgrounds and interests within the college community. The ratio of women to men is virtually 1:1 with minorities comprising five percent. Of the class of 1992, 100 percent obtained their undergraduate degree in the state.

Placement Records

In 1989 a full 70 percent of the graduating class was matched with their first choice of placement for residency. Ninety-three percent received one of their top four choices. Out of 90 graduates, 44 remained within the commonwealth. The remainder of the class opted for residency programs in

California, Connecticut, Pennsylvania, Maine, Rhode Island, New York, and nine other states.

Costs

Tuition is currently $6,500. The school does offer the option of deferring two-thirds of the full-time cost until after graduation. At that time the student may begin to repay on a schedule or to pay by agreeing to practice medicine within the state for one year.

Financial Aid

Seventy-five percent of the students receive some type of financial aid.

Faculty

The University of Massachusetts faculty consists of 504 full-time instructors.

Curriculum

The four years of study are divided into three cohesive sections beginning with two years of basic sciences. In the first year students concentrate on the normal structure and function of cells, tissues, and organs. A three-week family and community clerkship introduces the prospective doctor to clinical work. Physical abnormalities are explored in the second year, as well as pathological processes and the development of disease states. There will be the opportunity to examine "standardized patients" who will offer individualized attention. The final two years include hospital rotations as well as 24 weeks of elective work chosen by the student with the help of an advisor.

Facilities

The facilities at UMass abound with state-of-the-art equipment. The Sciences Building is the main site for the basic sciences, clinical sciences, and clinical laboratories. It houses three amphitheaters with audiovisual capabilities. Also on campus is Lamar Soutter Library, which holds over 100,000 volumes. For relaxation, there are weight rooms, a cardiovascular fitness course, and basketball courts. The University does not offer housing on campus. Many students find housing within the community and use public transportation.

Special Programs

Medical students may simultaneously earn a Ph.D. through the Graduate School of Biomedical Sciences. Applications for the M.D./Ph.D. program must be received before matriculation or during preclinical training. Usually after the second year, such candidates take a one-year leave of absence to complete grad school requirements and thesis research. The university also offers a summer enrichment program, which allows premedical students a taste of life at UMMC.

Application Procedures

Required of all applicants are: a completed application form,

MCAT scores (from up to three years ago), and a letter of evaluation from a premedical advisory committee from the student's undergraduate institution. If one is not available, two letters of recommendation from instructors, preferably in prerequisite fields are required. Also required is a notarized application for classification as a Massachusetts resident. Selected students are invited for personal interviews.

Contact

University of Massachusetts Medical School
Office of Admissions
55 Lake Avenue North
Worcester, Massachusetts 01655
(508) 856-2323

MAYO MEDICAL SCHOOL

200 First Street, S.W.
Rochester, Minnesota 55905
(507) 284-3671

Accreditation	AMCAS
Degrees Offered	M.D., M.D./D.M.S.
# Students Applied	1,400
Enrollment	40 / class
Mean GPA	3.57
% Men / % Women	54% / 46%
% Minorities	Not Available
Tuition	$8,200 In-State
	$17,650 Out-of-State
Application Fee	$40
Application Deadline	November 15

The University

The Mayo Medical School is a part of one of the world's largest medical group practices, the Mayo Clinic. Faculty members are on the staff of the clinic, which operates closely with two neighboring hospitals. Combined, the three centers care for 280,000 patients annually. The Mayo Medical School, the Mayo Clinic, and the two hospitals are under the governance of the Mayo Foundation, and students have access to all of its resources and research opportunities. The city of Rochester, Minnesota has a safe and comfortable environment with the diversity of a large city.

Admissions

The mean GPA for 1989 was 3.57 and mean MCAT scores were above 10 in all categories. A baccalaureate degree is required, but as long as academic prerequisites are met, applicants are encouraged to follow their personal choice in other premedical studies.

Undergraduate Preparation

Prerequisite courses include a minimum of one year of biology and/or zoology, two years of chemistry (including organic chemistry), one year of physics, and a course in biochemistry. No one major field of undergraduate study is preferred over another. Mayo Medical School encourages students with other than traditional premedical education to apply, as a wide range of talents will contribute to a physician's many societal responsibilities.

Student Body

Forty out of 1,400 applicants were accepted, of these, approximately 46 percent were women and 54 percent were men. The students, with 20 different majors, came from 29 colleges and universities in 13 states.

Placement Records

A great many graduates choose to practice at the Mayo Clinic itself. In recent years, 89 percent of Mayo students have received one of their top three choices.

Costs

Tuition for 1990-1991 was $8,200 for Minnesota residents; for nonresidents, $17,650. In addition, there is a general fee of $500. Books, supplies, and equipment for the first year cost between $550 and $750. For the second year, the costs are between $220 and $540. The cost of room and board varies, but a minimum of $6,500 is typical for single students. Substantial health care coverage is included in the tuition and fees.

Financial Aid

Financing a medical education is primarily the responsibility of the student and his or her family. Students are admitted to Mayo Medical School regardless of their financial circumstances. Mayo has loan funds available to supplement federally sponsored loan and grant programs. The school recommends students research private and governmental sources that provide aid to medical students who demonstrate a need for assistance. Approximately 90 percent of students receive financial aid.

Student Organizations

The Mayo Medical School supports branches of many national medical organizations, such as the American Medical

Women's Association, the American Medical Students Association, Student National Medical Association, Zumbro Valley Medical Society, Minnesota Medical Society, and the American Medical Association. Medical students, their spouses and children are also welcome to take part in the many social, recreational, and cultural activities. Sponsored sports include softball, touch football, volleyball, basketball, soccer, hockey, and broomball. There is also a dance band whose members include staff and students.

Faculty

The Mayo Medical School has one of the highest faculty/student ratios in the country. The faculty is drawn largely from the more than 800 men and women on the professional staff of the Mayo Clinic. Medical students also will have preceptorship experience with about 70 practicing physicians in southern Minnesota and northern Iowa, most of whom hold faculty appointments at Mayo Medical School.

Curriculum

At Mayo, after a concentrated period in the first year, the basic sciences are integrated with all segments of the remaining curriculum. Clinical application of the fundamentals and principles introduced in the basic science and body systems courses of the freshman year is continued and expanded throughout the curriculum. Second-year introductory clerkships prepare the student for responsibilities involving the care of hospital patients; third-year clerkships for patient care in an ambulatory setting. A research semester in the third year provides an in-depth experience in one aspect of science chosen by the student to best complement his or her career goals. The senior year is almost totally elective, allowing the student to refine skills and explore opportunities.

Facilities

Scholarships and authorship are encouraged at Mayo and appropriate help is provided. Mayo Clinic Proceedings is a monthly publication of papers presented at meetings of the Mayo staff that reaches a domestic and foreign readership of 86,000. The Mayo Medical Library receives more than 3,400 medical and scientific journals. Historic medical writings are among the library's 250,000 volumes.

Grading Procedures

Students receive honors, satisfactory, marginal, or unsatisfactory evaluations. Faculty are encouraged to add comments that describe the student's personal growth, behavior, and attitude in reference to professional goals. Evaluations strengthen the student's educational experience.

Special Programs

The M.D./Ph.D. program in biomedical sciences is intended for those students who wish to be trained as both physicians and independent investigators. M.D./Ph.D. students

receive an annual $13,000 stipend and tuition waiver for each year in the program. As part of the extramural clerkship opportunity, Mayo students may, for a portion of their third and fourth years, with appropriate approval, participate in electives at other medical schools.

Application Procedures

All applicants must submit scores from the MCAT. Students taking the test in the spring of the year of application may have an advantage over those who wait until fall. The deadline for applications is November 15 of the previous year. A $40 application fee is required. Interviews are arranged at the request of the admissions committee; no applicant is accepted without one. Mayo Medical School does not accept students with advanced standing or as transfers from other medical colleges. Only rarely is a post-baccalaureate degree (including a doctorate) helpful in accelerating undergraduate medical education.

Contact

Admissions Committee
Mayo Medical School
200 First Street, SW
Rochester, Minnesota 55905
(507) 284-3671

MEDICAL COLLEGE OF GEORGIA SCHOOL OF MEDICINE

1120 Fifteenth Street
Augusta, Georgia 30912
(404) 721-2231

Accreditation	AAMC, AMA
Degrees Offered	M.D.
# Students Applied	860
Enrollment	180 / class
Mean GPA	Not Available
% Men / % Women	Not Available
% Minorities	Not Available
Tuition	$3,942 In-State
	$11,826 Out-of-State
Application Fee	None
Application Deadline	November 1

The University

The Medical College of Georgia is the health sciences division of the University of Georgia system. The School of Medicine, founded in 1828, is the 11th oldest medical school in the United States. The college campus, situated in the approximate center of Augusta, is convenient to the downtown business district.

Admissions

Admissions preference is given to Georgia residents, with only a limited number of spaces available for out-of-state students. The admissions committee selects applicants on the basis of demonstrated level and pattern of academic ability and achievement, MCAT scores, letters of recommendation, and personal interviews.

Undergraduate Preparation

Specific coursework required for admission to the School of Medicine includes one academic year each of biology or zoology; physics; and general inorganic chemistry, all with lab; and one academic year of advanced chemistry, two quarters or one semester of which must be organic chemistry with lab. One academic year of English is required and biochemistry is recommended. At least three years of undergraduate work must be completed (a minimum of 90 semester or 135 quarter hours). Preference is given to applicants who have completed their baccalaureate degree.

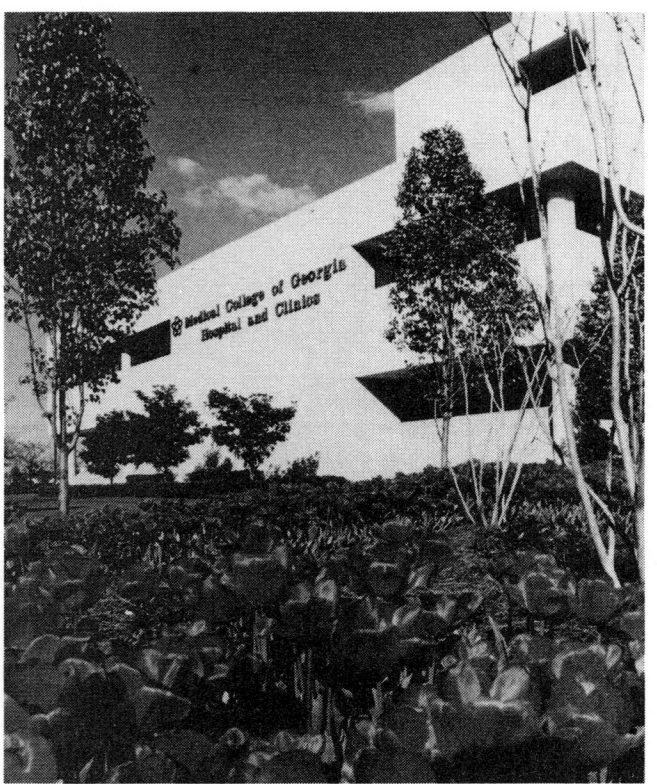

Placement Records

The college claims a "truly outstanding" track record of job placement with almost 100 percent of each year's graduates able to obtain jobs immediately or soon after graduation. Graduates practice in every state in the nation.

Costs

Tuition and fees at the School of Medicine total $1,335.50 per quarter for in-state students, while nonresident students are charged $3,861.50 per quarter. A variety of housing arrangements, both on- and off-campus, are available and rates vary with the option selected.

Financial Aid

Information on and applications for financial aid may be obtained from the Office of Student Financial Aid, 174 Administration Building, Medical College of Georgia, Augusta, Georgia 30912-7320.

Student Organizations

Members of Alpha Omega Alpha, the honorary scholastic fraternity of medicine, are selected on the basis of both peer and faculty recommendations and academic excellence. Alpha Omega Alpha sponsors two lectures each year.

Faculty

The college has a full-time faculty of nearly 650 and a part-time faculty of 800. More than 96 percent of professors and faculty have the highest degree appropriate for their fields. The student/faculty ratio is less than 4:1.

Curriculum

The curriculum at the School of Medicine consists of three phases. During Phase I (the first year), students study the function and structure of the human body through courses in the basic medical sciences. Contact with patients begins with physical diagnosis during the winter quarter of the first year. During Phase II (the second year), students begin courses in the clinical sciences, including pathology, pharmacology, genetics, community medicine, psychiatry, radiology, and laboratory medicine, which provide the didactic basis for the clinical studies of the third and fourth years. Opportunities for elective courses are also available during the first two years. Phase III consists of 72 weeks of required clinical clerkships during the third and fourth years, with the balance of the fourth year spent in elective courses in advanced medical subjects. Electives may also be taken during this time at other institutions and community hospitals.

Facilities

The Medical College of Georgia Hospital is a 540-bed teaching facility that offers a number of specialized medical services including pain management, comprehensive diabetes care, epilepsy surgery, and oncology. The MCG Hospital also serves as the designated Shock-Trauma Center for the East Central Georgia Health District. The MCG Hospital also includes a 90-bed Children's Medical Center. The Robert B. Greenblatt, M.D. Library collection consists of approximately 1,700 current journal titles and has an overall collection of approximately 130,000 volumes of books, journals, and audiovisual materials. The Medical College of Georgia is also affiliated with numerous hospitals and medical centers in the immediate Augusta area.

Grading Procedures

The School of Medicine issues letter grades; in order to be promoted or graduated, a student must have a grade of "C" or better in every required course.

Application Procedures

Because the School of Medicine participates in the AMCAS program, students must first submit an application to this service by November 1 for regular decision and by August 1 for early decision. In addition, students must submit supplemental information to the School of Medicine, including MCAT scores, two personal references, one of which must be from an individual active in the health sciences, and one letter of recommendation from the applicant's premedical advisor. The MCAT must be taken no later than the fall of the year prior to desired enrollment in medical school; scores from tests taken more than three years prior to application will not be accepted. Interviews, which are required prior to acceptance, are held by invitation of the admissions committee.

Contact

Office of Associate Dean for Admissions
School of Medicine
Medical College of Georgia
1120 Fifteenth Street
Augusta, Georgia 30912
(404) 721-4792

MEDICAL COLLEGE OF OHIO

P.O. Box 10008
Toledo, Ohio 43699
(419) 381-4229

Accreditation	LCME
Degrees Offered	M.D.
# Students Applied	1,907
Enrollment	135 / class
Mean GPA	3.35
% Men / % Women	64% / 36%
% Minorities	14%
Tuition	$7,749 In-State
	$10,536 Out-of-State
Application Fee	$30
Application Deadline	December 1

The University

The Medical College of Ohio (MCO) is a state-assisted academic health-science center that includes a School of Medicine, a Graduate School, a School of Allied Health, and a School of Nursing. The college was established in 1964 as the state's only free-standing medical college.

The college's first class of 35 medical students graduated in 1972. Today, a total of about 2,000 students attend classes on the MCO campus each year.

Toledo, the "Glass Capital of the World" and the home of MCO, has a population of about 340,000. The city has numerous shopping centers; and major cultural assets, including the Toledo Zoo, the Toledo Symphony Orchestra, and the Toledo Opera.

Admissions

The college considers a wide range of factors in the admissions process. These factors include academic grades; general scope of the academic background; understanding of the physical, chemical, biological, and social sciences; and sensitivity to the humanities. Completion of the bachelor's degree is strongly recommended. All applicants must take the MCAT.

The college favors applicants with motivation as well as those that meet the physical and emotional standards needed for the medical school program. Applicants are assessed with regard to skill in observation and communication, intellectual and qualitative abilities, motor function, and behavioral and social attributes. Preference is given to Ohio residents.

Undergraduate Preparation

Minimum requirements are one year each of biology, math, English, and physics, and two years of chemistry, including organic chemistry. Additional biology courses are strongly encouraged.

Student Body

Each year 135 students are admitted to the four-year M.D. program.

Costs

For Ohio residents, yearly tuition is $7,749 (1992-93). Nonresidents pay $10,536. The microscope rental fee is $47. Books and equipment are estimated to cost about $1,300 for the first year.

Financial Aid

Financial assistance is available from a number of sources within and outside the college. Students must submit a GAPSFAS needs analysis application, an MCO financial aid application, income tax records, and a financial aid transcript from every school attended prior to MCO.

Loans administered by the college include Perkins Loans, Health Professions Student Loans, and MCO Low-Interest Loans. Forms of assistance administered from outside agencies include Stafford Loans and SLS Loans.

All accepted students will receive a financial aid information manual from the college in February of each year.

Curriculum

The four-year curriculum is organized into four quarters per year. The first and second years consist of courses in most of the basic medical sciences—anatomy, embryology, biochemistry, physiology, and neurosciences. Students are also introduced to the behavioral sciences, clinical medicine, and physical diagnosis. Students can also choose some electives during these years, and are introduced to clinical medicine and physical diagnosis.

The third year consists of required clinical clerkships, including medicine, surgery, pediatrics, and psychiatry. The fourth year consists primarily of elective clerkships.

MCO students receive clinical experience in community hospitals, physicians' offices, and clinics in some 25 communities in northwest Ohio. They are supervised by more than 200 preceptors who are practicing health professionals.

Facilities

Facilities on the 350-acre campus include health science and health education buildings, the Medical College Hospital (a 260-bed acute care teaching hospital), the Child and Adolescent Psychiatric Hospital, the MCO Health Center, Glendale Medical Center, and the Eleanor N. Dana Center for Continuing Health Education. Instruction is given at several community-based teaching hospitals as well.

The Raymon H. Mulford Library houses more than 100,000 volumes and 2,400 periodicals. No on-campus housing is available.

Grading Procedures

The grading system is honors, high pass, pass, and fail. A passing grade on Part I of the National Boards will be required for graduation.

Special Programs

The college offers a combined M.D./Ph.D. program, which offers students the opportunity to conduct medical research that incorporates the skills obtained in clinical medicine.

Application Procedures

The School of Medicine participates in the AMCAS program. Processing of AMCAS applications occurs mid-July through November. On the basis of information provided in the preliminary AMCAS application, the school may ask applicants to fill out a secondary application. With the secondary application, the applicant must supply a photograph, recommendations, transcripts, and a $30 nonrefundable application fee. The admissions committee may request a formal interview before making a recommendation on acceptance. Offers of acceptance are sent to candidates starting October 15.

Contact

Medical College of Ohio
Office of Admissions
PO Box 10008
Toledo, Ohio 43699
(419) 381-4229

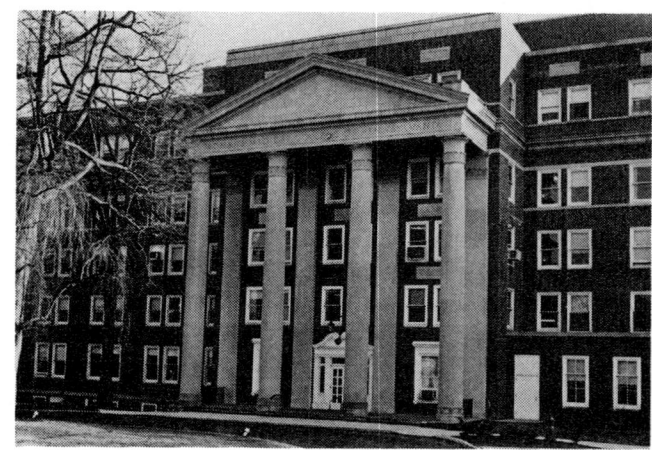

MEDICAL COLLEGE OF PENNSYLVANIA

3300 Henry Avenue
Philadelphia, Pennsylvania 19129
(215) 842-6000

Accreditation	LCME
Degrees Offered	M.D., M.D./Ph.D., M.D./ M.S., M.D./M.B.A.
# Students Applied	3,400
Enrollment	113 / class
Mean GPA	3.40
% Men / % Women	Not Available
% Minorities	20%
Tuition	$15,590
Application Fee	$55
Application Deadline	December 1

The University

Founded in 1850, the Medical College of Pennsylvania was the first medical school for women. Today it is open to all students. MCP was one of the first medical schools in the country to introduce courses in the humanities and bioethics. Located in an area with five medical schools, many hospitals, and numerous biomedical research institutes, MCP is part of an exciting medical community. The campus is located in a residential area next to Philadelphia's Fairmount Park. It offers the comfort of an attractive environment and the opportunities of a large and lively city.

Admissions

Residents and nonresidents are equally considered. Applications are welcome from students who are just completing college as well as from those who are in other careers or in advanced study programs. The MCAT is required. The 113-member freshman class this year had an average GPA of 3.40 and MCAT scores at or above the 75th percentile.

Undergraduate Preparation

Applicants are required to have completed four semesters of chemistry (inorganic or general chemistry and organic chemistry), two semesters of biology, and two semesters of physics, all with lab, and two semesters of English.

In addition, students are encouraged to take two semesters each of mathematics, humanities, and the social sciences.

Placement Records

Eighty percent of graduates are placed in one of their first three choices for residencies.

Costs

Tuition for all students is $15,590 for the school year. Room, board, books, instruments, health insurance, and personal expenses cost about $9,000 to $10,000. Microscopes are provided for MCP students, as are room, board, and transportation to rotations at Allegheny General Hospital in Pittsburgh.

Financial Aid

Ten entering freshmen receive merit scholarships, which can extend through all four years. MCP also administers a variety of programs based on financial need that offer loans, grants, and work opportunities. The financial aid office determines the distribution of funds, most of which are loans from the federal and state government as well as from private sources. Eighty-five percent of MCP students receive financial help.

Student Organizations

Student representative organizations include the Faculty-Student Relations Committee, the Curriculum Committee, the College Committee of the Board, the Student Government Association, and the Organization of Student Representatives. There are also many professional, social, and volunteer groups that students may join.

Faculty

There are 800 faculty members who have won numerous local and national teaching awards. In a research program that has tripled in size since 1981, faculty members lead internationally known research projects in the neurosciences and psychiatry, atherosclerosis, and geriatrics.

Curriculum

The first year consists of the basic sciences and clinically oriented courses in bioethics, nutrition, human sexuality, emergency medicine, cardiopulmonary resuscitation, gerontology, epidemiology, and oncology. In the second year, abnormal structure and function are studied, and physical and clinical laboratory diagnosis is taught. Courses include microbiology and immunology, community and preventive medicine, and introduction to clinical medicine. The third year consists of five required clerkships, which can take place either at the main campus in Philadelphia or the Allegheny campus in Pittsburgh. The fourth year involves 36 weeks of study, 16 of which are devoted to a four-week rotation in internal medicine, primary care, critical care, and a surgery subinternship. The remaining 20 weeks are electives.

Facilities

The 445-bed Hospital of The Medical College of Pennsylvania serves a very diverse population. Students work with

280 residents and fellows in 28 specialty and subspecialty programs. It was the first hospital in the country to introduce a Board-approved residency program in emergency medicine. MCP is now a level II trauma center.

In 1981, the college took over management of the Eastern Pennsylvania Psychiatric Institute, on campus. Here, students learn psychiatry and the neurosciences in one of the area's most comprehensive facilities.

At Allegheny General Hospital in Pittsburgh, a tertiary care hospital, students assist some of the hospital's 500 physicians. MCP students also do clinical rotations at other area hospitals.

Grading Procedures

An honors/pass/fail grading system is used. Grades are determined by both objective and subjective measures. There are four evaluations committees, one for each year of medical school. Students must take the NBME exams, Parts I and II, and have results reported to the registrar. Beginning with the Class of 1994, students must post a passing score on Part I of the exam in order to graduate.

Special Programs

The college offers a combined M.D./Ph.D. program, which can be completed in six years. Also offered are an M.D./M.S. five-year program, an M.D./D.M.D. for students interested in hospital dentistry or maxillofacial surgery, and an M.D./M.B.A. program offered by the College of Medicine and Drexel University.

Application Procedures

Applications should be made through the American Medical College Application Service (AMCAS). Applications are accepted from June 15 to December 1 for matriculation in the fall of the following year. After the AMCAS application is received, the school will send an activation request, which must be returned with a $55 nonrefundable application fee. Letters of recommendation are required. Interviews include a full orientation day.

The Medical College participates in the Early Decision Plan.

Contact

Admissions Office
The Medical College of Pennsylvania
3300 Henry Avenue
Ann Preston Hall, 2nd Floor
Philadelphia, Pennsylvania 19129
(215) 842-7009

MEDICAL COLLEGE OF WISCONSIN

8701 Watertown Plank Road
Milwaukee, Wisconsin 53226
(414) 257-8296

Accreditation	LCME
Degrees Offered	M.D., M.D./Ph.D., M.S./M.D.
# Students Applied	2,700
Enrollment	187 / class
Mean GPA	3.53 In-State
% Men / % Women	60% / 40%
% Minorities	33%
Tuition	$7,674 In-State
	$17,500 Out-of-State
Application Fee	$45
Application Deadline	December 1

The University

The history of the Medical College of Wisconsin dates to the 1890s. Once part of Marquette University, today the college is a private institution whose mission involves education, research, patient care, and community service. The college is the academic heart of the Milwaukee Regional Medical Center, a major academic center that includes the college and six other health care institutions.

The college is among the top third of medical schools in the nation for receiving federal research funding support. Its faculty attracts more than $35 million annually in research funding support from the federal government and other sources.

The 240-acre campus is located in western Milwaukee. The "City of Festivals" is situated on the shore of Lake Michigan, and is known for its culture and arts, high-tech industry, sports and recreational opportunities, and ethnic festivals, including Oktoberfest. Milwaukee is the 18th largest city in the country.

Admissions

The selection of candidates for admission is based upon a careful evaluation of individual suitability for the profession of medicine. Undergraduate academic achievement and MCAT scores are carefully reviewed; however, academic excellence alone does not assure acceptance. Personal characteristics are sought, including a mature sense of values, sound motivation, and willingness and ability to assume responsibility.

The AMCAS application, the candidate's personal statement, academic recommendations, and results of personal interviews are all essential parts of the admissions evaluation. The mean GPA of Wisconsin residents is 3.53, with a science/math GPA of 3.45. The mean GPA of nonresidents is 3.30, with a science/math GPA of 3.25. The new MCAT is required and must be taken not more than three years before matriculation.

Undergraduate Preparation

A minimum of three years of undergraduate work (90 semester hours) is required for admission. The following courses are required as a prerequisite for admission: eight semester hours of biology, organic chemistry, inorganic chemistry, and physics; six semester hours of English (with emphasis in composition); and completion of a course in algebra in high school or college. Electives in the liberal arts (language, literature, history, music, philosophy, and/or the social sciences) are strongly recommended.

Student Body

The total student body numbers almost 800. The college admits about 200 new students each year. In the Class of 1993, 104 are Wisconsin residents and 97 are nonresidents.

Costs

Tuition for residents for the 1989-90 academic year was $7,674. Tuition for nonresidents was $17,500. Student fees and activities fees totaled about $250, and books and supplies were estimated to cost approximately $1,300.

Financial Aid

All financial assistance offered through the college is awarded on the basis of need. This includes federal and institutional scholarships and loans.

Minority Programs

The college has a variety of services offered through its Minority Outreach Program. Full-tuition dean's scholarships are awarded each year to minority students who are residents of the state of Wisconsin. These awards are based on merit as well as need.

In 1986, together with the University of Wisconsin, MCW initiated a premedical curriculum for up to 25 undergraduate minority students, who are tutored at the university during the summer prior to the start of their freshman year and thereafter. Students participate in special seminars and occasionally visit the Medical College. Those who satisfactorily complete the UMW program may be offered admission to the Medical College.

The college is also involved in recruitment of minority students at local high schools.

Faculty

The college has approximately 680 full-time faculty, 70 part-time faculty, and 1,600 voluntary faculty members.

Curriculum

The college offers a solid foundation in the basic life sciences during the first two years of the four-year M.D. program. These years are spent in classroom, office, and laboratory settings, and provide students with the opportunity to participate with faculty in research projects.

During the third and fourth years, students are exposed to clinical care settings through clinical rotations. During this time, students develop their skills and confidence in dealing with patients.

Facilities

The collections at the Medical College of Wisconsin Libraries rank among the largest health sciences library collections in the Midwest. The main library is the Todd Wehr Library; there are three branch libraries. Altogether, the collection numbers some 200,000 volumes. The libraries maintain subscriptions to approximately 2,800 biomedical journal titles. The libraries have direct on-line access to more than 200 bibliographic databases. Students also have access to several medical databases, including MEDLINE.

The campus maintains an eye bank, a temporal bone transplant bank, and an organ procurement organization.

The college is affiliated with 20 health care institutions in Wisconsin, where faculty practice medicine and train physicians in residency programs.

Facilities available to students include Froedtert Memorial Lutheran Hospital, a 285-bed tertiary care facility; Children's Hospital of Wisconsin; the Milwaukee County Medical Complex, which includes the Eye Institute, a regional center for specialized eye care, vision research, and physician training; and the Milwaukee Mental Health Complex. There are numerous other centers and institutes, including the MACC Fund Research Center, which conducts primarily cancer-related research; the Diabetes Care Center; the Center for the Study of Bioethics; the Marcus Center for Allergy and Immunology Research; and the Koss Audiology Center for Research and Treatment.

Special Programs

The Medical Scientist Training Program is a seven-year scholarship program leading to the M.D. and Ph.D. degrees; two students per year are selected for this program.

Other special programs include dual-degree programs leading to master's or doctoral degrees in addition to the M.D. degree. Students in these dual degree programs should apply for admission to both the M.D. program and to the graduate studies division. Programs leading to an M.S. degree in biostatistics/epidemiology and an M.P.H. (Master of Public Health) are offered.

Application Procedures

The college participates in AMCAS. Applications can be submitted to AMCAS from July 1 to December 1 of the year prior to the year of intended enrollment. Early application is encouraged, and the college participates in the early decision plan of AMCAS (applications must be submitted to AMCAS by August 1).

The college must receive a nonrefundable $45 application fee by December 1. Interviews will be granted to qualified applicants beginning in November, pending completion of the application.

Contact

Office of Admissions and Registrar
Medical College of Wisconsin
8701 Watertown Plank Road
Milwaukee, Wisconsin 53226
(414) 257-8246

MEDICAL UNIVERSITY OF SOUTH CAROLINA COLLEGE OF MEDICINE

171 Ashley Avenue
Charleston, South Carolina 29425
(803) 792-2300

Accreditation	LCME
Degrees Offered	M.D., Ph.D.
# Students Applied	1,447
Enrollment	129 / class
Mean GPA	Not Available
% Men / % Women	Not Available
% Minorities	Not Available
Tuition	$4,140 In-State
	$8,820 Out-of-State
Application Fee	$25
Application Deadline	December 1

The University

A four-year, state-supported medical college for men and women, the Medical University of South Carolina is the oldest medical institution in the southern United States. For over six generations, the university has provided quality education for health professionals, biomedical scientists, and other health care personnel. The College of Medicine sits among five other medical education institutions of the university, including the College of Dental Medicine, the College of Graduate Studies, the College of Health Related Professionals, the College of Nursing, and the College of Pharmacy.

More than a half million people in the Charleston metropolitan area benefit from the beauty of the well-preserved 18th century buildings and historic charm. There is a host of cultural and historic museums including the Charleston Museum, considered the nation's oldest. Plenty of theaters, concerts, and opera houses provide entertaining pleasure for student and faculty alike. With an average temperature of 65 degrees, the climate is conducive to outdoor recreational activities.

Admissions

South Carolina residents have admissions preference; therefore, nonresidents must possess superior credentials for consideration. The Medical College Admission Test (MCAT) scores and a minimum of three years' college work are the basic requirements for admission. Although no specific course requirements exist, students who possess a baccalaureate degree take preference.

Undergraduate Preparation

Students who have chosen a major in science should also have a selection of courses from a wide range of learning disciplines. The admissions board looks for applicants who have taken courses that are intellectually interesting. All credentials must have been obtained from an accredited institution.

Student Body

The College of Medicine comprises about 16 percent of the total makeup of the student body. The Medical University itself is made up of approximately 2,200 students. The vast majority of these students are South Carolina residents.

Costs

For the 1990-91 school year the College of Medicine reported a tuition of $4,140 for in-state residents and $8,820 for nonresidents. The university does not provide any on-campus dormitories; however, an office of off-campus housing has a list of available Charleston housing and costs. Additional fees and expenses should range around $800 for the first year.

Financial Aid

The College of Medicine participates in a variety of scholarships, loan funds, and awards that assist in the financial responsibilities by designated stipends and restrictions. The university utilizes the American College Testing Service in determining the financial need of the student. Among the available scholarships are the Manning Simons Scholarship and the Kellogg Loan Fund.

Minority Programs

Incentive fellowships are offered to minority students of South Carolina for up to $5,000 per year with the condition that they agree to pursue their professional career in the state. Since 1976, the minority affairs office at the Medical University has been dedicated to encouraging minority students to apply to the Medical School.

Faculty

The professional teaching staff for the Medical University consists of 760 core and 1,460 part-time faculty members. This puts a student/faculty ratio for the university at 1:1.

Curriculum

Four major objectives are addressed during the first two years: basic science concepts, development of skills, performance of physical examination, and the role of the physician in society. The junior year consists of five core clerkships. Senior year entails a minimum of seven four-week rotations including clinical externship and a primary care ambulatory rotation. The academic years run an average duration of 34 weeks.

Facilities

The Medical University of South Carolina Medical Center is a 565-bed facility that includes the Medical University Hospital, the Albert Florens Storm Memorial Eye Institute, the Children's Hospital, and the Institute of Psychiatry. The Medical University of South Carolina Library estimates a volume collection of over 190,000. In addition, the library contains 2,900 serial subscriptions. The university also provides experimental laboratories at the Walton Research Building.

Grading Procedures

Different grading systems are used for different courses depending on the particular program of study, ranging from raw, T-score, and merit grades. During the introduction to clinical medicine (I.C.M.) program, a pass/fail system is utilized. A student progress committee reviews all students on their academic performance to ensure that a GPA of 2.0 or better is maintained and that all levels of academic requirements are met.

Application Procedures

The application period runs from June 15 to December 1. The College of Medicine participates in the American Medical College Application Service (AMCAS) to conduct preliminary admission screening. There is a fee for the AMCAS application as well as a nonrefundable fee for the Medical College supplementary application. The registrar and director of admissions will notify applicants of interview appointments. Applicants respond to the acceptance offer by sending in a $50 matriculation fee.

Contact

Office of the University Registrar and Director of Admissions
Medical University of South Carolina
171 Ashley Avenue
Charleston, South Carolina 29425
(803) 792-3281

UNIVERSITY OF MEDICINE AND DENTISTRY OF NEW JERSEY NEW JERSEY MEDICAL SCHOOL

185 South Orange Avenue
Newark, New Jersey 07103
(201) 456-4538

Accreditation	LCME
Degrees Offered	M.D.
# Students Applied	1,893
Enrollment	170 / class
Mean GPA	3.35
% Men / % Women	56% / 44%
% Minorities	22%
Tuition	$10,457 In-State
	$13,723 Out-of-State
Application Fee	$25
Application Deadline	December 15

The University

New Jersey Medical School is part of the University of Medicine and Dentistry of New Jersey (UMDNJ-NJMS), situated in Newark, New Jersey since 1977. The $250-million school complex comprises a medical school, a dental school and comprehensive teaching facilities. Clinical education is carried out at a host of community-based hospitals in northern New Jersey as well as the University Hospital.

Admissions

Students are evaluated for admission based on a variety of academic and personality factors. The school seeks students who have the aptitude and motivation to study and practice medicine. The school considers academic achievement, MCAT scores, communication skills, mechanical skill, and level of perseverance and stamina. The school gives preference to residents of New Jersey.

Undergraduate Preparation

A broad academic and cultural background is encouraged. Students must have at least three years (90 semester hours) of undergraduate coursework in order to be considered for admission.

Pre-professional coursework must include the following (minimum guidelines): eight semester hours of biology or zoology (with lab); eight semester hours of organic chemistry (with lab); eight semester hours in another category of chemistry (with lab), which could be inorganic, physical, or biochemistry; eight hours of general physics (with lab); and six semester hours of English. The school recommends, but does not require, students to take a math course. Students may pursue any undergraduate major but must demonstrate a high level of achievement in the required courses.

Student Body

Of the 1989 entering class, 44 percent were women. The mean GPA was 3.35. Of the 170 students in the 1990 entering class, 156 were New Jersey residents and 14 were nonresidents.

Costs

For the 1990-91 academic year, resident tuition was $10,457. Nonresidents paid $13,723. The yearly student fees totaled $600.

Financial Aid

About 70 percent of UMDNJ-NJMS students receive financial assistance in some form. The Financial Aid Office assists students in assessing their financial need and filling out the necessary forms. All financial assistance is awarded on the basis of need.

Minority Programs

The school provides a summer program for economically and educationally disadvantaged students who have been accepted into UMDNJ-NJMS. Other summer programs are offered to those who are still in undergraduate school.

Curriculum

The first two years of the curriculum give the student a thorough education in the basic medical sciences correlated with clinical subjects. During these years, the student is introduced to clinical science courses, as well as physical diagnosis, psychiatry, public health, and preventive and community medicine. During the third year, students participate in supervised clinical rotations that increase the student's clinical knowledge and technique. Instruction is individualized or conducted in small groups.

The fourth-year curriculum is comprised of advanced study and elective experiences. During this year, students become involved in the ethical and legal aspects of medical practice. Required fourth-year subjects include emergency medicine, neurology, and an acting internship.

Facilities

The $250-million complex that constitutes UMDNJ-NJMS includes the Biomedical Science Building, a hospital, a library, a community mental health center, and a dental school. Students participate in clinical education at University Hospital, any of about a dozen hospitals in northern New Jersey, including East Orange Veterans Administration Hospital, St. Michael's Medical Center (Newark, NJ), Beth Israel Hospital (Newark, NJ), St. Joseph's Hospital of Paterson, the Eye Institute of New Jersey, and Jersey City Medical Center.

Special Programs

UMDNJ-NJMS participates with various regional colleges and universities in a joint liberal arts/medical education program. The school is currently offering this seven-year joint-degree program in conjunction with Boston University, Stevens Institute of Technology (Hoboken, NJ), New Jersey Institute of Technology (Newark, NJ), and Trenton State College (Trenton, NJ).

Application Procedures

The school participates in AMCAS. Students must file the AMCAS application between June 15 and December 15 of the year preceding the year of intended enrollment. The school has an early decision plan for exceptional New Jersey residents (the filing dates are from June 15 to August 1). The school's application fee is $25. There is a $100 deposit required upon acceptance, which is applied toward tuition.

Contact

UMDNJ-New Jersey Medical School
Director of Admissions
185 South Orange Avenue
Newark, New Jersey 07103
(201) 456-4631

UNIVERSITY OF MEDICINE AND DENTISTRY OF NEW JERSEY ROBERT WOOD JOHNSON MEDICAL SCHOOL

675 Hoes Lane
Piscataway, New Jersey 08854-5635
(908) 463-1966

Accreditation	LCME
Degrees Offered	M.D., M.D./Ph.D.
# Students Applied	1,955
Enrollment	Not Available
Mean GPA	3.29
% Men / % Women	61% / 39%
% Minorities	Not Available
Tuition	$10,547 In-State
	$13,723 Out-of-State
Application Fee	$25
Application Deadline	December 15

The University

The Robert Wood Johnson Medical School, with divisions in Piscataway and Camden, was named for a former president of the Johnson & Johnson Company. The school has extensive facilities adjacent to the campus of Rutgers, the State University of New Jersey. Its teaching hospitals are Robert Wood Johnson University Hospital (New Brunswick) and Cooper Hospital/University Medical Center (Camden). All students, whether matriculated in Camden or Piscataway, receive their basic training at the Piscataway facility.

Admissions

Admission is competitive. Factors considered in the evaluation process are academic achievement, a well-rounded college education, MCAT scores, level of motivation, character, recommendations, and the results of a personal interview. Preference is given to residents of New Jersey; nonresident applicants must exhibit unusually high credentials.

Undergraduate Preparation

Applicants must have at least three years (90 semester hours) of undergraduate education in order to be considered for admission. The college seeks a balanced undergraduate curriculum that includes coursework in the liberal arts, humanities, and behavioral sciences. The following are required for entry: two semesters of biology or zoology (with lab); two semesters of inorganic chemistry (with lab); two semesters of organic chemistry (with lab); two semesters of physics (with lab); one semester of math; and two semesters of English (one semester must be college-level composition).

Candidates must have taken the MCAT within four years preceding the date of application, but no later than the fall of the year of application.

Student Body

Out of an applicant pool of almost 2,000, the school admitted 143 students for its 1990-91 class. Ten were from out of state and 133 were New Jersey residents. All students admitted held a bachelor's degree. Women made up 39 percent of the class. The mean GPA of the class was 3.29.

Costs

For the 1990-91 year, residents paid tuition of $10,547. Nonresidents paid $13,723. Student fees for that year were $790.

Financial Aid

During the 1990-91 academic year, about 80 percent of the student body received some form of financial assistance. The school offers freshmen scholarships, renewable yearly, that are based on merit. Other forms of financial aid include loans and grants, which usually come as part of a total financial aid package.

Minority Programs

The university and the medical school encourage applications from both resident and nonresident minorities. Special financial aid and support services are offered, including a summer pre-enrollment program for accepted minority students. The school also reaches out to undergraduate minority students through its biomedical careers program, offered over the summer to minority undergraduates wishing to learn more about health care careers.

Curriculum

Basic science instruction in the first two years is conducted in small groups, using a multidisciplinary approach. Students receive a high degree of individual attention in this teaching format. In addition to the traditional basic science courses, students take courses such as environmental medicine, human sexuality, and psychiatry. The first two years also include exposure to hospital settings and classroom discussion of patient care.

In the third year, students take basic clinical clerkships in areas such as medicine, pediatrics, and surgery, and attend lectures on the various subspecialties. A good deal of the fourth year is devoted to a choice of electives. The fourth year also provides the opportunity to choose a subinternship, neurology, or ambulatory care experience. Students are required to take a course in environmental forces medicine in the fourth year.

Facilities

The school complex in Piscataway comprises a basic science building; the Institute of Mental Health Sciences; and a host of facilities shared with Rutgers University, including the Library of Science and Medicine, the Center for Advanced Biotechnology and Medicine, and the Environmental and Occupational Health Science Institute. In addition to the Robert Wood Johnson University Hospital, community hospitals in central New Jersey provide comprehensive clinical teaching facilities.

Grading Procedures

Students are evaluated using grades of honors, high pass, pass, low pass, and fail.

Special Programs

A seven-year M.D./Ph.D. program is offered through the school and also in cooperation with Rutgers University.

Application Procedures

The school participates in AMCAS. Students must file their applications with AMCAS between June 15 and December 15 of the year preceding the year of desired enrollment. For early decision, applications must be submitted to AMCAS between June 15 and August 1. The school's application fee is $25.

Upon acceptance, students must pay a $50 deposit to hold their place in class; the fee is applied toward tuition.

Contact

Office of Admissions
UMDNJ-Robert Wood Johnson Medical School
675 Hoes Lane
Piscataway, New Jersey 08854-5635
(908) 463-4576

MEHARRY MEDICAL COLLEGE SCHOOL OF MEDICINE

1005 D.B. Todd, Jr., Boulevard
Nashville, Tennessee 37208
(615) 327-6111

Accreditation	AMA, AAMC
Degrees Offered	M.D., Ph.D., M.S.
# Students Applied	2,143
Enrollment	80 / class
Mean GPA	Not Available
% Men / % Women	52% / 48%
% Minorities	86%
Tuition	$13,300
Application Fee	$25
Application Deadline	December 15

The University

Located on a 26-acre campus in Nashville, the capital of Tennessee, Meharry Medical College was founded in 1876 and is one of the largest educators of black health care professionals in the nation. Approximately half of all black physicians and dentists in the United States are Meharry graduates, while close to 40 percent of the country's black medical school professors studied at the School of Medicine.

Admissions

The School of Medicine seeks to offer low-income and high-risk students from socially, economically, or educationally underprivileged backgrounds an opportunity for advanced medical training that would perhaps be unavailable otherwise.

Undergraduate Preparation

A minimum of three years of undergraduate study must be completed before enrollment at Meharry. Required courses include eight semester hours each of general biology or zoology, inorganic chemistry with qualitative analysis, general physics, and organic chemistry, all with lab. Also, six credits of English composition must be completed. The MCAT is required and must be taken no more than three years prior to the anticipated date of entrance to the School of Medicine.

Placement Records

Approximately 75 percent of Meharry graduates practice in inner city and rural areas where the nation's unmet health needs are concentrated.

Costs

Tuition and fees at Meharry Medical College total approximately $13,300 annually.

Financial Aid

Eighty-five percent of all medical students at Meharry receive financial aid of some kind, which is appropriated on the basis of need. The college maintains a small loan fund from which financial aid may be given. Also, Meharry participates in the Health Professions Student Loan Program. More specific information regarding sources of monetary support can be obtained from the financial aid office.

Curriculum

Meharry Medical College offers two curricular sequences leading to the M.D. degree. The first, the Regular Academic Program, is a four-year combination of basic and clinical science. The second option, the Special Academic Program, offers a five-year curriculum to students pursuing the M.D. In this program, the normal nine-month course of the first year program is extended over 15 months, beginning in June of the summer prior to the regular academic year and ending in August before the beginning of the second year. At this point, students may choose either to transfer to the regular sophomore class or move ahead with a decreased academic load, taking two years to complete the second-year course of study.

Special Programs

The School of Medicine has a Medical Scholars Program, offered jointly by the medical school and the graduate school, in which the student may receive a Master of Science degree as well as the M.D. degree. There is also a joint M.D./Ph.D. program open to students who demonstrate superior research potential prior to entering medical school and conduct sophisticated laboratory research projects in one or more of the basic science areas.

Application Procedures

Students must first submit a general application with the AMCAS. Candidates for admission who pass a preliminary screening process are then required to submit a supplemental application directly to Meharry along with a $25 application fee. The application deadline is January 31 of the year in which admission is sought.

Contact

Office of Admissions and Records
Meharry Medical College
1005 DB Todd Boulevard
Nashville, Tennessee 37208
(615) 327-6223 or (615) 327-6520

MERCER UNIVERSITY SCHOOL OF MEDICINE

1400 Coleman Avenue
Macon, Georgia 31207
(912) 744-2780

Accreditation	LCME
Degrees Offered	M.D.
# Students Applied	585
Enrollment	42 / class
Mean GPA	Not Available
% Men / % Women	50% / 50%
% Minorities	1%
Tuition	$12,960
Application Fee	$25
Application Deadline	December 1

The University

The School of Medicine sees as its mission educating physicians to meet the health care needs of rural and other underserved areas of Georgia. Located in the heart of central Georgia, Macon is a thriving, medium-sized city with museums and parks, and it is within easy reach of Ocmulgee National Monument State Forest and a host of outdoor activities. Macon is within easy driving distance of Atlanta and the beautifully restored Savannah.

Admissions

A faculty committee decides on applicants based on their potential for achievement in medical school and their motivation to meet Mercer's mission. No particular major is prescribed.

Undergraduate Preparation

All students must have completed at least three years of coursework leading to a baccalaureate degree. Mercer requires MCAT scores no more than three years old and taken no later than the fall of the application year. The college requires one year of laboratory courses in biology, general or inorganic chemistry, organic chemistry or biochemistry, and physics.

Student Body

The entering class consists of 42 students.

Placement Records

Graduates of Mercer typically practice primary care

throughout Georgia in family medicine, internal medicine, pediatrics, obstetrics and gynecology, general surgery, and psychiatry.

Costs

Tuition is $12,960 yearly.

Financial Aid

Research efforts are supported at Mercer. Besides institutional support, funds are available to medical students from federal and state grants, foundations, private donors, scholarships, service-payback programs, and loans. About 87 percent of Mercer medical students receive financial aid. Some 23 percent receive funds from mission compliant service-payback programs. For more information write to the office of financial aid.

Curriculum

Students learn the basic sciences for medical practice and then learn to apply them to clinical problems, allowing for new knowledge to be assimilated into the basic science core. Throughout the first two years of training, students begin clinical experiences within the first few weeks of school, in the offices of primary care physicians. Required third-year clerkships include family medicine, internal medicine, obstetrics and gynecology, pediatrics, psychiatry, and surgery. The senior year program includes clerkships in acute/critical care, substance abuse, and community-based primary care medicine. Students may take electives in their chosen area of practice in the senior year.

Facilities

Students work at the Medical Center of Central Georgia, The Center for Health Care, The Family Practice Center, and affiliated hospitals in Macon, Savannah, and Rome.

Application Procedures

Applications must be made through AMCAS. The deadline is December 1. An early decision program is available. Mercer encourages applications from all qualified persons.

Contact

Admissions Office
School of Medicine
Mercer University
Macon, Georgia 31207
(800) 342-0841 (Georgia residents)
(912) 752-2542 (out-of-state)

UNIVERSITY OF MIAMI SCHOOL OF MEDICINE

Miami, Florida 33101
(305) 547-6792

Accreditation	LCME
Degrees Offered	M.D., M.D./Ph.D.
# Students Applied	685
Enrollment	128 / class
Mean GPA	Not Available
% Men / % Women	Not Available
% Minorities	Not Available
Tuition	$18,050
Application Fee	$50
Application Deadline	December 1

The University

The University of Miami School of Medicine, the oldest medical school in the State of Florida, was founded in 1952. The school has grown considerably since its founding, especially in the area of research funding. The school places in the top 10 to 15 percent of all medical schools in terms of biomedical research.

Admissions

The Committee on Admissions evaluates an applicant's scholastic aptitude, integrity, maturity, motivation and activities, both community and academic. Preference is given to residents of Florida. Only a few nonresident candidates are selected. Applicants must be either U.S. citizens or permanent residents of the United States. Applications from women and members of minority and economically disadvantaged groups are welcomed. Those with advanced degrees or those who have worked for several years are also encouraged to apply.

Undergraduate Preparation

Applicants must have completed at least 90 semester hours of college work (not including military science or physical education courses). Only 60 credit hours of junior college credit will be accepted, and most of the required courses must be taken at the senior college level. Courses taken in any special school such as pharmacy, dentistry, or nursing may be accepted toward the hour requirement for admission to medical school. Completion of two semesters of the following courses is required (including necessary laboratory work): English, chemistry, organic chemistry, physics, biology or zoology and other science courses (in the biological sciences, chemistry, physics, or mathematics). A course in biochemistry is strongly recommended. These requirements must be graded credits (advanced placement credit is not applicable for required courses). The Committee on Admissions prefers candidates with a broad educational background. Courses in the humanities and social sciences are recommended. All academic requirements must be completed by August 1 of the year of matriculation.

A limited number of transfer students are accepted to the second and third years of the program. Contact the Admissions Office for further information.

Student Body

Students at the School of Medicine represent a wide variety of backgrounds, age, and experience.

Placement Records

Students obtain the residency positions of their choice in many of the nation's best hospitals.

Costs

Tuition costs per year amount to $18,050, plus $50 for student fees and $1,000 for books and supplies. All fees are subject to change.

Financial Aid

The School of Medicine participates in a variety of federal and state programs. Several tuition scholarships are also awarded through the Scholarship Committee.

Faculty

The 827-member faculty of the School of Medicine combine their teaching responsibilities with patient care and research.

Curriculum

The school emphasizes the importance of small group teaching and communication between students and faculty. Many classes offer a favorable student-faculty ratio. The curriculum is currently being revised to place more emphasis on problem solving, small group learning, computer interactive teaching, extensive early clinic patient contact, and self-paced learning.

The first two years include the basic sciences, as well as early patient contact. Students learn interviewing techniques and are able to follow their patients' progress. The third and fourth years consist of clinical training, including 48 weeks of required clinical rotations as well as 34 weeks of electives. This training is supported by small group conferences. The clinical facilities and large numbers of patients at the UM/JMH Medical Center offer students a wide variety of experiences.

Facilities

The UM-JMH Medical Center includes: the UM School of Medicine's Rosentiel Medical Sciences Building (where teaching facilities are located); the Kathleen and Stanley Glaser Medical Research Building, Jackson Memorial Hospital, which has 1,250 beds; the Veterans Administration Medical Center (870 beds); the Bascom Palmer Eye Institute; the Mailman Center for Child Development; the Magnetic Resonance Imaging Center; the Ambulatory Care Center; the William McKnight Vision Research Institute; the Medical Training and Simulation Laboratory, home of "Harvey," the cardiology patient simulator; the Fox Cancer Research Building and Annex, and the Ronald McDonald House of South Florida. The Sylvester Cancer Clinic and the Gautier Molecular and Biological Research Building are currently under construction. Teaching relationships are maintained with Mount Sinai Medical Center and other private hospitals throughout the country.

The Calder Memorial Library offers a large collection of journals and books and many modern technical materials and services.

Special Programs

A combined M.D./Ph.D. program is available. The program usually is completed in six to seven years. For more information, contact the Physician Scientist Program, (R 123), UM School of Medicine, P.O. Box 016960, Miami, Florida 33101; telephone: (305) 547-6851.

Application Procedures

Applications may be obtained by contacting the Admissions Office from June 1 to December 1 of the year preceding planned enrollment. Candidates are advised to apply early. Completed applications should be received from July 1 to December 31. It is the responsibility of the applicant to be sure that all necessary application materials have been received by the school. There is an application fee of $50. The MCAT is required and should be taken in the spring (or no later than the fall) of the year of application. Interviews are arranged by invitation of the Committee on Admissions.

Contact

Office of Admissions
University of Miami
School of Medicine
P.O. Box 06159
Miami, Florida 33101
(305) 547-6791

MICHIGAN STATE UNIVERSITY COLLEGE OF HUMAN MEDICINE

East Lansing, Michigan 48824-1317
(517) 353-1730

Accreditation	LCME
Degrees Offered	M.D.
# Students Applied	1,958
Enrollment	109 / class
Mean GPA	3.46
% Men / % Women	49% / 51%
% Minorities	23%
Tuition	$7,823 In-State
	$16,823 Out-of-State
Application Fee	$25
Application Deadline	December 1

The University

The College of Human Medicine at Michigan State blends a small class size with the resources of a large university. The college uses 17 affiliated community hospitals to serve as clinical training sites, rather than having a university hospital. MSU is spread over 5,000 acres on what is considered one of the most beautiful campuses in the nation. Crossing throughout the campus are the Red Cedar River and miles of bicycle and foot paths.

Admissions

Selection is based on factors including the GPA and MCAT scores, an autobiographical statement, relevant work experience, and state of residence.

Undergraduate Preparation

The state of Michigan specifies the following requirements for admission: English, nine credits; biological sciences, nine credits (including three hours or five credits of lab); chemistry (inorganic and organic), 12 credits (including three hours or five credits of lab); physics, nine credits including lab; psychology or sociology, nine credits; general nonscience coursework, 27 credits, which can include English and social science requirements. MSU gives preference to candidates who plan to practice in Michigan or other areas with physician shortages, who wish to pursue creative medical scholarship in both research and teaching, and who seek leadership roles in developing and implementing health care programs in Michigan.

Student Body

Eighty percent of the students are from Michigan, due to the fact that MSU is a state-assisted institution. Fifty-one percent of the students are women, 23 percent are minorities.

Costs

Tuition and student fees for the 1989 entering class were $7,823 for residents and $16,823 for nonresidents.

Financial Aid

The Health Professions Unit of the MSU Office of Financial Aid prepares financial aid packages specifically for medical students. Application is made on a yearly basis. Family Financial Statements from American College Testing are distributed to students in January and must be filed by April. Students may then be eligible for institutional grant money and/or government guaranteed loans. The college offers scholarships beginning in the second year. Graduation assistantships are also available. Special financial aid programs exist for underrepresented students.

Minority Programs

The College of Human Medicine offers the Summer Orientation and Retention (SOAR) Program, which includes an introduction to the basic science curriculum and study skills development seminars. The college also offers a postbaccalaureate program, Advanced Baccalaureate Learning Experience (ABLE). Black, Mexican American, mainland Puerto Rican, and Native American students are represented.

Student Organizations

Some of the student organizations represented on campus are the Student Council, the American Medical Student Association, the Minority Medical Student Association, the American Medical Women's Association, and Physicians for Social Responsibility. Student representation is required on all standing committees of the College, involving students in curriculum development, college evaluation, and other internal areas.

Faculty

Students have extensive contact with clinical faculty members, about 2,000 in all, from the community hospital affiliates. Each student chooses a member of the faculty as an advisor. The school has an active mentoring group matching students with faculty.

Curriculum

The curriculum comprises three "Blocks." Blocks I and II (40 and 33 weeks, respectively) make up the preclinical curriculum. Block I explores the fundamental biological, behavioral, and social science concepts and principles. In Block II, advanced concepts are organized in a problem-based format with emphasis on small group instruction and clinical context.

Clinical skills and a clinical correlations course in both blocks expose students to training in real and simulated medical settings, and integrates basic biological and social science information. Block III is a series of required and elective clerkships. This takes place in the student's third and fourth years, in one of the affiliated Michigan communities.

Facilities

The Clinical Center, Life Science Building, and Fee Hall contain the medical school's research facilities and laboratories. Extensive outpatient facilities and specialized clinics are also based in the Clinical Center. Seventeen affiliated community hospitals in six Michigan communities serve as training sites.

Application Procedures

The school will only review applications submitted through the American Medical College Application Service. MCATs must be taken by the fall prior to the year the student plans to matriculate. MCAT scores must appear on the AMCAS application. Students are encouraged, however, to apply before their MCAT results are in. There is an early decision plan for candidates whose first choice is the College of Human Medicine. AMCAS applications should be submitted by August, and notification will be given by October 1. The regular admission process is for students who apply between June 15 and December 1 and who plan to apply to other schools.

Contact

Director of Admissions
College of Human Medicine
A-239 Life Sciences
Michigan State University
East Lansing, Michigan 48824-1317
(517) 353-9620

UNIVERSITY OF MICHIGAN MEDICAL SCHOOL

1301 Catherine Road
Ann Arbor, Michigan 48109-0010
(313) 764-8175

Accreditation	LCME
Degrees Offered	M.D., M.D./Ph.D.
# Students Applied	3,279
Enrollment	170 / class
Mean GPA	3.5
% Men / % Women	Not Available
% Minorities	Not Available
Tuition	$10,000 In-State
	$18,902 Out-of-State
Application Fee	$10
Application Deadline	November 15

The University

The University of Michigan Medical Center ranks as one of the leading medical centers in the nation. Located in Ann Arbor, the center comprises the University of Michigan Medical School and the University of Michigan hospitals. While medical study is the main focal point on the 84-acre campus, cultural and recreational opportunities are also available. From lectures and symposiums to concerts and baseball games, Ann Arbor offers the medical community the unique combination of small-city atmosphere and large-city facilities.

Admissions

All applications are screened by a panel of medical students and faculty members from the basic science and clinic departments. Applicants are evaluated on their talents, skills, interests, and attributes. Candidates who meet the requirements necessary for the successful practice of medicine are then interviewed. This interview permits candidates to emphasize any important points in the application as well as solicit information about the school. The interview also permits the panel to further evaluate the motivation, competence, character, and personal fitness of the candidates.

Undergraduate Preparation

All applicants must have had at least a four-year high school education or its equivalent, as well as at least 90 semester hours of study at a college or university in the United States or Canada. The undergraduate education should include subjects that help to broaden the applicant's background rather then fulfill credits for medical school. These subjects include 11 hours of general inorganic and organic chemistry with at least three hours each of lab work and biochemistry, six hours of biology (including three hours of lab), six hours of physics (including lab work), six hours of English composition and literature, and 18 hours of nonscience courses. A biochemistry placement exam will be given to freshman medical students.

Costs

Tuition for Michigan residents is approximately $10,000 per academic year, while nonresidents pay an annual tuition of approximately $18,902. Additional fees for books, supplies, and lab usage are estimated at $600 for both residents and nonresidents. Living expenses depend on the type of accommodations preferred, but single students should expect to spend approximately $6,000 per year.

Financial Aid

Financial aid, in the form of scholarships, loans, and grants-in-aid, is available to qualified students. The university offers four-year, merit-based scholarships, which can be used to cover tuition and living expenses. Federally sponsored loans, such as National Direct Student Loans and Guaranteed Student Loans, are available to those students who qualify.

Minority Programs

Minorities and financially disadvantaged groups are given serious consideration by the admissions department. Special funds are available for minorities in the form of loans and scholarships. There are also two organizations that help provide strong networking and support for minority students. The medical school offers a Health Careers Opportunity Program for applicants who did not successfully gain admittance to the medical program but are still interested in a medical career.

Curriculum

The standard four-year curriculum begins with the basic science phase. The first year is devoted to the study of normal human biology, such as anatomy, chemistry, human genetics, and physiology. During this time, students will also be introduced to methods of conducting medical interviews and physical examinations.

The second year of the basic science phase is a concentration on disease processes and the correlation between basic science material and patient care. Students attend classes in pathology, microbiology, and pharmacology. By the end of this year, students will be prepared to begin assuming responsibility for patient care in the hospital setting.

In May, at the completion of the second year, students participate in interphase, a two-week course that prepares students for clinical rotation.

The third and fourth years comprise the clinical phase.

This phase consists of 22 four-week periods, with 13 of those weeks spent in junior clerkship. There are eight clerkships, which focus on such varied topics as internal medicine, pediatrics, surgery, and gynecology. These clerkships range from three months to eight weeks.

The remaining nine periods constitute the senior year. Students work with counselors to develop a senior year program pertinent to their individual career goals. Time can be spent in area hospitals while taking academic courses in other schools of the university. This final year gives students the opportunity to explore many medical interests.

Facilities

There are many facilities for medical students at the University of Michigan. The University of Michigan hospitals have a total of 888 beds and treat over one-half million patients, offering students many opportunities for patient contact.

Many research and service units are also available. The Epilepsy Laboratory, the Nuclear Medicine Clinic, and Physical Medicine and Rehabilitation Clinical units are a few of those facilities available for use.

Grading Procedures

The main focus in grading is on professional behavior as well as academic proficiency. At the completion of each course and clerkship, students are given a grade of honors, high pass, pass, marginal fail, or fail. These grades are assessed through observation, practical examinations, and tests of factual knowledge. Narrative evaluations also play a key role in summarizing students' work in the patient care setting. At the beginning of the last academic year, Dean's letters of recommendation are given out to assist students in obtaining resident or internship positions. Students are also required to take both parts of the National Board of Examiners examination as a comprehensive test of their medical and scientific knowledge.

Special Programs

The college offers many special programs. Each of the basic science departments and several of the clinical departments have graduate programs for students working toward master's and doctoral degrees. A student may pursue a dual M.D./Ph.D. degree either as a Fellow in the Medical Scientist Training Program (MSTP) or through an individualized combined degree program. MSTP Fellows usually receive full tuition and fees, plus an annual stipend of at least $8,000; this program typically takes six or seven years to complete. Students in the combined degree program must be admitted to both the medical and graduate schools; financial assistance is available through stipend, scholarship, research fellowships, and loans. A student customarily completes formal education via this route in seven to eight years. Residency programs are conducted to prepare physicians for practice in medical and surgical disciplines. Students also have the opportunity to study in fields allied to medicine such as dentistry, pharmacy, and nursing.

Application Procedures

The University of Michigan Medical School participates in the American Medical College Application Service. Students interested in applying should obtain an application request form from their premedical counselor or participating medical college. The application should be returned to AMCAS by November 15. AMCAS will forward the application as well as the two most recent Medical College Admission Test (MCAT) scores to the university. Upon receipt, the admissions committee will evaluate the application, and those under serious consideration will be asked to forward additional items.

Students interested in applying for early decision will be asked to sign a pledge that they will not apply to any other schools before a decision has been reached. Applicants to the early decision program must have received a bachelor's degree prior to matriculation in medical school. Nonresidents are encouraged to apply through early decision. Applicants should submit their applications by August 1 of the year prior to the year of admission. These applicants will be interviewed during August and September. The committee will make its decision by October 1. Successful applicants will be notified of acceptance. No more than 20 percent of the spaces in the entering class will be filled through the early decision process.

Those applicants who do not apply through the early decision program are free to proceed with the admissions process at other schools and to accept other offers. The students offered positions in the next entering class are required to accept or decline the offer within a specified time. A $100 deposit, refundable until May 1, must accompany acceptance of a position.

Contact

The Committee on Admissions
University of Michigan Medical School
1301 Catherine Road
Ann Arbor, Michigan 48109-0010
(313) 764-6317

UNIVERSITY OF MINNESOTA— DULUTH SCHOOL OF MEDICINE

10 University Drive
Duluth, Minnesota 55812
(218) 726-7571

Accreditation	LCME
Degrees Offered	M.D.
# Students Applied	479
Enrollment	49 / class
Mean GPA	3.4
% Men / % Women	80% / 20%
% Minorities	10%
Tuition	$2,502 In-State (per quarter)
	$5,005 Out-of-State (per quarter)
Application Fee	None
Application Deadline	November 15

The University

The University of Minnesota-Duluth (UMD) became a coordinate campus of the University of Minnesota in 1947. It is administered by a chancellor who reports directly to the president of the university. In 1969, the UMD School of Medicine was established to provide adequate health care facilities and personnel in northern Minnesota and Wisconsin. It is accredited as a free-standing two-year medical school by the Liaison Committee on Medical Education.

The city of Duluth, located on the westernmost shore of Lake Superior, offers many cultural activities, including the Duluth Art Institute, the Duluth Light Opera Company, the Civic Ballet, and the Junior Symphony. The Spirit Mountain ski area, within the city limits, is one of the country's newest and most well-equipped recreational facilities. In addition, many major ski areas, hunting, and fishing sites are located in the area.

Admissions

Preference is given to residents of Minnesota. Applicants who are residents of rural counties of neighboring states are also considered. Other United States residents and citizens of other countries are not considered for admission. The admissions committee considers an applicant's academic record, MCAT scores, letters of evaluation, personal interviews, and supplemental information. The committee also considers motivation, personal characteristics, and background traits that indicate a high potential for becoming a family physician in a small-town rural setting. Applicants accepted to the 1990 entering class had a mean GPA of 3.4. Applicants for advanced standing will not be considered.

Undergraduate Preparation

Applicants must have completed all requirements for a baccalaureate degree by the time of planned matriculation. The following prerequisite courses (including necessary laboratory work for all physical science courses) must be completed by the time of enrollment: general biology, one year; general physics, one year; chemistry, including organic chemistry, one year; English composition, or a combination of courses with a considerable writing component, one year; one semester of mathematics through calculus (differential and integral); eight semester credits of humanities, including at least one upper-division course; and eight semester credits of behavioral sciences, including at least one upper-division course. Applicants are encouraged to pursue interests in nonscience areas.

Student Body

Approximately 95 percent of students attending the School of Medicine are Minnesota residents. Women make up about 20 percent of the student body.

Costs

Tuition for resident students amounts to $2,502 per quarter; for nonresidents, $5,005 per quarter. Student fees of about $111 per quarter are required for residents and nonresidents. Textbooks cost approximately $250 to $300 per year, and the cost of supplies for first-year medical students amounts to approximately $325 to $400.

Financial Aid

Financial aid is available from a variety of federal, state, and private offices, including the Minnesota Medical Foundation, which offers scholarship aid based solely on need. With few exceptions, only students who are accepted for admission and are regularly enrolled qualify for financial aid. Most financial assistance is administered by the university's office of financial aid or by the Minnesota Medical Foundation. Students are strongly discouraged from seeking outside employment while enrolled at the School of Medicine.

Minority Programs

Native Americans into Medicine (NAM) is a six-week summer program that enables Native American undergraduate students to accurately assess their motivation for medicine. For more information, contact the Co-Director, American Indian Programs, 112 School of Medicine, University of Minnesota—Duluth, 10 University Drive, Duluth, MN 55812.

Student Organizations

Medical students have representatives to national organizations, including the Association of American Medical Colleges and the American Medical Student Association.

Faculty

There are approximately 45 full-time basic and clinical science faculty members. Part-time voluntary clinical science faculty includes over 280 area physicians representing all the major medical specialties.

Curriculum

During the two years at the School of Medicine in Duluth, students study the basic, behavioral, and clinical sciences in preparation for continuing studies in Minneapolis. Transfer to the Medical School in Minneapolis is guaranteed upon successful completion of the program in Duluth. The first year includes instruction in the basic sciences, which is correlated, whenever possible, with clinical instruction. The second year consists of clinical material which is again correlated with the basic science presentations and behavioral sciences. During this year, students spend more time in clinical settings and receive more intensive didactic instruction in clinical medicine.

During both years, students participate in the family practice preceptorship program. In the first year, each student is assigned to a family practitioner, who introduces him or her to the practice of medicine. The second-year preceptorship involves the student with physicians who practice in rural areas of northern Minnesota and Wisconsin.

Facilities

In 1979, the UMD School of Medicine moved into a new building that houses classrooms, seminar rooms, teaching and research laboratories, faculty and administrative offices, and the Learning Resources Center. The School of Medicine is affiliated with St. Luke's Hospital and Miller Dwan and St. Mary's medical centers of Duluth, giving students access to patients from the northern regions of Minnesota, Wisconsin, and Michigan.

The UMD Health Science Library, a department library within the campus library system, is one of 30 resource libraries in the greater Midwest regional medical library network. The Health Science Library contains more than 66,000 books and bound journal volumes, subscribes to 600 current English language medical journals and over 60 other serials in the biomedical sciences, and covers the basic and clinical sciences and their specialties. Computer information retrieval, as well as computer searching of medical databases such as MEDLINE, TOXLINE, and CANCERLIT, is also available. The general campus library contains more than 405,000 volumes and is a selective depository for federal documents, particularly those in the biomedical subject areas.

On-campus housing is available.

Grading Procedures

Grades are reported as O (outstanding), E (excellent), S (satisfactory), I (incomplete), or N (no credit).

Application Procedures

The UMD School of Medicine participates in the American Medical College Application Service (AMCAS). The AMCAS application should be completed and returned to AMCAS after June 15 and no later than November 15 of the year preceding planned enrollment. The new MCAT is required and should be taken by the spring of the year preceding planned enrollment. Applicants must also request that transcripts be sent to AMCAS. Applicants who are being considered for admission will then receive a request for supplemental information from the School of Medicine. A supplemental application form, a personal history, a prerequisite coursework form, and letters of evaluation must be mailed to the college. Applicants who receive favorable evaluations will be invited to come to the school for two personal interviews.

The School of Medicine participates in the early decision plan (EDP).

Contact

Office of Admission, Room 107
University of Minnesota-Duluth
School of Medicine
10 University Drive
Duluth, Minnesota 55812
(800) 762-1262

UNIVERSITY OF MINNESOTA MEDICAL SCHOOL—MINNEAPOLIS

420 Delaware Street SE
Minneapolis, Minnesota 55455-0310
(612) 626-4949

Accreditation	LCME
Degrees Offered	M.D., M.D./Ph.D.
# Students Applied	1,409
Enrollment	180 / class
Mean GPA	3.44
% Men / % Women	54% / 46%
% Minorities	Not Available
Tuition	$2,379 In-State (per quarter)
	$4,647 Out-of-State (per quarter)
Application Fee	None
Application Deadline	November 15

The University

The University of Minnesota Medical School is located centrally in the Twin Cities of Minneapolis and St. Paul. The School of Medicine was founded in 1888 and now enrolls nearly 900 students. The Twin Cities is a major metropolitan area near nature and wildlife.

Admissions

The Medical School considers undergraduate GPA and MCAT scores, but states that "neither high grades nor high MCAT scores alone are adequate to gain admission." The school also evaluates ethical standards, motivation, intellectual curiosity, ability to work with other professionals, and ability to deal with the ill.

Undergraduate Preparation

Although a bachelor's degree is required for admission, the admissions committee has no preference regarding an undergraduate's major. The Medical School does require candidates to have taken general courses in biology, inorganic chemistry, organic chemistry, physics (including labs in each), one year of introductory calculus, one year of courses in English literature, and at least 18 semester credits in the social and behavioral sciences and humanities.

Costs

Annual first-year tuition and fees total $11,440 for Minnesota residents and $22,440 for nonresidents. Second-, third-, and fourth-year tuition and fees for residents are $8,580, $11,440, and $5,942, respectively; for nonresidents, $16,830, $22,400, and $11,442. The Medical School estimates that annual living costs, including books and supplies, room and board, local transportation, and medical and personal expenses, will average $10,222 for both residents and nonresidents.

Financial Aid

The Medical School participates in several federal, state, and institutional loan and grant programs and offers several scholarships on the basis of merit and/or need. The school provides a number of student research grants for vacation or free time work in several medical departments through the Minnesota Medical Foundation (MMF). The MMF also offers loans (averaging $1,000) in coordination with the Medical School. The MMF makes awards of $1,000 to students of exceptional accomplishment in academics, community service, or student leadership.

Minority Programs

The Medical School awards two minority scholarships annually. Minority students may also gain financial aid through the University's central administration. Minority student facilities at the University of Minnesota include the Women's Center, International Student Association, and Asian-American Student Cultural Center.

Student Organizations

Student organizations include medical organizations such as the national honor medical society, Alpha Omega Alpha. The Medical Student Council, composed of representatives from each class and from several minority groups, presents medical students' interests to the administration and faculty and enforces an honor code covering medical exams.

Faculty

The Medical School staffs 900 full-time faculty.

Curriculum

M.D. candidates must complete 14 quarters of study over four years. During the first two years of study, students take courses in basic and behavioral sciences (anatomy, biochemistry, physiology, pharmacology, microbiology, pathology), with some introduction to clinical work; in the final two years, students do mostly clinical work and coursework in hospitals, clinics, and offices. The curriculum has recently added courses in medical ethics, health care economics, preventive medicine, and new health care systems. Most clinical training takes place in Twin Cities hospitals.

Facilities

Facilities include the University Hospital, Variety Club Heart Hospital, Masonic Cancer Center, Veterans of Foreign Wars Cancer Research Center, and Children's Rehabilitation Center. The University of Minnesota Hospital and Clinic treats 210,000 outpatients and 18,000 inpatients daily, more than half of which come from outside the Twin Cities. The Biomedical Library holds over 400,000 volumes and periodicals. The Learning Resources Center offers models, viewing areas for motion pictures and videotapes, and microcomputers. Two departmental libraries supplement the Biomedical Library.

Grading Procedures

Grades are reported as O (outstanding), E (excellent), S (satisfactory), I (incomplete), and N (no credit). Students are graded with examinations and written evaluations.

Special Programs

Students may pursue a six- to seven-year joint M.D./Ph.D. program in medicine and a basic science. The Medical School's advanced admission program enables undergraduate sophomores with a GPA of at least 3.75 to gain admission to the Medical School upon satisfactory completion of the undergraduate degree.

Application Procedures

Students must apply through AMCAS between June 15 and November 15 of the calendar year preceding entry into the Medical School. It is strongly suggested that students take the MCAT in the spring before applying. The University of Minnesota does not ordinarily consider transfer applications from other schools but is required to accept transfer applications from the accredited two-year branch of the University of Minnesota Medical School in Duluth.

Contact

University of Minnesota Medical School
Office of Admissions and Student Affairs
Box 293
420 Delaware Street SE
Minneapolis, Minnesota 55455-0310
(612) 624-1188

UNIVERSITY OF MISSISSIPPI SCHOOL OF MEDICINE

2500 North State Street
Jackson, Mississippi 39216-4505
(601) 984-1010

Accreditation	AMA, AAMC
Degrees Offered	M.D.
# Students Applied	462
Enrollment	100 / class
Mean GPA	3.6
% Men / % Women	Not Available
% Minorities	Not Available
Tuition	$6,000 In-State
	$12,000 Out-of-State
Application Fee	None
Application Deadline	December 1

The University

The University of Mississippi Medical Center is located on a 155-acre campus in the heart of Jackson. It comprises the schools of dentistry, medicine, nursing, health-related professions, graduate studies in the medical sciences, and the University Hospital.

Admissions

The first evaluation of candidates for admission is made on the basis of academic records and MCAT scores. Applicants who are favorably evaluated are then considered on the basis of character, motivation, and promise of fitness for the practice of medicine. Applicants must have three years (90 semester hours) of undergraduate coursework; however, preference is given to those who hold bachelor's degrees. The MCAT should be taken in the spring of the year preceding the year of enrollment.

Strong preference is given to Mississippi residents.

Undergraduate Preparation

Required courses include eight semester hours each of biology or zoology, inorganic chemistry, organic chemistry, and physics, all with lab; and six semester hours of English, mathematics (including at least one semester each of college algebra and trigonometry), and advanced science.

Costs

Tuition for Mississippi residents is $6,000 per year (non-residents pay $12,000 per year). This includes registration fee, laboratory charges, and library fees. There is an activity fee of $55 per year.

Financial Aid

The School of Medicine offers a limited number of merit scholarships. Loans and assistance from various federally sponsored programs are also available. Further information can be obtained from the Division of Student Services and Records.

Curriculum

The first two years of study consist of basic courses in the sciences. Third-year rotations include family medicine, obstetrics-gynecology, pediatrics, psychiatry, medicine, and surgery. The students select clerkships in the senior year for further intensive study. A unique feature of the curriculum is the Introduction to Clinical Medicine course, which is taught during the last six weeks of sophomore year. This course is designed to prepare students for work with patients in a clinical setting.

Facilities

The main teaching facility is the 531-bed University Hospital.

Application Procedures

Applications are made through AMCAS. Completed applications must be received by AMCAS between June 15 and December 1 of the year preceding the desired date of admission (deadline for early decision is August 1).

Contact

University of Mississippi Medical Center
Division of Student Services and Records
2500 North State Street
Jackson, Mississippi 39216-4505
(601) 984-5010

UNIVERSITY OF MISSOURI— COLUMBIA SCHOOL OF MEDICINE

Columbia, Missouri 65211
(314) 882-1566

Accreditation	LCME
Degrees Offered	M.D., M.D./M.S., M.D./Ph.D.
# Students Applied	789
Enrollment	110 / class
Mean GPA	3.4
% Men / % Women	49% / 51%
% Minorities	6%
Tuition	$7,130 In-State
	$11,165 Out-of-State
Application Fee	None
Application Deadline	November 15

The University

Founded in 1872, the University of Missouri-Columbia School of Medicine was originally a two-year medical institution. In 1956, the school began to offer a four-year program. The University Hospital and Clinics draw patients from all areas of Missouri. The atmosphere at the university is a blend of academics, social activities, and cultural events.

Admissions

Preference is given to residents of Missouri, although a limited number of well-qualified nonresidents are considered. The admissions committee evaluates an applicant's academic qualifications as well as nonacademic attributes, such as motivation, maturity, and leadership. The successful applicant usually has a GPA above 3.35, and most score eight or above in each subject area of the MCAT.

Undergraduate Preparation

Applicants must have completed a minimum of 90 semester hours of coursework (excluding physical education and military science) at an accredited college or university. This coursework must include English composition (two semesters), two semesters of college algebra and trigonometry, eight semester hours of general biology with lab, six semester hours of advanced biology, eight semester hours of organic chemistry with lab, eight semester hours of inorganic chemistry with lab, and eight semester hours of general physics with lab. Students are encouraged to pursue a strong foundation in the humanities and are also encouraged to develop their communication skills. Students should try to avoid overlapping undergraduate courses with medical school courses.

Student Body

Fifty-one percent of the entering class of 1990 were women, six percent were minorities.

Placement Records

Seventy-five percent of graduates receive their first or second choice of specialties and residency programs (60 percent receive their first choice).

Costs

Tuition for resident students is $7,130 per year; for non-residents, $11,165.

Financial Aid

Financial aid is available from federal, state, and private sources. The university provides loans to students on the basis of need. Financial aid forms are mailed with the notice of acceptance. Emergency loans are also available.

Minority Programs

The school is committed to recruiting minority, disadvantaged, and nontraditional applicants. Interested applicants should review the chapter "Information for Minority Group Students" in the AAMC publication *Medical School Admission Requirements*, and may wish to submit their names to AAMC's medical minority registry.

Student Organizations

Organizations of interest to medical students include the local chapter of the American Medical Student Association, the Student National Medical Association, the American Medical Women's Association, Alpha Omega Alpha, the Christian Medical Society, and the UMC Medical Student Section. The Organization of Student Representatives encourages student participation in the advancement of medical education, biomedical research, and health care.

Faculty

There are approximately 290 faculty members in the clinical and basic science departments, and 300 residents in 46 specialties and subspecialties.

Curriculum

Students have the opportunity to work with a wide variety of patients who are referred to the health-sciences complex from throughout the entire state. The basic sciences are taught during the first two years. Students also gain experience in interviewing patients and diagnosing illnesses. During the third year, students gain clinical experience while caring for patients at the health sciences complex, and work with a family practice physician in a rural area during a four-week preceptorship. The fourth year consists of 24 weeks of electives, including rotations in ambulatory care, critical care, or emergency medicine; chronic rehabilitative or geriatric care; and medical and surgical subspecialties. Electives are offered in a variety of subjects and settings. Students have many opportunities to take part in collaborative interdisciplinary research.

Facilities

The University Hospital features a helicopter emergency service that transports patients to its facilities, which include neonatal and pediatric intensive-care units and mid-Missouri's only Level 1 trauma center. The health-sciences complex also contains the University Clinics, Rusk Rehabilitation Center, Mid-Missouri Mental Health Center, Truman Veteran's Hospital, Cosmopolitan International Diabetes Center, and the Mason Institute of Ophthalmology. The school is affiliated with many other hospitals in the state.

The university's research reactor supplies radioactive isotopes for medical research and cancer treatment. Medical student education and residency training are given in the health-sciences complex.

The J. Otto Lottes Health Sciences Library contains more than 167,000 volumes. It regularly receives more than 1,900 periodicals and most of the indexes and abstracts pertaining to medicine and related fields. Through MEDLINE, the library also provides access to all National Library of Medicine databases.

Grading Procedures

Students must pass Part I of the NBME to be promoted to the third year of study. Part II must be passed in order to graduate. A five-level grading system is supplemented by narrative commentary from faculty.

Special Programs

The School of Medicine offers a combined M.D./M.S. degree or a combined M.D./Ph.D. degree. Graduate studies offered include anatomy, biochemistry, microbiology, and pathology. The program is usually completed in six to eight years.

Application Procedures

The School of Medicine participates in the American Medical College Application Service (AMCAS). Applications should be received by AMCAS after June 15 but no later than November 15 of the year preceding planned enrollment. The new MCAT is required. Each applicant must submit a letter of recommendation from his or her premedical advisory committee or from three former professors. Nonacademic and personal letters of recommendation also help the admissions committee. The admissions committee invites approximately 40 percent of all applicants for interviews. The School of Medicine participates in the early decision program. Applicants

not accepted as early decision candidates may apply to other schools as a regular candidate.

Contact

Office of Student Affairs
School of Medicine
MA 202 Medical Sciences Building
University of Missouri-Columbia
Columbia, Missouri 65212
(314) 882-2923

UNIVERSITY OF MISSOURI— KANSAS CITY SCHOOL OF MEDICINE

4825 Troost
Kansas City, Missouri 64110
(816) 276-1800

Accreditation	LCME
Degrees Offered	M.D., B.A.
# Students Applied	455
Enrollment	102 / class
Mean GPA	Not Available
% Men / % Women	45% / 55%
% Minorities	Not Available
Tuition	$10,990 In-State
	$14,960 Out-of-State
Application Fee	$25 In-State, $50 Out-of-State
Application Deadline	December 1

The University

The University of Missouri-Kansas City School of Medicine was founded in 1971 with a unique educational concept at its core. Instead of first attending four years of college at the undergraduate level and then proceeding to a separate four-year M.D. program, students in the UMKC medical program combine their undergraduate and medical training work in a six-year sequence of intensive study. Since its inception, the Kansas City program has graduated over 1,000 students.

Kansas City has a wealth of leisure time activities to offer, many within a medical student's budget. Crown Center offers free festivals and events, and on Sunday afternoons the Nelson-Atkins Museum of Art charges no admission. Loose Park, site of a historic Civil War battle, is a scenic place for jogging, kite flying, and picnicking; the 12-block-square shopping plaza welcomes window shoppers; and Westport Square is where nightlife happens in Kansas City.

Admissions

Students apply to the medical school directly from high school. Applicants must submit high school transcripts and ACT scores. Because of the early application procedure, the MCAT is not required. Missouri residents receive admissions preference, although applicants from out of state are regularly accepted.

Undergraduate Preparation

A strong high school background in science, including courses in biology, chemistry, physics, and mathematics, is recommended. Personal qualities, such as leadership, stamina, reliability, motivation for medicine, interpersonal skills, and previous work experience, are also considered.

Placement Records

Many students continue their postgraduate training at Truman Medical Center, the main teaching hospital of UMKC, as well as at other affiliated hospitals in the Kansas City area.

Costs

Tuition and fees vary depending on how far a student has progressed through the six-year M.D. sequence. During the first two years, annual tuition for residents is $10,990, while nonresidents pay $14,960 annually. Room and board during these years is estimated at $3,730 for all students. In years three through six, in-state tuition is $11,415, while out-of-state students pay $17,225. Room and board during these years is approximately $5,775. Books and supplies are estimated to cost $580 during each of the six years of the M.D. program.

Financial Aid

The School of Medicine offers a variety of academic scholarships based on scholastic excellence rather than financial need. However, the financial aid office also assists students in obtaining state- and federally-funded grants, scholarships, and loans on the basis of financial need.

Student Organizations

Extracurricular groups available to students at the School of Medicine include the Medical Student Advisory Council, the Student National Medical Association, the American Medical Women's Association, and the American Medical Student Association.

Curriculum

Curriculum at the School of Medicine is structured around something called the "docent system." With this approach, first-year students are grouped into teams of students and faculty members led by one coordinating faculty member, the "docent." This group remains the focal point of the student's learning activity through the six-year M.D. program. Coursework is flexible due to the integration of undergraduate studies with medical training. The curriculum allows students to design an educational approach that best suits their interests and needs. Generally speaking, however, year one includes an introduction to basic medical vocabulary and skills, the concept of a career in the health professions, and medical ethics and philosophy. Year two introduces the student to the clinical environment as well as reinforces basic medical sciences and the undergraduate coursework. During the final four years of the M.D program, the student focuses on more traditional medical subjects, including clerkships and a preceptorship, while also taking undergraduate liberal arts courses.

Facilities

Perhaps the most unique facility of the School of Medicine are the personal "offices" issued to all students in the final four years of the M.D. program. These spaces are open to students for study and personal use 24 hours a day and are in close proximity to labs, discussion rooms, computer terminals, and testing sites. The School of Medicine also offers students the Audiovisual Medical Library, a collection of over 3,000 audiotapes, models, films, slides, and videotapes (but no books). The Academic Development Center provides tutoring, supplemental teaching sessions, individual counseling, and special workshops in response to student needs and interests. The university is affiliated with 10 different hospitals in the Kansas City area.

Grading Procedures

Students are evaluated within their docent teams by their docent through written comments and on the basis of objective examinations. Passing scores in Parts I and II of the National Board Examination are required for graduation.

Special Programs

Medical students may select an undergraduate area of concentration or major. Ninety semester hours of nonmedical liberal arts courses must be completed (30 semester hours toward this degree are awarded toward medical courses), including courses in English, fine arts, government, history, humanities, literature, natural science, philosophy, physical education, and social/behavioral science. The students receive both a baccalaureate and M.D. degree.

Application Procedures

Students must submit application materials, including high school transcripts and ACT scores, between August 1 and December 1 of the year prior to desired entrance into the six-year M.D. program. After an initial evaluation, certain well-qualified applicants are invited to on-campus, personal interviews. A $25 application fee is required of Missouri residents, while nonresidents pay a $50 application fee.

Contact

Admissions Office
University of Missouri-Kansas City
4825 Troost
Kansas City, Missouri 64110-2499
(816) 235-1111

MOREHOUSE SCHOOL OF MEDICINE

720 Westview Drive, S.W.
Atlanta, Georgia 30310-9814
(404) 752-1500

Accreditation	LCME, SACS, AAMC
Degrees Offered	M.D.
# Students Applied	1,250
Enrollment	33 / class
Mean GPA	Not Available
% Men / % Women	48% / 52%
% Minorities	97%
Tuition	$12,700
Application Fee	$40
Application Deadline	December 1

The University

After becoming independent of its parent school, Morehouse College, Morehouse School of Medicine (MSM) is now a four-year degree-granting institution fully accredited by the LCME and the SACS, and is a member of the AAMC. The National Medical Association endorsed the development of the new school of medicine (1973) to help resolve the critical health-services shortage in Georgia as well as in medically underserved areas of the nation. MSM is the newest member of the Atlanta University Center, a consortium of six independent institutions constituting the largest predominantly black private educational complex in the world. Located in the heart of Atlanta, MSM has access to all the social and cultural amenities of a growing urban center.

Admissions

Students from Georgia, New York, and Alabama are given high priority. The MCAT is required, and applicants are urged to take it in the spring of the calendar year before the year of entry. Applicants may take the test again. The ability to finance a medical education is not a factor in student selection. Approximately 15 to 20 percent of all applicants will be asked to visit MSM for interviews.

Undergraduate Preparation

Most entering students will have completed a four-year undergraduate degree. MSM admits a few well-qualified students who complete 90 semester hours or 135 quarter hours in the arts and sciences. Undergraduate study must include one year each (with laboratory) of biology, general and organic chemistry, and physics. One year of college-level mathematics and English are also required. MSM prefers standard grading, not pass/fail, in undergraduate marking systems.

Student Body

The entering class size is 33. For the class of 1994, 48 percent were male and 52 percent female. Minorities constitute 97 percent of the accepted entering class. All together, the school enrolls 140 medical students. About 70 percent of the students come from Georgia, but the rest are from a wide geographical area. The Graduate Medical Education Program enrolls 15 residents; the Preventive Medicine Residency enrolls six.

Placement Records

MSM alumni have obtained appointments in hospital residency training programs affiliated with some of the nation's most prestigious medical schools, from Baylor, Columbia, and Tulane to Emory, Drew/UCLA, Howard, and the Mayo Clinic. Of the 234 graduates of MSM, 110 have completed their residencies and begun practice. Over 90 percent are located either in inner cities or rural areas, and about 75 percent practice primary care medicine.

Costs

For the 1990-91 academic year, tuition was $12,700. Associated fees total $1,270, not including the $100 acceptance deposit. The medical school does not have student housing. Inquire at the fiscal affairs office for available city housing.

Financial Aid

Students who have documented financial need that cannot be met by family and personal resources may apply for scholarships, loans, grants, and student employment. The fiscal affairs office assists students in preparing financial aid applications. Approximately 92 percent of MSM students receive some form of financial aid during part or all of their four years of study. About 46 school scholarships and six academic prizes and awards are available. The financial aid prospectus distributed to interviewed applicants offers full information.

Minority Programs

The Morehouse School of Medicine is the first predominantly black medical institution established in the United States in the 20th century; it is one of only four in the country. The school actively supports the education of minority groups regardless of race, ethnic origin, handicap, sex, or nationality.

Student Organizations

Besides the Student Government Association, active organizations at MSM include the Student National Medical Association, Medical Student Section of the AMA, Student American Medical Association, Family Practice Interest Group, American Medical Women's Association, Alpha Omega Alpha honor medical society, and the Pre-alumni Association.

Faculty

The faculty consists of 90 full-time faculty supplemented by 30 part-time members and 100 physician volunteers. The faculty/student ratio is approximately 1/2. Faculty members continue to compete successfully for research and training grants from a host of federal and private agencies.

Curriculum

The first year covers the basic medical sciences and includes clinical preceptorships, anatomy, biochemistry, physiology, human values in medicine, neurobiology, human behavior, and community medicine and family health. The second year, which begins in mid-August, includes coursework in clinical medicine and concludes after 10 months with Part I of the National Board of Medical Examiners test. The third year includes surgery, psychiatry, family practice, obstetrics and gynecology, internal medicine, and pediatrics. The fourth year comprises four required clerkships and five electives.

Facilities

The Basic Medical Sciences Building, where most instruction in basic sciences takes place, is a 91,000-square-foot facility. The newly completed 70,000-square-foot Medical Education Building is attached to the basic sciences building and has effectively doubled the size of the library. An additional nearby structure of about 30,000 square feet has repair shops and central stores. Area hospitals and clinics affiliated with the school provide facilities for clinical instruction.

Grading Procedures

MSM uses a letter grading system.

Special Programs

Morehouse offers three residency programs accredited by the ACGME—family practice (three years), preventive medicine (one year), and psychiatry (four years)—and currently enrolls 15 students. Some joint programs at Clark Atlanta University and Georgia State University are available for graduate students who wish to pursue the Ph.D. and work with qualified MSM faculty. Individual courses and continuing medical education (AMA category 1 credit) are available.

Application Procedures

First-year applications must be submitted through AMCAS. The School of Medicine begins accepting applications June 15 of the year prior to enrollment. The deadline for all credentials is December 1 of the year before admission. The fee is $40. After evaluation, an interview may follow. Early decision admissions are possible by October 1 if the applicant applies to Morehouse only. Within two weeks after acceptance, applicants must submit a letter of intent. A $100 reservation deposit is then required.

Contact

Morehouse School of Medicine
Office of Admissions and Student Affairs
720 Westview Drive, S.W.
Atlanta, Georgia 30310-9814
(404) 752-1650

MOUNT SINAI SCHOOL OF MEDICINE OF THE CITY UNIVERSITY OF NEW YORK

One Gustave L. Levy Place
New York, New York 10029
(212) 241-6500

Accreditation	LCME
Degrees Offered	M.D., M.D./Ph.D.
# Students Applied	2,323
Enrollment	115 / class
Mean GPA	3.4
% Men / % Women	53% / 47%
% Minorities	39%
Tuition	$16,000
Application Fee	$50
Application Deadline	November 1

The University

The Mount Sinai School of Medicine, incorporated in 1963, is an integral part of the Mount Sinai Medical Center, which was founded in 1852. The medical center occupies a four-block area on upper Fifth Avenue across from Central Park in Manhattan. The school is an affiliate of the City University of New York but is financially autonomous and self-supporting under its own Board of Trustees.

Mount Sinai was one of the first general hospitals in the nation to establish a School of Nursing and a program of postgraduate medical instruction. Members of the hospital's staff instructed students at other medical schools for more than 50 years before the medical school was established.

Admissions

Candidates must be capable of meeting the physical and emotional demands of the medical curriculum. An undergraduate degree from an accredited college or university is recommended, although exceptionally well-qualified students will be admitted after having completed three years of undergraduate work. Applicants are required to take the MCAT test.

Undergraduate Preparation

Minimum subject requirements are one year (including necessary laboratory work) of inorganic chemistry, organic chemistry, biology, college-level mathematics, English, and physics.

Students majoring in nonscience disciplines who meet the basic requirements above are encouraged to apply. Facility in oral and written communication is expected of all students.

Costs

Annual tuition for both residents and nonresidents is $16,000; fees total approximately $800; room and board, $6,500; books and supplies, $1,000; and microscope rental, $200. Total expenditures for all students are estimated at $24,500.

Financial Aid

Admission to the School of Medicine is completely independent of financial requirements or status. Students who wish to apply for financial aid must submit information to the Graduate and Professional School Financial Aid Service (GAPSFAS). The service provides graduate and professional schools with complete financial data on each student so that each applicant can be reviewed individually. Some loans and awards are given through the university, others are granted from a variety of federal, state, and private offices. During the 1987-88 academic year, financial aid was awarded to 288 students. Part-time positions may be available, but the school does not encourage outside employment, as this may interfere with academic performance.

Minority Programs

Strongly motivated students from underrepresented minority and educationally deprived backgrounds are encouraged

to apply. A pre-entrance summer program is available for students accepted to the freshman class.

Student Organizations

Student organizations include Alpha Omega Alpha and the Student Council. Students are represented on the Faculty Council Committees, Committees of the Dean and the Board of Trustees, and the Committee on Student Affairs.

Curriculum

The close interrelation of the basic sciences with clinical medicine is emphasized. The first two years can be divided into two periods. During the first period, the language and principles of the basic sciences are emphasized. The second-period courses consist of pharmacology, pathology, and interdepartmental teaching of organ systems or clinical disciplines, including early exposure to clinical medicine. First-year students are required to take a minimum of 87 hours of elective time. A minimum of 105 hours of elective time is required for second-year students.

The third- and fourth-year programs permit more intensive study of organ system diseases through direct patient contact. Students rotate through various specialties in clinical and community medicine. There is a required rotation in geriatric medicine. A large portion of the fourth year is devoted to electives, which may be taken at the School of Medicine or any formal or informal educational setting approved by the department chairman and the Dean for Student Affairs.

Facilities

The basic science departments and many clinical departments are housed at the medical center, as is student housing. The complex also includes the Annenberg Building, which contains first- and second-year teaching facilities including 128 individual work and study multidisciplinary laboratories; the Division of Environment and Occupational Medicine, where extensive research is conducted in chemical carcinogens, environmental pollutants, and industrial health hazards; and the Gustave and Janet W. Levy Library, which contains over 140,000 bound volumes, 2,500 audiovisuals, and 2,000 current journals. Also available are a wide variety of databases.

The hospital has established numerous programs for diagnosis and treatment including the Gerald H. Ruttenberg Cancer Center, the Lucy Moses Cardiothoracic Center, and a Clinical Genetics Center. Mount Sinai patients are drawn from the surrounding community, the rest of the nation, and many foreign communities. Mount Sinai's facilities also include a coronary intensive care unit (ICU), a neonatal ICU, a surgical ICU, modern radioactive scanning equipment, a 36-bed cancer center, a hematology center, and a leukemia research lab, among many other facilities and programs.

Grading Procedures

The school uses a pass-fail grading system for the first two years and an honors-pass-fail system for the last two years. Student evaluation in clinical courses emphasizes performance in the clinic and at the bedside, as well as performance on objective examinations. All students are required to pass Part I of the NBME for promotion to the third year and Part II as a requirement for graduation.

Special Programs

Approximately 40 students are enrolled in the Medical Sciences Training Program, a combined M.D./Ph.D. training program. Applicants interested in this program should indicate this on the medical school admission supplemental form. The school also offers an honors research track.

Application Procedures

The Mount Sinai School of Medicine participates in the American Medical College Application Service (AMCAS). Applicants should file their AMCAS application no later than November 1. Upon receipt of the AMCAS application, the Mount Sinai School of Medicine will request additional information. A letter of recommendation from the applicant's college premedical advisory committee is required (individual faculty recommendations are acceptable only if there is no premedical advisory committee at the applicant's college). Interviews are required.

Transfer students who have completed one or two years of medical school at an approved school and are in good academic standing are eligible for admission at advanced standing. Formal applications should be filed between January 1 and April 30.

Contact

Office of Admissions
Mount Sinai School of Medicine
Room 5-04 Annenberg Building
Box 1002
One Gustave L. Levy Place
New York, New York 10029
(212) 241-6696

UNIVERSITY OF NEBRASKA COLLEGE OF MEDICINE

600 South 42nd Street
Omaha, Nebraska 68198
(402) 554-2800

Accreditation	LCME
Degrees Offered	M.D., M.D./Ph.D.
# Students Applied	925
Enrollment	126 / class
Mean GPA	3.53
% Men / % Women	65% / 35%
% Minorities	Not Available
Tuition	$7,028 In-State
	$12,640 Out-of-State
Application Fee	None
Application Deadline	November 15

The University

In 1980, the College of Medicine celebrated its centennial year. Students began attending Omaha Medical College in 1880. To expand its scope and utility, the college merged with the University of Nebraska in 1902. Omaha is a sprawling, western urban center with a population of about 320,000. The largest city in the state, it offers attractions including the Henry Doorly Zoo, the Old Market Shopping Area, Opera/ Omaha, the Omaha Symphony, Omaha Royals AAA baseball, the College World Series, the Joslyn Art Museum, the Omaha Community Playhouse, and an extensive parks and recreation system.

Admissions

Students must take the MCAT and submit scores for consideration. Applicants for admission in 1992 are advised to submit scores from the 1991 MCAT test. The GPA of the 1990-91 class was 3.5 overall. The admissions committee will not accept pass-fail grades. Advanced placement and CLEP Subject Examination credit are accepted. Preference is given to residents. Foreign students with a permanent resident visa are considered for admission. The university offers transfer or advanced standing only to students attending medical schools that are accredited by the Liaison Committee on Medical Education. The deadline date for application with advanced standing is May 15.

Undergraduate Preparation

Students must have a minimum of 90 semester hours at an accredited college. However, completing an undergraduate degree is strongly recommended. The undergraduate program should include one year each of biology, inorganic chemistry, organic chemistry, and physics, all with lab.

Two years each of humanities and social sciences are also required. Courses in English composition/writing and introductory calculus or statistics are expected. Students are encouraged to study a well-rounded curriculum.

Student Body

Out of 925 applicants in 1990-91, 210 were Nebraska residents and 715 were from out of state. Of these, 126 were accepted for the entering class, of which 112 were residents and 14 were from outside Nebraska. Sixty-five percent of the applicants were male and 35 percent were female. For the entering class, 65 percent were men and 35 percent were women.

Placement Records

In the past six years, 65-70 percent of graduates have received their first choice of residency placement. Ninety percent of graduates have received one of their top three choices.

Costs

Tuition for the 1989 first year class was $7,028 for residents and $12,640 for nonresidents. Student fees were estimated at $645.

Financial Aid

Some scholarships based on academic achievement are available each year. A few are awarded to entering students. About 60 percent of the students receive some financial aid. In recent years, no student in good academic standing has been denied aid.

Minority Programs

The College of Medicine is committed to increasing the number of physicians who are from ethnic groups underrepresented in the health professions. Applications are encouraged from Black Americans, American Indians, mainland Puerto Ricans, and Mexican Americans. If tutorial assistance is deemed necessary or required, it will be provided by the college. For more information contact the Minority Student Affairs Officer.

Student Organizations

Student organizations on campus include the Medical Center Student Senate, the Organization of Student Representatives, the American Medical Student Senate, the Student National Medical Association, the Student Association for Rural Health, and Alpha Omega Alpha.

Faculty

There are approximately 395 full-time faculty members, 20 part-time members, and 1,071 volunteer faculty, representing more than 50 specialty and subspecialty disciplines.

Curriculum

The first and second years include the teaching of the basic sciences and clinical science. Courses on the legal and ethical issues of medicine are introduced. The third year consists of four-, eight-, and 12-week primary clerkships. The fourth year includes a community preceptorship in family practice and electives. Students get early experience in medical problem-solving through preceptorships and clinical case study in small groups.

Facilities

The Medical Center includes University Hospital, a 382-bed teaching hospital that, in conjunction with the College of Medicine, has developed leading programs in cancer treatment and research, transplantation, and human genetics; University Medical Associates, a 50-specialty group practice that serves more than 200,000 patients a year; and Meyer Rehabilitation Institute, provides specialized diagnostic and rehabilitative services for handicapped children. The college also has direct teaching affiliations with the Veterans Administration Hospital and eight private hospitals. The Leon S. McGoogan Library of Medicine contains about 180,000 volumes with a current journal titles list of about 3,300. On-line, computer-based bibliographic services are available.

Grading Procedures

A letter grading system is used. Students must maintain a "C" average for each academic year to be promoted. To be promoted to the second and third years, students must pass comprehensive exams in each of the courses taken.

Special Programs

The College of Medicine offers a combined M.D./Ph.D. program. Individualized scheduling options are available. Ph.D. programs available on the UNCM campus include anatomy, biochemistry, physiology, and biophysics. Students may also pursue doctoral programs in other fields by enrolling at the University of Nebraska at Lincoln or other institutions.

Application Procedures

Students must apply through AMCAS and may begin requesting applications after June 15. All completed applications, including transcripts, must be received by November 15. The University of Nebraska does not take part in the early decision plan. Before submitting an AMCAS application, students must send a complete set of transcripts directly to AMCAS from the Registrar of each U.S. and Canadian college and/or university attended. Applicants must also submit two references from faculty members including one in premedical science or an official report from their premedical committee. Applicants must also send a recent photograph (2 x 2). Interviews are required.

Contact

Officer of Academic Affairs
Room 5017C Wittson Hall
University of Nebraska College of Medicine
600 South 42nd Street
Omaha, Nebraska 68198-6595
(402) 559-4205

UNIVERSITY OF NEVADA SCHOOL OF MEDICINE

Reno, Nevada 89557-0046
(702) 784-6001

Accreditation	LCME
Degrees Offered	M.D., M.D./Ph.D.
# Students Applied	419
Enrollment	48 / class
Mean GPA	3.4
% Men / % Women	75% / 25%
% Minorities	Not Available
Tuition	$5,566 In-State
	$13,189 Out-of-State
Application Fee	$35
Application Deadline	November 1

The University

The School of Medicine was established in 1969 and is one of a small number of community-based medical schools in the United States. Located on the western border of Nevada and on the edge of Lake Tahoe, the School of Medicine is set in Reno (pop. 100,756), Nevada. This city is a center for tourism, legalized gambling, and resort facilities. Students are not far from excellent skiing in California and in Sun Valley, and the huge national preserves of Plumas, Tahoe, Eldorado National Forests, and Yosemite National Park are less than a day away.

Admissions

Applications will be accepted only from individuals in good standing at accredited U.S. schools. Scores from MCAT tests taken before 1991 will not be considered due to the change in the test. High priority is given to residents of Nevada, although a few out-of-state students (primarily those from western states without medical schools, such as Alaska, Wyoming, Montana, and Idaho) are considered each year. Non-U.S. citizens must have permanent resident visas for consideration. The mean GPA for the class of 1994 was 3.4, and the mean MCAT score was 8.7. Applications from minority groups are encouraged. For early decision applications, the GPA should be 3.5, and the MCAT must average 9.5.

Undergraduate Preparation

In addition to the MCAT, at least three years or 90 semester hours of college work are required before matriculation. The school strongly recommends a complete baccalaureate degree. No specific major is considered superior to another. People-oriented activity and health care work are encouraged. Courses must include chemistry, 16 hours (eight hours organic); biology and physics, eight hours each; behavioral sciences, six hours (three hours of which must be upper-division credit). Students are generally expected to have satisfied the undergraduate school's requirements for English composition. Strongly recommended supplementary courses include history, literature, philosophy, ethics, and computer science. CLEP or A.P. credit is not acceptable.

Student Body

The estimated size for the entering class is 48, suggesting an overall student body of about 200 students. Ninety percent of students entering in 1990 had majored in science or mathematics as undergraduates.

Placement Records

Most graduates serve and develop practices in the rural and underserved areas of Nevada and the nearby territory.

Costs

In-state tuition for 1991-92 is $5,566; out-of-state tuition is $13,189. Room and board are about $5,400, and books and supplies (including microscope) are $2,700.

Financial Aid

A limited number of loans and scholarships are available. Awards are made on the basis of need and merit. Over 80 percent of Nevada's medical students receive some financial assistance. Further information may be obtained from the financial aid office.

Curriculum

The first two years of the program take place on the Reno campus, where students learn the behavioral and biomedical sciences basic to medicine. Study of the basic sciences is often integrated with clinical problems and applications. Courses include anatomy, behavioral science, biochemistry, microbiology, pharmacology, physiology, pathology, and community health. Third- and fourth-year study includes a combination of required rotations and elective time in family medicine, internal medicine, obstetrics and gynecology, pediatrics, psychiatry, and surgery. Some electives may be done out of state.

Facilities

Besides the Reno campus, the School of Medicine works in close affiliation with a number of local hospitals and clinics.

Special Programs

The School of Medicine also offers the M.D./Ph.D.

Application Procedures

Applications can be obtained from either AMCAS or the school's own Office of Medical School Admissions. File applications between June 1 and November 1. The fee is $35. The earliest notification of acceptance is January 15. The early decision application period is June 15 to August 1 of the year prior to entry. Early applicants are notified by October 1. Students must reply within two weeks of notification, and no deposit fee is necessary to reserve the student's class place.

Contact

Office of Medical School Admissions
127 Savitt Medical Building/332
University of Nevada School of Medicine
Reno, Nevada 89557-0046
(702) 784-6001

UNIVERSITY OF NEW MEXICO SCHOOL OF MEDICINE

Albuquerque, New Mexico 87131
(505) 277-2321

Accreditation	LCME
Degrees Offered	M.D., M.D./Ph.D.
# Students Applied	570
Enrollment	73 / class
Mean GPA	3.4
% Men / % Women	57.5% / 42.5%
% Minorities	16.5%
Tuition	$3,032 In-State
	$8,468 Out-of-State
Application Fee	$10
Application Deadline	November 15

The University

The School of Medicine at the University of New Mexico was established in 1961. The first class of 24 students was enrolled in September 1964, and progress to a full four-year program was approved by the New Mexico State Legislature in 1966. The School of Medicine is a professional and graduate school that provides education in the basic and clinical sciences for the Doctor of Medicine degree, as well as providing medical education at the resident and postgraduate levels.

Admissions

Residents of New Mexico are given primary consideration. The University is a member of the Western Interstate Commission for Higher Education (WICHE). Secondary consideration is given to residents of participating states that have no medical schools: Alaska, Montana, and Wyoming.

WICHE applicants and residents of other states (including former New Mexico residents) must apply under the early decision plan. Longstanding former state residents who do apply under the early decision plan will be given equal consideration with the in-state residents.

Undergraduate Preparation

Each applicant must have completed the following required courses: eight credit hours each of general biology or zoology, general chemistry, and organic chemistry; six credit hours of general physics. Other science classes that may be helpful include biochemistry, physical chemistry, genetics, cell physiology, embryology, and comparative vertebrate anatomy. Competence in spoken and written English is necessary. A broad educational background is encouraged.

Student Body

Over the past few years, over 90 percent of accepted applicants have been from New Mexico. Forty-two percent of the applicants accepted in 1989 were women, and 16 percent were minorities. The average GPA of students admitted in recent years was 3.4.

Placement Records

Nearly three-fourths of the graduates from underrepresented groups are practicing medicine in New Mexico.

Costs

Tuition is $3,032 for residents, $8,468 for nonresidents. Books and supplies were estimated at $750. There is an additional $1,000 fee for first-year medical students for the purchase of microscopes and medical equipment.

Financial Aid

Financial aid is available from a variety of federal, state, and private offices. Loans, scholarships, and grants are awarded on the basis of need and/or ability. All financial aid is awarded on the basis of established need and within limitations of existing resources.

Minority Programs

The university sponsors an active minority recruitment program which encourages applications from minority students who are residents of New Mexico. In evaluating minority applicants, the admissions committee makes some allowances for educational and cultural disadvantage and places particular emphasis on GPA trend, rather than overall GPA.

Faculty

There are approximately 505 faculty members, with 320 full-time appointments.

Curriculum

The School of Medicine offers the opportunity for students to choose between a conventional curriculum and an innovative Primary Care Curriculum. The conventional curriculum employs an integrated approach, teaching basic medical sciences in the first and second years with an emphasis on interdepartmental cooperation. The Primary Care Curriculum is a problem-based program. During the first year, groups of five to six students work together with one faculty facilitator (tutor), who uses actual patient problems to direct students into the concepts of the basic, clinical, and behavioral sciences. At the end of the first year, students then spend four months in a non-urban clinical preceptorship in New Mexico.

The last two years of both tracks are devoted to clinical problems presented by patients in the hospital and outpatient settings. The senior year is devoted primarily to electives.

Facilities

The medical school facilities include a basic medical sciences building, biomedical research facility, medical center library (including a new computerized on-line catalog), the University of New Mexico Mental Health Center, the UNM Children's Psychiatric Hospital, Family Practice Center, Center for Non-Invasive Diagnosis, and an International Cancer Center. The 300-bed UNM Hospital serves as the major teaching hospital of the medical school, with additional teaching at the 413-bed Regional Federal Medical Center in Albuquerque.

Grading Procedures

Under the Primary Care Curriculum, grades are awarded as pass/fail. On a twice-yearly basis, students take comprehensive multiple-choice examinations in all seven basic sciences. On a quarterly basis, students work individually with a patient problem and are assessed on their clinical skills, scientific reasoning process, and ability to integrate new scientific information.

Special Programs

The School of Medicine offers a combined M.D./Ph.D. program. Applicants for this program must submit two separate applications, one through the AMCAS for the M.D. program and one through the Graduate Committee at the School of Medicine for the Ph.D. program.

Application Procedures

Applicants are advised to take the undergraduate MCAT in the spring of their junior year, or in the fall preceding the year of desired enrollment. Interviews are required. Strong preference is given to residents. Foreign students are considered for admission if they have a permanent resident visa, are state residents, have had at least two years of college in the U.S., and have a good command of English.

Applications for transfer to the second year will be considered from New Mexico and WICHE residents in approved foreign medical schools. Students in four-year U.S. medical schools who have a compelling need to transfer to the school will be considered for transfer at the second- and third-year levels.

Contact

Office of Student Affairs and Admissions
School of Medicine
The University of New Mexico Medical Center
Albuquerque, New Mexico 87131
(505) 277-4766

NEW YORK MEDICAL COLLEGE

Valhalla, New York 10595
(914) 993-4000

Accreditation	LCME
Degrees Offered	M.D., M.D./Ph.D.
# Students Applied	3,409
Enrollment	190 / class
Mean GPA	3.14
% Men / % Women	62% / 38%
% Minorities	Not Available
Tuition	$22,400
Application Fee	$50
Application Deadline	December 1

The University

The New York Medical College was chartered by the state of New York in 1860. It was the first medical school to own its own teaching hospital, to admit women, and to establish a scholarship program specifically for minority students.

Originally established in New York City, the college accepted an invitation from Westchester County to develop a campus in Valhalla. In 1978, the college established a rela-tionship with the Archdiocese of New York, which broadened the college's range of clinical affiliations through the Catholic-sponsored hospitals in New York City and the metropolitan region. A range of cultural and entertainment activities is located nearby for students in Westchester County, including on-campus sports facilities and outdoor trails.

Admissions

It is strongly recommended that the applicant successfully complete a baccalaureate degree from an accredited college of arts and sciences in the United States or Canada. Well-qualified students may be admitted after the completion of three years of undergraduate courses. Most students have graduated, on the average, in the top 25 percent of their undergraduate classes. Residents and nonresidents are equally considered. The MCAT must be taken prior to the application deadline of December 1. Foreign students will only be admitted if, by July 1 of the year of matriculation, the accepted student can deposit funds sufficient to meet tuition charges for the total period of enrollment in a designated account. Transfer students are admitted from U.S. or Canadian schools to the second- or third-year class, and from foreign medical schools to the first-year class.

Undergraduate Preparation

Each student's undergraduate credentials must include two semesters each of general and inorganic chemistry, organic chemistry, physics, and general biology, all with lab. Two semesters of English are also required. The admissions committee has no preference for a major field of undergraduate study.

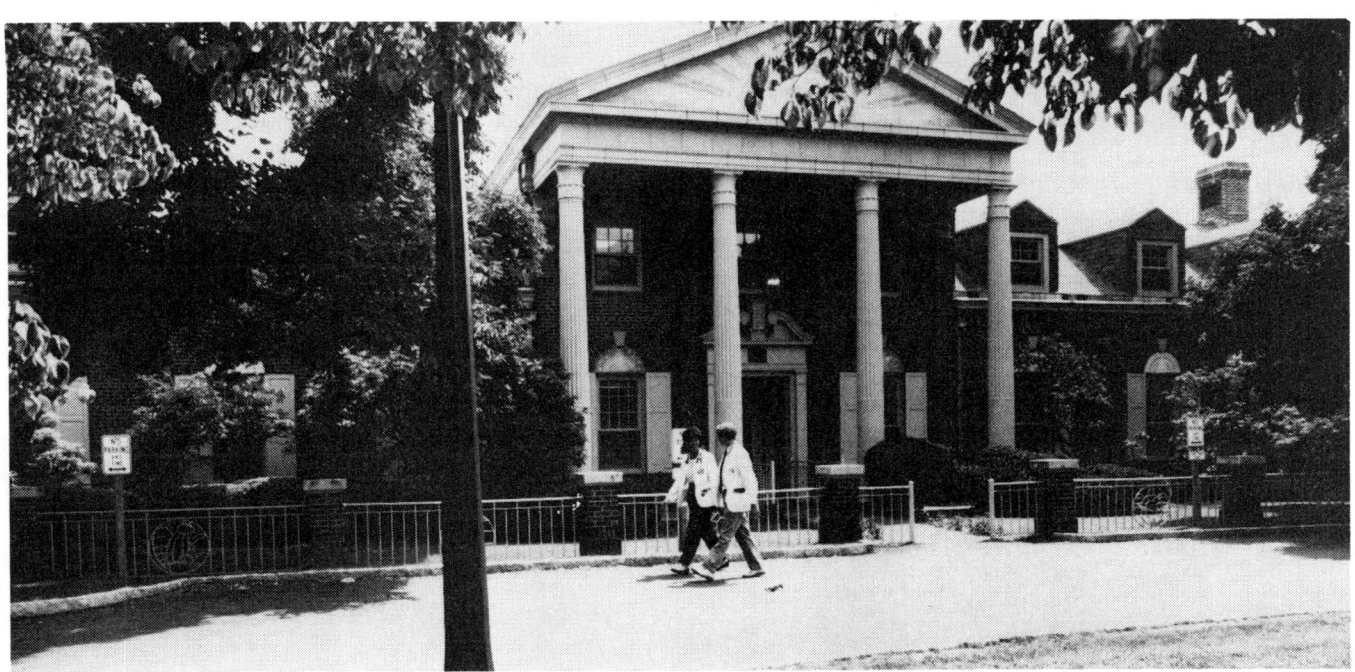

Placement Records

Each year approximately three-quarters of the fourth-year medical class are consistently placed in their first or second residency choices.

Costs

Tuition for the 1989 first-year class was $22,400, with student fees of $340.

Financial Aid

Financial aid is awarded from a variety of private, state, and federal offices on the basis of need and/or ability. Federally funded loans include the Health Education Assistance Loan Program, Perkins Loans, and Federal Health Professions Loans. New York State programs include the Tuition Assistance Program and the Regents Health Care Scholarship. Forgivable loans include the Altman Medical Scholars Service-Intensive Program and the Trustee Loan and Scholarship Programs. Foreign students are not eligible for financial aid.

Minority Programs

The college actively recruits applicants of both sexes and members of disadvantaged minority groups. The college conducts a special program to recruit and retain underrepresented minority students.

Student Organizations

Student organizations include a chapter of the American Medical Student Association, Alpha Omega Alpha, and the Student Senate.

Faculty

There are over 2,800 faculty at New York Medical College teaching 760 medical students and 500 graduate students. Approximately 1,000 of the faculty members work full-time.

Curriculum

The first year includes study of the basic sciences, including a unique behavioral science class that combines lectures with student-patient contact. Electives are also offered. The second year consists of advanced basic sciences and clinical work. The third year includes required clinical clerkships. Students are rotated through a variety of teaching hospitals. The fourth year consists of three months of required clinical clerkships. An elective program is planned by the student with the aid of a faculty advisor and a member of the Dean's office. Opportunities for research also exist.

Facilities

The college is affiliated wtih 32 area hospitals. The Medical Sciences Library holds approximately 120,000 volumes and 1,400 journals, including the collection of the Westchester Academy of Medicine.

Grading Procedures

Promotion from one grade to the next is determined by one of the three standing faculty committees on student promotions. Students must take both parts of the NBME exam.

Special Programs

The New York Medical College offers an M.D./Ph.D. program. A medical student may apply to the Graduate School of Basic Medical Sciences during the first two years of basic medical study. Students are not formally admitted until they have completed all of their preclinical subjects and Part I of the NBME exam.

Application Procedures

The applicant must file an application with AMCAS. Applicants must include a letter of recommendation from the college premedical advisory committee. If the college does not have a premedical advisory committee, letters of evaluation from three professors (preferably two in the physical sciences) are required. Applicants must also submit a signed personal photograph, and an application fee of $50 (nonrefundable).

All applications must be postmarked no later than December 1. Interviews are required. Applicants can be reviewed under the Early Decision Plan.

For transfer students, application for admission with advance academic standing are available after January 1 from the Office of Admissions. Applicants must also submit two letters of evaluation from medical school faculty as well as a certificate of good academic standing.

Contact

Admissions Office
New York Medical College
Valhalla, New York 10595
(914) 993-4507

NEW YORK UNIVERSITY SCHOOL OF MEDICINE

New York, New York 10011
(212) 340-5372

Accreditation	LCME
Degrees Offered	M.D., M.D./Ph.D.
# Students Applied	2,327
Enrollment	156
Mean GPA	3.5
% Men / % Women	62% / 38%
% Minorities	Not Available
Tuition	$19,325
Application Fee	$65
Application Deadline	December 15

The University

New York University was founded in 1831 as a private institution. The School of Medicine opened 10 years later. The first president of the University, Albert Gallatin, and his co-founders stated that New York University would be a "national university" that would provide a "rational and practical education." Today New York University is one of the 26 members of the Association of American Universities. Located in New York City, NYU offers its students a wide variety of cultural and recreational activities.

Admissions

The Committee on Admissions expects applicants to have achieved excellence in the sciences, as well as all aspects of college study, regardless of major. An applicant's work in the later years of college, and possible improvement over earlier years, is given extra consideration. All candidates are urged to select advanced courses and to examine indepth some special aspects of the course material. Candidates are evaluated on the basis of academic achievement, college faculty evaluations, the personal interview, and the results of the MCAT.

Undergraduate Preparation

Applicants must have completed at least three years of study at an accredited college or university, although the baccalaureate degree is preferred. At least six semester hours of the following courses are required for admission: English, inorganic chemistry, organic chemistry, physics, and general biology or zoology, all with lab. Although only six semesters of English are required, two years are recommended. Applicants should take the more rigorous of the basic science courses offered in college. One year's work in organic and inorganic chemistry and general physics should be completed. Additional courses in mathematics (including calculus), quantitative and physical chemistry, biochemistry, embryology, and genetics are recommended. Applicants are also advised to take one course or more in college-level conversational Spanish.

Student Body

Most of the students are residents of the eastern part of the United States, although applicants from all areas of the country are welcomed. Approximately 38 percent of students at the School are women.

Costs

Tuition costs and student fees amount to $19,325. Additional costs for supplies, books, clothing, etc. amount to $1,200. Costs for on-campus housing can range from $2,880 per year for single-room dormitory accommodations to $1,242 per month for a furnished, two-bedroom apartment.

Financial Aid

Students who have been accepted for admission are eligible to file a GAPSFAS application for financial aid. Loans and scholarships are available through the university, as well as from a variety of federal, state, and private offices.

Application fees may be waived if need is demonstrated.

Student Organizations

Organizations of interest to medical students include the Students' Association of the School of Medicine and a chapter of Alpha Omega Alpha fraternity.

Curriculum

The first year consists of the study of the basic sciences, given through interdepartmental correlations that present the relevance of the basic science materials to clinical medicine. The second year includes the study of human disease and a continuation of the introduction to clinical science, as well as studies of special pathology. The principles of physical diagnosis and the introduction to medicine complete the second year. The third year consists of clinical clerkships on hospital wards. The fourth year includes a required two-month subinternship and an elective program through which students may pursue approved research or clinical science programs.

Facilities

The School of Medicine is located in the New York University Medical Center. The Tisch Hospital (726 beds) and the Rusk Institute of Rehabilitative Medicine (152 beds) are also located at the Center. The Medical Science Building houses research laboratories, the library, and classrooms for the first two years of medical study. The Henry W. and Albert A. Berg Institute for Experimental Physiology, Surgery and Pathology is also part of the Medical Science Building. Most clinical instruction takes place at Bellevue Hospital Center, a large metropolitan hospital with a wide variety of patient needs.

The eight libraries at the University contain over three million volumes. The Frederick L. Ehrman Medical Library at the Medical Center contains more than 160,000 volumes and 1,900 periodicals. Bellevue Hospital Center, the Veterans Administration Medical Center, and the Institute of Environmental Medicine at Sterling Forest, NY, also maintain medical research libraries.

Special Programs

A combined M.D./Ph.D. degree (the Medical Scientist Training Program) is offered. This program is completed in a minimum of six years and may be taken in the basic medical sciences or in one of the social sciences related to health care. Candidates must have a bachelor's degree or the assurance that it will be granted after one year of medical school, and be U.S. citizens or have permanent-resident status. Previous research experience is important in evaluating candidates for the program. Applicants to the program should request a supplementary application form for the M.D./Ph.D. program to be submitted along with their regular application form. Unsuccessful candidates for the program will be considered for regular admission to the School of Medicine and will also be considered for application to the Medical Scientist Training Program at a later date.

Application Procedures

Application forms are available by late July. Completed forms should be received between August 15 and December 15. Applications postmarked later than December 15 are not accepted. There is a $65 nonrefundable application fee. The MCAT should be taken in the spring, and no later than the fall of the year of application. Applicants are responsible for confirming that transcripts of all college and graduate-level work, including summer school, and a college faculty evaluation are sent to the School of Medicine. Interviews are arranged by invitation of the Committee on Admissions.

Students who have failed in another medical school are not eligible for admission. Applicants who do not hold a permanent-resident visa may be considered for admission.

Contact

Office of Admissions
New York University
School of Medicine
P.O. Box 1924
New York, New York 10016
(212) 263-5290

UNIVERSITY OF NORTH CAROLINA AT CHAPEL HILL SCHOOL OF MEDICINE

CB #7000, 121 MacNider
Chapel Hill, North Carolina 27599-7000
(919) 966-4161

Accreditation	LCME
Degrees Offered	M.D., M.D./Ph.D., M.D./M.P.H.
# Students Applied	2,286
Enrollment	160 / class
Mean GPA	Not Available
% Men / % Women	Not Available
% Minorities	Not Available
Tuition	$1,344 In-State
	$12,132 Out-of-State
Application Fee	$35
Application Deadline	November 15

The University

The School of Medicine of the University of North Carolina at Chapel Hill was established in 1879 and expanded to a four-year school in 1952. Schools of dentistry, nursing, pharmacy, and public health are adjacent to the medical school on the university's campus.

Admissions

Admissions preference is given to North Carolina residents. The Admissions Committee is very selective about interviewing out-of-state residents. Applicant's scholastic records as well as their motivation, maturity, industry, and integrity are considered. Completion of the MCAT is required, and the AMCAS application is used for initial screening. All information is considered without priority to any single factor. The undergraduate major is not an important consideration, but excellence in the chosen field is expected. Early decision is available.

Undergraduate Preparation

Students must complete a minimum of 96 semester hours of accredited college work. Proficiency in the natural sciences is expected. In addition, eight semester hours each of biology (including vertebrate zoology with labs), inorganic and organic chemistry, and general physics, all with labs, are required, as well as six semester hours of English. Preparation showing serious and mature use of the undergraduate years is valued by the School of Medicine.

Costs

In 1989-90, tuition and fees were $1,344 for in-state residents and $12,132 for nonresidents. Books and supplies are expected to cost approximately $960. Food and housing is approximately $3,385 for on-campus residents and $3,735 for off-campus residents.

Financial Aid

Loans and scholarships are available from the School of Medicine, although students are encouraged to seek assistance from outside sources. Priority will be given to students applying for financial aid before March 1. Each year two students receive stipends of $9,000 for the first year and $10,000 for years two, three, six, and seven.

Minority Programs

The Admissions Committee will nominate some minority students to participate in the Board of Governors Medical Scholars Program. These students will receive annual stipends of $5,000 plus tuition and fees.

Curriculum

During the first two years, students study the scientific basis of clinical practice. In the third year, students rotate through clinical services of five major disciplines: medicine, obstetrics and gynecology, pediatrics, psychiatry, and surgery. In the fourth year, students take seven electives, two of which must be an acting internship at an AHEC hospital and a preceptorship in family medicine. Students may design individual research projects under faculty direction.

Facilities

The North Carolina Memorial Hospital is a 650-bed facility committed to education, research, patient care, and community service. A partnership between the university health science centers and the community is provided by The North Carolina Area Health Education Centers (AHEC) Program. It offers off-campus education and training opportunities for medical students and residents as well as ready access to continuing education and teaching activities for health professionals and practitioners throughout North Carolina. The health sciences library houses 233,770 printed volumes, 3,855 audiovisual programs, 31,000 microfilm pieces, and subscriptions to 4,500 periodicals.

Special Programs

The School of Medicine offers combined M.D./Ph.D. and M.D./M.P.H. degree programs.

Application Procedures

The MCAT must be taken no later than the fall prior to the class for which the student is applying. Applications must be received by November 15 of the year prior to admission, accompanied by a nonrefundable $35 fee. Either an evaluation by the student's campus premedical committee or letters of recommendation from two faculty members are required. Supplementary applications and residency forms are also required.

Contact

Admissions Office
CB# 7000, 121 MacNider
School of Medicine
The University of North Carolina at Chapel Hill
Chapel Hill, North Carolina 27599-7000
(919) 962-8331

UNIVERSITY OF NORTH DAKOTA SCHOOL OF MEDICINE

501 Columbia Road
Grand Forks, North Dakota 58203
(701) 777-2516

Accreditation	LCME, AAMC
Degrees Offered	M.D., M.D./Ph.D.
# Students Applied	124
Enrollment	57 / class
Mean GPA	3.49
% Men / % Women	60% / 40%
% Minorities	Not Available
Tuition	$7,800 In-State
	$22,015 Out-of-State
Application Fee	$25
Application Deadline	November 1

The University

The University of North Dakota is a coeducational, state-supported institution established in 1884. Today, the university complex comprises eight colleges and enrolls more than 11,000 students. Grand Forks, home of the university, is located in the Red River Valley and has a population of 60,000.

The School of Medicine was established in 1905, and by 1973 was authorized to grant the M.D. degree through a program of study that sent students out of state to complete part of the degree. By 1984, the entire curriculum was offered at the School of Medicine for the first time, giving North Dakota a complete, in-state medical education program. The school's emphasis is on rural primary care for North Dakota residents.

The school encompasses four campuses: the northwest campus, based in Minot; the southwest campus, based in Bismarck; the southeast campus, based in Fargo; and the northeast campus, based in Grand Forks. Each campus spans health facilities in a number of counties.

Admissions

Admissions decisions are based on MCAT scores, transcripts, and autobiographical information, including commitment to a medical career, motivation, ability to work with people, compassion and empathy, and ability to deal with everyday problems. The student's participation in research projects or health-related employment is also considered.

Preference is given to residents of North Dakota. Applicants certified by the Western Interstate Commission for Higher Education (WICHE) receive equal preference for up to four of the positions in each entering class. Residents of Minnesota also are considered for admission on a very limited basis, and Native Americans (regardless of residence) may apply through the school's minority program, Indians Into Medicine.

Undergraduate Preparation

A minimum of 90 semester hours of credit from an approved college or university is required. Preference is given to those with a bachelor's degree and a broad background in the sciences and humanities. Computer literacy is recommended. Minimal prerequisites are: 16 semester hours of inorganic and organic chemistry; eight of biology; eight of physics; three of psychology/sociology; six of language arts; and three of college algebra. A minimum GPA of 3.0 is expected.

Costs

Tuition and fees are $7,800 for the first three years of study; in the last year, tuition and fees drop to approximately $6,100. Books and supplies are estimated to cost about $1,100 for the first two years and $600 for the last two years.

Financial Aid

Financial assistance may be based on need or academic achievement. There are numerous loan funds, scholarships, and awards available. More information can be obtained by contacting the Student Financial Aid Office at the School of Medicine.

Minority Programs

The Indians Into Medicine (INMED) program became operational in 1973. Through its comprehensive recruitment program, INMED seeks to identify and encourage Native American students with aptitude for and interest in health careers as early as the junior high school level. A variety of support services are available throughout the student's medical school career.

Student Organizations

Students are encouraged to become members of the American Medical Student Association (AMSA). Students participate in the Association of American Medical College's Organization of Student Representatives.

Faculty

There is a full-time faculty of about 120 and a part-time or voluntary clinical faculty of about 750 who serve in community hospitals throughout the state.

Curriculum

The M.D. degree program offers a foundation in the basic sciences followed by individualized clinical instruction from practicing physicians who serve as faculty at the four regional campuses. The need for physicians in rural areas of the state is a factor influencing the curriculum.

First- and second-year courses include biochemistry, histology and organology, microbiology, human behavior, and introduction to clinical medicine. Also during these years the student is introduced to the hospital-based practice of medicine as well as primary care in North Dakota. A unique aspect of the program is the placement of students with physician-preceptors in 26 rural communities throughout North Dakota for periods of training during the four-year course of study.

Facilities

The Medical Center includes the School of Medicine, the USDA Human Nutrition Research Center, and the Rehabilitation Hospital. Other units include the North Dakota Lions Diabetes Ocular Research Center, a biomedical research facility, and the Ireland Research Laboratory.

The Harley E. French Library houses more than 67,000 books, journal volumes, and audiovisuals. The library also heads a statewide hospital library system which, together with its own collection, provides more than 130,000 volumes. The library serves as an information network via literature databases and interlibrary loan arrangements with the National Library of Medicine and other sources.

Grading Procedures

Student performance is graded as honors, satisfactory, or unsatisfactory. The faculty also evaluates and documents aspects of each student's general performance.

Special Programs

The M.D./Ph.D. program allows students enrolled in the School of Medicine to be admitted to the graduate school in the basic science departments that offer the Ph.D. degree.

First- and second-year medical students may apply to the program, which requires six years to complete.

The graduate school offers the opportunity for students to obtain an M.D. degree together with a master's or doctoral degree in a variety of fields, including anatomy and cell biology, biochemistry and molecular biology, and microbiology and immunology. Applications for graduate work should be submitted directly to the graduate school.

Application Procedures

School of Medicine application should be submitted no later than November 1. The application packet must contain the written application form, four letters of recommendation, MCAT scores, official academic transcripts, and a nonrefundable $25 application fee. Applicants being considered for admission are invited for a personal interview.

The School of Medicine participates in the Professional Student Exchange Program administered by the Western Interstate Commission for Higher Education (WICHE), under which legal residents of western states without a medical school may receive preference in admission.

Contact

Office of Student Affairs and Admissions
University of North Dakota School of Medicine
501 Columbia Road
Grand Forks, North Dakota 58203
(701) 777-4221

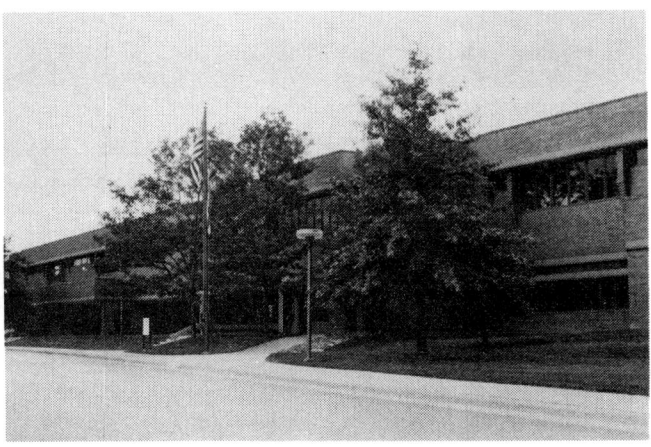

NORTHEASTERN OHIO UNIVERSITIES COLLEGE OF MEDICINE

4209 State Route 44
Rootstown, Ohio 44272
(216) 325-2511

Accreditation	LCME, AAMC, AMA
Degrees Offered	B.S./M.D., M.D., M.D./Ph.D.
# Students Applied	400
Enrollment	400
Mean GPA	Not Available
% Men / % Women	50% / 50%
% Minorities	Not Available
Tuition	$6,840 In-State
	$12,840 Out-of-State
Application Fee	$20
Application Deadline	December 15

The University

Northeastern Ohio Universities College of Medicine (NEOUCOM) is a public institution offering medical education through a unique consortium of three universities—the University of Akron, Kent State University, and Youngstown State University.

Founded in 1973, NEOUCOM was established to promote the education of physicians capable of entering any field but specifically oriented to family practice and community-based care.

In 1981, NEOUCOM received full accreditation and graduated its first class of 42 physicians. Today, the college graduates 100 physicians each year.

The basic campus is located in Rootstown on a 55-acre site. Rootstown is a small community in northeastern Ohio located 35 miles southeast of Cleveland.

Admissions

Criteria for admission to the M.D. program include demonstrated proficiency in appropriate coursework, MCAT scores, recommendations, a commitment to the field of medicine, and extracurricular and employment activities. The results of a personal interview are also considered in the admissions decision. Applicants must have completed at least three years of undergraduate study.

The MCAT should be taken no later than the fall prior to the year of anticipated enrollment.

Admission to the six-year B.S./M.D. program is a function of the consortium universities as well as the College of Medicine; application is made to one of the three universities in the fall of the senior year of high school. ¶NEOUCOM gives preference to Ohio residents.

Undergraduate Preparation

Students applying to the B.S./M.D. program come directly from high school and are not expected to have taken any college coursework. They should have a full background in science and should also take the ACT or SAT.

Students applying to the M.D. program should have attended undergraduate school for three years. Coursework should include one year of organic chemistry and physics.

Student Body

There are about 105 students per class year in the B.S./M.D. program, approximately half of whom are women.

Placement Records

NEOUCOM graduates have consistently scored above the national average (50th percentile) on the NBME test, and at times averaged at the 70th percentile.

Each year, more than 75 percent of College of Medicine graduates are placed in one of their top three residency choices. About 53 percent of graduates have been offered chief residency positions. More than half pursue primary care practice and, of the graduating class of 1990, 54 percent remained in Ohio.

Costs

Tuition for Ohio residents is approximately $6,840 for the first, second, and fourth years of the medical curriculum. The third year of the medical program costs $9,120. Tuition for nonresidents is approximately double.

Miscellaneous fees range from $550 to $1,000 per year (the first two years of medical school are the most costly). Books and supplies cost approximately $1,000 for the first year, but these costs drop significantly during the last three years.

Financial Aid

NEOUCOM awards most financial aid on the basis of need and uses the GAPSFAS as its need analysis service. Need-based sources of aid include Stafford Loans, Exceptional Financial Need Scholarships, Health Professions Student Loans, and Perkins Loans.

The GAPSFAS form, federal income tax forms, and a NEOUCOM financial aid application must be received by April 15 prior to the beginning of the academic year of matriculation into the M.D. program.

Minority Programs

The College of Medicine has an Office of Minority Affairs, which promotes support for minority students and a general awareness of minority issues among the student population. The office also visits high schools to encourage bright minority students to pursue careers in medicine and sponsors "Project Boost," which helps prepare undergraduate minority students in math and science.

Student Organizations

More than 500 student organizations are registered at the three consortium universities combined. Organizations specifically for medical students include the American Medical Student Association, American Medical Women's Association, Alpha Omega Alpha, Family Practice Club, Physicians for Social Responsibility, Christian Medical/Dental Society, the Student National Medical Association, and medical student sections of the American Medical Association and the Ohio State Medical Association.

Faculty

The College of Medicine has more than 50 full-time faculty members involved in teaching and research on the Rootstown campus. In addition, 1,200 clinical instructors are based at the university's associated teaching hospitals.

Curriculum

The overall goal of the medical program is to graduate well-qualified doctors of medicine capable of excelling in any specialization but oriented largely toward the principles and practices of primary care in the community setting. The first two years of the six-year B.S./M.D. program (the undergraduate curriculum) are carried out at the consortium university, and include a strong preparation in the physical and life sciences as well as introductory studies in humanities and social sciences.

The four-year medical curriculum includes basic medical sciences, clinical sciences, and community health sciences. Humanities and ethics are also part of the curriculum. While there is extensive clinical exposure in the sophomore year of the M.D. program, the primary clinical experience takes place in the junior year. Electives are chosen in the senior year.

Facilities

Among the facilities at the Rootstown Basic Medical Sciences Campus are classrooms, laboratories, a conference center, the basic sciences library, and student exercise and recreation centers. Rootstown is about 15 miles east of Akron (University of Akron), 35 miles west of Youngstown (Youngstown State University), and 35 miles southeast of Cleveland. It is also located in close proximity to Kent State University.

The Oliver Ocasek Regional Medical Information Center/Consortium Libraries comprise a 30,000 square-foot facility located on the Rootstown campus. The libraries house more than 73,000 books and bound journals and subscribe to nearly

1,100 journals. There is also a media center and a complete microcomputer laboratory. All teaching hospital and consortium universities have computer access to the library's holdings.

Grading Procedures

Students are evaluated using grades of honors, satisfactory, conditional unsatisfactory, and unsatisfactory. All medical students are required to achieve satisfactory scores on both parts of the NBME in order to graduate.

Special Programs

Medical students can enroll in the summer fellowship program, which offers the chance to develop research skills in the basic medical, clinical, or community health sciences.

Those wishing to pursue the doctorate can enroll in the M.D./Ph.D. degree program. The Ph.D. is obtained from the University of Akron or Kent State University. Ph.D. studies are offered in biomedical engineering and several of the traditional life sciences, such as physiology and microbiology.

Application Procedures

Application to the B.S./M.D. program is made to the undergraduate university in the fall of the senior year of high school. All applications must be received by December 31 of the year preceding anticipated enrollment.

For admission to the M.D. program, application must be filed with AMCAS. The deadline for receipt of the AMCAS application is December 15 of the year preceding anticipated enrollment. Applicants must take the MCAT no later than the fall prior to the year of enrollment. After a favorable review of the AMCAS application, the candidate will receive a NEOUCOM supplementary application. The deadline for submission of the NEOUCOM application with supplementary materials is December 30 prior to the year of anticipated enrollment.

NEOUCOM also has an early decision program. The deadline for submission of the AMCAS application under this program is August 1, and the deadline for submission of NEOUCOM supplementary materials is September 1.

Contact

Northeastern Ohio Universities
College of Medicine
4209 State Route 44
PO Box 95
Rootstown, Ohio 44272
(216) 325-2511

NORTHWESTERN UNIVERSITY MEDICAL SCHOOL

303 East Chicago Avenue
Chicago, Illinois 60611-3008
(312) 908-8186

Accreditation	LCME
Degrees Offered	M.D., B.A./M.D., B.S./M.D., M.D./Ph.D., M.D./M.M.
# Students Applied	4,492
Enrollment	168 / class
Mean GPA	3.51
% Men / % Women	62% / 38%
% Minorities	Not Available
Tuition	$19,965
Application Fee	$50
Application Deadline	November 15

The University

Northwestern University is an independent private institution founded in 1851. The university enrolls about 18,000 students annually on the Chicago and Evanston campuses.

The Medical School, which dates back to the mid-19th century, was one of the first schools offering an extended medical education with hospital instruction, rigorous graduation requirements, selective admission standards, and courses in bacteriology. The Medical School was the first to perform antiseptic surgery and to use microscopes in surgery, and among the earliest to use laser surgery. Among the school's other achievements are the production of a vaccine for whooping cough and the construction of electric-powered prosthetic limbs for children.

The headquarters of the American Medical Association, the American Hospital Association, and the American College of Surgeons are located in Chicago. The area is also home to quite a few other medical schools, professional academies, societies, and boards of specialty fields. The city has a population of about seven million and is the cultural, industrial, and commercial center of the Midwest.

Admissions

The Medical School seeks students who are liberally educated and who exhibit emotional maturity, motivation, achievement, and academic excellence. Desirable in applicants are observation, communication, and reasoning skills. Necessary motor skills are also important, as are emotional health and demonstration of compassion and integrity.

All students must take the MCAT. The Medical Schools seeks to fill about half its openings with Illinois residents. About 50 to 60 positions are generally open for out-of-state residents.

Undergraduate Preparation

The equivalent of three years of undergraduate college coursework at an accredited college is the minimum needed to gain entry into the Medical School. The following subjects are recommended: modern biology, one year; general biology, one year; general physics, one year; inorganic and organic chemistry, two years; and English, one year.

Placement Records

The Medical School, with the five-member hospitals of the McGaw Medical Center of Northwestern University, offers 23 fully approved residency programs and a number of advanced-level fellowships. Seventy-five percent of the school's graduating seniors are accepted to at least one of their top three residency selections.

Costs

Yearly tuition is $19,965. Books and instruments cost about $1,400 per year. Most students rent a microscope for $170.

Financial Aid

Financial aid is granted on the basis of need as determined through GAPSFAS needs analysis. All applicants who are invited for interviews may apply for aid. There are numerous aid funds administered by the Medical School. Loan funds available include the Northwestern University Parent-Student Loan Program, Health Professions Student Loans, Perkins Loans, and Supplemental Loans for Students. A host of named awards are granted on the basis of scholastic or other achievements.

Student Organizations

Student organizations include the Student Senate, the Organization of Student Representatives to the Association of American Medical Colleges, the American Medical Student and American Medical Women's associations, and the Asian Medical Student Organization. Fraternity chapters at the Medical School include Alpha Omega Alpha and Phi Rho Sigma.

Faculty

The Medical School faculty currently totals 2,200. Full-time faculty teach almost all the basic science courses, and much of the core material in the clinical clerkships is taught by both full-time and part-time faculty. Physicians who are in private practice provide a substantial portion of clinical instruction.

Curriculum

The curriculum affords opportunities to prepare for careers in virtually any field of medicine. Northwestern students typically perform well on the NBME exams relative to national norms.

The first two years build a foundation in the basic biomedical sciences and fundamental clinical skills. The third year consists of required clinical clerkships. The fourth year prepares students for postgraduate training in particular disciplines. There are 135 electives offered in the fourth year.

A host of clinical opportunities are offered, even in the first two years, when students may choose ambulatory care experiences at affiliated family health centers.

The senior elective emphasizes the delivery of comprehensive care in different settings in the United States and abroad, as well as preventive medicine and community health approaches.

Facilities

Located on the shoreline of Lake Michigan, the Medical School borders the five McGaw Medical Center hospitals on the university's Chicago campus. The McGaw Medical Center includes Evanston Hospital, Children's Memorial Hospital, Northwestern Memorial Hospital, Rehabilitation Institute of Chicago, and Veterans Administration Lakeside Medical Center. These hospitals serve as clinical instruction sites for medical students and also conduct cooperative research ventures. One major collaborative effort is the Heart/Lung Transplant and Mechanical Assist Program, which serves the Midwest with transplantation services.

City hospitals where students can obtain experience include Columbus-Cabrini Medical Center and St. Joseph Hospital and Health Care Center. Ambulatory care experience is provided by the Northwestern Medical Faculty Foundation and at various other facilities.

The Jack and Dollie Galter Health Sciences Library houses more than 250,000 bound volumes and receives more than 2,600 serials. Students have access to the National Library of Medicine's MEDLARS/MEDLINE database, as well as Psychological Abstracts, Chemical Abstracts, Biological Abstracts, ERIC, and more than 300 other databases.

The Barnes Learning Resources Center, separate from the library, houses various types of nonprint media—videocassettes, slides, films, and other instructional aids.

Grading Procedures

The Medical School uses an honors/pass/fail grading system. At the end of the second year, medical students must take Part I of the NBME; promotion to the third year is not contingent upon passing the exam, however.

Special Programs

The Baccalaureate/M.D. Program (Honors Program in Medical Education) is a seven-year course of study for Northwestern students wishing to pursue the B.A. or B.S. in addition to the medical degree. Information can be obtained from the office of the honors program at the Medical School or from the university office of undergraduate admission in Evanston.

The medical and graduate schools offer a combined degree program leading to the M.D. and the Ph.D. in a six- to seven-year period. The program is designed to prepare selected students for careers in biomedical research or academic medicine coupled with clinical practice. The Medical School offers a joint M.D./M.P.H. (Master of Public Health) program and an M.D./M.M. (Master of Management) program.

Other special programs include a post-baccalaureate physical therapy curriculum and a short-term prosthetic-orthotic education.

Application Procedures

Applications for admission must be filed with AMCAS by the AMCAS application deadline and 12 to 15 months before the date for which admission is sought. MCAT scores must have been earned during the three years prior to the date of admission in order to be accepted.

After reviewing the AMCAS materials, the Medical School sends supplemental materials to competitive applicants. The school will review the supplemental materials along with appropriate letters of recommendation. Interviews will be requested of all candidates who are seriously being considered for admission.

Contact

Office of Admissions
Northwestern University Medical School
303 East Chicago Avenue
Morton Building 1-606
Chicago, Illinois 60611-3008
(312) 503-8206

OHIO STATE UNIVERSITY COLLEGE OF MEDICINE

1800 Cannon Drive
Columbus, Ohio 43210-1200
(614) 292-0926

Accreditation	LCME
Degrees Offered	M.D., M.S., Ph.D.
# Students Applied	2,279
Enrollment	210 / class
Mean GPA	3.0
% Men / % Women	48% / 52%
% Minorities	Not Available
Tuition	$5,994 In-State
	$18,147 Out-of-State
Application Fee	$20
Application Deadline	November 15

The University

As the major comprehensive university in the state, Ohio State is a four-year, public university for men and women that operates on five campuses in Columbus, Lima, Mansfield, Marion, and Newark. The Ohio legislature established the College of Medicine in 1913. The school consists of 19 departments in medicine. Students and faculty are exposed to the multiple resources available in the city of Columbus and the surrounding area. The College of Medicine has affiliations with several institutions including Children's Hospital, Columbus State Hospital, Mt. Carmel Hospital, and the Veterans Administration Clinic.

Admissions

All applicants are reviewed by the College of Medicine Admissions Committee. A bachelor's degree is required, and every applicant must take the Medical College Admissions Test (MCAT). It is recommended that students take the exam at the end of the last quarter or semester of their sophomore year in college.

Undergraduate Preparation

Although no specific undergraduate curriculum or college major is required, the admissions committee seeks students who display backgrounds of diverse interests. Students are encouraged to take philosophy, literature, writing, history, arts, and languages in their premedical curriculum. Each student is required to take one full academic year of general chemistry, organic chemistry, physics, and biology (including vertebrate anatomy), all with lab. Preference is given to Ohio residents.

Student Body

Eighty-five percent of the students hail from Ohio. The remaining of each class is made up of out-of-state students.

Placement Records

The Office of Student Affairs maintains pertinent information and keeps credential files that can be sent out to potential employers at the request of the student.

Costs

Tuition for the 1990 entering class was $5,994 for residents and $18,147 for nonresidents. Students should allow $11,000 annually for other expenses.

Financial Aid

Financial aid is offered through a variety of scholarships and loans. Scholarships for the 1988-89 school year ranged from $800 to $1,000. Some loans pay as much as $18,000 a year. The programs available include the Health Professions Student Loan, the Perkins Loan, the Stafford Loan, and the Supplemental Loan for Students, the Alternative Loan Program, and Health Educational Assistance Loan.

Minority Programs

The Office of Minority Affairs is committed to a "3 R's Model." This stands for Recruitment, Retention, and Release (of minority students with diplomas to their respective communities). The OMA sponsors many initiative programs including Upward Bound and the Prelude Scholarship Recognition Program.

Student Organizations

Student organizations include the College of Medicine Student Council, American Medical Student Association, Student National Medical Association, and the American Medical Women's Association.

Faculty

The College of Medicine has a faculty of doctors and professional faculty that totals close to 1,700.

Curriculum

The curriculum is constructed of two years of preclinical study and two years of clinical experience. During the normal human and pathophysiology period of the first two years, students study cell structure and function, the cardiovascular system, gastrointestinal system, pathological mechanism, infectious diseases, and epidemiology. The scheduled outline for the third and fourth years calls for 80 weeks of required clerkships including surgery, pediatrics, and critical care.

Facilities

The university libraries are made up of the Main Library and several other college libraries and departments. The Health Sciences Library houses approximately 155,000 bound journals, and subscribes to over 2,000 journals and medical periodicals. The College of Medicine complex consists of several lecture halls, the School of Allied Medical Professions building, the Davis Medical Research Center, University Hospitals Clinic, and the Arthur G. James Cancer Hospital and Research Institute.

Grading Procedures

The College of Medicine uses a letter grading system that corresponds to a point value.

Special Programs

Awards for medical research are offered by the Samuel J. Roessler Memorial Medical Scholarship Fund. Depending on academic standing students can participate in a dual M.D./Ph.D. degree which takes seven years to complete. Joint M.D./Ph.D. students are encouraged to apply for the Medical Scientist Program (MSTP), which pays tuition and fees for the full seven years.

Application Procedures

Applications are processed through the American Medical College Application Service (AMCAS). There is a $20 application fee. AMCAS applications are accepted from June 15 through November 15. Students must include official transcripts from undergraduate colleges, and two or more letters of recommendation from professors.

Contact

Admissions Office
Third Floor, Lincoln Tower
1800 Cannon Drive
Columbus, Ohio 43210-1200
(614) 292-7137

UNIVERSITY OF OKLAHOMA COLLEGE OF MEDICINE

PO Box 26901
Oklahoma City, Oklahoma 73190
(405) 271-2265

Accreditation	LCME
Degrees Offered	M.D., M.D./Ph.D.
# Students Applied	875
Enrollment	158 / class
Mean GPA	3.4
% Men / % Women	67% / 33%
% Minorities	22%
Tuition	$5,370 In-State
	$12,840 Out-of-State
Application Fee	$10 In-State, $15 Out-of-State
Application Deadline	November 1

The University

The College of Medicine is located in Oklahoma City, Oklahoma, and was founded as a two-year school in 1900. In 1910 it merged with the Epworth Medical College, and its first degrees were granted in 1911.

Admissions

The school has admission requirements of a minimum 3.0 GPA, and a composite score of 7 on the MCAT. About 500 applicants are requested to interview for 150 positions in the freshman class; only 15 percent of each class may be from out of state.

Undergraduate Preparation

In order to apply, students must have completed a minimum of 90 semester hours at an accredited college, but must have completed their baccalaureate degree. Required undergraduate courses include one semester of general zoology/biology (including lab); two semesters each of general and organic chemistry; three semesters of English; two semesters of physics; two semesters of anthropology, psychology, or sociology, and one semester of histology, genetics, embryology, cellular biology, or comparative anatomy. Additional courses in the social sciences, humanities, mathematics, fine arts, computer science, and English are also encouraged.

Student Body

In the most recent entering class, 139 were Oklahoma state residents and 11 were nonresidents; one-third were women and two-thirds were men.

Placement Records

For students on both campuses, 56 percent were matched with in-state residencies, and 44 percent with out-of-state residencies.

Costs

As of 1989, tuition costs were $5,370 for residents and $12,840 for nonresidents for the academic year. Room and board is estimated to cost around $4,757, transportation to cost $720, and personal expenses to cost around $1,279. Books, supplies, instruments, and equipment for medical students should cost around $1,950 the first year, $1,230 the second, $425 the third, and $650 the fourth year.

Financial Aid

A number of federal programs provide aid to medical students. In addition, the Association of American Medical Colleges sponsors a consolidated loan program. There are also a number of local, county, state, and national organizations that offer limited financial aid to medical students.

Minority Programs

The University of Oklahoma Health Sciences Center offers a Health Careers Pathway Program that recruits, admits, retains, and graduates students from economically disadvantaged and ethnic backgrounds who have an interest in and aptitude for a health career in medicine. The Health Sciences Enrichment Institute is an eight-week summer program for 20 undergraduate freshmen and sophomores. The program gives these students a chance to experience the levels of academic excellence and personal commitment required of medical students. The three-week summer pre-admission workshop is designed to improve the reading rate, comprehension, and study skills of 20 college-level juniors and seniors, who also get classroom instruction in math, biology, and chemistry. Room and board is provided at no cost in both programs, and students are given a weekly stipend in the enrichment institute program. The school is a member of the Medical Minority Applicant Registry (Med-MAR).

Curriculum

In the first year, students are required to take courses in biochemistry, gross anatomy, physiology, microanatomy, and neuroanatomy. Second-year students take pathophysiology, pathology, microbiology, and pharmacology. In the third year students take clerkships in medicine, surgery, pediatrics, psychiatry, family medicine, and obstetrics, as well as required courses in otorhinolaryngology, dermatology, and neurology. Fourth-year students take an ambulatory care experience and four separate one-month externships in medicine, pediatrics, surgery, and psychiatry, a gynecology clerkship, and a rural preceptorship.

Facilities

The OUHSC library contains approximately 70,000 monographs, 2,500 journal titles, and over 4,000 audiovisual programs and microcomputer software programs in the fields of medicine, nursing, pharmacy, dentistry, public health, and allied health. The library is the medical resource library for the state of Oklahoma.

Special Programs

The College of Medicine allows enrollment in combined M.D./Ph.D. programs. Students also have the option of completing their last two years of medical school in either Oklahoma City or Tulsa. Both campuses have essentially the same course requirements, objectives, and methods of evaluation. Oklahoma City is larger, more academic and research oriented; the Tulsa program is smaller and more oriented toward community practice.

Application Procedures

Applications are processed through the American Medical College Application Service (AMCAS), and must be filed by October 15. A supplementary application will then be sent and must be completed by November 1. With the application students should include MCAT scores, four 2x2-inch glossy photographs, two letters of evaluation, and a $10 application fee for Oklahoma residents or a $15 fee for nonresidents. An interview is required, and will be conducted between October 15 and January 15.

Contact

Admissions and Student Affairs
University of Oklahoma
College of Medicine
Health Sciences Center
PO Box 26901
Oklahoma City, Oklahoma 73190
(405) 271-2339

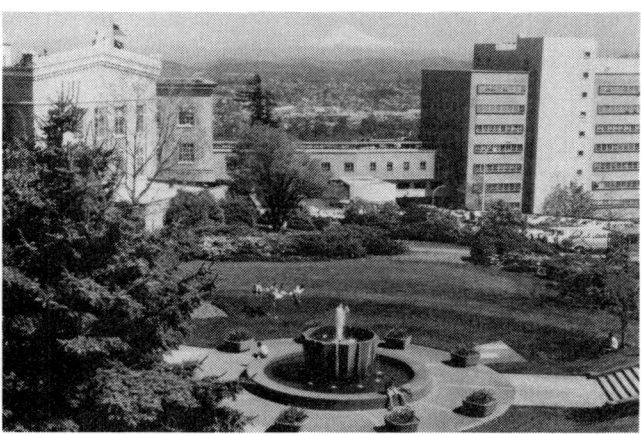

Photo by L.R. Lewton, Oregon Health Sciences University

OREGON HEALTH SCIENCES UNIVERSITY SCHOOL OF MEDICINE

3181 SW Sam Jackson Park Road
Portland, Oregon 97201-3098
(503) 279-8220

Accreditation	LCME, AAMC
Degrees Offered	M.D., Ph.D.
# Students Applied	802
Enrollment	94 / class
Mean GPA	3.5
% Men / % Women	55% / 45%
% Minorities	11%
Tuition	$5,166 In-State
	$11,958 Out-of-State
Application Fee	$40
Application Deadline	November 15

The University

The Oregon Health Sciences University is part of the Oregon State System of Higher Education and is one of the few independent academic health centers in the United States. Located on a 116-acre campus in a wooded section of Portland, the university's main purpose is to serve as a teaching center and training ground for health professionals and biomedical researchers. The city of Portland is just two miles away and may be reached via the jogging and cycling paths that weave in and around the campus.

Admissions

The School of Medicine strives to admit students with exceptionally capable minds who possess the compassion to use their talents wisely. Candidates for admission must exhibit evidence of strong motivation and the capacity to acquire the knowledge, skills, and attitudes necessary to practice medicine. Admissions preference is given to residents of the state of Oregon and other neighboring western states that are members of the Western Interstate Commission on Higher Education and do not have medical schools.

Undergraduate Preparation

A minimum of three years of undergraduate academic work must be completed before a candidate can be considered for admission to the School of Medicine. Specific requirements include the following: at least two years of college chemistry, including 10 to 16 quarter hours of general chemistry and eight to 12 hours of organic chemistry, with lab experience in qualitative techniques and methods; at least nine quarter hours of general biology/zoology including basic genetics; 12 quarter hours of physics with lab work covering the division of mechanics, heat and sound, and light and electricity; 12 quarter hours of college mathematics including calculus; and a minimum of six quarter hours of general psychology. The MCAT is also required.

Costs

Tuition is $5,166 for residents and $11,958 for nonresidents. Student fees are $1,149.

Financial Aid

The School of Medicine offers financial assistance to accepted students who demonstrate need. To apply for financial aid, students must submit the financial aid form to the College Scholarship Service.

Minority Programs

The medical school's office of multicultural student affairs provides a close, cooperative working relationship among students, faculty, and administration in developing programs and services that reflect the diversity of cultures and support academic development for minority students. Services include classes in learning skills, the development of English as a foreign language, cross-cultural counseling, and workshops in the development of ethnic sensitivity.

Curriculum

The first two years of the medical program consist of required courses in the basic and preclinical medical sciences. In the third and fourth years, students participate in required clinical clerkships. A number of elective courses are available in the fourth year.

Special Programs

The School of Medicine offers a combined M.D./Ph.D. program in biochemistry and molecular biology, cell biology and anatomy, medical genetics, medical psychology, microbiology and immunology, pathology, pharmacology, and physiology. Advanced research training is also available through the Vollum Institute for Advanced Biomedical Research, Veterans Affairs Medical Center, Oregon Regional Primate Research Center, Shriner's Hospital for Crippled Children, and the Neurological Sciences Institute of Good Samaritan Medical Center. Also, the Oregon legislature has established a "Rural Health Service Program," which offers extensive financial assistance to students who agree to practice in rural areas of Oregon after graduation.

Application Procedures

Students must first apply through AMCAS. Applications and supplemental materials are accepted no later than November 15 of the year prior to desired admission to medical school. Preliminary evaluations are made on the basis of scholarship, MCAT scores, and personal recommendations by the student's premedical advisers. Selected students are invited to on-campus interviews.

Contact

Director of Admissions
Oregon Health Sciences University
School of Medicine
3181 SW Sam Jackson Park Road
Portland, Oregon 97201-3098
(503) 494-7800

UNIVERSITY OF PENNSYLVANIA SCHOOL OF MEDICINE

Suite 100 — Medical Education Building
Philadelphia, Pennsylvania 19104-6056
(215) 898-5181

Accreditation	LCME
Degrees Offered	M.D., Ph.D., M.S.
# Students Applied	4,721
Enrollment	154 / class
Mean GPA	3.6
% Men / % Women	Not Available
% Minorities	11%
Tuition	$18,334
Application Fee	$55
Application Deadline	November 1

The University

Established in 1765 as the College of Philadelphia, the University of Pennsylvania School of Medicine was the first medical college in colonial America and has since consistently been at the forefront of American medicine. When the American Medical Association was organized in 1847, Nathaniel Champman, a professor of medicine at Penn, was chosen as the group's first president. Located in Philadelphia on a campus west of the Schuylkill River, the medical school strives to uphold its pioneering tradition today.

Admissions

There are no specific minimum GPA or MCAT requirements for admission to the School of Medicine. Instead, Penn looks for applicants who demonstrate the qualities of motivation, intellect, and character essential to success as a physician. Consideration will be given to experience or special aspects of a candidate's background that contribute to his or her potential for a medical career. Applicants must be able to deal effectively with people, organize their activities, set priorities, accept responsibility, and function under stress.

Undergraduate Preparation

Students are encouraged to pursue any rigorous course of undergraduate study that corresponds to their individual academic interests. A science major is not required, although an undergraduate degree must be earned prior to enrollment. All applicants are required to have a firm foundation in biology, chemistry, physics, and mathematics, and possess the corresponding laboratory skills. Also, candidates for admission to the School of Medicine must be proficient in writing, speaking, and reading the English language. Basic computer literacy is also strongly recommended.

Placement Records

Over the past several years, through the National Residency Matching Program, approximately 35 percent of Penn medical students entered residency positions in internal medicine, 12 percent entered pediatrics, 10 percent entered surgery, five percent entered obstetrics and gynecology, and five percent entered family practice. Other positions secured by students included programs in dermatology, neurology, ophthalmology, orthopedics, otorhinolaryngology, radiology, and psychiatry.

Costs

For the 1990-91 academic year, tuition at the School of Medicine was $48,334 and is expected to rise. Living expenses, which vary according to the type of living accommodations chosen, are estimated at $12,000 for a single, first-year student.

Financial Aid

Accepted students who require financial assistance must request financial aid forms from the office of admissions. Students requesting aid must submit tax data for themselves and their parents as well as other information requested by the GAPSFAS. Types of financial assistance include School of Medicine grants, School of Medicine loans, and a variety of federally and state-funded loan programs.

Minority Programs

In order to increase the number of minorities who are underrepresented in academic and clinical medicine, the School of Medicine maintains an office of minority affairs. Established in 1968, this office works to recruit potential candidates for admission, facilitate applications, serve as an advocate for admission applicants and enrolled students, and aid in retention through counseling. Currently, minority groups make up 11 percent of the total enrollment of the medical school.

Curriculum

The curriculum of the medical school is divided into three stages: Stage I, the 10-month first year emphasizing basic science; Stage II, the first six months of the second year emphasizing the pathophysiology of disease and introduction to clinical medicine; and Stage III, the remainder of the curriculum emphasizing clinical medicine. Stage I provides the student with the vocabulary, habits of thought, and core facts and principles in the basic sciences. The material of Stage II, organized and presented around organ systems, conveys a body of knowledge of disease and prepares the student for clinical experiences with programs on physical diagnosis and laboratory medicine. Stage III, finally, provides students with a broad base of clinical experience that will give them skills in diagnosis and patient management that will qualify them for postgraduate house officer training.

Grading Procedures

Grades are given on an honors/pass/fail system and are based on examinations as well as observation of student performance and professional qualities.

Special Programs

The School of Medicine offers students many opportunities to pursue independent research and other advanced degrees. The Office of Special Research and Combined Degree Programs maintains a directory of faculty research activities and offers interested students advice on how to pursue different options. Generally, qualified students may apply to pursue the M.D. as well as either a master's or a Ph.D. degree simultaneously in any subject related to medicine. Most students are able to obtain the M.D. and the master's degree in five years while the M.D. and the Ph.D. usually takes seven years to complete. Penn participates in the National Institutes of Health National Scientist Training Program and offers six to eight places annually in this program. Students interested in pursuing an advanced degree along with the M.D. must apply for admission to both through the Graduate School of the university.

Application Procedures

Applicants must submit the generalized application form to AMCAS no later than November 1 of the year prior to desired enrollment. In addition, the student must submit a supplemental application to the School of Medicine along with a $55 application fee no later than December 15. This application must also be accompanied by one letter of recommendation from the premedical advisory committee of the undergraduate college or, if no such committee exists, at least two letters of recommendation from professors who have taught the student (one in a science-related subject). The MCAT is required and must be taken during the calendar year preceding desired entrance into medical school.

Contact

Director of Admissions
University of Pennsylvania
School of Medicine
Suite 100
Medical Education Building
Philadelphia, Pennsylvania 19104-6056
(215) 898-8001

PENNSYLVANIA STATE UNIVERSITY COLLEGE OF MEDICINE

PO Box 850
Hershey, Pennsylvania 17033-0850
(717) 531-8521

Accreditation	LCME, AAMC
Degrees Offered	M.D.
# Students Applied	2,408
Enrollment	112 / class
Mean GPA	3.53
% Men / % Women	66% / 34%
% Minorities	19%
Tuition	$13,544 In-State
	$19,442 Out-of-State
Application Fee	$40
Application Deadline	November 15

The University

The school that Milton S. Hershey, the chocolate king, established for orphan boys in 1909 has become a campus of 10,000 acres for the nearly 1,200 students enrolled. The Milton S. Hershey Medical Center was founded from a trust Hershey established in 1935. In 1963, $50 million from this trust was set aside for the medical center, and ground was broken in 1966. The site is 12 miles east of Harrisburg, the state capital, and 103 miles from the University Park campus. The College of Medicine campus occupies 550 acres of a field along Route 322 on the western edge of Hershey, a thriving resort town of

about 18,000. Tourism is a major industry. Hersheypark, a local community theater, and restaurants offer ample entertainment.

Admissions

All candidates must take the MCAT and are urged to take the test the spring before the fall in which they apply. Applicants may take the test more than once. The mean GPA is 3.57, and MCAT mean scores are as follows: biology, 9.43; chemistry, 9.1; physics, 9.01; science prob., 9.01; reading, 8.85; quant., 8.36. Preference is given to qualified Pennsylvania residents.

Undergraduate Preparation

An applicant must have a baccalaureate from an accredited institution earned under residence and credit requirements similar to Penn State. Undergraduate preparation should include one year of biology and physics, two years of chemistry, familiarity with calculus and statistical methods, humanities that encourage moral choice and communications skills, and courses in psychology, sociology, and cultural anthropology. Laboratory exercises in all sciences are important, and library skills are essential. Applicants must complete all prerequisites before matriculation into the College of Medicine.

Student Body

Enrollment in 1989 at the university was 70,031, 1,200 in the College of Medicine. For the first-year class of 112, the Medical Center received 2,408 applications. Of these, 66 percent were male, 34 percent female, eight percent minority, 43 percent Pennsylvania residents, and 57 percent out-of-state residents. The entering class is composed of 69 percent Pennsylvania residents. The class includes 59 percent men and 41 percent women, and represents 30 Pennsylvania counties.

Costs

Tuition for Pennsylvania residents is $13,544; for out-of-state applicants, $19,442. All medical students attend school full time. Penn State estimates nine months' living expenses at $8,664, including health insurance, instruments and supplies, lodging, and food.

Financial Aid

The College of Medicine awards funds, except for a few academic awards, based solely on the student's financial need as documented by the GAPSFAS. Students' needs are reviewed annually. In 1989-90, the university awarded approximately 300 students scholarship aid out of its own resources. Federal programs, university loans, and some awards from external agencies are also available.

Student Organizations

Third- and fourth-year students may become part of Alpha Omega Alpha honor society. The American Medical Student

Association has a chapter on campus. Other groups include the Christian Medical Society, the Emergency Medical Society, Family Physicians, Medical Student Obstetrics and Gynecology Society, Physicians for Social Responsibility, Student National Medical Association, Student Psychiatric Society, Student Surgical Society, and Student Women's Group.

Faculty

The graduate faculty of Penn State University is 1,700, suggesting a student/faculty ratio of about 35:1.

Curriculum

The curriculum consists of four years' work. The first year focuses on the biology of the normal human organism. Courses include neurobiology, biochemistry, physiology, human anatomy, microanatomy/embryology, clinical correlation, molecular genetics, behavioral science, human genetics, statistics, and radiobiology. The second year introduces the student to human disease and pathology. The majority of students begin full-time clinical study in the summer after the second year. The third and fourth years are a continuum for required clerkships and electives. Required clerkships include medicine, neurology, obstetrics and gynecology, pediatrics, psychiatry, surgery, and family and community medicine.

Facilities

The George T. Harrell Library houses 125,000 volumes, 100,000 journal volumes, texts, and monographs. The department of educational resources offers graphics and audiovisual equipment, and operates a learning center on the ground floor.

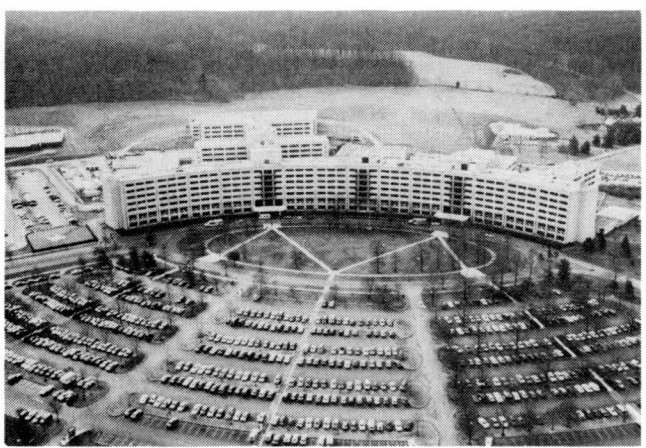

The computer learning center offers software packages for word processing, statistical analysis, and other research. Several nearby hospitals offer further opportunity for study.

Grading Procedures

The medical school awards final grades of honors, high pass, pass, or fail for each course. In addition, students must pass the National Board of Medical Education, Part I, to graduate. If students receive unsatisfactory/incomplete in a course(s), they may continue based on a faculty restructuring of their curriculum or course. Students may also repeat or suspend a year; otherwise, they may face a final dismissal.

Special Programs

The College of Medicine offers the M.D./Ph.D. A special research version is also offered to interest students in careers in clinical investigation as medical school faculty. The M.S. degree is available, along with residencies in graduate medical education. Students may pursue associate degrees and full-time certificate programs in radiologic technology and cardiovascular profusion technology. An extended nursing program leads to the B.S. About five students each year participate in the overseas electives program in countries in Africa, Asia, and Latin America.

Application Procedures

Applicants should request applications from AMCAS. The fee is $40. The deadline for submission, including transcripts, is November 15. The office of student affairs must receive supplemental applications by January 15. Letters of recommendation are required from each institution that granted the applicant a degree or in which a program was pursued. Otherwise, submit one letter each from faculty members in biology, chemistry, physics, and humanities. An interview may follow. Students are notified of acceptance starting after October of the year before entry. After acceptance, a student deposit ($100) is required by March 1.

Contact

Office of Student Affairs
Pennsylvania State University
College of Medicine
The Milton S. Hershey Medical Center
PO Box 850
Hershey, Pennsylvania 17033-0850
(717) 531-8755

UNIVERSITY OF PITTSBURGH SCHOOL OF MEDICINE

518 Sciafe Hall
Pittsburgh, Pennsylvania 15621
(412) 648-9891

Accreditation	LCME
Degrees Offered	M.D., Ph.D.
# Students Applied	2,920
Enrollment	138 / class
Mean GPA	Not Available
% Men / % Women	Not Available
% Minorities	Not Available
Tuition	$14,500 In-State
	$19,960 Out-of-State
Application Fee	$50
Application Deadline	November 15

The University

The School of Medicine was founded in 1886 as the Western Pennsylvania Medical College. In 1892, the school affiliated itself with Western University of Pennsylvania, which later became the University of Pittsburgh. Today, Pitt is a major research institution located in the Oakland section of Pittsburgh close to Carnegie Mellon University, the Carnegie Museum of Natural History, and the Sciafe Gallery of Art.

Admissions

Candidates for admission to the School of Medicine must demonstrate academic excellence as well as creativity, responsibility, and self-discipline. The admissions committee considers an applicant's college board scores, undergraduate academic record, MCAT scores, independent and advanced study, extracurricular activities, letters of recommendation, and personal essay. The School of Medicine seeks students who have integrity, maturity, and the ability to interact with people.

Undergraduate Preparation

Courses required for admission to Pitt include one year each of biology, general chemistry, organic chemistry, and physics (all with laboratory), as well as one year's work in English. Students are also required to have a strong background in mathematics, including calculus or calculus-based courses, while work in biostatistics and computer science is also recommended. No specific major is required and students are encouraged to study subjects in the social and behavioral sciences and humanities. A minimum of 120 semester hours of undergraduate coursework must be completed prior to enrollment.

Costs

Since the School of Medicine receives significant financial support from the state of Pennsylvania, tuition for students who are state residents is $14,500 annually, while out-of-state students are charged $19,960 per year. Pitt estimates that living expenses, including room and board, laundry, books, instruments, health insurance, and incidentals, will be between $9,000 and $11,000.

Student Organizations

Extracurricular groups for medical students include the student executive council, the American Medical Student Association, the Student National Medical Association, the Christian Medical Society, Pitt Women in Medicine, the American Medical Association, and the History of Medicine Society. Also, Phi Delta Epsilon, a social fraternity for all medical students, and Alpha Omega Alpha, a national medical honor fraternity, each have chapters at Pitt.

Curriculum

The first two years of the M.D. program familiarize students with the basic medical sciences. Students get their first introduction to patient interviewing, physical diagnosis, and specialty examinations in a series of interdisciplinary clinical sessions in the second year. In the third year, students spend 48 weeks in a sequence of clinical clerkships providing students with practical clinical experience in each of the major disciplines. The fourth year consists of 36 weeks of electives, the only required rotation being a four-week subinternship in medicine, pediatrics, or surgery. This structure allows the student to develop individual interests while also providing additional clinical experience in one area and significantly more responsibility for patient care.

Facilities

The School of Medicine is mainly housed in Sciafe Hall, a 13-story building that contains lecture rooms, labs, a library, and an auditorium. Adjacent to this building is the recently completed Biomedical Tower, which houses a variety of technologically advanced research labs. The School of Medicine is affiliated with Presbyterian-University Hospital of Pittsburgh, the Pittsburgh Cancer Institute, the Western Psychiatric Institute and Clinic, Eye and Ear Hospital of Pittsburgh, and the Falk Clinic, as well as other hospital and health care facilities in the greater Pittsburgh area. The collection of the Falk Library of the Health Sciences included more than 220,000 volumes and 1,500 journal subscriptions.

Grading Procedures

The School of Medicine uses an honors/satisfactory/unsatisfactory grading system. An honor code governs student academic behavior. Students are required to pass Parts I and II of the National Board Examination before graduating.

Special Programs

Pitt, in conjunction with nearby Carnegie Mellon University, offers a limited number of students the opportunity to simultaneously pursue the M.D. and Ph.D. degrees in preparation for careers in academic medicine. Admission to the program is made concurrently with admission to the medical school, and financial support is available on a competitive basis. The Western Pennsylvania Health Preceptorship Program offers summer experience in primary care to students who have completed the second year of medical training. Participating students spend eight weeks in a community hospital and in the office of a primary-care physician. A $1,000 stipend is offered with this program.

Application Procedures

Students must first make application with the AMCAS and then submit a secondary application to Pitt, along with a $50 application fee. Supporting materials required by the School of Medicine include a brief personal essay, MCAT scores, academic transcript, record of extracurricular activities, and letters of recommendation. Deadline for the receipt of these materials is December 15. The early decision deadline is September 1.

Contact

Office of Admissions
University of Pittsburgh
School of Medicine
518 Sciafe Hall
Pittsburgh, Pennsylvania 15261
(412) 648-9891

PONCE SCHOOL OF MEDICINE

PO Box 7004
Ponce, Puerto Rico 00732
(809) 840-2511

Accreditation	AMA
Degrees Offered	M.D., Ph.D
# Students Applied	409
Enrollment	40 / class
Mean GPA	3.15
% Men / % Women	65% / 35%
% Minorities	Not Available
Tuition	$14,000 In-State
	$21,000 Out-of-State
Application Fee	$50
Application Deadline	December 15

The University

The Ponce School of Medicine was formerly part of the Catholic University of Puerto Rico. In 1980, the school was reorganized by the Ponce Medical School Foundation and became an independent medical school. Emphasis at the school is on primary care and community medicine for underserved communities of Puerto Rico and areas of the mainland U.S. that have large Hispanic populations. Instruction is offered in both Spanish and English. The School of Medicine has an implied obligation to educate students who are likely to serve in Puerto Rico.

Admissions

The admissions committee considers MCAT scores, letters of recommendation, undergraduate achievement, and results of the personal interview in the admissions process. Preference is given to residents of Puerto Rico. Students are required to be bilingual in English and Spanish. Candidates are encouraged to obtain a broad cultural background.

Undergraduate Preparation

A minimum of 90 credit hours of undergraduate coursework from an accredited institution is required. Required courses include eight hours each of biology, organic and inorganic chemistry, and physics, 12 hours of Spanish, six hours of algebra, trigonometry, and/or advanced mathematics, six hours of humanities, and 12 hours of English. The MCAT should be taken in the year prior to the year of application.

Student Body

The graduating class of 1988 consisted of 43 students. The 1990 entering class had an average GPA of 3.15. Ninety-six percent of the entrants were from Puerto Rico, 35 percent were women. Eighty-three percent had baccalaureate degrees.

Placement Records

The students of the class of 1988 went on to practice at hospitals all of the mainland U.S. as well as Puerto Rico.

Costs

Tuition is $14,000 annually for residents of Puerto Rico and $21,000 annually for nonresidents. Nonresidents, however, can obtain resident status after successfully completing the first two years of medical school. Other fees total approximately $1,500.

Financial Aid

Loan programs include Guaranteed Student Loans and Health Education Assistance Loans. Armed Forces scholarships are also available. The school requires the Ponce School of Medicine application for financial aid as well as the GAPSFAS form. Some direct grants and emergency loan funds may be available on a limited basis.

Student Organizations

Student organizations include the student council. The office of student affairs represents the students, helps with housing and financial aid, and assists with clinical training at U.S. mainland hospitals.

Curriculum

The four-year program consists of basic and clinical sciences, clerkships and electives. First- and second-year courses include anatomy, embryology, physiology, basic psychiatry, community medicine, pathology, and medical ethics. The third year provides training in surgery, pediatrics, obstetrics/gynecology, and other basic medical skills. Required clerkships in the last three quarters of the year include medicine, surgery, pediatrics, and psychiatry. Required clerkships of the fourth year are in the same disciplines as those mentioned above, plus emergency medicine, family medicine, electives, and several other areas.

The school also offers a five-year extended M.D. degree program. In this program, the first two years of the regular four-year program are extended over a three-year period. Candidates for admission may request the five-year program.

Facilities

For clinical education, the school uses a network of affiliated institutions that include clinics and hospitals in Puerto Rico and a U.S. mainland hospital, St. Michael's Medical Center in Newark, New Jersey. The medical library houses reference, research, and general materials in print and nonprint formats; produces instructional materials for lectures and conferences; offers interlibrary loan services; and provides access to MEDLINE and other databases.

Grading Procedures

Students' work is graded according to an honors/pass/fail/incomplete/extended system.

Special Programs

The school offers a Ph.D. degree program in the biomedical sciences, intended for students who wish to pursue careers in research. Students can specialize in anatomy, biochemistry, medical microbiology, pharmacology-toxicology, or physiology.

Application Procedures

The Ponce School of Medicine participates in AMCAS. Applications should be filed with AMCAS by November 15 of the year prior to the year of desired enrollment. Three letters of recommendation from three college professors or one letter from the premedical committee must be submitted directly to the school's office of admissions. There is a $50 application fee.

Contact

Admissions Office
Ponce School of Medicine
University Street
PO Box 7004
Ponce, Puerto Rico 00732
(809) 840-2511

UNIVERSITY OF PUERTO RICO SCHOOL OF MEDICINE

PO Box 365067
San Juan, Puerto Rico 00936-5067
(809) 758-2525

Accreditation	LCME
Degrees Offered	M.D., M.S., Ph.D.
# Students Applied	313
Enrollment	93 / class
Mean GPA	3.54
% Men / % Women	51% / 49%
% Minorities	Not Available
Tuition	$2,500 – Resident
	Pays according to a standardized fee scale – Nonresident
Application Fee	$15
Application Deadline	December 1

The University

Established in 1949, the University of Puerto Rico School of Medicine is part of the university's medical sciences campus. The campus also comprises the School of Dentistry, the College of Allied Health Professions, the Faculty of Biosocial Sciences, the School of Pharmacy, and the Graduate School of Public Health.

Admissions

The school considers a wide range of factors in the admissions process, including academic record, MCAT scores, letters of recommendation, personality, extracurricular activities, and other relevant information. Personal interviews are granted by invitation to selected applicants. In some cases, interviews can be conducted on the mainland. The school gives preference to U.S. citizens who are legal residents of Puerto Rico. All students of the 1990 entering class were residents of Puerto Rico. The mean GPA of the class was 3.54; the mean science GPA was 3.46.

Undergraduate Preparation

Applicants must have had at least 90 semester hours of undergraduate coursework from an accredited institution. Students should take the MCAT on or before September of the year prior to enrollment. Required undergraduate courses are eight semester hours of biology; eight hours of inorganic chemistry (with lab); eight hours of organic chemistry (with lab); eight hours of physics (with lab); 12 hours of English; 12 hours of Spanish; and six hours of behavioral and social sciences. Students should be fluent in both English and Spanish.

Student Body

The 1990-91 first-year class numbered 93 students. All students took the MCAT, and 69 percent held the bachelor's degree. The class comprised 51 percent men and 49 percent women.

Costs

For the 1990-91 academic year, resident tuition was $2,500. Nonresident students who are U.S. citizens pay a tuition equal to the amount they would pay in their home state. Student fees for the year were $285.

Financial Aid

Over half of the student body receives some form of financial aid during the course of the four-year program. Scholarships and loans are granted primarily on the basis of need. Students can apply for scholarships at the same time they file their applications for admission, or any time before April 30.

Student Organizations

Medical students may join the American Medical Student Association. Alpha Omega Alpha, the national medical honor society, is also active on campus.

Faculty

The School of Medicine employs more than 400 faculty members.

Curriculum

Basic sciences and clinical sciences are the focus of the first two years of the program. During the second year courses in pathology, physiology, physical diagnosis, and basic clerkship are added. Other subjects studied during this part of the curriculum include collective human behavior, environmental factors in medicine, and public health. The third year focuses on clinical clerkships in medicine, pediatrics, surgery, obstetrics and gynecology, and psychiatry. The fourth year includes both required clerkships and elective experiences, a six-week rotation, and a one-week course in legal, ethical, and administrative aspects of medicine.

Facilities

The main facility used in the clinical education of students is the University District Hospital. The hospital, located near the campus, provides a high level of integration of the basic and clinical components of the program. Other affiliated institutions include the Puerto Rico Medical Center and the Hospital Consortium, which has health care units in Ponce, Mayaquez, Carolina, and Caguas. The library collection totals more that 110,000 volumes; an audiovisual center contains nonprint materials for student use.

Grading Procedures

Students are evaluated using a letter-grade system.

Application Procedures

Applications should be filed with the school between July 1 and December 1 of the year prior to year of intended enrollment. The school does not participate in an early decision plan. Students are notified of acceptance between February 15 and March 15. Upon acceptance, students must submit a $100 deposit, which is applied toward tuition.

Contact

Central Admissions Office
University of Puerto Rico
School of Medicine
Medical Sciences Campus
PO Box 365067
San Juan, Puerto Rico 00936-5067
(809) 758-2525

UNIVERSITY OF ROCHESTER SCHOOL OF MEDICINE AND DENTISTRY

Rochester, New York 14627
(716) 275-3407

Accreditation	AAMC
Degrees Offered	M.D., Ph.D., M.S.
# Students Applied	1,812
Enrollment	96 / class
Mean GPA	3.52
% Men / % Women	51% / 49%
% Minorities	10%
Tuition	$17,300
Application Fee	$50
Application Deadline	November 1

The University

The University of Rochester was originally founded in 1850 as a small liberal arts college for men. It is now a coeduca-

tional, independently supported, nonsectarian institution. The university is accredited by the Middle States Association of Colleges and Secondary Schools and is a member of the prestigious Association of American Universities. The School of Medicine and Dentistry itself was founded in 1920. The medical school, the School of Nursing, and Strong Memorial Hospital are the principal components of the University of Rochester Medical Center. This center was one of the first in the country to house both a medical school and hospital in a single building. Special care was taken in its design to promote interdepartmental cooperation in teaching and research. Since its opening, the original 560,000-square-foot complex has grown to its present 2,444,351 square feet. Rochester is a culturally sophisticated, medium-sized city south of Lake Ontario and north of the glacier-formed hills of the Finger Lakes region of New York. It has been rated among the East's most livable cities: small and clean enough to be comfortable, but large and cosmopolitan enough to afford a variety of diversions. The cost of living is moderate and because of its reasonable size, the metropolitan area is easy to negotiate by car or public transportation. Housing is affordable, generally of high quality, and readily available.

Admissions

The MCAT can be a helpful addition to the right undergraduate coursework. Applicants who have taken the examination should request that a score report be sent to Rochester. However, the MCAT is not required and applicants who have not taken the test receive full and careful consideration.

Undergraduate Preparation

Students are advised to obtain an undergraduate degree unless there are compelling reasons for seeking admission to medical school at an earlier date. However, at least three years of study in an approved university or college are required. At least one year of college English is required, which must include major expository writing. One year of physics (with lab) is required; students are assumed to be familiar with atomic and nuclear physics. One full year of biology, with lab, is required. Two years of college chemistry, including one year of organic chemistry (with laboratory) or one semester of organic chemistry and one semester of biochemistry, are required. Courses in genetics, embryology, comparative anatomy, and cellular physiology are recommended, as are courses in statistics and calculus and experience in research, clinical practice, public health, or health policy issues. Additional requirements warrant a minimum of four courses in the humanities or social sciences. Advanced placement courses may be used to satisfy one semester of the physics requirement as well as one semester of the chemistry requirement. Advanced placement courses will not satisfy the biology, English, or non-science requirements.

Costs

Tuition for the 1990-91 academic year is $17,300. The

tuition fee covers all instructional and collateral costs, such as the use of recreational facilities, graduation charges, etc. Costs for second-, third-, and fourth-year students are similar, but vary somewhat depending upon the length of the academic period and different curricular requirements. The first-year fixed costs can be broken down as follows: tuition $17,300, health fee $648, microscope fee (first and second years only) $160, locker fee $12, activity fee $30. Variable costs include books and equipment $800, housing and food $5,000, personal expenses $1,750, and transportation allowance $1,500. Each student is issued two white jackets to be returned upon graduation. New uniforms may be purchased at a cost of $16 to $20 per set and four sets are the minimum number suggested for each student. Laundry will be provided upon the purchase of cards through the cashier's office.

Financial Aid

The base of any financial aid package is a self-help component. Students must come up with $11,000 through loans or other non-school sources before school aid is awarded. Students usually meet this need by obtaining a Stafford (formerly Guaranteed Student) Loan of $7,500 and a combination of additional loans, outside scholarships, or part-time employment. If the student's need exceeds the self-help index, then university scholarship and loan assistance is awarded to fully meet the remaining financial need. In addition, the school awards grants under two federal programs administered by the Department of Health and Human Services: the Exceptional Financial Need Program and the Program of Financial Assistance for Disadvantaged Health Professions Students (FADHPS). There are also numerous loan programs, college work-study programs, and New York State assistance for those with residency of one year in the state. More information can be obtained through the Medical School Financial Aid Handbook.

Minority Programs

Since an office of minority affairs was established in 1981, the number of minority students increased from nine to 40 in 1989. A foreign national may be considered for admission to the school, but must have a permanent resident visa in the United States and should have spent at least two years studying in an undergraduate college in this country, including premedical coursework. Special help is available for applicants to make arrangements for visiting Rochester, settling in, and locating housing, volunteer opportunities, and student employment. Numerous programs and fellowships are available. More information can be obtained through the office of minority affairs.

Student Organizations

The University of Rochester houses a chapter of the Alpha Omega Alpha honor medical society to which students are elected in their fourth year based on scholarship and professional excellence. The Society of Sigma Xi annually elects students who show unusual promise of becoming able scientific investigators. For the medical student with an interest in history, there is the George W. Corner History of Medicine Society, which promotes activities in the history of medicine at the school. Popular organizations include the Medical Student Senate, Student National Medical Association, American Medical Student Association, and the Graduate Student Society. The Medical Alumni Association is comprised of approximately 7,000 alumni. Over 50 percent are medical degree holders, 20 percent are graduate degree holders, and the balance are those who have completed at least one residency program at the Medical Center.

Curriculum

In the first year of study, mastery of the basic science principles and information required for understanding human body and human behavior is coupled with the study of illustrative patients and clinical problems. In the second year, emphasis shifts to the study of mechanisms of human disease and students learn how to work directly with the sick, which prepares them for intensive clinical training in the third and fourth years. At the beginning of the third year, students work with patients under close faculty supervision in the general clerkship. Thereafter, students rotate through clinical specialty services, participating fully in the evaluation and management of patients. Through the fourth year, the clinical program expands to involve the study and care of ambulatory and hospitalized patients.

Facilities

The Edward G. Miner Library offers of full range of library services, including access to a variety of computer databases and the collections total more than 200,000 volumes. A medical education wing provides multidisciplinary teaching laboratories, and a medical media center has available all the audiovisual services at the school. The primary teaching hospital for the school is Strong Memorial Hospital, with approximately 28,000 admissions and 237,000 patient days each year. It is the largest acute general hospital in Rochester and is both a community hospital and specialized referral center for the region. The University of Rochester Cancer Center is one of 56 centers approved and funded by the National Cancer Institute. The Center on Aging promotes curriculum development in basic and clinical areas dealing with geriatrics. The Clinical Research Center is one of about 78 located at academic health science centers in the United States. Additional area hospitals have become major teaching affiliates of the medical school, and specialize in several disciplines.

Grading Procedures

Various courses are graded on different scales. They range

from a satisfactory/fail basis to a three-point scale of honors/satisfactory/fail, to a five-point system of honors/good/satisfactory/poor/fail.

Special Programs

There are many special programs available to medical students, such as the "In-Depth" Experience, Student-Faculty Program, First Year/Fourth Year Program, medical student research day, community programs, and student teaching days. Through the school's program in international medicine, students may work in the health care system of another country during the summer following the first or second year, or in an elective period during the clinical years. In addition, students can participate in summer fellowships or a full-year student fellowship, which carries a stipend of $9,000 per year. Combined degrees can also be obtained through the M.D./M.S. or M.D./Ph.D. program, for which students can apply at the time of initial application or after a year or more of study at the school.

Application Procedures

Applications should be filed between June and October of the year preceding the date of enrollment, and must be received by November 1. A nonrefundable application fee of $50 is required.

Contact

Medical Admissions Committee
University of Rochester
School of Medicine and Dentistry
Box 601
Rochester, New York 14642
(716) 275-4539

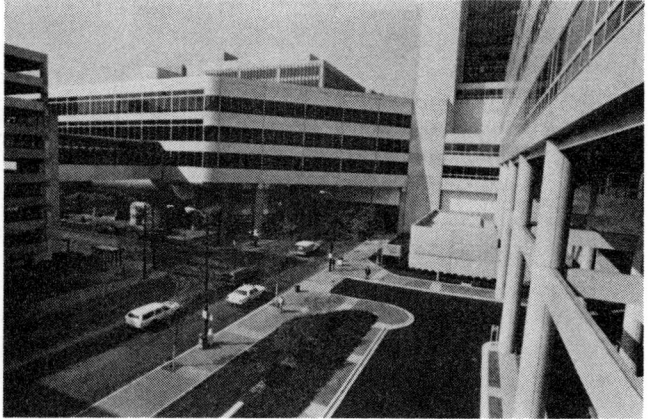

RUSH MEDICAL COLLEGE OF RUSH UNIVERSITY

Chicago, Illinois 60612
(312) 942-5099

Accreditation	LCME
Degrees Offered	M.D., M.D./Ph.D
# Students Applied	2,528
Enrollment	119 / class
Mean GPA	Not Available
% Men / % Women	76% / 24%
% Minorities	Not Available
Tuition	$17,520
Application Fee	$35
Application Deadline	November 15

The University

Rush University has expanded from one college and fewer than 100 students to four colleges and over 1,000 students. It includes Rush Medical College, the College of Nursing, the College of Health Sciences, and the Graduate College. Rush is located on the west side of Chicago near the Loop, in an area undergoing much redevelopment. There are several other health care facilities in the Medical Center district.

Admissions

The admissions committee considers both the academic and nonacademic qualifications of applicants in making its decisions. The committee also takes into account such factors as the degree of difficulty of the applicant's academic program, the need to be employed while in school, the applicant's social and cultural background, outside interests, motivation, and nonacademic achievement. Applicants with three years of college but no baccalaureate degree who meet the necessary requirements will be considered. The MCAT is required. Although there is no absolute numerical cutoff for GPA and MCAT scores, applicants are not likely to be admitted if they were not in the upper third of their college class. The medical college is currently expanding the number of positions available to nonresidents. Only U.S. citizens or applicants who have permanent residency status are considered for admission.

Undergraduate Preparation

The following coursework (including all necessary laboratory work) is required: physics, eight semester hours; biology, eight semester hours; inorganic chemistry, eight semester hours; organic chemistry, eight semester hours, or four semester hours of organic chemistry and four semester hours of biochemistry. Survey courses in the premedical sciences will not fulfill these requirements. Courses in mathematics, social sciences, and English are strongly recommended. The committee advises that additional science courses be taken.

Student Body

Rush Medical College students come from a wide variety of educational and social backgrounds. Students range in age from 19 to 57. In 1989, over 80 percent of students lived in Illinois prior to entering Rush. The 1,112 students include 24 Hispanic, 110 Asian/Pacific Islander, 55 black, three American Indian, and 29 foreign students.

Placement Records

Graduates practice in all 50 states and in 11 foreign countries.

Costs

Tuition was $17,520 for the 1990-91 entering class.

Curriculum

Students of the college are encouraged to develop habits of self-education and enthusiasm for the lifelong study of medicine. For the first two years of study, the medical college offers students a choice between a conventional curriculum and the Rush Alternative Curriculum. The first year of the conventional curriculum consists of basic sciences, emphasizing the structure, function, and behavior of the normal person. During the second year, students study the causes and effects of disease and therapeutics while initiating their work with patients in programs that emphasize interviewing, history-taking, and the physical examination. The content of the alternative program is similar to the conventional program, but the learning format is different. Units within the curriculum are integrated across the preclinical disciplines rather than taught as separate courses. Specially designed "learning guidebooks" outline the basic science content to be learned in each unit, and provide appropriate reference material and learning exercises. A major emphasis of the curriculum is the discussion of clinical problems, which are developed to illustrate the underlying basic science principles. Specially trained clinicians help groups of six students with their studies of the basic and behavioral sciences, preventative medicine, and the clinical skills of physical examination. The alternative program is limited to 28 students. The third and fourth years include 54 weeks of required core clerkships; a four-week sub-internship in family practice, pediatrics , or medicine; and 20 weeks of elective study. Students are encouraged to complete their required courses early to make better use of the elective options offered in the fourth year.

Facilities

Rush Medical College students receive training in a variety of clinical settings, including the academic medical center and community hospitals located in the inner city and in suburban and rural areas of Illinois. Students receive their clinical training primarily at Rush-Presbyterian-St. Luke's Hospital, a voluntary, not-for-profit hospital with a professional staff of 758 physicians and scientists and 435 house staff in graduate medical education in over 30 specialty areas. There are over 30,000 patients admitted annually to the hospital. Christ Hospital, a major teaching hospital associated with Rush, has 873 beds and is located in a south suburb of Chicago. It participates in the teaching of required core clerkships. On-campus housing is available for about 25 percent of university students.

Grading Procedures

A letter-grading system is used. Under the Rush Alternative Curriculum, performance in group and individual problem-solving is assessed. Examinations are given. Students must pass Part I of the NBME exams and complete Part II in order to graduate.

Special Programs

Rush offers a combined M.D./Ph.D. program. The Graduate College offers the Ph.D. degree in anatomical sciences, biochemistry, immunology/microbiology, pharmacology, physiology, and clinical psychology. Applications and information for Ph.D. programs may be obtained by designating an interest on the Rush Medical College supplemental application.

Application Procedures

All formal applications to Rush must be initiated through AMCAS. AMCAS strongly recommends that an applicant's college forward his or her transcript at least two weeks prior to processing an application. The deadline for regular application is November 15 of the year preceding matriculation. An information packet outlining the Rush application procedure and timetables will be sent to each applicant upon receipt of the processed AMCAS application. There is an application fee of $25. Applicants are encouraged to take the MCAT in April of the year of application. Interviews are required, and are given only by invitation from the committee on admissions.

Contact

Office of Admissions
Rush Medical College
Room 524H
600 S Paulina Street
Chicago, Illinois 60612
(312) 942-6319

SAINT LOUIS UNIVERSITY SCHOOL OF MEDICINE

1402 South Grand Boulevard
St. Louis, Missouri 63104
(314) 517-8000

Accreditation	LCME
Degrees Offered	M.D., M.D./Ph.D.
# Students Applied	1,547
Enrollment	148 / class
Mean GPA	3.49
% Men / % Women	78% / 22%
% Minorities	Not Available
Tuition	$18,700
Application Fee	$50
Application Deadline	December 15

The University

Founded in 1818, St. Louis University is a private institution enrolling 6,900 undergraduate and 1,500 graduate students. It was the first university chartered west of the Mississippi River, and was founded by the Jesuits. The School of Medicine was established in 1836 as the medical department of the university. Today, the school's mission is to educate physicians and biomedical scientists, conduct basic and applied medical research, and provide health services on a local, national, and international level. St. Louis is a modern city in the heart of the Midwest, with a population of more than 2.4 million people. More than 100 hospitals and clinics employ approximately 65,000 individuals in a variety of medical fields, making the city a hub of health care and medical research.

Admissions

Most accepted applicants complete a baccalaureate degree of at least 120 semester hours from an accredited college or university. The 1989 entering class had an overall GPA of 3.4, and science/math GPA of 3.4. The mean score on the MCAT was 57. All candidates for the M.D. degree must demonstrate satisfactory communication, behavioral, and social skills and possess the proper visual, motor, and tactile skills needed to become a physician.

Undergraduate Preparation

Undergraduate courses required for admission are eight semester hours each of general biology or zoology, inorganic chemistry, organic chemistry, and physics. Six semester hours

of English and 12 semester hours of other humanities and behavioral sciences are also required. The study of biochemistry is highly recommended but not required.

Student Body

The School of Medicine enrolls 600 medical students, directs the training of 360 medical residents and fellows, and teaches 80 graduate students in the biomedical sciences. Twenty percent of the students are Missouri residents. Twenty-two percent are women.

Placement Records

The School of Medicine participates in the National Residency Matching Program (NRMP). In recent years, 80 percent of the school's graduates participating in NRMP have matched with one of their first three residency program choices.

Costs

Tuition for the 1990-91 first-year class was $18,700. The student fee is $450. Books and equipment in the first year total approximately $700.

Financial Aid

The School of Medicine gives priority assistance to those students who demonstrate the greatest relative need, in the form of loans or grants. Federally funded loans include Stafford Loans, Health Education Assistance Loans, and Supplemental Loans to Students. Programs administered by the university include university scholarships, health professions student loans, Perkins loans, and various restricted student scholarship and loan funds. Other sources of aid may come from the private sector. The school also maintains a medical student revolving loan fund.

Student Organizations

Students may become representatives of the student council and the student executive council of the Medical Center. The school has chapters of Alpha Omega Alpha and other honors societies. Students can also join the American Medical Students Association, the American Medical Women's Association, the Family Practice Club, or the Christian Medical Society. There are also coeducational fraternities on campus.

Faculty

There are 460 full-time faculty members and 875 part-time/voluntary faculty members who are practicing physicians.

Curriculum

The curriculum follows the classical structure of two years of training in the basic and behavioral sciences followed by two years of both structured and elective experiences in the core clinical disciplines. The first two years include formal instruction in basic medical science with lectures, demonstrations, laboratories, discussion groups, and preceptorships. The third year consists of 48 weeks of instruction through rotating clerkships. The fourth year consists partly of required instruction and clinical experiences and partly of electives offering both clinical and research opportunities.

Facilities

In addition to the medical school, St. Louis University Medical Center comprises the School of Allied Health Professions, the School of Nursing, the Graduate Program in Orthodontics, and the Center for Health Services Education and Research. Clinical, teaching, and research facilities include St. Louis University Hospital, a 362-bed institution, Cardinal Glennon Children's Hospital, Bethesda Eye Institute, and an ambulatory care facility staffed by St. Louis University clinical faculty and house officers from various departments within the medical school. The medical center also includes the Institute for Molecular Virology and the Pediatric Research Institute. The Medical Center Library provides medical literature searches and MEDLINE. In addition to the library's on-site collection, the resources of 30 major health science libraries and the National Library of Medicine collection are made available through interlibrary loans.

Grading Procedures

The School of Medicine uses an honors/pass/fail grading system.

Special Programs

Research fellowships are available for students in basic or scientific research, and behavioral and epidemiologic investigations. Fellowships are available primarily during the summer after the first year of medical school. The combined M.D./Ph.D. program is designed for students interested in research careers in medicine, and enables the student to complete both degrees in a six- to seven-year period.

Application Procedures

The school reviews AMCAS application materials (including transcripts) and asks applicants to provide supplementary information including letters of evaluation, a photograph, and a $45 application fee. The deadline for submission of all materials is December 15. All candidates must take the MCAT, preferably during the spring of the junior undergraduate year. Interviews are granted only to selected applicants. Accepted applicants must make an advance tuition deposit of $100 to hold their place. The school also has an early decision plan, under which all required credentials must by submitted to AMCAS by August 1.

Contact

Saint Louis University
School of Medicine
1402 South Grand Boulevard
St. Louis, Missouri 63104
(314) 577-8205

UNIVERSITY OF SOUTH ALABAMA COLLEGE OF MEDICINE

2015 Medical Sciences Building
Mobile, Alabama 36688
(205) 460-7187

Accreditation	AAMC, AMA, SACSS
Degrees Offered	M.D., M.D./Ph.D.
# Students Applied	777
Enrollment	64 / class
Mean GPA	3.1
% Men / % Women	60% / 40%
% Minorities	Not Available
Tuition	$5,280 In-State
	$10,560 Out-of-State
Application Fee	$25
Application Deadline	November 15

The University

The University of South Alabama College of Medicine was chartered in 1969 as a public, state-sponsored school by the Alabama legislature in response to the health care needs of southern Alabama. The school occupies 13 buildings on the university's 1,200 acre wooded campus in the Springhill section of Mobile and operates a 400-bed medical center. Total university enrollment is approximately 11,000 students. The campus adjoins the 750-acre municipal park with its extensive recreational facilities as well as a municipal golf course.

Admissions

Candidates for admission to the College of Medicine are required to present an undergraduate GPA of 3.0 or better. Applicants from out of state or for the early decision option are expected to have a GPA of at least 3.5. The MCAT exam is also required. Special accomplishments and the substance of an applicant's overall academic program are also considered.

Undergraduate Preparation

To be considered for admission, an applicant must present 90 semester hours of academic work, with completion of a B.A. degree preferred. Required courses are eight semester hours each of general biology, general chemistry, organic chemistry and general physics, all with lab. Six semester hours of humanities, eight of English composition or literature, and eight of college mathematics are also required. Calculus is highly recommended. A science major is not a prerequisite for admission to the College of Medicine but an applicant must have sufficient scientific training to show "superior aptitude." Pass/fail grades for undergraduate courses are not acceptable.

Student Body

A large number of students in the College of Medicine are Alabama state residents and have attended universities in the southern United States. However, students are regularly admitted from out of state and come from major colleges and universities all around the country. Sixty percent of the student body are men, 40 percent women.

Placement Records

Because the student body is predominantly southern, the majority of graduates seek and obtain residency appointments to major southern hospitals and medical centers.

Costs

Tuition is $5,280 per year for state residents and $10,560 per year for nonresidents. A recent change in Alabama law grants in-state status for tuition purposes to residents of certain counties on the Mississippi Gulf Coast and the Florida Panhandle. Other fees for services such as student health, activities, and laboratory equipment total approximately $500 annually.

Financial Aid

Loans and scholarships are available to students on the basis of need. Application for these funds must be made to the University of South Alabama office of financial aid and a family financial statement must be submitted to the American College Testing Service by April 1. Students in the College of Medicine are discouraged from working part time during the academic year and are advised not to depend on such income to finance their education.

Minority Programs

Under the National Medical Fellowship, minority students may receive grants based on eligibility criteria.

Student Organizations

Interested students may participate in activities sponsored by the American Medical Student Association, the Student National Medical Association, the Student Business Section of the American Medical Association, the Family Practice Club, and the Military Medical Students Society. Alpha Omega Alpha, an honor society, also has a chapter on campus. The university is governed by a student assembly to which the College of Medicine elects members.

Faculty

The College of Medicine has 539 affiliate full- and part-time faculty members.

Curriculum

During the first two years students of the M.D. program must take required courses in general medical topics. The third year consists of six clinical clerkships in medicine, obstetrics and gynecology, pediatrics, surgery, family practice, and psychiatry, as well as electives. The fourth year is composed of 12 four-week rotations within selected clinical areas with each student required to participate in a minimum of nine. The semester between the second and third year is devoted to a clinical clerkship while the summer between the third and fourth year is reserved for fourth-year electives.

Facilities

The biomedical library of the College of Medicine has a permanent collection of over 77,500 volumes of books and journals and approximately 2,300 medical/scientific periodicals. The 400-bed Medical Center is the major physician-staffed emergency facility in south Alabama. The College of Medicine also boasts a 10,000-square-foot primate research facility and a forensic laboratory operated in conjunction with the state of Alabama.

Grading Procedures

Grades are numerical with 94-100=outstanding, 86-93=above average, 78-85=average, 70-77=below average, and below 70=failure. In addition, grades are accompanied by written comments from professors.

Special Programs

In conjunction with the Graduate School of the University of South Alabama, the College of Medicine offers a seven-year program leading to a combined M.D./Ph.D. The Graduate School also offers a five-year Ph.D. program in basic medical sciences.

Application Procedures

Applicants must submit an application to both the Association of American Medical Colleges and directly to the College of Medicine. The College of Medicine application must be accompanied by the $25 application fee, three faculty letters of recommendation, one personal reference, and a photograph of the applicant. The applicant should take the MCAT previous to April of the year before desired entrance into medical school; however, scores from the past three years will be considered. After evaluation of these materials is complete, certain students will be invited to the university for personal interviews.

Contact

Office of Admissions
University of South Alabama
College of Medicine
2015 Medical Sciences Building
Mobile, Alabama 36688
(205) 460-7176

UNIVERSITY OF SOUTH CAROLINA SCHOOL OF MEDICINE

Columbia, South Carolina 29208
(803) 733-3200

Accreditation	LCME
Degrees Offered	M.D., M.D./Ph.D.
# Students Applied	1,133
Enrollment	72 / class
Mean GPA	3.33
% Men / % Women	64% / 36%
% Minorities	12%
Tuition	$4,800 In-State
	$11,000 Out-of-State
Application Fee	$20
Application Deadline	December 1

The University

The School of Medicine is one of the newest academic units of the University of South Carolina. The first class of 24 medical students was admitted in the fall of 1977. Class size has almost tripled since then. In the summer of 1983 the school's administrative offices and basic science departments moved to a new campus. Most clinical departments are located at affiliated hospitals in the Columbia area.

Admissions

Preference is given to applicants who hold a bachelor's degree upon enrollment. Well-qualified applicants who have completed 90 semester hours of undergraduate work will be considered. Although the school requires that the MCAT be taken no more than two years prior to the time of application and no later than the fall of the year of application, applicants who plan to enter the class of 1992 are encouraged to take the 1991 revised MCAT. As a matter of policy, the School of Medicine will not admit students from other health science schools or graduate degree programs until such students have completed the degree program for which they are enrolled. Transfer students will be considered for second- and third-year classes if positions are available. Preference for admission is given to state residents.

Undergraduate Preparation

Undergraduate coursework must include eight semester hours each of physics, organic chemistry, and inorganic chemistry (all with labs), six semester hours of English (composi-tion and literature), mathematics (college level algebra is required, calculus is suggested), and biology, with lab, which may be satisfied with general biology, general zoology, or botany (but no more than four hours may be botany). The admissions committee recommends that students take more than the minimum requirements in the natural sciences. College Level Placement (CLEP) and advanced placement credits are accepted if they do not represent more than 25 percent of undergraduate credit awarded.

Costs

Annual tuition for residents is $4,800; nonresidents pay $11,000. Books and supplies for the first year cost about $3,000; second year, $1,500; third year, $1,200; and fourth year, $1,800.

Financial Aid

Some financial aid specifically earmarked for medical students is available from the School of Medicine. Eligibility for all aid except some academic scholarships is based on an applicant's financial circumstances. Aid is available from federal, state, and private sources. The financial statement of the American College Testing Service is used to determine the amount of assistance each applicant is eligible to receive. Outside employment is available, but the academic responsibilities of the first year of medical school preclude outside employment.

Student Organizations

Student organizations include the USC School of Medicine Student Association, the American Medical Student Association, the American Medical Women's Association, the Medical Student Section of the AMA, the South Carolina Medical Student Section, the Student National Medical Association, the Family Practice Club, and the Behavioral Science Society. Religious activities are available on the Carolina campus.

Faculty

There are over 680 faculty members.

Curriculum

The first two years consist of a core curriculum of basic sciences and clinical disciplines necessary for an understanding of human systems. During the second year, emphasis is placed on pathology and general therapeutic principles. Interdisciplinary material on such subjects as nutrition, human values, and geriatrics is presented. The third year comprises eight-week clerkships in medicine, surgery, obstetrics/gynecology, psychiatry, family medicine, and pediatrics. The fourth year requires rotations on medicine, surgery and neurology. The remainder of the year is dedicated to a selective/elective program, enhanced by direct contact with patients.

Facilities

The new campus of the School of Medicine is located

approximately 4.5 miles from the university campus. The complex provides teaching and research facilities. The School of Medicine Library has a collection of more than 67,000 volumes and subscribes to more than 1,200 periodicals. Through its participation in various networks, students are assured of rapid access to major collections of books and journals from national and international sources. Clinical training is given at the affiliated hospitals, which include: Richland Memorial Hospital, a 611-bed unit with a large family practice center; and Dorn Veterans Center, one of the busiest VA hospitals in the South Carolina-Georgia region, which has 580 beds. A new 90-bed psychiatric unit is scheduled to open in 1992; William S. Hall Psychiatric Institute, which is conducting research into childhood affective disorders. A limited number of housing units are provided for married couples. They are assigned on the basis of application receipt.

Grading Procedures

Letter grades are given. A student must be recommended for promotion or continuation by the promotions committee. To continue in the third-year clerkships, a student must pass Part I of the NBME examination. Part II must be passed before graduation.

Special Programs

The School of Medicine offers a combined M.D./Ph.D. program. Participants are able to earn both the M.D. degree and the Ph.D. degree in biomedical sciences in approximately six years. Applicants must be admitted separately to each degree program.

Application Procedures

The School of Medicine participates in the American Medical College Application Service (AMCAS). Application forms should be returned directly to AMCAS for forwarding to the School of Medicine. Application forms are available after May 1. All basic application materials must reach AMCAS by December 1. All supplementary materials must be received by the School of Medicine by January 15. A $20 fee is requested from all applicants. Through AMCAS, the university participates in the early decision plan (EDP). EDP applicants are required to take the MCAT prior to application and are required to have interviews on campus. EDP applicants not admitted under the early decision plan will be considered as regular candidates and will have time to apply to other schools.

Contact

Office of Admissions
University of South Carolina
School of Medicine
Columbia, South Carolina 29208
(803) 733-3325

UNIVERSITY OF SOUTH DAKOTA SCHOOL OF MEDICINE

Vermillion, South Dakota 57069-2390
(605) 339-6648

Accreditation	LCME
Degrees Offered	M.D., M.S., Ph.D.
# Students Applied	383
Enrollment	46 / class
Mean GPA	3.39
% Men / % Women	57% / 43%
% Minorities	Not Available
Tuition	$6,670 In-State
	$13,780 Out-of-State
Application Fee	$15
Application Deadline	November 15

The University

The first class at the University of South Dakota enrolled in 1882. Today, the university comprises eight schools and enrolls 5,520 students. The university is located in Vermillion on the bluffs of the Missouri River in southeastern South Dakota. It is a community of approximately 10,000. The School of Medicine was established in 1907 and, after 68 years as a two-year medical school, recently established a full clinical program and graduated its first M.D.'s in 1977. Accreditation by the Liaison Committee on Medical Education (LCME) was granted in 1974. The program emphasizes family medicine and primary care and is dependent upon the participation of physicians and community hospitals throughout the state. Through residency-training programs and continuing medical education programming, the school ensures quality health care for the state's population.

Admissions

The School of Medicine is guided by the LCME in its evaluation process. The school examines an applicant's character, personal qualities, motivation, physical health, and emotional stability as well as his or her sense of dedication and desired to serve others. The faculty places strong emphasis on the academic achievements of applicants in the sciences relevant to medicine and seeks students who are broadly educated. The candidate must also demonstrate ability in the following areas: observation, communication, motor, conceptual, integrative and quantitative skills, and behavioral and social skills.

Undergraduate Preparation

Although academic excellence is important, the school emphasizes that high GPA and MCAT scores alone are not sufficient for admission. The school seeks students with a broad education and other life experiences that demonstrate the applicant's potential as a physician. There are no preferred undergraduate majors. All applicants must have earned at least 64 semester credits of college coursework. All students must take the MCAT. Prior to matriculation, students must have submitted transcripts of all college credits earned, indicating at least 90 semester credit hours, or preferably a bachelor's degree from an accredited institution.

Students are encouraged to take college courses in the humanities and in the natural and social sciences. Good communication skills are essential. Required prerequisites include one year (with lab) in biology, general chemistry, organic chemistry, mathematics, and physics.

Costs

Tuition for 1990-1991 is $6,670 per year for residents of South Dakota. Nonresidents pay $13,780. Fees are approximately $700 for the first year, and they include a general university fee and a medical liability insurance premium. One-bedroom, on-campus apartments cost $140 monthly.

Financial Aid

Loans are available on the basis of demonstrated financial need. They include the David A. Gregory Loan Fund, Health Professions Loan Fund, South Dakota State Medical School Endowment Association Loan Fund, and Supplemental Loans to Students.

The school also awards scholarships and grants on the basis of scholastic ability, dedication, aptitude for the study of medicine, and financial need. Numerous grants and scholarship awards are available, but they are usually reserved for upperclassmen and second-semester freshmen. Financial aid applications from first-year medical students are considered only after fall matriculation.

Student Organizations

The school maintains a chapter of the American Medical Student Association. Honor societies include Alpha Omega Alpha and Alpha of South Dakota.

Faculty

Of the full-time faculty, 100 hold the M.D. degree and 40 hold the Ph.D. or other professional degree. There are also more than 480 part-time or voluntary community practicing physicians who participate in the education of medical students.

Curriculum

The need for physicians in South Dakota, particularly in the smaller, rural communities, is reflected in the school's orientation toward primary care.

The first two years cover the basic medical sciences, providing fundamental knowledge of the human body and a rational approach to diagnosis and treatment. In the second year, students are introduced to patient care in the school's affiliated hospitals. The basic science courses include gross anatomy, microscopic anatomy, biological chemistry, introduction to clinical medicine I through IV, medical pharmacology, and general and special pathology.

The third year consists of six major clerkships. Required studies for the fourth year include rural family practice, emergency medicine, and an introduction to specialties. A variety of other clerkships are available on an elective basis.

Facilities

The Lee Medical Building in Vermillion houses the basic teaching and research facilities. Clinical education is carried out in several community hospitals located in Sioux Falls, Yankton, Rapid City, and Fort Meade. Numerous other hospitals throughout the state provide fourth-year education. The Christian P. Lommen Health Sciences Library, located on campus, is part of the Greater Midwest Regional Medical Library Network and is responsible for serving the needs of all health professionals in South Dakota. The library provides access to MEDLINE. Students also have access to libraries at the affiliated hospitals. There are also rural-area health-education centers for regional medical education.

Grading Procedures

The school uses letter-grading system of A,B,C,D, and F to evaluate student performance. A minimum score of 350 must be attained on Part I of the National Board of Medical Examiners test, taken after completion of the sophomore year. To graduate, students must pass Part II of the NBME.

Special Programs

The school offers the Master of Medical Science degree (open to those who hold the M.D. degree), Master's, and Ph.D. degrees in the basic sciences, the Bachelor of Science in Medicine degree, the Bachelor of Science in Medical Technology degree, and the Bachelor of Science in Anesthesia.

Application Procedures

The School of Medicine participates in AMCAS. For South Dakota residents, the deadline for submission of the AMCAS form plus transcripts and other required materials is November 15. It is recommended that the MCAT be taken no later than October of the year prior to the year of intended admission. Supplemental materials, including three references and a photograph, are also required. All resident applicants are interviewed by members of the admissions committee. There is a $15 application fee.

Although South Dakota residents are given preference in admissions, there may be vacancies for nonresidents in any given year. Completed nonresident applications are reviewed by the admissions committee after all resident applications have been evaluated. Non-residents follow the same application procedure as residents.

In addition to the 50 full acceptances recommended for entry into the first-year class, the admissions committee recommends an additional 10 to 15 applicants for consideration as alternative candidates.

Contact

Office of Student Affairs
University of South Dakota
School of Medicine
414 E Clark Street
Vermillion, South Dakota 57069-2390
(605) 677-5233

UNIVERSITY OF SOUTH FLORIDA COLLEGE OF MEDICINE

12901 Bruce B. Downs Boulevard
Tampa, Florida 33612-4799
(803) 974-4066

Accreditation	LCME
Degrees Offered	M.D.
# Students Applied	565
Enrollment	96 / class
Mean GPA	3.5
% Men / % Women	66% / 34%
% Minorities	24%
Tuition	$6,264 In-State
	$15,307 Out-of-State
Application Fee	$75
Application Deadline	December 1

The University

The College of Medicine, one of the three colleges of the University of South Florida Health Sciences Center, admitted its first class in 1971. The University of South Florida (USF) is now the 35th largest university in the nation, with more than 30,000 students. Located on a 1,672-acre site in the northeast section of Tampa, USF is in the heart of an expand-

ing metropolis of more than 2 million people. The university is a short drive to beaches, parks, the Sundome, the Performing Arts Center, historic Ybor City, and Busch Gardens.

Admissions

USF prefers Florida residents; nonresidents are discouraged from applying. Residents should have a GPA of 3.0 or better, and score at least an 8 in each MCAT category. The new MCAT is a must, to be taken no later than the fall of the year preceding the date for which admission is sought. Early admission is possible for as many as 29 applicants who meet certain guidelines. For further information contact the office of admissions.

Undergraduate Preparation

Some preference may be given to students with a completed bachelor's degree from a liberal arts college approved by one of the national accrediting agencies. At a minimum, students must have three years of college work (90 semester or 135 quarter hours). CLEP credit is strongly discouraged. USF requires two semesters or three quarters each (including laboratory) of biology, general and inorganic chemistry, mathematics, and physics. In addition, two semesters or three quarters of English are required.

Student Body

The freshman class consists of 96 students each year, suggesting a student body of about 400. The applicant pool for admission in 1990 increased 40 percent.

Placement Records

USF students have done well on National Board examinations and graduates have obtained excellent positions in residencies at prestigious institutions.

Costs

Resident tuition is $6,264; nonresident tuition is $15,307. Health fees come to $117.43. Room and board is a minimum of $5,600, and books and supplies cost about $1,360.

Financial Aid

So far, students have not had to withdraw from the College of Medicine because of financial need. Limited funds are available for loans and scholarships. Financial aid is, however, available to all students with demonstrated need. Part-time employment is available in local hospitals to academically qualified students. Several sources of aid are available only to minorities.

Minority Programs

Qualified minority students (with a GPA of 3.0 or better) are encouraged to apply. Minority medical student recruiters, in conjunction with the director of admissions, periodically visit undergraduate colleges and universities to recruit minority students and speak to them about the University of South Florida College of Medicine's admission policies and procedures.

Student Organizations

Students are able to effect changes in curriculum, student health policies, and all other medical aspects of their education through student government. National medical and educational organizations are well represented at USF.

Faculty

The College of Medicine employs 522 faculty members.

Curriculum

The course of study lasts four years. The first two years (74 weeks) are devoted to the basic medical sciences. The third year (48 weeks) is devoted to academic clerkship programs, which provide clinical experience in medicine, surgery, obstetrics and gynecology, pediatrics, and psychiatry. The fourth year (44 weeks) is given over to electives in clinical and basic medical sciences.

Facilities

The primary teaching facility is the Tampa General Hospital. TGH has a Level 1 Trauma Center and a Regional Cardiovascular Center, and is the base for airborne adult and pediatric emergency teams. On-campus facilities include the USF Medical Clinic, the USF Eye Institute, the H.L. Moffitt Cancer Center and Research Institute, the Shriners Hospital for Crippled Children, the USF Psychiatry Center, and the University Diagnostic Institute.

Special Programs

Some students become involved in indigent care through the Judeo Christian Clinic. A Shadow Program allows students to spend time with community physicians. Many medical students go to local public schools to educate students about AIDS and substance abuse. A mini-internship program allows USF undergraduate students to spend several days with third-year medical students in the hospital to get a sense of what medical school entails.

Application Procedures

Applicants must file through AMCAS. A secondary application may be sent to qualified applicants. The deadline for all application materials is January 1 of the year for which the student is applying for entry. The fee is $15 and is not refundable. Interviews may follow. Within two weeks of acceptance, students must file a written statement of intent.

Contact

Office of Admissions, Box 3
University of South Florida
College of Medicine

12901 Bruce B. Downs Boulevard
Tampa, Florida 33612-4799
(813) 974-2229

UNIVERSITY OF SOUTHERN CALIFORNIA SCHOOL OF MEDICINE

1975 Zonal Avenue
Los Angeles, California 90089
(213) 224-7001

Accreditation	LCME
Degrees Offered	M.D., M.D./Ph.D.
# Students Applied	3,000
Enrollment	136 / class
Mean GPA	3.42
% Men / % Women	54% / 46%
% Minorities	22%
Tuition	$20,600
Application Fee	$50
Application Deadline	November 1

The University

The School of Medicine at the University of Southern California was established in 1885. It is located in Northeast Los Angeles, on the 30-acre Health Science Campus.

Admissions

Members of the committee on admissions include full-time and voluntary faculty, alumni, and students. When evaluating candidates, the committee on admissions considers academic achievement and MCAT performance, as well as personal characteristics. Although the school does not require a minimum MCAT score for applicants, admission is highly selective.

Undergraduate Preparation

At least three years of college (90 semester hours of college work) is required for admission. Completion of a bachelor's degree is preferred. Each applicant must have completed at least two semester hours (three quarter hours) of the following required courses, including necessary laboratory work: biology, inorganic chemistry, organic chemistry, and general physics. The study of biochemistry, developmental biology, genetics, and calculus is strongly recommended. A broad background in the humanities, arts, and behavioral sciences is encouraged.

Student Body

Almost half of the students accepted to the 1990-91 entering class were women. All of the students accepted to this class had completed their baccalaureate degrees at the time of admission.

Costs

Estimated tuition costs amount to $20,600 per year for residents and nonresidents. Student fees total $266.

Financial Aid

Financial aid is available from a variety of federal, state, and private offices. Loans, scholarships, and grants are awarded on the basis of need and/or ability. The university also provides financial assistance. The school discourages students from seeking outside employment.

Minority Programs

The office of minority affairs encourages applications from members of minority groups underrepresented in the health professions. The office provides tutorial assistance, counseling services, and interdepartmental communications.

Student Organizations

There is a branch of Alpha Omega Alpha, the medical honors society, on campus.

Curriculum

The study of basic sciences is combined with early exposure to patient care. During the first two years, groups of six to seven students work together with one faculty member (tutor) who uses actual patient problems to direct students into the concepts of the basic, clinical, and behavioral sciences. The first-year basic science courses are presented through the study of organ systems. Further investigation of the material being taught is offered through the introduction to clinical medicine course, which provides contact with patients. The second year consists of the study of disease and pathology. This is taught through integrated basic and clinical studies of eight major human organ systems. During this year, students may also begin a research project. The last two years are devoted to providing an in-depth study of clinical problems presented by patients in the hospital and outpatient setting. Each student's program is individually designed with the assistance of faculty advisors and includes 42 weeks of required clinical clerkships, 18 weeks of selective clerkships, and 18 weeks of free elective clerkships. The free electives may be taken on campus, at hospitals affiliated with USC, or at more distant medical schools or medical centers.

Facilities

The main teaching hospital, the Los Angeles County-USC Medical Center, is located across the street from the campus. The USC Medical Center is one of the largest teaching facilities in the nation. Additional clinical opportunities available to students include the newly constructed USC University Hospital; the Doheney Eye Hospital; the Children's Hospital of Los Angeles; Rancho Los Amigos Hospital; the Kenneth T. Norris, Jr. Cancer Hospital and Research Institute, which provides a number of core facilities; the Orthopedic Hospital; the Hospital of the Good Samaritan; California Hospital; Presbyterian Intercommunity Hospital; and Eisenhower Medical Center. The school is currently developing plans for an interdisciplinary Center for Molecular Medicine, which will house new programs in molecular biology, genetics, and neurobiology.

Grading Procedures

Grades are awarded as honors, satisfactory, and unsatisfactory. Near honors may be awarded when a student has performed outstanding work in a clinical clerkship. Faculty instructors establish evaluation criteria appropriate for each course, and must specify how these evaluations will be made.

Special Programs

The School of Medicine offers a combined M.D./Ph.D. program, which is open to well-qualified candidates. The program enrolls a maximum of six students per year. Participants must be accepted to the USC School of Medicine. Interested applicants are encouraged to request information about the program at the time of application. The following departments participate in the program: anatomy and cell biology, biochemistry, microbiology, pathology, pharmacology and nutrition, physiology and biophysics, and preventative medicine. The program is usually completed in seven years. For more information, contact the office of the Associate Dean for Scientific Affairs, USC School of Medicine, 1975 Zonal Avenue (KAM 300), Los Angeles, California 90033, Phone (213) 224-7480.

Application Procedures

The School of Medicine participates in the American Medical Colleges Application Service (AMCAS). Applications should be filed between June 15 and November 1 of the year prior to entry. The school participates in the early decision plan. The new MCAT is required and should be taken in the spring of the year before planned enrollment. There is an application fee of $50. After receipt of the AMCAS application, the school requests that qualified candidates complete a supplemental application and submit letters of recommendation. Interviews are required, and are arranged only by the committee on admissions. Foreign students who have completed at least one year of study at an accredited university or college in the United States will be considered for admission.

Contact

Office of Admissions
University of Southern California
School of Medicine
1975 Zonal Avenue
Los Angeles, California 90033
(213) 342-2552

SOUTHERN ILLINOIS UNIVERSITY SCHOOL OF MEDICINE

PO Box 19230
Carbondale, Illinois 62901
(217) 782-3318

Accreditation	LCME
Degrees Offered	M.D., M.D./J.D.
# Students Applied	872
Enrollment	74 / class
Mean GPA	3.28
% Men / % Women	61% / 39%
% Minorities	19%
Tuition	$7,892 In-State
	$22,164 Out-of-State
Application Fee	None
Application Deadline	November 15

The University

Southern Illinois University has campuses at Carbondale (SIUC) with a School of Medicine at Springfield, and Edwardsville (SIUE) with a School of Dental Medicine at Alton and a center in East St. Louis. The school was chartered as Southern Illinois Normal University, a teachers college, in 1869; the School of Medicine was established in 1969. Students spend the first year of the program at the medical education facilities on the Carbondale campus, and the remaining three years at the medical education center in Springfield. SIUC serves a total of 35,000 students in a rustic setting perfect for many outdoor activities. The Carbondale area boasts seven lakes, a 240,000-acre national forest, a national wildlife refuge, and a state park. Springfield is the capital of Illinois and serves as the tourism, retail, wholesale, and agricultural center for much of the mid-state region. The 6.6-mile Lake Springfield

has 57 miles of shoreline. The city is home to eight libraries and has abundant educational and cultural opportunities.

Admissions

Applicants are considered on the basis of overall and science GPAs, MCAT scores, quality of education, recommendation letters, and interview results. Applicants should present credentials equivalent to better than a B average and MCAT science and reading scores of 8 or better. Preference is given to applicants who have achieved a baccalaureate degree by the time of matriculation in medical school, who are residents of central or southern Illinois, and who have recent academic activity that demonstrates the potential for successful completion of the medical curriculum.

Undergraduate Preparation

The MCAT and a minimum of 90 semester hours of undergraduate work are required. Applicants should have a good foundation in the natural sciences, social sciences, and the humanities.

Student Body

Students at Southern Illinois University School of Medicine are from a variety of cultural and academic backgrounds.

Placement Records

As of May 1989, 893 students had earned the M.D. degree. These graduates are pursuing a variety of medical careers in numerous specialties, with the highest percentage (26 percent) in family practice and the second highest (21 percent) in internal medicine.

Costs

Tuition and student fees: resident, $7,892; nonresident, $22,164. Estimated annual cost for room and board total about $6,000; books and supplies, $1,158; and personal expenses, $2,834. Fees decrease for the sophomore and junior years. The senior year is tuition free.

Financial Aid

Approximately 85 percent of the student body receives financial aid. Most financial need is met by a combination of various loan funds, and scholarships, when available.

Minority Programs

The School of Medicine sponsors the Medical Education Preparatory Program (MEDPREP) for minority and economically disadvantaged students. MEDPREP consists of developmental and enrichment tutorials in small classroom format, preparation for the MCAT, and medical school application assistance. For further information on MEDPREP, contact Director: MEDPREP, Southern Illinois University School of Medicine, Carbondale, Illinois 62901.

Student Organizations

Among the organizations medical students may participate in are the American Medical Students Association, the Student National Medical Association, the American Medical Women's Association, and the med students' section of the American Medical Association. The state and county medical societies are open to students, and the School of Medicine sponsors a Family Practice Club. A chapter of Alpha Omega Alpha was established in 1985.

Faculty

The faculty includes over 95 full-time and 115 part-time physicians in Springfield and Carbondale. There are more than 400 other faculty members and researchers in clinical, basic science, and other academic departments.

Curriculum

During the first semester, students are involved in clarifying and solving actual medical problems. Basic sciences, including anatomy, physiology, biochemistry, and behavioral science are taught. The student also studies probability and genetics, introductory pharmacology, community health, and clinical reasoning. The second year begins in Springfield with a six-week introduction to microbiology and immunology followed by a 10-week multidisciplinary, case-oriented block that focuses on infectious and immunologic disease. The second semester of the second year deals with the organ system structure for the delivery of pathology, pharmacology, radiology, and clinical medicine. Third-year students begin clinical clerkships in the six specialties and medical humanities. Elective study completes the program.

Facilities

Three community hospitals and clinics in Springfield and Carbondale and the Veterans Administration Medical Center in Marion are used for clinical instruction. Both campuses provide study carrels, audiovisual tutorial rooms, and computer terminal areas for individual study, and seminar areas for group study. The Springfield Combined Laboratory Facility, completed ion 1988, provides 75,000 square feet of space with controlled environment areas and oncology and virology laboratories.

Grading Procedures

The grading system is honors/pass/fail.

Special Programs

The Southern Illinois University School of Medicine offers a six-year M.D./J.D. program. Students must meet the admissions standards of both the School of Medicine and the School of Law. A limited number of places are available in the combined M.D./J.D. program. Eighteen freshmen each year may elect to participate in a problem-based learning track. In this program, students learn basic science content in a clinical setting, through exploring and evaluating patient problems within tutorial groups.

Application Procedures

The AMCAS application is accepted between June 15 and November 15. There is no application fee. Applicants with competitive academic credentials and MCAT scores will be sent the SIU School of Medicine supplementary application and a request for four letters of recommendation. Application files, including interviews, must be completed by March 15 to be eligible for consideration for the August term. Early application is suggested. Letters of recommendation may be submitted before the applicant takes the MCAT.

Contact

Office of Student and Alumni Affairs
Southern Illinois University
School of Medicine
PO Box 19230
Springfield, Illinois 62794-9230
(217) 782-2860

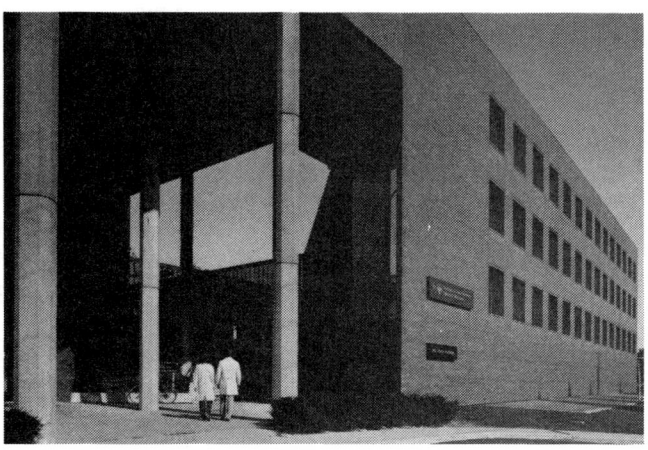

STANFORD UNIVERSITY SCHOOL OF MEDICINE

Stanford, California 94305
(415) 723-6436

Accreditation	LCME
Degrees Offered	M.D., M.D./Ph.D., M.S./Ph.D.
# Students Applied	4,189
Enrollment	86 / class
Mean GPA	3.6
% Men / % Women	60% / 40%
% Minorities	20%
Tuition	$17,925
Application Fee	$55
Application Deadline	November 1

The University

Stanford University ("The Farm") was founded in 1885. In 1959, the university opened a new medical center adjacent to Stanford's main building. Today, the school is recognized as one of the finest in the country. The 8,800-acre campus was once the Stanford family farm and racehorse breeding ground and borders on Palo Alto, Menlo Park, Los Altos, and Portola Valley. Recreational, cultural, and social opportunities abound in California. San Francisco is just 35 miles north of the campus.

Admissions

An undergraduate major in any field is acceptable provided that the applicant has an outstanding academic record and high achievement in the required basic sciences. A baccalaureate degree is preferred but not required. The mean GPA has been about 3.6. Students must take the MCAT. No preference is given to California residents.

Undergraduate Preparation

Undergraduate course requirements include one year each (with lab) of the biological sciences, physics, and organic and inorganic chemistry. Courses must be consonant with the requirements of the state of California for purposes of licensure. Stanford highly recommends students have a knowledge of a foreign language and coursework in the behavioral sciences, calculus, biochemistry, and physical chemistry.

Student Body

The entering class size numbers 86. Classes in recent years have typically had representatives from more than 40 undergraduate institutions. About 50 percent pursued biological sciences as undergraduates; about 25 percent physical sciences and math; social and behavioral sciences, 15 percent; and literature and philosophy, five percent. The median age of the entering class has been 22-23. About 95 percent are usually between 20 and 30. Approximately 40 percent of the students are women and nearly 20 percent are minorities.

Costs

Tuition and fees for the 1990 entering class totaled $17,925.

Financial Aid

About 75 percent of the students receive some financial aid. Most aid is offered in the form of grants, loans, and part-time employment. Awards are granted based upon financial need, as documented through the GAPSFAS form. Students must participate with a level of self-help. For 1990, the self-help requirement was $4,300 per quarter.

Minority Programs

The School of Medicine is committed to an affirmative action program for identifying, recruiting, and matriculating qualified minority students. A number of medical school and university officers dedicate themselves specifically to minority concerns. Counseling, networking, lists of minority faculty, and access to ongoing minority activities are all offered through these officers.

Student Organizations

Student organizations that support the needs of minorities include the Stanford National Medical Association (SNMA), the Stanford Raza Medical Association, Chicanos in Health Education (CHE), and the Stanford American Indian Association.

Faculty

Stanford has about 602 full-time faculty for a medical student body of 450, as well as about 1,200 voluntary clinical faculty who practice in nearby communities.

Curriculum

The program of study usually lasts four years, but may be spread out over five or six years. The preclinical part of the program covers six or more quarters in the biomedical sciences. The first two preclinical years include courses in cell biology, biochemistry, surgery, genetics, neurobiology, physiology, microbiology, pathology, pharmacology, and psychiatry. Clinical clerkships begin in the third year and continue into the fourth. Electives begin in the fourth year. Students are encouraged to plan for a five-year course of study in order to include research activities, teaching assistantships, and elective courses both in the medical school and in other schools of the university in their educational plans.

Facilities

The Lane Medical Library houses a comprehensive selection of volumes and periodicals in medical literature. The Cecil H. Green Library is devoted to the social sciences and humanities, and other libraries specialize in engineering, chemistry, biology, mathematics, computer science, law, and music. Affiliated teaching hospitals include Kaiser Permanente Hospital, Santa Clara Valley Medical Center, Palo Alto V.A. Hospital, and Children's Hospital at Stanford.

Grading Procedures

Students are graded on a pass/fail system. Narrative evaluations are incorporated into the student's record. Students must pass both Parts I and II of the National Board Examinations to graduate, as well as complete 13 quarters of academic work.

Special Programs

Stanford also offers a combined M.D./Ph.D. program under the aegis of the Medical Scientist Training Program (MSTP). The M.S./Ph.D. is also available as well as the M.S. in health research and policy.

Application Procedures

Students should take the MCAT in April, but no later than the fall of the year in which application is submitted. Students must apply through AMCAS. Applications are available from March 1 and may be filed beginning June 1. Following receipt and review of the AMCAS application, Stanford requires a supplementary application including three letters of evaluation. The deadline is November 1. Selected candidates may then be invited for an interview. The early decision plan is available.

Contact

Director of Admissions
Office of Admissions
Stanford University
School of Medicine
851 Welch Road
Palo Alto, California 94304
(415) 723-6861

STATE UNIVERSITY OF NEW YORK HEALTH SCIENCE CENTER AT BROOKLYN COLLEGE OF MEDICINE

450 Clarkson Avenue
Brooklyn, New York 11203
(718) 270-2057

Accreditation	LCME
Degrees Offered	M.D., M.D./Ph.D.
# Students Applied	2,596
Enrollment	203 / class
Mean GPA	3.36
% Men / % Women	Not Available
% Minorities	Not Available
Tuition	$5,850 In-State
	$13,250 Out-of-State
Application Fee	$50
Application Deadline	December 15

The University

The Health Science Center at Brooklyn evolved out of the Long Island College Hospital in 1860 as the nation's first teaching hospital. Today, the Health Science Center has a student body of over 1,400, a full-time and clinical faculty of nearly 2,500, and support staff of 3,500. Located on a 13-acre campus in the East Flatbush section of Brooklyn, the Health Science Center and the College of Medicine currently strives to address the modern health care problems of traditionally underserved urban communities, including AIDS, drug addiction, mother-infant relationships, and alcoholism. Brooklyn itself offers a variety of diversions, including beaches, museums, and parks. The school is a short subway ride from Manhattan.

Admissions

The commission on admissions considers the total qualifications of each applicant. Admission decisions are based on several factors, including academic records, the results of standardized tests, letters of recommendation, and personal interviews. Students from minority groups are encouraged to apply.

Undergraduate Preparation

A minimum of three years of undergraduate work is required in order to be considered for admission to the College of Medicine. Students are encouraged to pursue a broad, liberal arts course of study that best fits personal academic interests. Although a general competence in the physical and biological sciences is required, no specific undergraduate major is necessary. Specific required courses include one academic year each, with lab, of biology, general physics, inorganic chemistry, and organic chemistry. One academic year of English is also required.

Student Body

The College of Medicine, as well as other schools of the Health Science Center, attracts many students from Brooklyn and the surrounding New York metropolitan area. Also, the College of Medicine makes a particular effort to recruit and maintain minority and disadvantaged students. The 1990 entering class had a mean total GPA of 3.36.

Costs

Tuition for state residents is $5,850 annually and $13,250 for nonresidents. Living expenses vary greatly; however, additional expenses for single first-year medical students are estimated to total another $9,700 annually.

Financial Aid

Students are encouraged to apply to the College of Medicine regardless of their ability to pay. The goal of the Health Science Center is to make educational opportunity available to all who can benefit from it. Loans, scholarships, and work-study assistance are available to eligible students demonstrating financial need. Applicants for financial aid are required to complete the financial aid form from the College Scholarship Service.

Minority Programs

Application fees for minorities waived by AMCAS are automatically waived by the school. A summer prematriculation program is available. First-year students are assigned a faculty advisor to serve as mentor. Peer support for minorities is provided by the Daniel Hale Williams Society.

Student Organizations

A variety of extracurricular student groups is available to medical students. These organizations include the student council, the College of Medicine student governing body, the university Council (which deals with the concerns of the entire university), the American Medical Student Association, the Family Practice Club, the Asian Students Club, the Daniel Hale Williams Society, and the American Medical Women's Association. Alpha Omega Alpha, the national medical honor fraternity, also has a chapter on campus.

Faculty

The Health Sciences Center at Brooklyn has a full-time clinical faculty of approximately 2,500.

Curriculum

During the first year, students focus on the basic medical sciences, including gross anatomy, biochemistry, the neurosciences, preventive medicine, physiology, cell biology, and histology. In the second year, students use this basic science foundation to study preclinical topics, such as human disease, diagnosis, prevention, and treatment, and the techniques of patient interviewing and examination. Clinical clerkships in each of the major clinical areas span the third year of medical study. During this time each medical student works as a member of a functioning health care team under the supervision of a faculty member. In the fourth year, after completing a required 12 weeks of courses, students are able to develop their own curriculum of elective courses that will best prepare them for future medical training. These courses may be taken at University Hospital, Kings County Hospital Center, or any affiliated institution.

Facilities

The main teaching facility of the College of Medicine is University Hospital, a 354-bed teaching and research hospital, which serves most of Brooklyn and Staten Island. Also, Kings County Hospital, a 1,284-bed facility, the largest hospital in New York City, is located adjacent to University Hospital and affiliated with the Health Sciences Center. The College of Medicine is affiliated with 19 other hospitals and health care facilities throughout New York City. The medical research library of Brooklyn combines the collections of the Academy of Medicine of Brooklyn and the Health Science Center, and contains over 254,000 volumes and 1,422 periodical titles.

Grading Procedures

Students at the College of Medicine are assigned grades of either satisfactory, unsatisfactory, or honors. Grades of incomplete are given with the approval of the dean of students when students have failed to complete course requirements in the allotted time.

Special Programs

The College of Medicine offers a Medical Scientist Training Program leading to a combined M.D./Ph.D. degree for students interested in careers in research, teaching, and academic medicine. Generally, six years are required to complete this program and the order of the curriculum is flexible, depending on a student's particular academic needs and interests. Topics available for Ph.D. study include anatomy and cell biology, biochemistry, biophysics, microbiology and immunology, neural and behavioral science, pathology, pharmacology, and physiology.

Application Procedures

The College of Medicine participates in the centralized application service of AMCAS. Students must submit this application between June 15 and December 15 of the year prior to desired entrance into medical school. Supplemental materials required include MCAT scores, letters of recommendation, and a $50 application fee. Students are advised to take the MCAT in the spring of the year prior to desired medical school entrance. One letter of recommendation from the premedical committee at the undergraduate college, or two letters from professors familiar with the student's academic work, is required.

Contact

Office of Admissions
State University of New York
Health Sciences Center at Brooklyn
Box 60M
450 Clarkson Avenue
Brooklyn, New York 11203
(718) 270-2735

STATE UNIVERSITY OF NEW YORK AT BUFFALO SCHOOL OF MEDICINE AND BIOMEDICAL SCIENCES

101 Farber Hall, South Campus
Buffalo, New York 14214
(716) 831-3436

Accreditation	LCME
Degrees Offered	M.D., M.D./Ph.D.
# Students Applied	2,217
Enrollment	135 / class
Mean GPA	3.51
% Men / % Women	59% / 41%
% Minorities	Not Available
Tuition	$5,850 In-State
	$13,250 Out-of-State
Application Fee	$50
Application Deadline	December 1

The University

The School of Medicine of the State University at Buffalo, founded in 1846, is among the oldest medical schools in the United States. Millard Fillmore, the 13th president of the United States, served as the first chancellor of the original

department of medicine. The school remained a private institution until it joined the SUNY system in 1962.

Admissions

Factors considered in the admissions process include scholastic achievement, aptitude, personal qualifications, and motivation toward medicine. College records, the MCAT results, letters of reference and evaluation, and a personal interview are required. Students with a bachelor's degree from an accredited college or university are preferred, although in exceptional cases students will be admitted after three years of undergraduate study.

Undergraduate Preparation

The minimum undergraduate requirements are two semesters of biology (with lab), three semesters of chemistry (with lab), and two semesters of general physics courses, in addition to coursework in the humanities. It is not necessary to major in the sciences to be admitted to the medical school.

Costs

Yearly tuition for state residents is $5,850; for out-of-state residents, $13,250. There is a microscope fee of $150 and an insurance fee of $155.

Financial Aid

Awards are based on financial need, and applicants must submit a FAF. Only full-time matriculated students are eligible for financial assistance. Grants and scholarships as well as loans are available, including Perkins Loans, Health Education Assistance Loans, and Supplemental Loans for Students (SLS). Financial aid forms should be submitted no later than April 16.

Minority Programs

The medical school provides special services for applicants from disadvantaged and minority backgrounds. A summer enrichment and support program is available to first-year educationally and socioeconomically disadvantaged students.

Student Organizations

Students with high academic records may be elected to membership during their third or fourth year to Alpha Omega Alpha, a national honor society.

Curriculum

Major emphasis is directed toward combining the elements of scientific preparation with an appreciation for the patient as a human being. Opportunities for clinical contact are provided early in the curriculum and students can work with basic science and clinical faculty throughout the four-year course of study. The first two years consist of required courses designed to furnish a comprehensive presentation of basic biomedical science and its application to the practice of medicine.

A variety of elective courses is also offered. The third year stresses clinical experience through clerkships at the school's teaching hospitals. The fourth year is individually planned by the student under the guidance of an advisor.

Facilities

The school consists of seven basic science departments, the Health Sciences Library, and the Educational Communications Center. A cluster of teaching hospitals provides the facilities for the clinical education of medical students. The library houses more than 260,000 volumes, subscribes to about 2,700 serials, and has over 1,500 audiovisual titles. Students have access to MEDLINE and the Bibliographic Retrieval Service.

Grading Procedures

During the preclinical years, the grading scale is honors/satisfactory/unsatisfactory/incomplete/withdrawal. The grading scale for the clinical years is similar except for the addition of "high satisfactory" after "honors."

Special Programs

The School of Medicine has an Early Assurance Program for undergraduate sophomores who have at least a 3.5 GPA and have completed at least half of the premedical course requirements. There is also an accelerated three-year program leading to the M.D. degree. The school's Medical Scientist Training Program (combined M.D./Ph.D. degree) is designed to provide students with an opportunity to combine intensive scientific training with medical school experience. The program requires six to seven years to complete. Applicants must meet the requirements of both the medical school and the graduate program in which they wish to enroll.

Application Procedures

Applicants must take the MCAT no later than the fall of the year preceding admission. Transcripts should be submitted to AMCAS for verification. Applicants are required to submit a letter of recommendation from their premedical committee or from two different required basic science departments at their undergraduate institution. Personal interviews are required in the final stage of the admissions process. Applications for admission to the first-year class must be submitted to AMCAS by December 1. Early submission of applications is recommended. There is a $50 application fee.

Contact

Office of Medical Admissions
State University of New York at Buffalo
Farber Hall, Room 138
Buffalo, New York 14214
(716) 831-3466

STATE UNIVERSITY OF NEW YORK AT STONY BROOK HEALTH SCIENCES CENTER SCHOOL OF MEDICINE

Stony Brook, New York 11794-2113
(516) 444-2080

Accreditation	LCME
Degrees Offered	M.D., M.D./Ph.D.
# Students Applied	2,755
Enrollment	100 / class
Mean GPA	Not Available
% Men / % Women	Not Available
% Minorities	Not Available
Tuition	$5,850 In-State
	$13,250 Out-of-State
Application Fee	$50
Application Deadline	December 15

The University

The School of Medicine opened in 1971 as part of the Health Sciences Center. The center consists of five professional schools and the University Hospital, the main teaching facility for the School of Medicine. Other professional programs offered at the center are allied health professions, dental medicine, nursing, and social welfare. Approximately 1,900 students are enrolled at the center, including more than 500 graduate professional students.

Admissions

Preference is given to New York state residents although qualified residents and nonresidents are encouraged to apply for the M.D./Ph.D. program. Students with a wide variety of backgrounds are actively sought. Grades, MCAT scores, letters of evaluation, and extracurricular work experience are among the elements evaluated as well as personal characteristics, motivation, and the personal interview.

Undergraduate Preparation

Applicants must have completed at least two years of college, although the school recommends that applicants complete the baccalaureate degree. Completion of at least one year of the following courses, including necessary laboratory work, is required: biology, physics, inorganic chemistry, organic chemistry, and English. Required courses should be completed before application.

Student Body

Most students are residents of New York state. Of the 1992-93 entering class, all students had taken the MCAT, and all had baccalaureate degrees.

Costs

Tuition is $5,850 per year for New York state residents and $13,250 for nonresidents. Student fees amount to approximately $120 per year.

Financial Aid

Financial aid includes programs administered by off-campus agencies to which the student applies directly, special funds administered by the center, and campus-based programs administered by the office of student services and the university office of financial aid. The office of student affairs helps students complete the financial aid process.

Student Organizations

There is a chapter of Alpha Omega Alpha, the national medical honor society, on campus.

Faculty

The Health Sciences Center employs more than 2,000 faculty members.

Curriculum

The first year consists of the basic sciences and introductory courses related to patient care. Introduction to clinical medicine is taught during the second semester of both the first and second years. The second year also includes basic and clinical sciences taught through the study of organ systems. The third year curriculum consists of 12-week clerkships in medicine and surgery and six-week clerkships in pediatrics, obstetrics-gynecology, psychiatry, and primary care. The fourth year curriculum includes four months of selectives and four-and-a-half months of electives. Students are expected to acquire laboratory and clinical skills, and to demonstrate competence at patient contact exercises and animal laboratories. The study of social and ethical issues involved in the practice of medicine is stressed.

Facilities

University Hospital, which opened in 1980, offers highly specialized services, using modern instrumentation and computerized physiological monitoring. The hospital has 494 beds, of which half are specialty beds. There are eight intensive care units and a transplantation service. The Health Sciences Cen-

ter has affiliations with many area institutions and agencies. The Health Sciences Library contains approximately 238,000 volumes, and subscribes to 4,394 periodicals and serial titles. Interlibrary loan services and microcomputer services are also available.

Grading Procedures

An honors/pass/fail grading system is used. Students must take Parts I and II of the NBME examination. Scores may be used to determine whether a student should be promoted.

Special Programs

The school offers a combined M.D./Ph.D. program, which usually requires six to eight years to complete. To receive the degree, students must satisfy the requirements of the Graduate School, basic health science graduate studies requirements, and requirements of the School of Medicine.

Application Procedures

The School of Medicine participates in AMCAS. Applications should be received between June 15 and December 15 of the year preceding enrollment. There is an application fee of $50. The MCAT should be taken no later than the year of admission. Candidates from foreign countries must have completed at least one year of academic studies in an accredited American college or university. Personal interviews will be arranged by the school.

Contact

Office of Admissions
State University of New York at Stony Brook
 School of Medicine
Health Sciences Center, Room 046, Level 4
Stony Brook, New York 11794-2113
(516) 444-2113

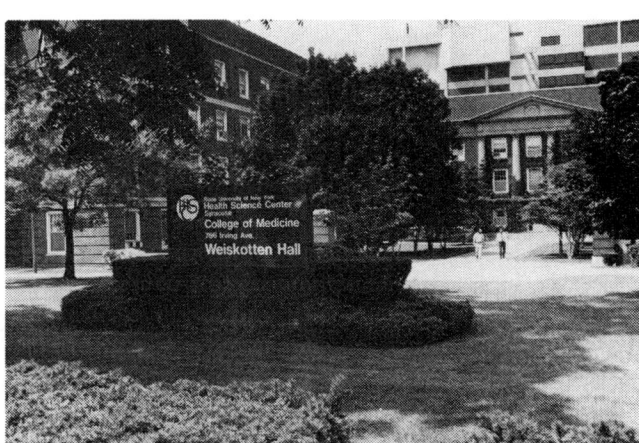

STATE UNIVERSITY OF NEW YORK HEALTH SCIENCE CENTER AT SYRACUSE COLLEGE OF MEDICINE

155 Elizabeth Blackwell Street
Syracuse, New York 13210
(315) 464-4570

Accreditation	LCME
Degrees Offered	M.D., M.D./Ph.D., M.D./M.B.A.
# Students Applied	2,652
Enrollment	150 / class
Mean GPA	Not Available
% Men / % Women	64% / 36%
% Minorities	Not Available
Tuition	$5,850 In-State
	$13,250 Out-of-State
Application Fee	$50
Application Deadline	December 1

The University

The College of Medicine Health Science Center at Syracuse was founded in 1834, making it the 14th oldest college of medicine in the country. Numbered among the graduates is Elizabeth Blackwell, the first woman graduate of a medical school in the United States. The college is located in Syracuse, an urban setting surrounded by countryside, which offers access to cultural as well as recreational activities.

Admissions

New York residents, students with baccalaureate degrees, and those who have fulfilled the undergraduate coursework prescribed for admission are given preference. Selected criteria include scholastic and scientific aptitude, communication skills, personal experiences, character, and motivation.

Undergraduate Preparation

Admission requirements include four to six hours each of organic and inorganic chemistry (both with lab), six to eight hours of biology or zoology with a lab, six to eight hours of physics with a lab, and six hours of English.

Student Body

The freshman class is typically composed of 150 students representing 50 to 60 colleges. The number of applicants each year is over 2,600. Thirty-six percent of the class of 1993 is female.

Costs

New York state residents pay $5,850 in tuition, while non-residents pay $13,250. Additional costs include a $25 college fee, a $65 student activities fee, $125 for microscope rental, $700 for books and supplies, and $490 for diagnostic equipment. Room and board in the dormitory ranges from $210 to $430 per month. Food is approximately $180 per month and personal expenses are about $160 per month. In all, New York state residents can expect to spend $14,915 per year and nonresidents $22,315.

Financial Aid

Students applying for financial aid directly from the college are required to include information about their parents' finances. The average total loan for a graduate of the class of 1990 was $35,600. Financial aid is given to over 80 percent of the students, the average being $13,330. Of this amount, grants or scholarships comprised $2,372; loans averaged $10,866.

Minority Programs

The Health Science Center has devised a program called Project 90 designed to encourage enrollment and the rate of graduation of minority and disadvantaged students. Students who belong to ethnic, social, and socioeconomic groups underrepresented in medicine as identified by the Association of American Medical Colleges and the state of New York are given admission preference.

Student Organizations

Co-curricular activities available for students on campus include the Student National Medical Association, the Christian Medical Society, the Jewish Student Association, Geri-Action, the local chapter of the Medical Society of New York State, American Medical Student Association, and the student branch of the American Medical Women's Association.

Faculty

The College of Medicine has a full-time and clinical faculty of 1,667. In addition, a staff of 169 professionals teaches health-related professional courses.

Curriculum

During the first year, students study the normal structure and functions of the human body through courses in embryology, cell and molecular biology, gross anatomy, microscopic anatomy, neuroscience, biochemistry, physiology, and genetics. Second-year students study the pathology of human disease in introduction to clinical medicine, and take classes in microbiology, pathology, immunology, pharmacology, behavioral science, family medicine, epidemiology, nutrition, and endocrinology. Clinical clerkships, which include medicine, surgery, pediatrics, obstetrics and gynecology, psychiatry, radiology, anesthesiology, otolaryngology, orthopedic surgery, and ophthalmology, plus electives, comprise the third year. In the fourth year, clinical clerkships continue with courses in preventive medicine, urology, neuroscience, and additional electives.

Facilities

Forty third-year students are assigned to clinical clerkships at the clinical campus at Binghamton. The facilities available in Binghamton include United Health Services, which include Binghamton General and Wilson Hospitals; Lourdes Hospital; Robert Packer Hospital in Sayre, Pennsylvania; Binghamton Psychiatric Center; and community agencies, physicians' offices, and local health care facilities. The Health Science Center Library located on the Syracuse campus houses a collection of over 130,000, with more than 1,700 serials, two on-line bibliographic services, and the Media Services/Instructional Computing Facility. University Hospital, a 358-bed teaching facility, is the Health Science Center's primary clinical facility. With 52 clinics, the University Hospital is staffed by the faculty of the College of Medicine.

Special Programs

The continuity of care program, geriatrics/gerontology program, perinatal program, and psychosocial program are part of the clinical campus programs at Binghamton. The medical student research program is available to 20 students who want to do medical research without entering a Ph.D. program. The combined M.D./Ph.D. program provides a way for eligible students to obtain both degrees within seven years. Students accepted to the medical school program at the College of Medicine may also apply to the M.D./M.B.A. program cosponsored by SUNY Binghamton School of Management.

Application Procedures

Applicants complete and send an application and official transcripts to the American Medical College Application Service (AMCAS) by December 1. A supplemental application will be sent upon receipt of the AMCAS application and should be submitted with a $50 application fee. Letters of evaluation by a premedical committee or letters from faculty in two different premedical science departments and MCAT results should be sent to the admissions committee. Nonscience majors should also send letters from instructors in the major department, and students who have done graduate work should send letters from graduate faculty members. Students who are invited for an interview are instructed to bring a recent, signed, unmounted photo (1-1/2"x 2-1/2"). Only qualified students are invited to be interviewed.

Contact

Admissions Office
College of Medicine
SUNY Health Science Center
155 Elizabeth Blackwell Street
Syracuse, New York 13210
(315) 464-4570

TEMPLE UNIVERSITY SCHOOL OF MEDICINE

Broad and Ontario Streets
Philadelphia, Pennsylvania 19140
(215) 787-7000

Accreditation	LCME
Degrees Offered	M.D., M.D./Ph.D.
# Students Applied	3,951
Enrollment	180 / class
Mean GPA	3.25
% Men / % Women	52% / 48%
% Minorities	12%
Tuition	$14,212 In-State
	$18,964 Out-of-State
Application Fee	$40
Application Deadline	December 1

The University

Located in Philadelphia, Temple University is in the unique position of being in the heart of a bustling city and having some of the best facilities—Temple University Hospital and Saint Christopher's Hospital for Children—to work with.

Admissions

Every application made to the first-year class is reviewed by at least one member of the admissions committee, which is made up of 14 faculty members and four upperclass medical students. The committee evaluates an applicant's undergraduate record, the college attended, MCAT scores, references, essay, extracurricular activities, work experience, and other credentials. No minimum MCAT scores are required.

Undergraduate Preparation

Applicants must have completed a minimum of 90 semester hours at an accredited college or university to be considered for admission. Students who have not completed a bachelor's degree, but who have exceptional academic qualifications (BCPM of 3.5 or better and high MCAT scores) and evidence of unusual maturity may apply. One academic year of the following required courses, with laboratory work and lectures, should be completed by the time of application: biology, inorganic chemistry, organic chemistry, and general physics. The admissions committee does not prefer science majors, though all applicants must demonstrate their capacity for excellent achievement in the sciences. Students should also have a broad education in the humanities (at least six semester hours) and have taken subjects requiring expository writing as well as courses in foreign languages, history, religion, philosophy, and the arts. Calculus is suggested but not required.

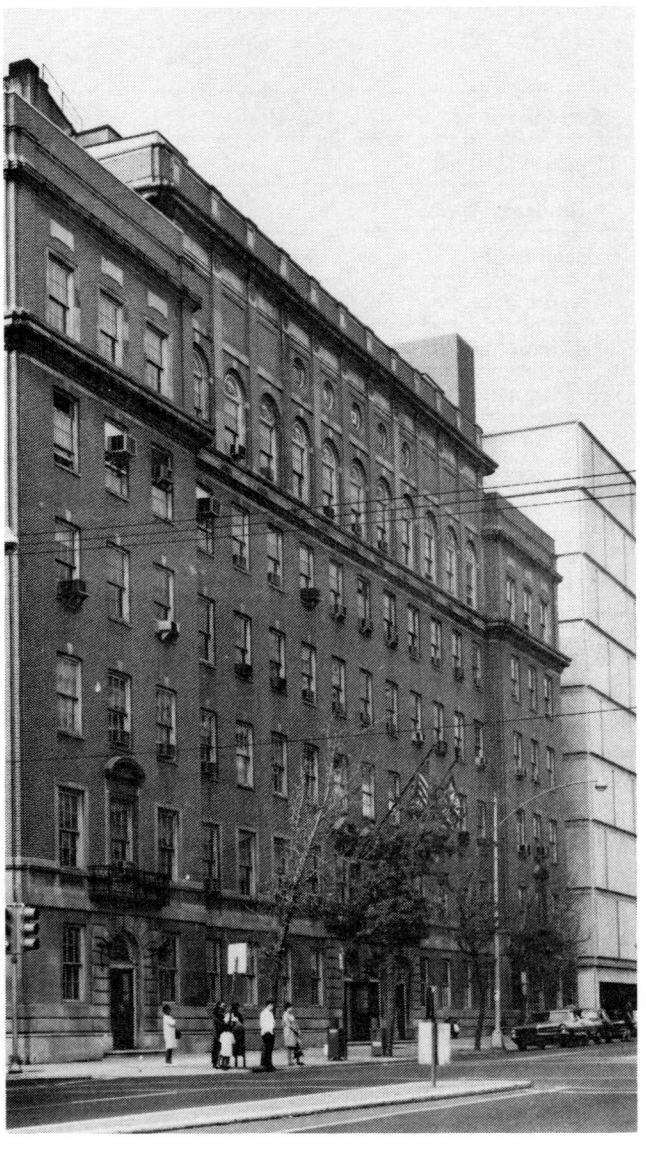

Student Body

Approximately 87 percent of graduating seniors chose university hospitals or major affiliates of university hospitals for their residencies.

Placement Records

Preference is given to Pennsylvania residents, although residents of other states are represented.

Costs

Tuition for residents of Pennsylvania is $14,212, while nonresidents pay $18,964.

Financial Aid

Except for limited scholarship funds (based on need and academic performance), all financial aid is in the form of loans and is given to students who demonstrate financial need.

Minority Programs

The Recruitment, Admissions and Retention Program (RAR) provides advice on premedical requirements and financial aid, pre-enrollment counseling, and summer educational reinforcement. Temple is among the top five medical schools with regard to the number of minority freshmen enrolled, and approximately 91 percent of these students complete their medical education at the School of Medicine.

Student Organizations

There is a Temple chapter of the Student National Medical Association.

Faculty

Many faculty members combine their work in research and teaching with their practice. Faculty members are familiar with the Socratic method of teaching, through which students are questioned and led to the correct answer through dialogue.

Curriculum

The School of Medicine offers a hands-on experimental approach and a tradition of problem solving and self-instruction. The introduction to clinical medicine course offers first-year students the chance to begin interaction with patients. Temple's innovative course in gross anatomy is taught virtually without lectures, and includes laboratory dissections, self-instruction, diagnostic imaging displays, and videotapes. At a clinical problem-solving conference, there is Socratic questioning in which each student must demonstrate knowledge of the body region studied and be able to think through the clinical applications of the anatomic information. The third and fourth years consist of clinical training.

Facilities

The new $130 million Temple University Hospital opened in 1986. It is a 500-bed facility staffed by faculty of the

School of Medicine and by many volunteer physicians. It attracts patients and referring physicians from a wide geographic area. St. Christopher's Hospital for Children is staffed by full-time Temple pediatric faculty and contains the region's only pediatric renal, cardiac, and liver transplant units as well as a cystic fibrosis center, a burn center, and a center for children with serious handicaps. Other facilities include the department of diagnostic imaging, the Functional Gastrointestinal Disease Center, the Heart Transplanation Program, the Laser Center, and the Department of Neurosurgery. Affiliated hospitals include the Albert Einstein Medical Center (formerly the Jewish Hospital of Philadelphia), the Abington Memorial Hospital, and the Philadelphia Psychiatric Center.

Special Programs

Temple University offers a combined M.D./Ph.D. program. Participating students spend the first two years in the medical school's basic science curriculum. The next three years are spent carrying out an original research project and completing coursework and other requirements for the Ph.D. degree. During the final two years, students return to the School of Medicine and its affiliated hospitals for clinical training.

Application Procedures

The School of Medicine participates in the American Medical College Application Service (AMCAS). Completed applications must be returned to AMCAS no later than December 1 of the year preceding planned enrollment. The MCAT is required and should be taken in the spring of the year before application. It must be taken no later than October of the year in which the candidate applies. MCAT scores that are more than three years old at the time of application will not be accepted. After the school receives the AMCAS application, an applicant is asked to forward supplementary materials (letters of recommendation from undergraduate premedical science faculty and a nonrefundable fee of $40). Applicants who have applied in previous years must resubmit all application materials. After review of the applications, approximately 800 Pennsylvanians and 400 non-Pennsylvanians will be interviewed. Of these, approximately 450 will be invited to be members of a class of 180 students. The school participates in the early decision plan.

Applicants for advanced standing to the second and third years will be considered. Applicants who are not currently enrolled or who have graduated from schools not approved by the Liaison Committee on Medical Education are not considered for advanced standing. Applicants for advanced standing must send a recommendation from the dean of the medical school in which the student is currently enrolled.

Contact

Assistant Dean for Admissions
Temple University
School of Medicine

Faculty-Student Union, Room 305
Broad and Ontario Streets
Philadelphia, Pennsylvania 19140
(215) 221-3656

UNIVERSITY OF TENNESSEE, MEMPHIS COLLEGE OF MEDICINE

800 Madison Avenue
Memphis, Tennessee 38163
(901) 528-5529

Accreditation	LCME
Degrees Offered	M.D.
# Students Applied	602
Enrollment	138 / class
Mean GPA	3.4
% Men / % Women	Not Available
% Minorities	Not Available
Tuition	$7,004 In-State
	$11,224 Out-of-State
Application Fee	$25
Application Deadline	November 15

The University

The University of Tennessee at Memphis, founded in 1851, is a 41-acre comprehensive health sciences campus consisting of the College of Medicine, the Graduate School of Health Sciences, and the colleges of dentistry, nursing, pharmacy, and allied health.

Admissions

Several factors are evaluated in the admissions process. Candidates are reviewed on the basis of MCAT scores, academic achievement, and preprofessional evaluations. The results of the personal interview are also important. The interview allows the school an opportunity to assess the applicant's personal background, character, and level of preparation for the study and practice of medicine.

Applications are accepted from nine states: Tennessee, Mississippi, Arkansas, Missouri, Kentucky, Virginia, North Carolina, Georgia, and Alabama. The college gives preference to residents of Tennessee.

Undergraduate Preparation

Applicants must have taken at least 90 semester hours of undergraduate coursework in order to be considered for admission. The college seeks broadly educated students who have a background in nonscience areas, such as humanities, fine arts, or social sciences. Evidence of independent study in the undergraduate years is sought. The following are required courses: eight semester hours of biology (with lab), including four hours of zoology; eight semester hours of inorganic chemistry (with lab); eight semester hours of organic chemistry (with lab); eight semester hours of general physics (with lab); six semester hours of English; and 52 semester hours of electives.

Student Body

There were 138 students in the 1990-91 first-year class. The mean GPA was 3.4. One hundred thirty enrollees were in-state residents. All students took the MCAT and 98 percent held baccalaureate degrees.

Costs

For the 1990-91 first-year class, resident tuition was $7,004. Nonresident tuition was $11,224. Student fees were $373.

Financial Aid

Accepted students receive a financial aid packet from the university. Students generally apply for a combination of both loans and scholarships. Federal scholarships as well as various loan funds are available for students who have demonstrated financial need. Several scholarships are awarded on a competitive basis, including the Doggett Scholarship and the Killeffer Scholarship.

Minority Programs

The policy of the university is to encourage applicants from minority groups who are traditionally underrepresented in the field of medicine. Scholarships of $10,000 are available to black students who are also residents of Tennessee. The college offers academic support programs for minority and disadvantaged students.

Curriculum

The academic program trains students with the skills, knowledge, and proper attitude for primary care specialties, other medical or surgical fields, or for research or academic careers. The program has two major components, biomedical science and clinical clerkships/electives. The first year includes the basic medical sciences: gross anatomy, histology, biochemistry, health promotion, and neuroanatomy. Second-year courses include microbiology, pharmacology, pathology, nutrition, and introduction to clinical skills.

The curriculum includes 20 months of required and elective clerkships. Clerkships begin in the third year with the standard areas like pediatrics, medicine, and obstetrics-gynecology. During the fourth year, students take several required clerkships along with three months of electives.

The college offers an expanded program in which students can elect to take the biomedical sciences in three years.

Facilities

The university is situated on a 41-acre campus. The campus hosts 15 affiliated hospitals and clinics that represent over 6,000 patient beds. These facilities include the University of Tennessee William F. Bowld Hospital, St. Jude Children's Hospital, Veterans Administration Hospital, and LePasses Rehabilitation Center. The college has clinical education centers in Chattanooga and in Knoxville.

Application Procedures

Students must submit applications to the college between June 15 and November 15 of the year prior to the year of desired enrollment. The school does not have an early decision plan. There is an application fee of $25. Applicants are notified of acceptance between October 15 and April 1. To hold a place in the class, accepted students must submit a $100 deposit, which is applied toward tuition.

Contact

Office of Enrollment Management
University of Tennessee, Memphis
College of Medicine
800 Madison Avenue
Memphis, Tennessee 38163
(901) 528-5560

TEXAS A&M UNIVERSITY COLLEGE OF MEDICINE

College Station, Texas 77843-1114
(409) 845-3432

Accreditation	LCME
Degrees Offered	M.D., M.D./Ph.D.
# Students Applied	904
Enrollment	48 / class
Mean GPA	3.41
% Men / % Women	62% / 38%
% Minorities	Not Available
Tuition	$5,463 In-State
	$21,852 Out-of-State
Application Fee	$35
Application Deadline	November 1

The University

The establishment of the College of Medicine in College Station, Texas, was authorized by the Texas state legislature in 1971. The first class of 32 students matriculated in 1977. Today, the college maintains a class size of 48 students. The college was accredited by the Liaison Committee on Medical Education in 1981.

Admissions

Factors considered in the evaluation process are the GPA, MCAT scores, college preprofessional committee evaluations, letters of recommendation, results of personal interviews, and physical and emotional health. Personal character, level of motivation, and a broad background in the humanities and social sciences are also important. Preference is given to residents of Texas.

Undergraduate Preparation

A minimum of two years (60 semester hours) at an accredited U.S. undergraduate institution is required for admission. The following coursework must be included in the undergraduate curriculum: eight hours (or one year) each of inorganic chemistry, organic chemistry, general physics, and general biology (all with lab). Three hours of additional biological sciences and calculus, and six hours (or one year) of English are also required.

Student Body

Of the 1989 entering class, 38 percent were women.

The mean GPA was 3.4, and the average MCAT score was 50.6.

Costs

Tuition for the 1992-93 academic year is $5,463 for residents and $21,852 for nonresidents. Fees are $820 per year. Books and supplies are estimated to cost from $1,000 to $1,500 for the year, and room and board is estimated at $5,000 to $6,000 for the year.

Financial Aid

Some scholarship and loan funds from local, state, and federal sources are available. Financial need of the applicant is not a consideration in the admission process; after acceptance, every effort is made to assist students in meeting their financial requirements. Approximately 90 percent of the students in the program are receiving some form of financial aid.

Curriculum

The curriculum is designed to provide a sound foundation in basic science as well as in clinical experience. Students are given the chance to participate in primary medical care, particularly in family practice, general internal medicine, and pediatrics.

The first two years are taken in residence on the Texas A&M campus. In addition to basic medical sciences (including physiology, biochemistry, microbiology, gross anatomy, and microscopic anatomy), students are exposed to behavioral science, humanities in medicine, and community medicine. The basic sciences are integrated with clinical experience in all courses, and regular clinical sessions are scheduled during the first two years. The third and fourth years are taken primarily on the Temple campus at the Scott and White Clinic and Hospital and the Olin E. Teague Veterans' Center. These years consist of traditional clerkships and a series of selective clerkships. Each student spends a minimum of four weeks in an approved family medicine clerkship.

Special Programs

The college has a joint degree program for those wishing to pursue the M.D./Ph.D. degree. Students can enroll in doctoral or masters' programs in areas such as bioengineering, food and nutrition policy, man and the sea, environmental sciences, and other fields offered elsewhere within the university.

Application Procedures

Applicants must submit an application form, an official transcript from each college or university the applicant has attended, MCAT scores (scores from tests taken earlier than 1989 will not be accepted for admission in 1992), a composite evaluation from a premedical advisory committee or letters of recommendation from at least three faculty members, and a nonrefundable application fee of $35. Applications can be submitted to the associate dean for student affairs as early as May 1 but no later than November 1.

Contact

Office of Student Affairs
Texas A&M College of Medicine
College Station, Texas 77843-1114
(409) 845-7743

UNIVERSITY OF TEXAS MEDICAL SCHOOL AT GALVESTON

Galveston, Texas 77550
(409) 761-2671

Accreditation	SACS
Degrees Offered	M.D., M.D./Ph.D.
# Students Applied	2,072
Enrollment	196 / class
Mean GPA	3.3
% Men / % Women	64% / 36%
% Minorities	30%
Tuition	$5,463 In-State
	$21,852 Out-of-State
Application Fee	$35
Application Deadline	October 15

The University

Celebrating its centennial year as a four-year, state appropriated, public institution, the college graduates some 475 students each year. In addition to the School of Medicine, the University of Texas Medical Branch (UTMB) includes the School of Nursing, the Graduate School of Biomedical Sciences, and the School of Allied Health Sciences. Located in the Gulf of Mexico, Galveston is a barrier reef island of approximately 47 square miles that hosts some 66,000 residents and 6 million annual visitors. Galveston offers a slower paced metropolis atmosphere than the major Texas cities of Dallas and Houston. A host of activities and attractions are available nearby, including NASA's Johnson Space Center, the Astrodome, the Houston Ballet, the Grand 1894 Opera House, and the February Mardi Gras.

Admissions

Of the 196 accepted applicants of 1990 the mean GPA was 3.3 and the mean MCAT score was 52.2. Students are urged to take the Medical College Admission Test in the spring of the year applying. A baccalaureate degree is highly desirable.

Undergraduate Preparation

Texas residents receive preference for admissions. A minimum of 90 semester hours of college work is required of all applicants. Mandatory coursework for entering students includes two years of biology, and one year each of inorganic chemistry, general physics, calculus, organic chemistry, and English. A broad background of the humanities is encouraged for all applicants.

Student Body

Of the accepted students for the 1990 entering class, 99 percent were Texas residents. Sixty-four percent were men, and 36 percent were women. Thirty percent were minorities.

Placement Records

Most graduates of UTMB are placed within Texas.

Costs

Tuition for the 1990 year was $5,463 for residents. The nonresident tuition was $21,852. In addition, student fees average $250 per year.

Financial Aid

A number of long-term, low interest loans as well as scholarships are available to students who demonstrate financial need. Approximately 45 percent of the students enrolled in the School of Medicine receive financial aid. Students are advised to contact the office of student fiscal planning and management for more information.

Minority Programs

UTMB is dedicated to increasing the number of minority students accepted into the schools of medicine. Minority applicants are reviewed by experienced members of the committee on admissions.

Faculty

The School of Medicine has 564 full-time faculty members, 46 part-time, and 335 volunteers. The student/faculty ratio is approximately 1:1.25.

Curriculum

The curriculum is divided into two core sections. One consists of the study of basic science and the other of clinical medicine. The basic science core typically makes up the first two years and is separated by four 16-week terms and completed with a 10-week introduction to clinical medicine. During the second two years the clinical medicine core is broken down into 50 weeks of clerkship experience and 36 weeks of electives.

Facilities

UTMB offers 234,000 square feet of designated space for research purposes. The multidisciplinary commitment of the university is demonstrated through the presence of two World Health Organization Centers. Located on the 64 acres of campus space are a major medical library, specialty centers, classroom buildings, and extensive research laboratories. In addition, the university is affiliated with seven hospitals.

Grading Procedures

The grading system for the first three years of the School of Medicine is A, B, C, and F. A pass/fail system is used for all elective courses.

Special Programs

Eligible candidates interested in pursuing careers in biomedical research and/or academic medicine can participate in a program to earn a combined M.D./Ph.D. degree. A competition by the National Student Research Forum is sponsored annually by the Medical Branch to encourage the spirit of research in future scientists.

Application Procedures

Students are accepted on the basis of the results of their aptitude and achievement tests, the college and professional committee evaluations, and the personal interview. The application period runs from April 15 to October 15. MCAT scores, official transcripts, and an application fee of $35 must be sent to the application center. Applicants have a maximum of two weeks to respond to the acceptance offer when notified sometime after January 15.

Contact

Office of Admissions
University of Texas
Medical Branch
G.210
Ashbel Smith Building
Route M-17
Galveston, Texas 77550
(409) 761-3517

UNIVERSITY OF TEXAS MEDICAL SCHOOL AT HOUSTON

Houston, Texas 77225
(713) 792-5000

Accreditation	LCME
Degrees Offered	M.D., M.D./Ph.D., M.D./M.P.H.
# Students Applied	2,111
Enrollment	189 / class
Mean GPA	3.41
% Men / % Women	60% / 40%
% Minorities	Not Available
Tuition	$5,463 In-State
	$21,852 Out-of-State
Application Fee	$35
Application Deadline	October 15

The University

The University of Texas formally opened in 1883. The university system today comprises numerous schools, colleges, divisions, and branches located throughout the state. The University of Texas Health Science Center at Houston, established in 1972, administers the Medical School, the School of Nursing, the Texas Dental College, the School of Allied Health Sciences, and several other health-related schools, centers, and institutes.

The Medical School was established in 1969. It is a member of the Texas Medical Center, a comprehensive medical complex in Houston with 41 member institutions.

Houston is a rapidly growing financial, commercial, and industrial center. The city hosts about 28 colleges and universities, and has an array of cultural and recreational attractions.

Admissions

In addition to MCAT scores and academic ability, consideration is given to the depth and breadth of the candidate's undergraduate education. Other factors considered include interest in the Medical School, evidence of leadership, achievement in a nonacademic field, and various personal qualities and characteristics. The school weighs the applicant's preprofessional committee evaluations and the results of personal interviews.

Admissions preference is given to Texas residents.

Undergraduate Preparation

Applicants must have completed at least 90 credit hours at an accredited U.S. or Canadian university; however, students should plan to complete the requirements for the bachelor's degree prior to admission. The following coursework is required for admission: one year of English; two years of biology; one-half year of calculus; one year of physics; and two years of chemistry (one in general chemistry and one in organic chemistry).

Student Body

The 1990-91 total Medical School enrollment is 774. Almost 50 percent of the 1990-91 class comes from Texas A&M, University of Texas at Austin, Baylor, Rice, and the University of Houston. The remaining students come from 58 different undergraduate schools.

Ninety percent of students enrolled at the Medical School are Texas residents. Women account for about 40 percent of the student body, compared to the national average of 36 percent. Of the 127 U.S. medical schools, UT Medical School ranks in the top quarter of schools with regard to the proportion of minority students.

Accepted students for the 1990 first-year class had a mean GPA of 3.41.

Placement Records

In 1990-91, the Medical School placed 570 resident physicians in 22 accredited training programs. Almost 60 percent of graduates have remained in Texas. The same approximate percentage has entered family practice, internal medicine, pediatrics, psychiatry, or general surgery.

Costs

The 1989-90 annual resident tuition was $5,463; tuition for nonresidents was $21,852. The annual student service fee ranges from $165 to $220. Laboratory fees, insurance charges, microscope fees, and other charges are minimal. The cost of books and equipment ranges from $500 to $1,000 per year.

Financial Aid

Scholarships and loans are available to students on the basis of proven financial need and/or academic exellence. The Medical School has limited loan and scholarship funds. Financial assistance is also available from state, local, and federal sources. Enrolling students can obtain financial aid application forms and information from the Office of Student Financial Aid, University of Texas, Health Science Center at Houston, P.O. Box 20036, Houston, Texas 77225.

Faculty

The faculty numbers nearly 2,000, and includes 560 full-time members, 70 part-time members, and approximately 1,330 voluntary instructors.

Curriculum

The Medical School endeavors to offer students the opportunity for personalized education that will encourage them to understand the biological and scientific bases of modern medicine, the cultural and social forces that shape its practice, and the role of physicians in society.

During the first two years of the four-year program, students prepare to embark on the clerkship experiences of the third academic year. During these primary years, students become familiar with the basic and applied biomedical sciences, including molecular and cellular biology, the structure and function of organ systems, and morphology. Students are also exposed to the techniques of interviewing, history-taking, and performance of physical and mental status examinations.

The third year consists of a series of clinical clerkships in the major disciplines. In the fourth year, the student takes two months of required clerkships, six periods of electives, and one period for additional instruction in medical jurisprudence and clinical epidemiology.

Facilities

The primary teaching hospital is Hermann Hospital, a private 650-bed facility connected to the Medical School buildings. The hospital offers a broad range of services and includes University Children's Hospital, the Texas Kidney Institute, and the Jesse H. and Mary Gibbs Jones Medical Surgical Center. Other affiliated hospitals include the M.D. Anderson Cancer Center, St. Joseph Hospital, the Harris County Psychiatric Center, San Jose Clinic, Southwest Memorial Hospital, and the Lyndon Baines Johnson Hospital.

Other centers and institutes affiliated with the University of Texas Health Science Center include the Center on Aging, the Center for Health Promotion Research and Development, the Human Nutrition Center, the Southwest Center for Occupational Health and Safety, and the Speech and Hearing Institute.

The Houston Academy of Medicine/Texas Medical Center Library is a cooperative resource center supported by 22 institutions within the Texas Medical Center. Considered one of the leading academic health sciences libraries in the nation, it ranks in the top 10 percent in terms of size and activity. The library subscribes to more than 3,000 journal titles and houses more than 229,000 bound volumes. Computer access is provided to current medical literature through TexSearch.

The Medical School's Learning Resource Center houses a collection of more than 3,500 titles and an audiovisual library.

Grading Procedures

The Medical School evaluates students using grades of honors, high pass, pass, marginal performance, and fail.

Special Programs

The Medical School and the Graduate School of Biomedical Sciences participate in a program that leads to the M.D.

and Ph.D. degrees. The program generally takes six years to complete.

The Medical School and the School of Public Health offer a joint program leading to the M.D. and M.P.H. (master of public health) degrees.

Application Procedures

Applications should be filed with the University of Texas System Medical and Dental Application Center, Suite 620, 702 Colorado, Austin Texas 78701. The application deadline is October 15. For Texas residents, the application fee is $35 for one school and $5.00 for each additional school. Applicants who are favorably considered are asked to participate in a personal interview.

Contact

Office of Admission, Room G-024
University of Texas
Medical School at Houston
PO Box 20708
Houston, Texas 77225
(713) 792-4711

UNIVERSITY OF TEXAS MEDICAL SCHOOL AT SAN ANTONIO

7703 Floyd Curl Drive
San Antonio, Texas 78284-7701
(512) 567-3000

Accreditation	LCME
Degrees Offered	M.D.
# Students Applied	2,052
Enrollment	202 / class
Mean GPA	3.38
% Men / % Women	60% / 40%
% Minorities	Not Available
Tuition	$5,463 In-State
	$21,852 Out-of-State
Application Fee	$35
Application Deadline	October 15

The University

The University of Texas Health Science Center at San Antonio (UTHSCSA) sits on 100 acres in the heart of the South Texas Medical Center. UTHSCSA is built on a hill in the northwest quadrant of the city and has been designed to preserve large areas of grass and trees, offering a view of the famous Texas Hill County. San Antonio offers a full range of cultural and social activities. The SPURS professional basketball team makes its home here, and Sea World of Texas is a major attraction. Nearby lakes, rivers, and parks make outdoor activities inviting and accessible.

Admissions

Over 50 percent of those admitted have GPAs over 3.5. Fewer than five percent have GPAs under 3.0. The MCAT is required. The admissions committee considers the student's overall academic record, health professions advisor or advisory committee recommendations, maturity, and motivation. By law, 90 percent of the entering classes must be Texas residents. Some outstanding nonresidents are considered.

Undergraduate Preparation

Although some students are admitted after 90 semester hours of college work, most enter with their bachelor's degree completed. Students must achieve a C or better in the following courses to be considered: one year each (with lab) of inorganic and organic chemistry, and physics. Two years of biology (with lab), one-half year of college calculus, and one year of English are also required.

Student Body

About 200 students are admitted to the entering class. The total university enrollment is 2,200 students. For the 1990 entering class, 40 percent of the students were women and 94 percent were Texas residents.

Costs

Tuition for the 1990 first-year class was $5,463 for residents and $21,852 for nonresidents. Required fees for the first year are $250. Books and manuals are $1,375. UTHSCSA has no on-campus housing, but apartments near the college rent from about $250 to $400 per month.

Financial Aid

Over 90 percent of UTHSCSA students who apply for aid receive assistance in the form of long-term loans, grants, and scholarships. Nonresident students are eligible for all forms of aid because most programs are federally funded. International students are not generally eligible for assistance.

Minority Programs

Minority students are supported by the office of special programs. A network of tutoring, study groups, mentors, resource materials, and referrals is available to assist minority members of the student body. Several minority student organizations are sponsored by special programs for group recreation and support.

Curriculum

The curriculum covers clinical and preclinical sciences in the first two years. Courses offered in the first year include gross anatomy and embryology, microscopic anatomy, biochemistry, psychosocial dimensions of health care, physiology, microbiology, and neurosciences. The third year is spent in the clinical setting in eight assignments of six weeks each. The fourth year consists mainly of electives.

Facilities

UTHSCSA's Dolph Briscoe Jr. Library is the fifth largest medical library in the nation, including over 191,000 books and journals. Worldwide computer access to information is available. A bookstore, large and complete recreational facilities, and a convenient Student Health Service clinic round out the practical campus facilities available.

Grading Procedures

A letter grading system is used.

Application Procedures

Students must apply between April 15 and October 15 of the year preceding entry and through the University of Texas, Medical and Dental Application Center. MCAT scores should be sent directly to the application center. Beginning in 1992, the new MCAT will be required.

Contact

Medical Admissions
Registrar's Office
UTHSCSA
7703 Floyd Curl Drive
San Antonio, Texas 78284-7702
(512) 567-2665

UNIVERSITY OF TEXAS SOUTHWESTERN MEDICAL CENTER AT DALLAS SOUTHWESTERN MEDICAL SCHOOL

Dallas, Texas 75235
(214) 688-7670

Accreditation	LCME
Degrees Offered	M.D., M.D./Ph.D.
# Students Applied	2,094
Enrollment	194 / class
Mean GPA	3.56
% Men / % Women	69% / 31%
% Minorities	Not Available
Tuition	$5,463 In-State
	$21,852 Out-of-State
Application Fee	$35
Application Deadline	October 15

The University

The University of Texas Southwestern Medical School is located on a 60-acre campus three miles north of downtown Dallas. Founded in 1943, the Medical School is now part of a larger medical center that contains the Graduate School of Biomedical Sciences and the School of Allied Health Sciences. The Howard Hughes Medical Institute, a molecular biology research facility, is located on campus. The Medical School supports an internship and residency program at Parkland Memorial Hospital, which provides a major forum for clinical instruction. An additional 15 affiliated health facilities conveniently located either on campus or in the Dallas area insure that students can take advantage of many clinical learning opportunities.

Admissions

Each applicant is judged worthy of admission based upon the combined package of grade-point average, Medical College Admission Test (MCAT) scores, difficulty of undergraduate curriculum, extracurricular activities, communication skills, motivation, and integrity.

Undergraduate Preparation

Applicants to the Medical School must have completed at least 90 semester hours of undergraduate work, including one year of English, one-half year of college calculus, two years of biology, one year of physics, one year of inorganic chemistry, and one year of organic chemistry. Formal lab work must accompany the lecture courses in physics, chemistry, and one year of biology.

Student Body

Two hundred freshmen are accepted each year, 90 percent of whom are Texas residents. Nonresidents are accepted if they are ranked among the top third of the entering class. Transfer students are accepted only if they are married to current students, faculty, or house staff completing training at Parkland Memorial Hospital or Children's Medical Center.

Costs

Annual tuition is $5,463 for Texas residents and $21,852 for nonresidents. The approximate cost of books over the four-year period is $3,527. Laboratory fees are $32 for the first year, $30 for the second year, and $24 for the third and fourth years. All students are required to pay a $180 student services fee for a nine-month term and a $25-per-year malpractice insurance fee. A graduation fee of $55 is required upon registration for the final term. Students may elect to pay tuition and certain fees in three installments. (The Medical School does not provide student housing.)

Financial Aid

Students desiring to apply for financial aid must file a financial aid form (FAF) with the College Scholarship Service. Available loans include the Stafford Guaranteed Student Loan, the Carl D. Perkins National Direct Student Loan, and the Health Professions Student Loan. Scholarship money is available from memorial funds maintained by the Southwestern Medical Foundation and other foundations.

Student Organizations

The university activities office sponsors intramural sports and special interest clubs, sells discount tickets to theaters and sporting events, and offers group travel opportunities. Social events and services are sponsored by campus chapters of the American Medical Student Association, the Student National Medical Association, the Mexican-American Student Organization, and the medical fraternities Phi Beta Pi and Phi Delta Epsilon. The Medical School also has a chapter of the medical honor society Alpha Omega Alpha.

Faculty

Seven hundred full-time faculty members teach at the Medical School.

Curriculum

First-year studies begin with the molecular and cellular processes at work in the healthy human body, and conclude with the more systemic picture presented by anatomy, physiology, and endocrinology. Second-year studies concentrate on immunology, pathology, and pharmacology in order to understand diseases and their treatment. Students also begin to

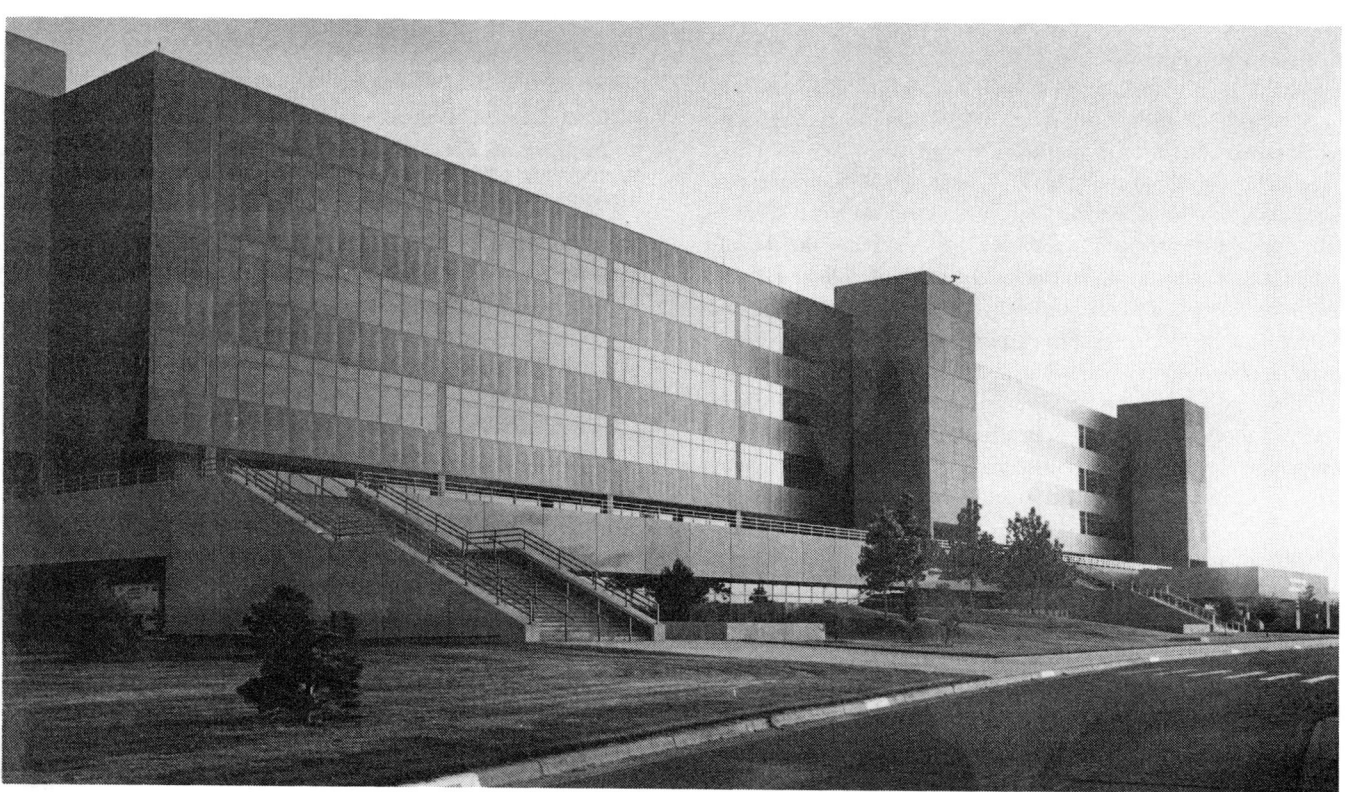

take patient histories and perform physical examinations under faculty supervision. Emphasis shifts in the third and fourth years to clinical studies. The 10-month junior year includes rotations in pediatrics, surgery, obstetrics, psychiatry, family medicine, and internal medicine. Senior year continues with a rotation in neurology, a four-week subinternship in internal medicine, and a series of clinical electives.

Facilities

Through the Academic Computing Services (ACS) students have access to a VAX 8800 research computer as well as Macintosh and PC labs. The campus library contains about 220,700 volumes and receives about 2,400 serials. Students perform MEDLINE searches directly, and the library staff performs searches on databases provided by agencies such as the National Library of Medicine. The Animal Resources Center (ARC) provides courses on animal experimentation for biomedical research. The Algur H. Meadows Diagnostic Imaging Center houses three state-of-the-art magnetic resonance imaging units for clinical diagnosis and research. The Charles Sprague Clinical Science Building on the main campus is interconnected with two teaching hospitals, Parkland Memorial Hospital and Zale Lipshy University Hospital.

Grading Procedures

All courses are graded on the traditional letter grading system. Students must achieve a grade of C or better in order to pass a course. Electives in the fourth year are graded on a pass/fail basis.

Special Programs

The Medical Scientist Training Program (MSTP) offers an opportunity to those interested in biomedical research and teaching to obtain both an M.D. degree from Southwestern Medical School and a Ph.D. degree from Southwestern Graduate School of Biomedical Sciences in six years. Acceptance into the program requires a baccalaureate degree and experience in laboratory research. One year of college calculus and one year of physical chemistry are recommended. A candidate may gain the necessary research experience while attending the Medical School and apply to the MSTP during the first two years. The Ph.D. may be earned in biochemistry, cell and molecular biology, immunology, microbiology, pharmacology, or physiology. All MSTP students receive stipends from available funds for tuition and fees.

Application Procedures

Applications for admission must be submitted between April 15 and October 15 preceding the fall semester of the first year and sent to the central application center of The University of Texas System. Student selection is based on college performance, MCAT scores, faculty recommendations, and a required interview. Students must take the MCAT during the year they apply. There is a $35 application fee.

Contact

The University of Texas System
Medical/Dental Application Center
Suite 620
Austin, Texas 78701
(512) 499-4785

TEXAS TECH UNIVERSITY HEALTH SCIENCES CENTER SCHOOL OF MEDICINE

3601 Fourth Street
Lubbock, Texas 79430
(806) 743-2900

Accreditation	LCME
Degrees Offered	M.D., M.S./M.D., M.D./Ph.D.
# Students Applied	902
Enrollment	100 / class
Mean GPA	3.2
% Men / % Women	79% / 21%
% Minorities	25%
Tuition	$5,463 In-State
	$21,852 Out-of-State
Application Fee	$35
Application Deadline	November 1

The University

The Texas Tech University Health Sciences Center, established in 1979, serves 108 counties, covers over 135,000 square miles, and has a population of 2.5 million people. In addition to the School of Medicine in Lubbock, the university has campuses in Amarillo, El Paso, and Odessa. All of the regional academic health centers are dedicated to the study and research of health medicine serving predominantly rural areas. The School of Medicine has affiliations with Northwest Texas Hospital and the Veterans Administration Hospital. Being the major Health Sciences Center for such a substantial geographic area enables the school to provide many diverse services.

Admissions

Scores from the Medical College Admission Test (MCAT) are required. Students are advised to take the MCAT in the spring prior to application. Most applicants possess a GPA of 3.2 or higher.

Undergraduate Preparation

Any incomplete courses should be removed from the official transcripts prior to application. Part of the mandatory course load for entrance includes biology, chemistry, physics, and calculus. Any other coursework that reflects a broad background of interests is viewed favorably.

Student Body

There are 79 male and 21 female students making a total enrollment of 100. Most of the accepted applicants are Texas residents. Twenty-five percent of the students are of minority backgrounds.

Placement Records

The School of Medicine offers residency programs through its regional academic health centers located on all of the related campuses. Students can participate in residencies in anesthesiology, dermatology, opthalmology, and orthopedics.

Costs

The Texas resident tuition fee is $5,463. Nonresidents pay $21,852.

Financial Aid

Over 65 percent of the accepted applicants receive some form of financial aid.

Curriculum

Students will receive a rotation schedule for their medical education and training courses. The first two years of study will take place primarily on the Lubbock campus. The third and fourth years are divided among the surrounding Amarillo, El Paso, and Odessa campuses. Residency training is offered in four different urban Texas areas.

Facilities

The School of Medicine uses a Mednet planned computer satellite network supported by $2.2 million in federal funding. This system links rural doctors with the technological expertise available in the Health Sciences Center. The research library links all four of the health sciences centers and contains over 170,000 volumes.

Application Procedures

Applications, along with a $35 application fee, are due no later than November 1. Supporting documents are due by November 30. Included in the supporting documents must be the student's official transcripts, letters of evaluation, and a recent passport-style photograph with signature. Students are advised to complete the admissions application thoroughly to avoid delays in the acceptance process.

Contact

Office of Admissions
Texas Tech University
Health Sciences Center School of Medicine
3601 Fourth Street
Lubbock, Texas 79430
(806) 743-3000

TUFTS UNIVERSITY SCHOOL OF MEDICINE

136 Harrison Avenue, Stearns 1
Boston, Massachusetts 02111
(617) 628-5000

Accreditation	LCME
Degrees Offered	M.D., M.D./Ph.D., M.D./ M.P.H.
# Students Applied	5,038
Enrollment	152 / class
Mean GPA	3.0
% Men / % Women	50% / 50%
% Minorities	Not Available
Tuition	$22,980
Application Fee	$55
Application Deadline	November 1

The University

Founded in 1850 as the Tufts Institution of Learning, Tufts University today is a major university offering a wide variety of undergraduate academic programs at three campuses in Massachusetts. The School of Medicine was founded in 1893 and has graduated more than 8,000 physicians since this time. The medical school is located in downtown Boston, amidst the city's Chinese community, and close to the New England Medical Center and Boston's theater district. The city runs an efficient public transportation system that connects greater Boston with its outlying areas.

Admissions

Admissions to Tufts School of Medicine is based not only on performance in the required premedical courses but also on the applicant's entire academic record and extracurricular experiences. Almost all admitted students have a GPA of at least 3.0.

Undergraduate Preparation

Specific coursework required includes: one year of biology (eight semester credits) including laboratory work (knowledge of classical genetics is essential); not less than 16 semester credits equally divided between general and inorganic chemistry, including lab work in both divisions; and a general introductory course in physics (eight semester credits) that covers mechanics, heat, light, sound, electricity, and nuclear radiation. Work in the areas of mathematics, such as calculus, statistics, and computer science, is encouraged. The ability to speak and write English correctly is required. All applicants must also take the MCAT.

Costs

For the 1990-91 academic year, tuition and fees for medical students at Tufts totalled $23,340. In addition, students are required to pay an annual health insurance fee of $1,100.

Financial Aid

Because resources for financial assistance are limited, it is Tufts' policy that the primary responsibility for the cost of a medical education belongs to the student and his or her family. All financial aid awards are based on financial need. Applicants are required to file the Graduate and Professional Student Financial Aid Service (GAPSFAS) form as soon as possible after January 1 of the year of desired medical school entrance. Available sources of aid include the Perkins, Health Professions, Massachusetts Medical Society, and Franklin Fund loans as well as Tufts' loans and scholarships.

Minority Programs

In honor of the first black female medical graduate of the TU School of Medicine, the Progressive Alliance of Minority Students has established the Dr. Ruth Marguerite Easterling Fund, which annually offers a four-year, $1,000 scholarship to a selected entering minority student. Also, a six-week prematriculation summer program is open to all minority and selected majority students; the program provides a comprehensive introduction to the first semester of medical school coursework.

Student Organizations

The medical student council serves as a liaison between the student body and the administration, and manages the affairs of medical students as a whole, supervising various lotteries and class elections as well as organizing occasional social events. The Progressive Alliance of Minority Students is the on-campus minority medical student association. The Student National Medical Association and Alpha Omega Alpha, the national medical honor fraternity, also have groups on campus.

Curriculum

As a result of a new curriculum plan implemented in 1985, all medical instruction at the School of Medicine is problem based, with students learning by examining case studies. The first two years of the curriculum is devoted to the study of preclinical and basic sciences; the first year focuses on the normal aspects of the human body, and the second concentrates on the abnormal. During this time students have the opportunity to participate in a preclinical elective program that allows them to work closely with faculty members on various clinical, laboratory, and community experiences. Third-year medical students at Tufts are required to spend 12 weeks each in clinical rotations of medicine and surgery, and six weeks each of obstetrics and gynecology, pediatrics, psychiatry, and an elective subject. During the fourth year of the medical program, students expand the basic clinical knowledge and skills acquired in the third year by participating in another series of clinical rotations.

Facilities

The USDA Human Nutrition Research Center on Aging is located on campus. Owned by the U.S. Department of Agriculture and operated by Tufts, this 200,000-square-foot facility studies human nutrition and metabolism emphasizing the relationship between nutrition and aging and the nutrition requirements of the aging. The Health Sciences Library offers a collection of 109,000 volumes and 1,500 serial subscriptions. The library has several medical databases available. Tufts students also have access to many academic and research libraries throughout Massachusetts.

Special Programs

In conjunction with the Sackler School of Biomedical Sciences, the School of Medicine offers a joint M.D./Ph.D. program. Students accepted into this program may simultaneously pursue their medical degrees while working in advanced areas of biochemistry and pharmacology; cellular, molecular, and developmental biology; cellular and molecular physiology; immunology; molecular biology and microbiology; and neuroscience. Normally both degrees can be completed within six years and special financial assistance programs may be available. Tufts also offers a combined M.D. and master of public health degree program. For an additional tuition charge of $2,000 per year, medical students selected to this program complete their medical degree while fulfilling the public health requirements during available elective time.

Application Procedures

The School of Medicine participates in the AMCAS application program. Students must submit an application to the AMCAS before November 1. Once this information is received by Tufts, the candidate is required to submit a $55 application fee along with a supplemental application information sheet and letters of recommendation. Selected applicants will be chosen to participate in an on-campus personal interview. The MCAT is also required and should preferably be taken in the spring prior to desired medical school admission.

Contact

Committee on Admission
Tufts University
School of Medicine
136 Harrison Avenue, Stearns 1
Boston, Massachusetts 02111
(617) 956-5000

TULANE UNIVERSITY SCHOOL OF MEDICINE

New Orleans, Louisiana 70112
(504) 588-5187

Accreditation	AAMC
Degrees Offered	M.D., M.D./M.P.H., M.D./M.S., M.D./Ph.D.
# Students Applied	4,343
Enrollment	148 / class
Mean GPA	Not Available
% Men / % Women	Not Available
% Minorities	Not Available
Tuition	$23,000
Application Fee	$55
Application Deadline	December 15

The University

Founded in 1834, Tulane School of Medicine is located in New Orleans. The Charity Hospital of New Orleans is a major hospital located next to the school, and it is their primary teaching hospital.

Admissions

Three years or 90 college credits are required for entrance to the school, however, a four year degree is strongly recommended. The MCAT is also required. Any major, as long as the basic science requirements have been fulfilled, is acceptable.

Undergraduate Preparation

Prospective students must have earned at least 90 semester hours of credit, and courses in biology or zoology with lab,

inorganic chemistry with lab, organic chemistry with lab, general physics with lab, and English are required. As stated above, a major in one of the sciences is not required.

Costs

Tuition and student fees for the 1991-92 entering class were $23,000 per year.

Financial Aid

There are several forms of financial aid available. Students can qualify for scholarships, long-term loans, and deferred tuition plans, depending on their financial status as determined by Tulane. More than two-thirds of students receive some type of financial aid throughout their medical education.

First-year students are strongly advised not to seek outside employment. Students wishing to seek outside, relevant employment might find a paid externship at a local hospital, or receive a summer research fellowship through the school.

Minority Programs

Summer enrichment programs, tutorial, and special counseling services are available for minorities.

Curriculum

The curriculum at Tulane is completed over four years. During the first two years, the basic sciences are covered in the classroom, although clinical aspects of the sciences are reviewed. In the third and fourth years, students gain valuable clinical experience through working in hospital and community health care settings. Approximately one-third of the curriculum in these years is in elective and advanced studies courses.

Facilities

The Tulane Medical Center Hospital and Clinic has recently been added into the medical school teaching program.

Special Programs

While studying for the M.D. degree, students may also earn a Master of Science, Master of Public Health, or Doctorate of Philosophy degree.

Application Procedures

The school uses the American Medical College Application Service, and applications are accepted beginning June 15. The latest date students can file with the AMCAS is December 15. Applications are reviewed starting October 15 with no set ending date. Scores received on an MCAT taken before 1991 will not be accepted. All applications are reviewed by a member of the Admission Committee. Interviews are held in New Orleans. After an interview is completed, the applicant's record is once again discussed during an admissions meeting. The committee then makes a final decision regarding acceptance. No early decision is available.

Contact
Office of Admissions
School of Medicine
1430 Tulane Avenue
New Orleans, Louisiana 70112
(504) 588-5187

UNIFORMED SERVICES UNIVERSITY OF THE HEALTH SCIENCES F. EDWARD HÉBERT SCHOOL OF MEDICINE

4301 Jones Bridge Road
Bethesda, Maryland 20814-4799
(301) 295-3101

Accreditation	LCME
Degrees Offered	M.D.
# Students Applied	2,624
Enrollment	162 / class
Mean GPA	3.45
% Men / % Women	78% / 22%
% Minorities	Not Available
Tuition	No Tuition
Application Fee	Contact School
Application Deadline	November 1

The University

The Uniformed Services University of the Health Sciences (USUHS) was created by Congress under the Department of Defense in 1972 to train career medical officers to serve in the Army, Navy, Air Force, and the U.S. Public Health Services. The university is located on the grounds of the National Naval Medical Center in Bethesda.

The School of Medicine is located on the grounds of the Naval Medical Command, National Capital Region, in Bethesda, Maryland. Bethesda is a suburb of Washington, D.C., a city with many historical and cultural attractions.

A wide variety of social and recreational activities is available at area military posts and bases for students and their families. Officers' clubs offer social activities for students and spouses; other facilities include bowling lanes, tennis courts, theaters, swimming pools, gymnasiums, and golf courses.

The historic areas of Fredericksburg, Williamsburg, Mount Vernon, Annapolis, and Baltimore are all within driving distance and each have museums, monuments, and a wide variety of cultural activities.

Admissions

Applicants to the School of Medicine must be citizens of the United States and have reached the age of 18 at time of matriculation. Civilians must not be older than 27 years old by June 30 in the year of admission. Any student who has served on active duty in the Armed Forces may exceed the age limit by a period equal to the time served on active duty, provided he/she has not reached age 34 by June 30 in the year of admission. Applicants must also meet the physical requirements for military commission, be of sound moral character, and be motivated for a military medical career. Academic accomplishments are important when evaluating an applicant, although extracurricular activities, military service employment, and graduate study are considered. The School of Medicine admits students only to the first-year class.

Undergraduate Preparation

An applicant must have completed the requirements for a bachelor's degree at an accredited college or university by June 30 of the year of planned matriculation. Required coursework comprises one academic year each of general or inorganic chemistry, organic chemistry, physics, and biology (all with labs), mathematics through calculus (computer sciences and statistics do not fulfill this requirement), and English.

Applicants who are not in the process of completing the last eight semester hours (or 12 quarter hours) of the required courses at the time of application will normally be ineligible for admission. CLEP and advanced placement credits will be accepted if the applicant has taken formal additional work in the same area. Applicants who have done college work in the humanities and social or behavioral science receive preference.

Student Body

The 1990 class had a mean GPA of 3.45 and a mean MCAT of 9.4. The mean age of applicants was 23. Twenty-two percent of the class were women. Thirty-nine percent majored in biology. Students represent every part of the country.

Placement Records

Graduates from the School of Medicine are required to spend the first year after graduation in internships in approved programs in teaching hospitals of the student's chosen branch of military service. Internships are competitive, and a graduate is not guaranteed his or her first choice.

Costs

The School of Medicine is a tuition-free institution. Books, equipment, and instruments are furnished to students either without charge or on a loan basis.

Financial Aid

Students enrolled in the School of Medicine serve on active duty as reserve commissioned officers, and receive all the pay and benefits of their rank (Second Lieutenant in the Army and Air Force, Ensign in the Navy and the Public Health Service). As active duty officers, students are eligible for a wide range of benefits, including medical insurance, a nontaxable monthly housing allowance, a uniform allowance, and reimbursement for relocation expenses. When medical education is completed, graduates must fulfill a service obligation of seven years. Time spent in an internship and time spent in a residency does not count toward satisfying the service obligation.

Minority Programs

The university encourages applications from groups underrepresented in the medical profession, including women, Blacks, American Indian/Alaskan natives, and Hispanics. Minority affairs activities are coordinated in the office of admissions.

Faculty

Approximately 326 full-time basic and clinical sciences faculty members and 2,017 part-time scientists and clinicians teach at USUHS. There is a mix of military and civilian faculty.

Curriculum

Students are taught both the traditional medical curriculum and courses of direct military medical relevance so that they will be as effective serving in a military field hospital as in a medical center. Prior to matriculation, all incoming students attend a four- to six-week officer's orientation program, which introduces them to the customs and traditions of military life in their respective services and the responsibilities of an officer. Students then begin their medical training in Bethesda.

The first and second years consist of the basic sciences, study of the psychosocial aspects of health and disease, and an introduction to military medicine and patient care techniques. Five weeks during the first summer are devoted to a course in military medical field studies. During the second year, study of the basic sciences and clinical problems and their management are integrated. The third year consists of required clinical clerkships. The fourth year begins with one week of instruction in military preventative medicine, followed by 40 weeks of required clerkships and electives. Elective courses are offered in both national and international clinical and research facilities.

Facilities

The university is affiliated with the National Naval Medical Center, Walter Reed Army Medical Center, Malcolm Grow USAF Medical Center, and Wilford Hall USAF Medical Center. These centers have large outpatient workloads and together have more than 3,000 teaching beds. The university complex and 15 affiliated teaching hospitals provide student study areas, departmental laboratories, and academic support units such as an electron microscopy suite, a vivarium, and a library. The Learning Resource Center (LRC) has more than 100,000 volumes, including books, journals, slides, videotapes, and microcomputer programs. The LRC computer system is linked into the university system and is also available for off-site use. Many local information sources are available, including the Library of Congress and the National Library of Medicine.

Grading Procedures

Letter grades are given for most classes, although a few classes are pass/fail. The student promotions committee determines if a student is eligible for promotion. Students must take and pass Parts I and II of the NBME in order to graduate. Part I is usually taken at the end of the second year and Part II in the fourth year.

Application Procedures

The School of Medicine participates in the American Medical College Application Service (AMCAS). Applications may be submitted beginning June 15. All required credentials must be received by AMCAS by November 1. It is advisable to apply during the summer months. Applicants must have taken the MCAT within three years of matriculation. The test must be taken by the fall of the year prior to planned enrollment. When the basic application materials have been received from AMCAS, the admissions office will send supplementary application materials to eligible applicants. Supplemental credentials include a personal statement, a passport-style photograph, and a premedical committee letter. If the applicant cannot provide a premedical committee letter, three individual academic recommendations from persons unrelated to the applicant are required. Letters of recommendation are extremely important in the selection process. Well-qualified applicants will be interviewed. Prior to admission, all interviewed entrants to the School of Medicine will be investigated by the National Agency Check Center of the Defense Investigative Service. The school does not participate in the AAMC Uniform Acceptance Dates program or the early decision plan.

Contact

Office of Admissions
Uniformed Services University of the Health Sciences
4301 Jones Bridge Road
Room A1041
Bethesda, Maryland 20814-4799
(301) 295-3101 (Collect calls accepted)

UNIVERSITY OF UTAH SCHOOL OF MEDICINE

308 Park Building
Salt Lake City, Utah 84112
(801)581-6436

Accreditation	LCME
Degrees Offered	M.D., M.S., Ph.D.
# Students Applied	532
Enrollment	100 / class
Mean GPA	3.6
% Men / % Women	Not Available
% Minorities	Not Available
Tuition	$4,896 In-State
	$10,953 Out-of-State
Application Fee	$25
Application Deadline	October 15

The University

A four-year, state-assisted educational institution for men and women, the University of Utah Health Sciences Center includes the University of Utah Hospital, the College of Pharmacy, the College of Nursing and Health, and the Spencer S. Eccles Health Sciences Library. The University of Utah Medical Center serves as a major research and training center of the six-state Intermountain region. Beside the 1,500-acre university campus, the School of Medicine is situated overlooking the Wasatch mountain range. At the heart of the Salt Lake City area a progressive population of almost 900,000 enjoys easy access to the alpine forests, the red-rock deserts, and a variety of spectacular sports and performing arts. The Utah Symphony, Dance Theater, Mormon Tabernacle Choir, and professional hockey and basketball are located within the city. In addition to the city's resources, the university is less than a day's drive from seven national parks.

Admissions

All applicants are required to take the Medical College Admissions Test (MCAT). Scores must be no more than four years old upon application. Contracts with Wyoming and Idaho reserve 13 percent of out-of-state admissions. The majority of students come from Utah.

Undergraduate Preparation

Before entrance into the School of Medicine, a completion of four years of college work is desired. The following coursework is mandatory: one year of English composition, two years of chemistry, one year of physics, and work in biology, the humanities, and social science.

Student Body

Because of its state assistance the School of Medicine accepts mostly Utah residents. Over 75 percent of the student body comes from within the state.

Placement Records

Most students find residency with one of the school's affiliated medical institutions. Of the many institutions is the Howard Hughes Medical Institute on the Health Sciences Center campus, which employs an investigative staff of eight and a research team of 100.

Costs

Tuition for the 1990 entering class is $4,896 for residents and $10,953 for nonresidents. Activity, computer, and acceptance fees are $450. Freshmen and sophomores must rent or purchase their own microscopes.

Financial Aid

The School of Medicine offers assistance through Perkins Loans, Stafford Loans, and the Health Professions Student Loan Program. A limited number of scholarships are awarded each year. Students are advised to contact the university financial aid office or consider an Armed Forces Duty Program for unconstrained support.

Minority Programs

The office of minority affairs is open for counseling and student assistance. Applications from minority students or black, Mexican American/Chicano, and American Indian persuasions are encouraged.

Student Organizations

A Student Advisory Committee (SAC) acts to organize the student body as a government with a constitution and executive commitment. In addition, several prominent organizations are in operation including the American Medical Student Association, the American Medical Women's Association, the Medical Student Section-American Medical Association, and the Western Student Med-Res. Comm.

Faculty

The clinical program of the School of Medicine is directed by a nationally recognized faculty. The full- and part-time staff totals over 800 professional members.

Curriculum

The first two years emphasize the areas of anatomic, biochemical, genetic, and microbiological study. Further study incorporates the principles of basic medicine. Pathophysiological processes, clinical manifestations, and treatment are also covered. The third year stresses the integration of basic science knowledge with acquisition of clinical diagnostic and problem-solving skills. Clinical clerkships are undertaken during the third year. The fourth year curriculum is entirely elective.

Facilities

The 372-bed University Hospital connects the School of Medicine classrooms with the laboratories and rehabilitation center. A great deal of training takes place at the nearby Veterans Administration Medical Center or the affiliated institutions including the Primary Children's Medical Center. The Spencer S. Eccles Health Sciences Library accommodates 300 patrons at various stations which include computer and media services, videotape players and slide and film projector carrels. The library is a resource for the Midcontinental Regional Medical Library Program.

Grading Procedures

The School of Medicine utilizes a pass/fail grading system. Numerical and narrative evaluations are presented during clinical clerkships, however, the transcript grade will be P or F.

Special Programs

Ten students are admitted each year to the Regional Dental Education Program. This extends dental education opportunities to Utah residents.

Application Procedures

The School of Medicine participates in the American Medical College Application Service (AMCAS). Applications accompanied by official transcripts should be filed no later than October 15. Supplementary application materials are due no later than December 15. Included with the supplementary materials should be letters of recommendation, a biographical sketch, a premedical course listing, and the $25 application fee. The dean's office will notify those eligible candidates about interview appointments.

Contact

Public Relations Office
University of Utah
308 Park Building
Salt Lake City, Utah 84112
(801) 581-7498

VANDERBILT UNIVERSITY SCHOOL OF MEDICINE

Nashville, Tennessee 37232-0685
(615) 322-2164

Accreditation	LCME
Degrees Offered	M.D., M.D./Ph.D.
# Students Applied	3,215
Enrollment	97 / class
Mean GPA	3.6
% Men / % Women	61% / 39%
% Minorities	Not Available
Tuition	$14,580
Application Fee	$50
Application Deadline	November 1

The University

Vanderbilt University was founded in the reconstruction period following the Civil War, and medical education has been part of the university's tradition since its inception. Today, Vanderbilt is a private university system consisting of 10 schools and a diverse student body of about 8,600 from all over the country. It is located about one-and-a-half miles from Nashville's downtown business district

The university issued its first medical diplomas in 1875. Today, the School of Medicine admits 100 students each year and has a threefold mission of education, research, and patient care. The school seeks to educate physicians at all levels of their professional experience: medical school; postgraduate education, including basic science and clinical experience; and continuing education in both formal and informal settings.

Nashville, the state capital, has a population of about 500,000. The city is located in the rapidly growing sunbelt region of the country and offers a wealth of professional, cultural, and recreational opportunities.

Admissions

The School of Medicine seeks students with a strong education in both the sciences and the liberal arts. Preferred candidates hold bachelor's degrees. The MCAT is required in order to predict success in preclinical coursework.

The school prefers candidates who have demonstrated academic excellence, leadership qualities, concern for others, and have participated in research and other extracurricular activities. Candidates must possess sufficient intellectual ability, emotional stability, and sensory and motor function. The applicant's essay, letters of recommendation, and the results of the personal interview are important factors in the admissions process.

Undergraduate Preparation

The following coursework is required for admission: eight semester hours of biology (with lab); a minimum of eight semester hours each of organic and inorganic chemistry (with lab; organic chemistry must cover aliphatic and aromatic compounds); six semester hours of English; and eight semester hours of physics emphasizing quantitative lab work. A broad liberal arts background is encouraged, especially post-introductory experience in the humanities, the arts, the social and behavioral sciences, and English.

Costs

Tuition for the 1990-91 academic year is $14,580. Student activity/recreation fees total $186 per year, and microscope fees for the first and second years total $100 per year. Student health insurance costs approximately $490 per year. The total annual expense for a medical student is estimated to be about $25,000.

Financial Aid

Both scholarships and loans are available through the university. They are based on demonstrated financial need and continued satisfactory academic progress. These types of aid, however, are considered supplementary to government and other sources of aid, which are considered the primary sources of financial assistance.

Financial aid to individual students usually comes from a combination of sources. Numerous scholarships (including honors scholarships) and revolving loans are available. Government assistance includes the Stafford Student Loan Program, the Health Education Assistance Loan Program, Supplemental Loans to Students, and other sources.

Applications for financial aid are sent to incoming first-year students in January, or, if invited after that date, along with the offer of admission to the School of Medicine.

Summer research fellowships offer stipends of $2,000 to $3,500, depending on experience.

Curriculum

The curriculum is divided into required courses and elective courses. Required courses constitute the basic medical sciences, including biochemistry, gross anatomy, physiology, cell and tissue biology, radiology, pharmacology, and psychiatry. Electives in the first year include courses on alcohol and drug abuse, human sexuality, medical ethics, and cancer biology The second year introduces the student to diagnosis, history taking, and physical examination.

The student's elective curriculum is developed to meet individual needs with the assistance of the faculty and approval of the associate dean for students or a designee. Electives include lecture or seminar series; specialty clinics, clinical clerkships,

or research experience at Vanderbilt or other approved institutions; and, in special circumstances, undergraduate or graduate courses elsewhere in the university.

Required ward clerkships are scheduled primarily during the third year. The fourth-year medical student takes seven academic units in clinical selectives and electives, including one ambulatory and two inpatient selective clerkships.

Facilities

The School of Medicine is part of the Vanderbilt University Medical Center, which also includes a school of nursing and the 661-bed Vanderbilt University Hospital. Other facilities include the Newman Clinical Research Center, the Cooperative Care Center, the Vanderbilt Child and Adolescent Psychiatric Hospital, the Vanderbilt Clinic, and the Stallworth Rehabilitation Center, and the Kim Dayani Human Performance Center. Also part of the school is the Center for Health Services, founded in 1971 to encourage and pursue improvements in health care, primarily in underserved communities.

The Medical Center Library holds more than 155,000 volumes. About two-thirds of these are bound periodicals, and about 2,000 periodicals and serial publications are currently received. The library provides a wide range of services, including MEDLINE. Students also have access to the Jean and Alexander Heard Library.

Grading Procedures

A letter grading system is used to evaluate student performance, except for electives in the first and second years, which are graded on a pass/fail basis.

Special Programs

The combined M.D./Ph.D. program is designed to develop investigators and teachers in the clinical and basic medical sciences. Students in the program have the opportunity to study a basic biomedical science in depth and to do research in some aspect of that subject while pursuing studies that lead to the M.D. degree. The program generally takes six to seven years to complete.

Application Procedures

The School of Medicine participates in AMCAS. The school evaluates the AMCAS application and sends a second application to candidates who have been reviewed favorably. AMCAS applications should be submitted between June 15 and November 1 prior to an anticipated fall semester enrollment date.

Contact

Office of the Associate Dean for Students
Vanderbilt University School of Medicine
203 Rudolph A. Light Hall
Vanderbilt University
Nashville, Tennessee 37232-0685
(615) 322-2145

UNIVERSITY OF VERMONT COLLEGE OF MEDICINE

Burlington, Vermont 05405
(802) 656-3390

Accreditation	LCME
Degrees Offered	M.D., M.D./Ph.D.
# Students Applied	2,728
Enrollment	93 / class
Mean GPA	3.3
% Men / % Women	52% / 48%
% Minorities	Not Available
Tuition	$10,150 In-State
	$21,700 Out-of-State
Application Fee	$50
Application Deadline	October 31

The University

Located in Burlington, Vermont, on the eastern shore of Lake Champlain, the University of Vermont has a total enrollment of approximately 10,000. The College of Medicine was established in 1822 and is the seventh oldest medical school in the nation. Today the College of Medicine graduates nearly 100 medical students every year and serves the health care needs of more than 400,000 residents of Vermont, upstate New York, and northern New Hampshire.

Admissions

The average GPA of successful applicants to the College of Medicine is 3.2 with MCAT scores averaging approximately 8.9 on each section. Admissions preference is given to residents of Vermont. Also, due to an agreement between the two states, a number of positions in each entering medical school class at the University of Vermont are reserved for students from Maine.

Undergraduate Preparation

While only a minimum of three years of undergraduate study must be completed before a student is eligible to apply to the College of Medicine, a baccalaureate degree is preferred. No particular major is required to apply to the medical school. One year each of biology, physics, general chemistry, and organic chemistry, all with laboratory, is required. Other recommended subjects for study include literature, mathematics, behavioral sciences, history, philosophy, and the arts. Above

all, an applicant's college record must demonstrate intellectual drive, independent thinking, curiosity, and discipline.

Student Body

Although the College of Medicine is part of a larger, state-sponsored university, approximately half of all medical students come from states other than Vermont. Of the 1989 entering class, 50 students were men and 43 were women. Thirty-five percent of the class was over the age of 25, and 63 percent of all medical students were "non-traditional" students, who took one to 14 years between graduating from college and entering medical school. Thirty-two percent of this group of students did their undergraduate work in the humanities or social/behavioral sciences, with the rest completing science majors.

Costs

For the academic year 1990-91 tuition for residents of Vermont was $10,150. Maine residents participating in the exchange program were charged $9,010. For out-of-state students, tuition was $21,700. Other costs include $380 in university fees, $600 for books and equipment, approximately $5,700 for housing, $2,800 for food, $1,680 for transportation, and another $2,500 for personal and miscellaneous expenses.

Financial Aid

The College of Medicine office of financial aid assists students in planning and financing the cost of a medical education. Financial awards are made on the basis of need as determined by the College Scholarship Service. Primary responsibility for meeting educational expenses at the College of Medicine rests with the student and his or her family, with the university considered as a supplemental source only. Available forms of aid include the Stafford Loan, the Perkins Loan, the Health Profession Student Loan, the Health Education Assistance Loan, and military service commitment scholarships.

Faculty

The College of Medicine presently has a total of 925 faculty members with 126 in the basic science areas and 799 in the clinical sciences. Currently, 209 of the clinical faculty have full-time appointments, while 590 are part-time faculty who maintain active practices.

Curriculum

The curriculum at the College of Medicine is divided into three main components which span the course of four years. The first section, the basic science core, covers the first one-and-one-half years of medical education. During this time students are instructed in the basic science subjects, including anatomy, biochemistry, medical microbiology, pathology, pharmacology, physiology, neuroscience, medical sexuality, and human behavior. The second phase of the curriculum is the clinical core. During this year students study and train in the clinical sciences of medicine, surgery, obstetrics and gynecology, pediatrics, and psychiatry under the supervision of house staff and attending physicians at the Medical Center Hospital of Vermont in Burlington as well as the Maine Medical Center in Portland, Maine, and the Champion Valley Physician's Hospital in nearby Plattsburgh, New York. Finally, students spend another one-and-one-half years in the Senior Selective Program. During this time students complete 16 months of clinical rotations, some of which are required and some of which are electives.

Facilities

The Medical Center Hospital of Vermont is the main clinical teaching facility of the College of Medicine. With 484 beds and 38 bassinets, this hospital is immediately responsible for the health care needs of the greater Burlington area and is a referral center for all of Vermont, upstate New York, and northern New Hampshire. The Medical Center was renovated in 1985. These redevelopments added 13 modern operating suites, and state-of-the-art medical, surgical, and neonatal intensive care units as well as emergency, radiology, and cardiology departments. Also, due to affiliation programs, medical students may opt to pursue a portion of their clinical training at either Maine Medical Center in Portland, Maine, or Champlain Valley Physician's Hospital in Plattsburgh, New York. The Charles A. Dana Medical Library subscribes to more than 1,650 journals and has a collection of approximately 86,000 volumes in the areas of biomedicine, nursing, and allied health. The audiovisual department maintains a collection of over 3,500 media titles in several different formats and provides facilities for their use.

Grading Procedures

Students at the College of Medicine are evaluated on an honors/pass/fail grading system. In clinical courses, this is combined with narrative evaluations from instructors evaluating the students' performance at the termination of each clinical rotation. Students are able to review and discuss these evaluations with faculty members as well as evaluate their courses and instructors.

Special Programs

Students interested in pursuing careers that combine basic science research and clinical care are able to pursue an integrated curriculum leading to both the M.D. and Ph.D. degrees. Normally this course of study lasts six years and is available in the departments of anatomy and neurobiology, biochemistry, medical microbiology, pathology, pharmacology, and physiology and biophysics. Students electing this option must be accepted separately by both the Graduate College and College of Medicine.

Application Procedures

Applicants must first submit an application form to AMCAS between June 15 and the end of October of the year prior to desired entrance into medical school. Once the College of Medicine receives this information from AMCAS, the college conducts a preliminary screening. Selected applicants will be required to submit a supplementary application and letters of recommendation along with a nonrefundable $50 application fee. At this point, another screening process takes place after which certain students will be invited to personal interviews on campus in Burlington. Final admissions will be made from this pool of interviewed applicants. The College of Medicine encourages students to apply as early as possible.

Contact

Office of Admissions
University of Vermont
College of Medicine
Burlington, Vermont 05405
(802) 656-2154

UNIVERSITY OF VIRGINIA SCHOOL OF MEDICINE

Charlottesville, Virginia 22908
(804) 924-5118

Accreditation	LCME
Degrees Offered	M.D., M.D./Ph.D.
# Students Applied	2,750
Enrollment	139 / class
Mean GPA	3.53
% Men / % Women	56% / 44%
% Minorities	Not Available
Tuition	$6,928 In-State
	$14,728 Out-of-State
Application Fee	$50
Application Deadline	November 15

The University

The University of Virginia was founded in 1819 by Thomas Jefferson. In 1825, the university enrolled its first 68 students. Today, the university enrolls well over 17,000 students and its campus covers more than 1,000 acres.

A survey conducted by *U.S. News & World Report* placed the University of Virginia 21st among the nation's universities, and in 1988 rated it first among the country's public institutions. The education editor of the *New York Times* rated the university as the nation's best public university and one of the three best overall.

The medical school was one of the eight original schools of the university. The four-year curriculum was established in 1900.

Settled in the 18th century, Charlottesville is located 120 miles from Washington, D.C., and 70 miles from Richmond. Among its historic sites are the homes of Thomas Jefferson, James Madison, and James Monroe. Downtown Charlottesville features a pedestrian mall with fine dining, distinctive shops, and night spots. The city and Albemarle County have a combined population of 115,000.

Admissions

The school seeks a diverse and talented student body. Admissions personnel seek those candidates who they believe will make the most significant contributions to society as members of the medical profession. Factors considered in the selection process include academic ability as reflected in the undergraduate transcript, MCAT score, and characteristics such as career goals, cultural background, ethnic and economic status, moral qualities, commitment to community service, and location of applicant's permanent residence.

Undergraduate Preparation

Preference in admissions is given to those students who, by the time of registration, will have received the bachelor's degree from an approved college of arts and sciences or an accredited institute of technology. Required undergraduate coursework is as follows: one year each of biology, general chemistry, organic chemistry, and physics, all with labs.

Costs

For 1990-91, Virginia residents pay $6,928 in annual tuition and fees. Nonresidents pay $14,728 in tuition and fees. The medical school activities fee is $70 for all students. For single students, rent for university housing can cost from about $1,650 to $1,850 per session. Books and instruments can cost about $1,100 for the first year, but these costs decrease considerably in subsequent years.

Financial Aid

The medical school helps qualified students obtain financial assistance from school-administered scholarships and loans; loans from federally regulated Stafford Loan, Supplemental Loan, and Health Education Assistance Loan programs; and minority student scholarships provided by the National Medical Fellowship Program.

Most financial aid is awarded on the basis of need. The school's scholarship and loan office determines need based on information supplied in the FAF. The office provides financial assistance information in January. The deadline for submitting applications for aid from the medical school's funds is March 1.

Minority Programs

The School of Medicine offers a six-week intensive medical academic advancement program each summer to encourage disadvantaged students to enter, remain in, and graduate from medical school. Level I is aimed at increasing acceptance rates into medical school; Level II is designed to help minorities remain in medical school.

Student Organizations

Medical student organizations include the Mulholland Society (the medical student body), the Mulholland Society Council (the medical student government), the Family Practice Club, the Spinal Chords singing group, Physicians for Social Responsibility, the Student Medical Society, and Share, an organization through which students offer volunteer services to the community. Medical students can also join the staff of the University of Virginia Medical Examiner. Fraternal and honorary societies include Alpha Omega Alpha, the Lychnos Society, and Omicron Delta Kappa.

Curriculum

The curriculum consists of preclinical sciences, clinical clerkships, and electives. The first two years introduce the student to the basic sciences that lead to an understanding of human biology, both its physical and psychological aspects. Normal body structure and function is emphasized during the first year. An introduction to physical examination, interviewing, and some clinical experience is also part of the first year. The second year emphasizes anatomical, physiological, and psychological deviations from normal structure and function. Among the second-year course topics are general principles of pathology, psychopathology, pharmacology, and physical diagnosis.

The third year consists of 12-week clerkships in a number of fields, including medicine and surgery, pediatrics, neurology, and obstetrics-gynecology. Emphasis is placed on prevention, diagnosis, and treatment, and integrating the basic sciences with clinical practice. The psychological factors that influence health are also emphasized during these clerkships. Teaching occurs in small tutorial seminars, lectures, and group discussion. Clerkships take place at the University of Virginia hospitals as well as several community-based hospitals.

The electives program in the fourth year provides the opportunity to pursue individual interests under the guidance of a faculty advisor. Students can choose clinical rotations, graduate courses, or research activities.

Facilities

The University of Virginia Hospital serves as one of the major acute-care referral institutions in central and western Virginia, providing care for almost 26,000 patients. Here, members of the teaching staff supervise all activities in the clinics where students learn methods of diagnosis and treatment. Other clinical facilities include Ambulatory Care Services, Kluge Children's Rehabilitation Center of the University of Virginia Hospital, the Surgical Oncology Clinic, and Blue Ridge Hospital.

Research facilities are located in the Medical School Building, Cobb Hall, Jordan Hall, and the Medical Education and Research Building and its annex. In total, over 240,000 square feet of space is dedicated to research in a variety of fields.

The Claude Moore Health Sciences Library maintains well-developed collections of books, journals, and audiovisuals. The library also houses numerous databases related to health care for easy citation retrieval. All basic services of the library are computerized for in-house and remote access.

Grading Procedures

Grades for preclinical courses and clinical clerkships are A (high honor), B (honor), C (passing), D (conditional), and F (failure). Plus or minus signs may be used with the letter grades at the discretion of the department that assigns the grade. Electives are graded as satisfactory or unsatisfactory. Students must take Parts I and II of the NBME; a passing score on Part II is necessary for graduation.

Special Programs

The Medical Scientist Training Program is designed for students wishing to pursue careers in teaching and research. In addition to the M.D., the program awards the Ph.D. in one of the biomedical sciences. The program is designed to be completed in six to seven years. Interested students must file a supplementary application with the office of interdisciplinary graduate studies.

Application Procedures

The School of Medicine participates in AMCAS. Applications may be submitted to AMCAS until November 15 of the year prior to enrollment. All applicants are required to pay a $50 application fee. Students are notified of acceptance on a rolling basis; early application is encouraged. All applicants must take the MCAT.

Selected individuals are asked to participate in a personal interview. Every student accepted to a place in the entering class must pay a $100 deposit, which is credited toward tuition.

Contact

Director of Admissions
University of Virginia
School of Medicine
Box 235
Charlottesville, Virginia 22908
(804) 924-5571

VIRGINIA COMMONWEALTH UNIVERSITY MEDICAL COLLEGE OF VIRGINIA SCHOOL OF MEDICINE

Richmond, Virginia 23298-0565
(804) 786-9788

Accreditation	LCME
Degrees Offered	M.D., M.S./M.D., M.D./Ph.D., M.P.H.
# Students Applied	2,688
Enrollment	168 / class
Mean GPA	3.21
% Men / % Women	70% / 30%
% Minorities	Not Available
Tuition	$6,600 In-State
	$14,500 Out-of-State
Application Fee	$50
Application Deadline	December 1

The University

Virginia Commonwealth University (VCU) is a public research university supported by the state. Founded in 1838, VCU today is Virginia's largest public urban university. It has a total enrollment of 20,000 students studying on two campuses in Richmond.

The Medical College of Virginia (MCV) comprises six professional schools and the Medical College of Virginia Hospitals, which together make up the fourth largest health care teaching complex in the country. The college, originally founded in 1838 as Hampdyn-Sydney College, today hosts some 3,500 students, interns, residents, and postdoctoral fellows studying the health sciences. MCV also hosts a comprehensive cancer treatment center and extensive research facilities where faculty conduct investigative projects funded at more than $63 million annually.

The MCV campus is near downtown Richmond in central Virginia. Richmond is a historic, cosmopolitan city located near the Atlantic seashore, the Appalachian Mountains, and Washington, D.C.

Admissions

The school reviews academic achievement as represented by the academic record, MCAT scores, evaluations, and the results of interviews. The character and personality of the applicant are also considered. Applicants may be admitted on the basis of 90 semester hours of outstanding achievement, but the majority of students admitted have completed their bachelor's degrees at the time of entrance. Priority is given to Virginia residents.

Undergraduate Preparation

The following undergraduate coursework is required for admission: two semesters of English, two semesters of mathematics, eight semester hours of biology, eight of general chemistry, eight of physics, and six of organic chemistry. Outside of these requirements, students are encouraged to pursue an undergraduate course of study according to their individual intellectual interests.

Student Body

The 1990 class totaled 168 students. The majority of students majored in the sciences with 34 percent concentrated in the arts or humanities. Eighty-two percent were from Virginia. The overall undergraduate GPA was 3.21 with an MCAT average score of 9.

Costs

Tuition is $6,600 per year for state residents and $14,500 for nonresidents. There is a university fee of $575 per year and a student health fee of $114 per year.

Financial Aid

The university assists students in obtaining grants, loans, and work-study opportunities. Grants and loans are available based on financial need. All students are eligible for work-study assistance.

Financial need is determined through the FAF. Applicants who are not Virginia residents are encouraged to inquire about state grant funds from their state of residence.

Minority Programs

Applicants from minorities underrepresented in the health sciences are encouraged to contact the Office of Health Careers Opportunity Program.

Student Organizations

The Student Body Organization on the MCV campus operates through the Student Government Association. Honor societies on campus include Phi Kappa Phi, Alpha Sigma Chi, and Sigma Zeta.

Faculty

The School of Medicine faculty consists of 169 basic scientists, 596 geographic full-time clinicians, including affiliates, assisted by 611 interns and residents, and 31 part-time and 714 volunteer clinical faculty.

Curriculum

During the first year, normal human structure, function, growth, and development are emphasized. Courses include cell biology, biochemistry, cellular physiology, and genetics. The second year stresses the abnormal aspects of human functioning and structure. During this time the student is introduced to neuroscience, pathogenesis, and clinical skills. Some electives are offered during these years.

The third year consists of clinical education and training. Rotating clerkships include internal medicine, surgery, pediatrics, and community practice. The fourth year consists of one-third required clinical education and training and two-thirds electives taken at MCV and at other approved medical schools elsewhere in the U.S. and abroad. Students are encouraged to consult with faculty members during the fourth year to develop a course of study that meets their individual needs.

Facilities

The Medical College of Virginia Hospitals is one of the largest university-owned teaching hospital complexes in the nation, with a 1,058-bed capacity. The hospitals serve the Richmond metropolitan area and operate an extensive array of general and subspecialty clinics in which nearly 160,000 patient visits occur annually.

Also part of MCV is the Massey Cancer Center, a basic and clinical cancer research center and health care provider. The center houses a bone marrow transplantation research facility and a human tissue acquisition and histopathology laboratory.

The Virginia Center on Aging, established in 1978, is a state-wide resource for aging-related research, education, service, training, and technical assistance.

The James Branch Cabell Library houses more than 610,000 volumes and over 6,100 journal titles. The Tompkins-McCaw Library houses more than 247,000 volumes and over 3,400 journals. Both libraries provide on-line catalogs. There are also three learning resource centers housing nonprint materials—tapes, microscopes, filmstrips, and similar study aids.

Grading Procedures

Students are graded on an honors/high pass/pass/marginal/ fail basis.

Special Programs

The M.D./Ph.D. program prepares students for careers in academic medicine or medical research. Applicants must be accepted to both the MCV School of Medicine and the School of Basic Health Sciences.

Application Procedures

The School of Medicine participates in AMCAS. Applications must be filed between June 15 and December 1 of the year preceding intended enrollment. Applicants who are screened for further consideration are asked to submit supplemental information along with a nonrefundable $50 application fee. Supplemental information must be submitted to the school by January 15 of the year preceding intended enrollment.

The school participates in the early decision plan. This plan permits an applicant to file a single application through AMCAS between June 15 and August 1.

The MCAT should be taken no later than the fall of the year of application.

Contact

Admissions Office
Virginia Commonwealth University
Medical College of Virginia
School of Medicine
Richmond, Virginia 23298-0565
(804) 786-9630

UNIVERSITY OF WASHINGTON SCHOOL OF MEDICINE

Seattle, Washington 98195
(206) 543-1515

Accreditation	LCME
Degrees Offered	M.D., M.D./Ph.D.
# Students Applied	512
Enrollment	165 / class
Mean GPA	3.53
% Men / % Women	59% / 41%
% Minorities	5%
Tuition	$4,926 In-State
	$12,513 Out-of-State
Application Fee	$25
Application Deadline	November 1

The University

The University of Washington School of Medicine was founded in 1945, and is the only medical school directly serving the states of Washington, Alaska, Montana, and Idaho (WAMI). The WAMI program, which began in 1971, provides a decentralized medical education and offers a broad range of educational opportunities. The states participating in the program share resources and responsibilities in the regional educational program. Through the program, basic science training and clinical training is offered in sites throughout the four states.

Admissions

Preference is given to legal residents of Washington, Alaska, Montana, and Idaho. Out-of-region minority students will be considered. A limited number of exceptionally well-qualified nonresident candidates will also be considered. Residents of foreign countries and those who have failed to meet minimum standards in another medical or dental school will not be considered. Candidates for admission are evaluated on the basis of academic performance, motivation, maturity, personal integrity, and demonstrated humanitarian qualities. Extenuating circumstances in an applicant's background are evaluated as they relate to these selection factors. Students selected for admission for the class of 1994 had a mean GPA of 3.53 and the following mean MCAT scores: biology, 10.6; chemistry, 10.2; physics, 10.2; science problems, 10.4; reading, 9.6; and quantitative, 9.5. Ninety-nine to 100 percent of entrants in recent years have earned bachelor's degrees. Transfer students will be considered for admission only in exceptional cases. Transfer applicants should correspond directly with the office of admissions.

Undergraduate Preparation

At least three years of coursework at an accredited college or university is required prior to matriculation. Nearly all successful applicants, however, have completed a bachelor's degree before enrollment in the School of Medicine.

The following premedical course requirements must be completed before matriculation (or, preferably, by the time of application): chemistry, 12 semester hours (includes any combination of inorganic, organic, biochemistry, or molecular biology courses); physics, four semester hours; biology, eight semester hours; and eight semester hours of other "open" science subjects, which can be fulfilled by taking other courses in any of the above three categories.

Under exceptional circumstances, certain course requirements may be waived for individuals who present unusual achievements and academic promise. Applicants should be proficient in the use of the English language and basic mathematics, and should also have a basic understanding of personal computing and information technologies, as well as some knowledge of health care delivery systems. The admissions committee does not prefer any specific major, but each candidate should demonstrate academic achievement in their major field.

Costs

Tuition costs are subject to change. Resident tuition amounts to $4,926 a year. Nonresident tuition is $12,513 per year. The average annual cost for books, supplies, equipment, and examination fees is $1,749.

Financial Aid

Financial aid is available from a variety of federal, state, and private offices. Applicants for aid must complete the needs analysis form from the College Scholarship Service. Application forms for financial aid may be obtained from the School of Medicine office of student financial aid. To be eligible for full financial aid, a student must submit the FAF on time regardless of whether he or she has been accepted to the schools listed. Special sources of financial aid are available to disadvantaged and minority students. Students are discouraged from taking outside employment.

Minority Programs

The minority affairs program offers information and assistance to minority students interested in pursuing a medical career through a six-week summer enrichment program conducted at the universities of Washington, Utah, North Dakota, Nevada-Reno, and California-Davis. Students accepted to the school may participate in a pre-enrollment summer program designed to teach useful skills and provide exposure to the medical curriculum. The minority affairs program also serves as a source of academic and nonacademic information and provides referrals to tutoring, counseling, and other area resources.

Faculty

There are more than 1,000 full-time faculty members at the School of Medicine.

Curriculum

The basic curriculum of the first two years (six quarters) consists of three phases (groups of courses) in the human biology series: pre-organ system courses in the sciences basic to medicine; organ systems taught by basic scientists and clinicians; and introduction to clinical medicine and health care. The introduction to clinical medicine course is taken throughout all six quarters. During these first six quarters, students will usually be able to take additional elective courses. Students who are residents of Alaska, Montana, and Idaho are expected to spend their first year of study at the university site in their particular state.

The clinical curriculum of the third and fourth years consists of prescribed clerkships to be completed by all students, a clinical selective series requiring at least 20 credits in three clinical areas (family medicine, rehabilitation medicine/chronic care, and emergency care/trauma), and a minimum of 28 credits of clinical clerkships elected by the student. Through the case-study method, students work as junior members of a medical care team headed by a faculty clinician.

In order to graduate, students must fulfill the independent study in medical science requirement. This planned program should include investigation in the basic medical science disciplines studied and results in a written paper acceptable to the student's advisor and faculty committee supervising this phase of the curriculum. The school also offers a medical student research training program to medical students interested in gaining valuable experience from training in medical research, and a voluntary medical thesis program.

Facilities

The school is located in the Warren G. Manguson Health Sciences Center, which provides educational opportunities for students from all schools and colleges within the University of Washington. Through the WAMI program, residents of Alaska, Montana, and Idaho receive part of their basic science education in their home-state institutions (the University of Alaska, Montana State University, or the University of Idaho). Clerkships are completed at the University of Washington and its affiliated hospitals, as well as in community clinical units located in the four-state region.

Grading Procedures

An honors/satisfactory/not satisfactory grading system is used. All students are required to pass Parts I and II of the National Board Examination in order to graduate.

Special Programs

The Medical Scientist Training Program (MSTP), which allows certain well-qualified students to obtain a combined M.D./Ph.D., is not restricted to residents of Washington, Alaska, Montana, and Idaho. Eight medical scientist trainees are admitted per year. Candidates are interviewed by a single MSTP committee for acceptance to both the School of Medicine and the Graduate School. The program is usually completed in seven years. An application for the program is mailed with an acknowledgement of the receipt of application materials. Applicants for the program should submit supplementary materials as soon as possible. For further information, contact the Medical Scientist Training Program, C516 Health Sciences, SM-30, Seattle, Washington 98195 (206) 543-4188.

Application Procedures

The university participates in the American Medical College Application Service (AMCAS). Applications must be submitted to AMCAS by November 1. Qualified applicants will then be asked to submit a $25 application fee and supplemental application materials, including a 300-word autobiographical statement, a premedical committee letter of recommendation, and a supplemental application form.

The MCAT is required and should be taken no later than the fall of the year prior to planned enrollment. Scores more than three years old will not be considered. The admissions committee may consider GRE scores during the application process (under exceptional circumstances). However, the applicant will be required to take the MCAT prior to matriculation.

Contact
Office of Admissions, SM-22
University of Washington
School of Medicine
Seattle, Washington 98195
(206) 543-7212

WASHINGTON UNIVERSITY SCHOOL OF MEDICINE

660 South Euclid Avenue
St. Louis, Missouri 63110
(314) 362-6830

Accreditation	LCME
Degrees Offered	M.D., M.A./M.D., M.D./ Ph.D.
# Students Applied	3,544
Enrollment	121 / class
Mean GPA	3.66
% Men / % Women	73% / 27%
% Minorities	Not Available
Tuition	$14,900
Application Fee	$45
Application Deadline	November 15

The University

The St. Louis Medical College, an independent institution, was founded in 1842. In 1891, it became the medical department of Washington University. The Missouri Medical College also became part of Washington University in 1899. The School of Medicine has established itself as an important research center, and was recently designated as a Specialized Center of Research in Coronary and Vascular Diseases.

The Washington University Medical Center is located on the eastern edge of Forest Park in St. Louis. The Hilltop Campus of the University is located along the western edge of the park. A regularly scheduled shuttle bus brings the campuses within 10 minutes of each other.

St. Louis offers many varied cultural activities, including the rich local traditions in jazz, blues, and ragtime music, the St. Louis Symphony, the Fox Theater, and the Opera Theater of St. Louis.

Admissions

The committee on admissions evaluates an applicant's intellectual achievements and ability, personal character, motivation, and extracurricular work. Students accepted to a recent class had a mean overall GPA of 3.66, and a mean science GPA of 3.66.

Undergraduate Preparation

Applicants must have completed at least 90 semester hours of college courses at an approved college or university. Completion of at least one year of the following courses is required before enrollment (including necessary laboratory work): physics, biology, mathematics (through integral and differential calculus), inorganic chamistry, and organic chemistry. The admissions committee may waive one or more prerequisites. Applicants are encouraged to pursue their interests in the sciences, humanities, and social sciences.

Student Body

Students attending the School of Medicine are residents of more than 41 states and three foreign coutries. More than 93 percent of the applicants accepted to the school were accepted by one or more other U.S. medical schools.

Placement Records

Of the students participating in an earlier national residency matching program, 83 percent matched one of their top three choices; 63 percent matched their first choice.

Costs

Tuition costs and fees for residents and nonresidents amount to $14,900 per year. Books, supplies, and instruments for a first-year student cost approximately $1,355. On-campus room and board for a single student amounts to $5,395. The total cost for the first year of study is approximately $21,650.

Financial Aid

The office of financial aid assists students in making financial aid arrangements. Students accepted to the school may request an application for financial aid. The financial aid form (FAF) requires detailed information about the applicant's financial resources. First- and second-year students are urged not to accept employment. Some fourth-year students find employment in hospitals within the medical center. The personnel office provides assistance to spouses seeking employment.

Student Organizations

Student organizations on campus include the American Medical Student Association, the American Medical Women's Association, the Medical Student Section of the American Medical Association, the Missouri State Medical Association, and the Organization of Student Representatives in the Association of American Medical Colleges.

Faculty

The school employs approximately 940 full-time faculty members. The 1,021 part-time faculty members are physicians who practice their medical specialties in St. Louis and staff one or more of the four hospitals in the Washington University Medical Center.

Curriculum

The first year consists of the basic sciences, including medical genetics, neural science, biomedical statistics, and electives. The second year includes the study of disease and pathology, and introduction to clinical medicine. The third year consists of clinical clerkships. The fourth year elective program allows students to decide where their major interests lie, and to select the areas they wish to explore or study in depth.

Facilities

The Medical Center includes the School of Medicine, Barnes Hospital, Jewish Hospital, St. Louis Children's Hospital, Barnard Hospital, and the Central Institute for the Deaf. The clinical departments of the School of Medicine are located on the west side of the Medical Center, next to the hospital and patient areas; the preclinical departments are located on the eastern side. The main preclinical teaching facility is the McDonnell medical sciences building, which includes research laboratories and classroom space. The newest research facility at the Medical Center is the 10-story clinical sciences research building, which houses research laboratories for the clinical departments, the Howard Hughes Institute, and modern animal care facilities.

Students take clinical training at the Barnard, Barnes, Jewish, and St. Louis Children's Hospitals, which offer a total of 1,788 patient beds. Clinical training is also offered at the St. Louis Regional Medical Center and St. Louis Veterans Administration Hospitals, which are both served by full-time and part-time faculty members of the School of Medicine.

The Institute for Biomedical Computing is an interschool facility that spans computing research activities at the School of Medicine and the School of Engineering and Applied Science. Its primary location is at the School of Medicine. The medical school library maintains a comprehensive collection of over 217,000 volumes and subscribes to over 3,200 current journals. Students can access a variety of information sources, including the book and journal holdings of 34 libraries in the area and MEDLINE.

Grading Procedures

A pass/fail grading system is used for the first semester of the first year. Afterwards, an honors/high pass/pass/fail system

is used. Each student's performance is evaluated periodically by a faculty committee.

Special Programs

Students may apply to the M.A./M.D. program in their first, second, or third year of medical school. In the program, students spend one year working in the laboratory of the faculty member they have selected. The program requires submission of a thesis (publication-quality manuscript) at the end of the year. Students who qualify for the program receive a stipend for the extra year of study.

Students interested in careers in academic medicine may apply to the Medical Scientist Training Program, which offers a combined M.D./Ph.D. degree. The program accepts 20 students per year. All students involved in the program receive a stipend and tuition remission. Only those students who have spent an equivalent of at least one semester in a research laboratory should apply for the program.

Application Procedures

The school participates in the American Medical College Application Service (AMCAS). The AMCAS application is distributed by the AMCAS and preprofessional advisors. Applications should be received by AMCAS from June 15 to November 15 of the year preceding planned enrollment. There is an application fee of $45. The MCAT is required. When the AMCAS application has been received, the school requests that applicants complete additional application materials. Interviews are arranged with selected applicants by the committee on admissions.

Eight to 12 transfer students are accepted each year to the third-year class. Transfer students who are enrolled in good standing in their current U.S. medical school and who have a cogent reason for requesting transfer will be considered. Transfer candidates must submit their applications by November 1 of the year preceding enrollment. Inquiries should be directed to the Third Year Class Transfer Program, Washington University School of Medicine, 600 South Euclid Avenue-Campus Box 8077, St. Louis, Missouri 63110.

Applicants who do not hold U.S. permanent residence visa status will be considered for admission, but before the school may issue a visa, an international student must document that the necessary funds are available to pay the costs of the student's education.

Contact

Office of Admissions
Washington University
School of Medicine
660 South Euclid Avenue #8107
St. Louis, Missouri 63110
(314) 362-6857

WAYNE STATE UNIVERSITY SCHOOL OF MEDICINE

540 East Canfield
Detroit, Michigan 48201
(313) 577-2424

Accreditation	LCME
Degrees Offered	M.D., Ph.D., M.S., M.D./Ph.D.
# Students Applied	1,954
Enrollment	264 / class
Mean GPA	3.35
% Men / % Women	70% / 30%
% Minorities	21%
Tuition	$7,286 In-State
	$14,517 Out-of-State
Application Fee	$25
Application Deadline	November 1

The University

Wayne State University School of Medicine was founded in 1868 and is conveniently located in the north-central area of Detroit. The Detroit Medical Center (DMC), with which the medical school is closely affiliated, is the largest of its kind in the United States, and comprises six health care institutions on 110 acres. The medical school's close partnership with the medical center provides the advantages of a comprehensive clinical education and a practicing faculty.

The university, in the heart of Detroit's cultural center, is within walking distance to the Detroit Institute of Arts—the country's fifth largest art museum, with more than 100 galleries. The institute also offers cultural programs in various other arts. Also near to the campus are the Detroit Science Center, the Children's Museum, the International Institute, the Renaissance Center (with more than 100 shops and eateries), and the riverfront Hart Plaza, which holds weekend ethnic festivals. A public minibus connects the main and medical campuses with each other and outlying areas of the city.

Admissions

Applicants are judged on the basis of grade point average, MCAT scores, three college recommendations, an interview rating, extracurricular activities, and work. The mean GPA for the 1989 freshman class was 3.35. Qualification to apply

through the early decision program includes a GPA of at least 3.5 and MCAT scores of 9 or higher on each subtest. Fifteen percent of the places in the incoming class are filled by early decision program applicants.

Undergraduate Preparation

Undergraduate academic requirements for admission include eight semester hours of English, 12 semester hours of general biology or zoology with lab, and eight semester hours each of inorganic chemistry, organic chemistry, and general physics, with their respective labs. In addition to a foundation in science, the medical school stresses the importance of a liberal arts background. The baccalaureate degree is usually required, but exceptional third-year students may be considered for admission.

Student Body

The medical school enrolls 256 freshmen each year, about 86 percent of whom are Michigan residents. Foreign students are considered if they have completed at least two years of undergraduate education at a United States or Canadian college and have a permanent visa. There are over 1,000 medical students in the school. About 30 percent are women and more than 21 percent are minority students.

Placement Records

Seventy percent of the graduates choose residency programs in Michigan hospitals, and half of them stay in Detroit. Over 50 percent of the graduates enter a primary care field, and a large number start practices in Detroit.

Costs

Annual tuition is $7,286 for Michigan residents and $14,517 for nonresidents. Students may elect to pay tuition in regularly scheduled payments over a 10-month period through a deferred payment plan. The additional cost for books, supplies, equipment, microscope rental, and living expenses is about $9,885 for the first year. The university has limited on-campus housing for graduate, professional, and handicapped students. Medical school students are responsible for finding their own living quarters.

Financial Aid

Students desiring to apply for financial aid must file a copy of the Financial Aid Form (FAF) with the College Scholarship Service. Based on need determined by the FAF, a student may be eligible for a Guaranteed Student Loan (GSL) of up to $7,500 per year. School administered loans include the Perkins Loan and Health Professions Loans. Other need-based aid from the medical school includes college work-study, Grant-in-Aid for Michigan residents, and medical school scholarships and loans. Armed Forces Health Professions Scholarships are also available.

Minority Programs

Minority students whose ethnic group is underrepresented in medicine may be eligible for grant assistance from National Medical Fellowships, Inc. Candidates from areas where there are not enough physicians receive special consideration.

Student Organizations

The student organizations office has guides, maps, and information to aid students in their search for housing. A self-instruction center makes all lectures and audio-visual material available to students for individual study. Students may join the student senate, the Association of Women Medical Students, the Black Medical Association, the Family Practice Club, and various nonmedical interest groups.

Curriculum

The first year of the medical curriculum consists of an overview of the normal workings of the human body. Studies include anatomy, biochemistry, physiology, histology, and embryology. Second-year studies concentrate on pathology, immunology, microbiology, pharmacology, and pathophysiology in order to understand diseases and their treatments. Intensive clinical instruction begins in the third year with a series of clerkships in internal medicine, surgery, gynecology/obstetrics, pediatrics, psychiatry, family medicine, opthalmology, and otolaryngology. During the fourth year, which is divided into eight clinical elective periods, students may choose from over 200 electives in 23 disciplines.

Facilities

All campus facilities currently in use were built within the last 20 years. The Shiffman Medical Library contains more than 150,000 volumes. The Kresge Eye Institute of Wayne State University, a major center for research and treatment of eye diseases, is part of the Detroit Medical Center. The Wayne State University Comprehensive Sickle Cell Center is one of 10 national centers that research sickle cell anemia and its treatment.

Special Programs

The medical school offers graduate training programs for those interested in research and teaching careers. Individuals may earn the Ph.D., M.S., or combined M.D./Ph.D. degrees in the areas of anatomy, biochemistry, immunology/microbiology, pathology, pharmacology, and physiology. The M.S. degree program is offered by the audiology, psychiatry, and radiology departments. A nine-month post-baccalaureate program prepares applicants who have not been admitted to the School of Medicine but show academic promise. The program consists of premedical science courses, study skill training, personal adjustment counseling and development, academic tutoring, and an introduction to the first-year medical school curriculum. Acceptance into the medical school is contingent on successful performance in the program.

Application Procedures

Applications must be sent through the American Medical College Application Service (AMCAS). Students should apply by November 1 and take the MCAT during the year that they apply, preferably in the spring. The selection process is done via rolling admissions, so candidates are advised to apply 12 to 15 months prior to the entrance date. Those who apply through the early decision program must do so between June 15 and August 1 before the year that they will enroll, and may not apply to any other schools during this time. Students who are accepted under this program are obliged to attend Wayne State University, and students who are not accepted are considered with the pool of regular applicants. Only candidates who are being seriously considered by the admissions committee are asked for letters of recommendation and an interview. Early decision applicants will be notified by October 1. All other selections are made by March 1.

Contact

Admissions Office
Wayne State University
School of Medicine
1310 Scott Hall
540 East Canfield
Detroit, Michigan 48201
(313) 577-1466

WEST VIRGINIA UNIVERSITY SCHOOL OF MEDICINE

Health Sciences Center
Morgantown, West Virginia 26506
(304) 293-4511

Accreditation	LCME
Degrees Offered	M.D., M.D./Ph.D.
# Students Applied	1,276
Enrollment	83 / class
Mean GPA	3.47
% Men / % Women	62% / 38%
% Minorities	Not Available
Tuition	$5,455 In-State
	$9,865 Out-of-State
Application Fee	$30
Application Deadline	November 1

The University

The West Virginia School of Medicine, established in 1902, was affiliated with the College of Physicians and Surgeons of Baltimore. In 1912, the school began giving instruction in the first two years of basic sciences. In 1960, the University Hospital opened, and the four-year curriculum began. In 1972, the Charleston Area Medical Center was affiliated with the university and became the West Virginia University Health Sciences Center, Charleston Division. The Wheeling Division of the Health Sciences Center was established in 1974.

Morgantown has a population of 45,000, and offers many recreational activities. It is within traveling distance of Pittsburgh, Baltimore, and Washington, D.C.

Admissions

Preference is given to residents, although outstanding nonresidents are considered. Applicants who have been suspended from the West Virginia University School of Medicine or other medical schools can be admitted only in very exceptional cases. The admissions committee evaluates academic performance, course load, letters of recommendation, MCAT scores, motivation, interpersonal skills, and the personal interview.

Undergraduate Preparation

A total of 90 credit hours (not including physical education or ROTC) is required for admission. Completion of the following courses is also required: eight semester hours each of biology, general chemistry, organic chemistry, and physics, all with labs; six semester hours of English composition and rhetoric; and six semester hours of social and behavioral sciences. College mathematics (including calculus) and a solid background in biology are recommended.

Student Body

Ninety percent of the 1990 entering class was from West Virginia. The mean overall GPA was 3.47. Thirty-eight percent of the class are women. Ninety percent majored in the sciences.

Placement Records

Graudates of the School of Medicine practice in communities throughout the state, more than half in underserved areas.

Costs

Tuition for residents is $5,455 and for nonresidents, $9,865.

Financial Aid

Financial aid is available from a variety of federal, state, and private offices. Grants, scholarships, and loans are granted on the basis of need and/or academic performances.

Minority Programs

The Health Careers Opportunity Program offers special classes, individual tutoring, and other support for minority and economically or socially disadvantaged students.

Faculty

There are approximately 360 faculty members.

Curriculum

The first year consists of basic science classes. Certain students are selected during their first year to spend their third and fourth years at the Charleston Division of WVU Health Sciences Center. There is an introduction to clinical medicine course during the second year, in addition to basic science classes and courses in the behavioral sciences and genetics. The third year consists of required clinical clerkships which give students a foundation in history taking, examination, patient relations, laboratory aids, diagnosis, treatment, and the use of medical literature. During the fourth year, each student works with an advisor to select the program best suited to his/her goals. Most students choose a broad selection of clinical rotations. Twenty-four weeks of the fourth year must be spent in the intramural program at the Morgantown campus or at the Charleston division campus.

Facilities

Facilities at the Health Sciences Center include the Ruby Memorial Hospital, built in the 1980s, which offers equipment such as magnetic resonance imagery, spectroscopy, lithotripsy, and laser surgery; the Mary Babb Randolph Center, devoted to cancer research, treatment, and education; the Ambulatory Care Center; and Chestnut Ridge Hospital, which deals with psychiatric and behavioral problems. A 70-bed rehabilitation center is planned. One-third of students complete their M.D. program at the Health Sciences Center, Charleston Division.

Grading Procedures

Classes are graded as honors (H), satisfactory (S), or unsatisfactory (U). The committee on academic standards determines the promotion and dismissal rules. Part I of the NBME exam is usually taken at the end of the second year. Part II is usually taken in September of the fourth year. Part II must be passed in order to graduate.

Special Programs

An M.D./Ph.D. program is available. The Ph.D. can be earned in biochemistry, microbiology, pharmacology, physiology, and the biomedical sciences.

Application Procedures

The school participates in the American Medical College Application Service (AMCAS). The deadline for filing an application is November 1. An applicant should be sure that recent MCAT scores, current transcripts, and three letters of recommendation are received on (or preferably before) the deadline. Applicants must have taken the MCAT within two years of applying. It is recommended that the MCAT be taken in the spring of the year before matriculation. There is an application fee of $30. Interviews are required for admission. All applicants who are residents of West Virginia are granted an interview. Qualified nonresidents are interviewed at the discretion of the admissions committee. Advanced standing positions are offered in very exceptional cases to students who can present certification of good standing from the LCME-accredited school he or she is attending.

Contact

Admissions and Records
West Virginia University
1170 Health Sciences North
Morgantown, West Virginia 26506
(304) 293-3521

UNIVERSITY OF WISCONSIN MEDICAL SCHOOL

1300 University Avenue
Madison, Wisconsin 53706
(608) 263-4910

Accreditation	LCME
Degrees Offered	M.D., M.D./Ph.D
# Students Applied	1,255
Enrollment	143 / class
Mean GPA	Not Available
% Men / % Women	62% / 38%
% Minorities	Not Available
Tuition	$9,700 In-State
	$14,200 Out-of-State
Application Fee	$20
Application Deadline	November 1

The University

The University of Wisconsin Medical School opened in 1907 as a two-year program. It became a traditional four-year program in 1924.

Admissions

Applicants are evaluated based on total GPA, science GPA, MCAT scores, difficulty of undergraduate course load, trend in academic performance, recommendations, extracurricular activities, personal accomplishments or disadvantages, and motivation. The approximate MCAT score for entering classes at UW is 10. The medical school considers the higher score from the two most recent exams. Wisconsin residents have the option of delaying matriculation for one year. A transfer program for qualified Wisconsin residents allows them to transfer from foreign medical schools and begin their third year at UW.

Undergraduate Preparation

An undergraduate science background is required for admission. The necessary science courses, with their respective labs, include one semester of general biology/zoology, one semester of advanced biology/zoology, and two semesters each of inorganic chemistry, organic chemistry, and general physics. There is a minimum math requirement of college algebra and trigonometry, and calculus is recommended. Courses in English composition, the humanities, and social sciences also weigh in a candidate's favor. Students with an outstanding record may be admitted after three years of undergraduate study.

Student Body

Wisconsin residents comprise 95 percent of each entering class. One hundred forty-three freshmen enrolled in UW Medical School in 1990. Out of a total number of 475 applicants, 222 were accepted. Thirty-eight percent of the class is female, and 72 percent of the class majored in biological or physical sciences.

Costs

Tuition is $9,700 for Wisconsin residents and $14,200 for nonresidents. Yearly costs for rent, food, transportation, health care, and other living expenses add up to about $6,460 per year.

Financial Aid

The ability of an applicant to pay for his/her medical education is not considered in the admission process. The major portion of total financial aid is available in the form of loans.

Minority Programs

UW Medical School's affirmative action program supports the recruitment of students whose ethnic groups are underrepresented in medicine. Students are also recruited from areas in Wisconsin that do not have enough physicians.

Curriculum

The curriculum provides early introduction to clinical experience, and up to 43 weeks of elective opportunities in the senior year. Also during the senior year, an eight-week preceptorship is available with physicians throughout Wisconsin.

Special Programs

The Medical Scholars Program (MSP) allows 50 Wisconsin high school seniors to pursue a liberal arts education at UW Madison as preparation for enrollment in the medical school. Students who are interested in careers in academic medicine or the biotechnology industry may apply to the UW Medical School M.D./Ph.D. program. Candidates must complete the graduate school application and may have to take the Graduate Record Exam (GRE). Students may also enter the program after the second year of medical school or after one or two years of graduate work. Financial support via stipend or full tuition remission is available to highly qualified applicants.

Application Procedures

Students must take the MCAT within four years of the year they plan to enroll and no later than the fall before enrollment. Applications accompanied by a transcript must first be filed through AMCAS by November 1. Upon receiving a candidate's AMCAS application, the Medical School sends a UW supplemental application. This application requires the candidates to write an essay and submit three academic letters plus one nonacademic letter of recommendation. A premedicine committee letter in addition to one academic letter may substitute for three academic letters. The supplemental application requires a $20 fee and must be received by January 15.

Contact

Admissions Committee
University of Wisconsin Medical School
Medical Sciences Center, Room 1205
1300 University Avenue
Madison, Wisconsin 53706
(608) 263-4925

WRIGHT STATE UNIVERSITY SCHOOL OF MEDICINE

Dayton, Ohio 45435
(513) 873-2933

Accreditation	LCME
Degrees Offered	M.D.
# Students Applied	1,304
Enrollment	91 / class
Mean GPA	3.3
% Men / % Women	48% / 52%
% Minorities	Not Available
Tuition	$7,035 In-State
	$9,960 Out-of-State
Application Fee	$25
Application Deadline	November 15

The University

Wright State University is a state-assisted institution, established in 1964. The university is a nationwide leader in making its campus facilities accessible to the handicapped.

Wright State University School of Medicine was established in 1974. Its four-year M.D. curriculum emphasizes primary care.

The university is located in Dayton, Ohio, in the state's Miami Valley area. The 557-acre campus includes a biological preserve. The city is known for its picturesque scenery and is also home to a variety of cultural and recreational attractions, including over 35,000 acres of parks, nature preserves, and golf courses. Museums, such as the United States Air Force Museum, ballet, theater, and art offer diversions to students.

Admissions

The school seeks a student body of diverse social, ethnic, and educational backgrounds. The admissions committee evaluates the student's academic load and undergraduate curriculum, GPA, extracurricular activities, MCAT scores, and work experience. Other important factors in the evaluation process are evidence of intellectual ability, maturity, motivation, ability to interact with others, dedication to human concerns, ability to learn independently, and potential for service.

Undergraduate Preparation

Ninety semester hours of preparation at an approved college or university in the U.S. or Canada is required for admittance. Most who are admitted have earned the bachelor's degree.

Prerequisite courses must include one year each of the following: biology, general chemistry, organic chemistry, physics, mathematics, and English. A broad background in the humanities is important.

It is recommended that applicants take the MCAT no later than the fall of the year in which the application is filed.

Placement Records

Over 65 percent of Wright State graduates receive their first or second choice of residency programs. Students are accepted into some of the most highly competitive residency programs in the country. In recent years, about 70 percent of the school's graduates have entered into family practice, internal medicine, and pediatric disciplines. The rest have entered a clinical specialty of their choosing.

Costs

Tuition for the 1992 entering class is $7,035 for residents and $9,960 for nonresidents. Student fees are $864.

Financial Aid

About 90 percent of the student body receives financial aid in the form of scholarships, grants, loans, and work-study opportunities. Financial aid eligibility is assessed by analyzing the student's financial resources. The school's financial aid office provides counseling in securing financial resources and managing debts.

Faculty

The School of Medicine has about 200 full-time faculty members, as well as about 1,000 practicing clinicians and researchers who volunteer their time and expertise.

Curriculum

The school offers a four-year curriculum with courses taken in 23 academic departments. Students receive a primary-care orientation in a community setting, with direct patient contact throughout all four years of the program.

The first two years introduce the student to the normal and abnormal conditions and functions of the human body at all levels of organization, from molecular and cellular levels through organ systems. Students can also explore medical topics from contemporary clinical perspectives through a wide variety of elective courses. Students study medical ethics and participate in community service projects.

In the third and fourth years, students rotate through clerkships in all the major clinical fields, providing the opportunity for students to participate on a medical team with faculty preceptors. Students run rounds, obtain patient histories, perform physical examinations, evaluate laboratory results, learn diagnostic procedures, and assist in developing treatment plans. During the fourth year, students can choose from over 150 electives.

Facilities

A variety of practice settings are available to students through the school's affiliates. Seven major affiliates are home for the medical school's clinical departments, providing classrooms, teaching laboratories, and research facilities.

The Fordham Health Sciences Library houses a comprehensive selection of reference materials, periodicals, audio-visual aids, and an extensive collection of computer software, while also providing access to the resources of an area consortium of 12 libraries and the National Library of Medicine's Regional Network.

Special Programs

Wright State University School of Medicine offers the only civilian aerospace medicine residency program in the country.

Application Procedures

The School of Medicine participates in AMCAS. Applicants must submit applications to AMCAS by November 15. Applications will be forwarded to the School of Medicine, which will request additional information from applicants, including letters of recommendation from a premedical advisory committee or three science faculty members. These supplementary materials must be submitted no later than January 15. Interviews are granted by invitation of the school's admissions committee.

Contact

Wright State University
School of Medicine
PO Box 1751
Dayton, Ohio 45401
(513) 873-2934

YALE UNIVERSITY SCHOOL OF MEDICINE

367 Cedar Street
New Haven, Connecticut 06510
(203) 785-4672

Accreditation	LCME
Degrees Offered	M.D., M.D./Ph.D., M.D./ M.P.H., M.D./J.D., M.D./ M.Div.
# Students Applied	2,219
Enrollment	Not Available
Mean GPA	Not Available
% Men / % Women	68% / 32%
% Minorities	Not Available
Tuition	$16,950
Application Fee	$50
Application Deadline	November 1

The University

The School of Medicine was established in 1810 when the Connecticut General Assembly passed a bill granting a charter for "The Medical Institution at Yale College." The Yale-New Haven Medical Center consists of the School of Medicine, the School of Nursing, and the Yale-New Haven Hospital.

Admissions

The committee on admissions evaluates an applicant's academic record, MCAT scores, record of activities and accomplishments, recommendations from premedical committees and individual science teachers, and personal interviews. Foreign students must have completed at least one year of study in an American college or university prior to application. Transfer students are only accepted in the second- or third-year class.

Undergraduate Preparation

Applicants must have completed at least three years at an approved college or institute of technology, although a baccalaureate degree is recommended. Six to eight semester hours of the following courses are required for admission: general biology or zoology, general chemistry, organic chemistry, and general physics, all with lab.

The admissions committee has no preference for a college major, but requires that a student be prepared to cope with chemistry and biology at a graduate level. Students who receive advanced placement credits for required courses are encouraged to substitute advanced science courses for those courses.

Student Body

Of the class of 1990, approximately 32 percent of the students were women. Students come from all areas of the country, as well as from foreign countries, although approximately 50 percent of the students attending the medical school are from the northeastern United States.

Costs

Tuition for the 1992 entering class is $16,950. Student fees total approximately $385.

Financial Aid

Financial aid is available from the School of Medicine, as well as from a variety of federal, state, and private offices. The amount of aid a student is eligible to receive is calculated by the Graduate and Professional School Financial Aid Service (GAPSFAS). The School of Medicine discourages extracurricular work.

Minority Programs

The school makes an effort to ensure that women and members of all minority groups are adequately represented in the student body. Applicants invited for interview have the opportunity to meet with minority students and faculty.

Curriculum

In order to graduate, a student must submit an approved dissertation based on original investigation, by March of the year of graduation. The student is encouraged to design his or her own research project and to select the faculty member with whom the work will be done.

The first three semesters consist of the basic sciences, as well as courses in biostatistics, epidemiology, public health, behavioral sciences, and the history of medicine. In addition, three hours a week will be devoted to clinical correlations. During the fourth semester, a major course, introduction to clinical medicine is offered, which includes history taking, clinical examination, laboratory medicine, pathophysiology, and mechanisms of disease. The final two years consist of the intensive study of clinical medicine. Students have clinical rotations in medicine, surgery, pediatrics, psychiatry, obstetrics and gynecology, and neuroscience. In addition, the student will spend time in a required ambulatory care experience, and participate in a variety of basic science and clinical electives.

Facilities

Facilities for clinical instruction and experience in patient care are provided by the Yale-New Haven Hospital as well as other area hospitals, including the Veterans Administration Medical Center in West Haven, the Connecticut Mental Health Center, and Bridgeport Hospital.

The Yale Medical Library's collections are among the country's largest, containing over 360,000 volumes. Over 2,500 current journals are received regularly.

Grading Procedures

Students are evaluated by faculty members, although no grades are given, and rank order is not established. The final decision of acceptable performance rests with the chairman of the department of the designated director of the course. Students must pass Part I and Part II of the NBME in order to graduate.

Special Programs

The Medical Scientist Training Program is a combined M.D./Ph.D. program for students who wish to obtain a research degree. The program requires at least six years of registration. An M.D./M.P.H. (master of public health) program is also available. Special arrangements may be made with the appropriate associate deans to receive an M.D./J.D. (doctor of jurisprudence) degree, or an M.D./M.Div. (master of divinity) degree.

Application Procedures

Application forms will be available on or after June 1, and should be submitted by November 1 of the year prior to planned matriculation. Applicants seeking admission under the early decision plan must submit their applications by August 1. Applications should also include complete official transcripts, and an evaluation from the premedical advisory committee (or individual letters from three of the applicant's teachers, two of whom should be in science). There is an application fee of $50. The MCAT is required. Scores should be sent directly to the school. Selected students will be invited for interviews with the committee on admissions.

Contact

Office of Admissions
Yale University
School of Medicine
Edward S. Harkness Hall
367 Cedar Street
New Haven, Connecticut 06510
(203) 785-2643

CANADIAN MEDICAL SCHOOLS AT A GLANCE

School	Accreditation	Degrees Offered	# Students Applied	Enrollment
University of Alberta Faculty of Medicine	LCME, CACMS	M.D., M.S., Ph.D.	814	118 / class
University of British Columbia Faculty of Medicine	LCME, CACMS	M.D., M.D./Ph.D.	571	120 / class
University of Calgary Faculty of Medicine	LCME, CACMS	M.D.	875	72 / class
Dalhousie University Faculty of Medicine	LCME, CACMS	M.D., M.D./Ph.D.	*	350
Université Laval Faculty of Medicine	LCME, CACMS	M.D.	1,785	140 / class
University of Manitoba Faculty of Medicine	LCME, CACMS	M.D.	191	82 / class
McGill University Faculty of Medicine	LCME	M.D.	1,339	149 / class
McMaster University Faculty of Health Science	LCME, CACMS	M.D.	2,068	400
Memorial University of Newfoundland Faculty of Medicine	LCME, CACMS	M.D., B.MS./M.D.	576	56 / class
University of Montreal Faculty of Medicine	LCME, CACMS	M.D., M.D./M.S., J.D., M.D./Ph.D.	1,974	170 / class
University of Ottawa School of Medicine	LCME, CACMS	M.D.	2,109	84 / class
Queen's University Faculty of Medicine	LCME	M.D.	2,162	72 / class
University of Saskatchewan College of Medicine	LCME, CACMS	M.D., B.S.	373	60 / class
University of Sherbrooke Faculty of Medicine	LCME, CACMS	M.D., M.S., Ph.D.	1,763	102 / class
University of Toronto Faculty of Medicine	LCME, CACMS	M.D., M.D./Ph.D.	2,300	250 / class
University of Western Ontario Faculty of Medicine	LCME, CACMS	M.D., M.D./Ph.D., M.D./M.S.	2,211	105 / class

* Not Available   ** Not Applicable   C/S – Contact School   I/P – In-Province   O/P – Out-of-Province

Mean GPA	% Male / % Female	% Minorities	In-State Tuition	Out-of-State Tuition	Application Fee	Application Deadline
8.0	64% / 36%	*	$2,047	$2,944	$30	November 1
3.0	55% / 45%	*	$2,900	$7,250	$50 I/P $75 O/P	January 15
3.62	63% / 37%	*	$2,336	$3,504	$25	November 30
*	*	*	$2,200	$3,900	$20	November 15
*	*	*	$1,644	$7,390	$15	February 1 Non-Canadian March 1 - Canadian
3.84	64% / 36%	*	$2,581	**	$35	November 15
3.7	*	*	$1,176	$5,800	$25	November 15 I/P February 1 O/P
2.5	30% / 70%	*	$3,169	$12,641	$50	November 1
*	*	*	$1,344	**	$25	December 15
*	42% / 58%	*	$1,198	$5,800	$15	March 1
3.2	*	*	$2,255	$9,975	$50	November 1
*	*	*	$2,083	$9,157	$50	November 1
*	*	*	$2,247	**	$25 I/P $50 O/P	January 15 I/P December 1 O/P
*	65% / 35%	*	$2,355	$8,700	$15	March 1
3.4	67% / 33%	*	$2,367	$10,072	$50	November 1
*	*	*	$2,157	**	$50	November 1

* Not Available   ** Not Applicable   C/S – Contact School   I/P – In-Province   O/P – Out-of-Province

UNIVERSITY OF ALBERTA FACULTY OF MEDICINE

Edmonton, Alberta
Canada T6G 2R7
(403) 492-6350

Accreditation	LCME, CACMS
Degrees Offered	M.D., M.S., Ph.D.
# Students Applied	814
Enrollment	118 / class
Mean GPA	8.0 on a 9.0 scale
% Men / % Women	64% / 36%
% Minorities	Not Available
Tuition	$2,047 – Canadian residents
	$2,944 – Nonresidents
Application Fee	$30
Application Deadline	November 1

The University

Founded in 1908, the University of Alberta represents Canada's third largest university campus. It is the oldest and largest university in the Province of Alberta. The university, located in Edmonton, Alberta's capital city, offers a full range of undergraduate- and graduate-level degrees, as well as professional programs in medicine, dentistry, law, and library science.

The Faculty of Medicine was established in 1913 and enrolled its first class of 26 students in 1914. The three-year program was expanded to a full M.D. program in the 1920s, and the first M.D. degrees were granted to the graduating class of 1925. With the graduating class of 1990, over 4,100 M.D.s have earned their degrees from the Faculty of Medicine.

Edmonton, with a population of about 700,000, is a cosmopolitan city known for sports, a rich cultural life, and its proximity to the Canadian Rockies.

Admissions

Factors considered in the evaluation process include the GPA from the best two full years of study, the GPA from prerequisite courses (see below), MCAT scores, results of the interview, letters of reference, and autobiographical essay ratings. The majority of class seats are reserved for residents of Alberta. Personal qualities are also important in the admissions process.

Undergraduate Preparation

Candidates for admission must have taken full-year courses or two single-term courses of the following: inorganic chemistry, organic chemistry, physics, biology, and English (English language proficiency is essential). In addition, a course in statistics is required. To be considered for admission, students must have achieved an average of 7.0 (Alberta residents) or 7.5 (nonresidents) on the University of Alberta 9.0 scale, in two full years of study. It is recommended that students complete the baccalaureate degree prior to admission.

Student Body

The Faculty of Medicine admits 118 new students each year.

Costs

Costs are in Canadian dollars.

For the 1989 first-year class, tuition was $2,047 for Canadian students and $2,944 for non-Canadians. Student fees were estimated at $225.

Financial Aid

Loans are available under the Canada Student Loan Plan or the Province of Alberta Loan Plan to Canadian citizens or permanent residents who have been in Canada and in Alberta for 12 months prior to the beginning of the academic term.

Minority Programs

The Faculty of Medicine has a special policy with regard to the admission of aboriginal candidates. The faculty may provide up to two positions over the regular quota of 118 for the M.D. program. Aboriginal students will be subject to normal minimum admission requirements and approval by the admissions committee.

Curriculum

The four-year program is divided into three phases. Phase I (first year) covers the basic sciences but also introduces the student to community medicine, medical ethics, nutrition, and basic clinical skills. Phase II (second year) covers the mechanisms of disease and allows more time in clinical settings. Phase III (third and fourth years) consists of 52 weeks of required rotations and a minimum of 10 weeks of electives. Rotation subjects include medicine, obstetrics and gynecology, surgery, and family medicine and geriatrics. There are opportunities for students to pursue research ranging from short summer programs to the M.D./Ph.D. program.

Facilities

The Walter C. Mackenzie Health Sciences Centre, completed in 1984, comprises the main hospital complex and a host of other facilities and student services. The John W. Scott Health Sciences Library houses a collection of 64,000 books and more than 4,000 periodicals, as well as a reference section including major medical indices. The computer search systems available include DIALOG, BRS, and MEDLINE.

Grading Procedures

Grades are assigned on the nine-point scale commonly used in Canadian post-secondary institutions.

Special Programs

Master's degrees and Ph.D.s are granted by the departments of anatomy, biochemistry, physiology, pharmacology, and surgery. The faculty offers a master's program and a post-graduate diploma in health services administration. The Ph.D. in medical sciences program is a special offering to honors students with the desire and motivation to pursue a research career. Candidates can choose from a variety of fields, including applied sciences in medicine, pathology, medical microbiology, pediatrics, and psychiatry. Coursework is tailored for the individual candidate and guided by a supervisor.

Application Procedures

The University of Alberta Faculty of Medicine has its own application form that must be filled out and submitted to the faculty's admissions officer no later than November 1 of the year prior to the year of intended admittance. MCAT results should also be submitted directly to the admissions officer (the MCAT must have been taken during the last two years and at the latest, in the autumn prior to admission). There is a nonrefundable $30 application fee. Qualified applicants will be invited for a personal interview. Letters of reference and a personal essay are also required. Upon acceptance, students must send a $50 deposit, which is applied toward tuition.

Contact

Admissions Officer
University of Alberta
Faculty of Medicine
2J2-11 Mackenzie Health Science Centre
Edmonton, Alberta T6G 2R7
Canada
(403) 492-6350

UNIVERSITY OF BRITISH COLUMBIA FACULTY OF MEDICINE

317-2194 Health Sciences Mall
Vancouver, British Columbia
Canada V6T 1W5
(604) 228-4482

Accreditation	LCME, CACMS
Degrees Offered	M.D., M.D./Ph.D.
# Students Applied	571
Enrollment	120 / class
Mean GPA	3.0
% Men / % Women	55% / 45%
% Minorities	Not Available
Tuition	$2,900 – Canadian residents
	$7,250 – Nonresidents
Application Fee	$50 In-Province, $75 Out-of-Province
Application Deadline	January 15

The University

Founded in 1950, the Faculty of Medicine at the University of British Columbia is the only medical school in the province. The goal of the faculty is to offer a stimulating and challenging curriculum that permits all students to acquire basic knowledge and skills suitable to proceed to further training in a variety of professional roles.

Admissions

Admissions preference is given to qualified students from British Columbia, although there are occasional openings for students from other provinces or countries. The minimum acceptable academic standing for admission is an overall average of 70 percent or the equivalent. The MCAT is also required and must be taken no later than the fall prior to the year in which matriculation in medical school is anticipated.

Undergraduate Preparation

A minimum of three years' work must be completed at an undergraduate institution before an applicant is eligible for admission to the Faculty of Medicine. Specific prerequisites include: one semester of English literature and composition; two semesters of college mathematics, through calculus; one semester of physics; two semesters of biology; one semester of chemistry; and one semester of biochemistry. There is no particular degree program or major required by the Faculty of Medicine.

Student Body

Most of the students in the Faculty of Medicine are residents of British Columbia.

Costs

Tuition for the 1990 first-year class was $2,900 for Canadian residents and $7,250 for nonresidents. Books and other academic supplies cost approximately $3,000 per year.

Financial Aid

The University of British Columbia offers numerous scholarships, prizes, and bursaries for which medical students may apply. Scholarships are awarded on the basis of academic achievement while bursaries are given on the basis of financial need. For information and application forms students may contact the awards office.

Curriculum

In the first year students are instructed in the basic medical sciences, taking correlated courses in anatomy, biochemistry, and physiology. Also during this time students are introduced to the basics of patient care through a course in family practice and a course in clinical skills. During the second year students take courses in pharmacology, pathology, medical microbiology, psychiatry, and medical genetics. The neurological sciences are also presented in the second year. The third year focuses on more in-depth clinical study and students are required to pursue electives in the clinical sciences. The fourth year is a clinical clerkship during which time students develop a working knowledge of medicine by studying at a number of affiliated clinical sites.

Facilities

The University of British Columbia Health Sciences Centre Hospital is a 600-bed facility located on campus that serves as the major clinical teaching facility for the Faculty of Medicine. The Woodward Biomedical Library houses on-campus library facilities including medical reference sections and study areas. There are also branch locations of the library at each of the major clinical teaching sites.

Grading Procedures

The Faculty of Medicine evaluates student performance as follows: 60 percent is the minimum passing mark; first class, 80 percent or more; second class, 65 to 79 percent; pass 60 to 64 percent.

Special Programs

A combined M.D./Ph.D. program is available to highly qualified students who are considering academic careers in the biomedical sciences. This course of study takes six or seven years to complete. To be eligible for application, a student must have completed his or her undergraduate work with first class honours or the equivalent academic distinction. Applicants to this program must be accepted separately into both the Faculty of Medicine and a Ph.D. program sponsored by the department of medicine in the Faculty of Graduate Studies. During the first three years of this program, the student will take all the courses required of the first year of medical study as well as complete all the required seminars, directed readings, and thesis work required for the Ph.D. Upon completion of this work, the student will be allowed to register for the second year of medical study and continue working toward the M.D.

Application Procedures

Applications are available from the Faculty of Medicine between August 15 and December 31 of the year prior to desired entrance into medical school, and all applications must be completed no later than the following January 15. An application fee of $50 is required as is a $25 surcharge for applicants from Canadian provinces other than British Columbia or from other countries. Students are required to submit transcripts of all undergraduate work, MCAT scores, and three letters of recommendation or evaluation. Selected applicants will be required to attend on-campus personal interviews and all final admissions decisions will be made by early July at the latest.

Contact

The University of British Columbia
Faculty of Medicine
2194 Health Sciences Mall
Vancouver, B.C. V6T 1W5
Canada

UNIVERSITY OF CALGARY FACULTY OF MEDICINE

3330 Hospital Drive NW
Calgary, Alberta
Canada T2N 4N1
(403) 220-6849

Accreditation	LCME, CACMS
Degrees Offered	M.D.
# Students Applied	875
Enrollment	72 / class
Mean GPA	3.62
% Men / % Women	63% / 37%
% Minorities	Not Available
Tuition	$2,336 – Canadian residents
	$3,504 – Nonresidents
Application Fee	$25
Application Deadline	November 30

The University

The University of Calgary campus is located in the northwest section of Calgary. The university began in 1945, and the Faculty of Medicine accepted its first students in the fall of 1970. Since 1972, facilities have been located at the Calgary Health Sciences Centre.

Admissions

Seventy-two positions are available for students entering the Faculty of Medicine. Preference is given to residents of Alberta, although applications from residents of other provinces are invited. For the class of '93, the mean GPA was 3.62 and the mean MCAT score was 10.1.

Undergraduate Preparation

Two years of university-level study are required for admission. No formal premedical program is required, but it is recommended that students take a full university course in general chemistry, organic chemistry, biochemistry, psychology (or sociology or anthropology), English, general biology, mammalian physiology or comparative physiology, calculus, and physics.

Student Body

The class of '93 was 63 percent male and 37 percent female. Out of 72 students, 55 were Albertans, 16 non-Albertans, and one was an international student. The mean age was 24.8.

Costs

For a single student living away from home, total expenses are expected to be about $7,500 per year, not including tuition, fees, books, and supplies. Books and supplies should cost about $1,585 for the first year and $1,040 for the second and the third years. For Canadian residents, tuition is $2,336 per year. Nonresidents pay $3,504 per year. (Canadian dollars)

Financial Aid

Both Province of Alberta and Canada Student Loan plans are available. Maintenance grants are available for special-needs groups such as single parents and disabled persons. Other sources of financial aid, such as bursaries and other funds, are also available.

Student Organizations

All medical students are automatic members of the Calgary Medical Students' Association. Students may also act as representatives on major faculty committees such as the curriculum committee and the admissions committee.

Curriculum

The introductory course deals with basic concepts essential to understanding human structure, function, and growth. The clinical skills course runs parallel to body system courses and continuity courses over the first two years. The third curricular course is the independent study program. Beginning in the first year, four hours each week are dedicated to the elective program, which allows students to gain practical experience applying the principles of problem solving, and to explore areas of individual interest in depth. In the third year, students engage in a clinical clerkship. After the three-year program, students elect one of three pathways: family practice, other specialties, or medical scientist.

Facilities

The health sciences library has 1,583 serials and 110,065 books and periodicals on hand. The Faculty uses the University of Calgary Medical Clinic, and takes advantage of the facilities of the Foothills Hospital, Calgary General Hospital, Alberta Children's Hospital, Holy Cross Hospital, and Rockview Hospital. The Bacs Medical Learning Resource Centre houses 12 areas, each of which contain audiovisual aids, anatomical models, reference books, computer-assisted learning programs, and more. The building also has a radiology museum, career room, and physical examination room.

Grading Procedures

Student performance is evaluated through the collection of data concerning each student's knowledge, skills, and behavior. The student may periodically obtain feedback on his or her performance, so that instructors may gain some measure of the efficacy of their teaching, and so the school may ascertain that its graduates are professionally competent in every respect.

Application Procedures

In order to apply, applicants must take the MCAT by the autumn before the term for which admission is sought. First, a preliminary application form including a list of courses taken and grades received, as well as MCAT scores, is used to screen applicants. This application must be received by November 30. A formal application is then mailed to candidates who pass the initial screening. This application is due by the first Friday in February, and must be accompanied by a $25 application fee, the names of three individuals writing letters of reference, an autobiographical narrative including employment history and extracurricular activities, and an essay. Candidates who pass this stage will be invited for an interview in March.

Contact

The University of Calgary
2500 University Drive Northwest
Calgary, Alberta T2N 4N1
Canada
(403) 220-6849

DALHOUSIE UNIVERSITY FACULTY OF MEDICINE

Halifax, Nova Scotia
Canada B3H 4H7
(902) 494-1874

Accreditation	LCME, CACMS
Degrees Offered	M.D., M.D./Ph.D.
# Students Applied	Not Available
Enrollment	350 / total school
Mean GPA	Not Available
% Men / % Women	Not Available
% Minorities	Not Available
Tuition	$2,200 – Canadian residents
	$3,900 – Nonresidents
Application Fee	$20
Application Deadline	November 15

The University

Dalhousie University enrolls 10,000 students from Canada

and from more than 60 other countries. The university, which has an international reputation in professional and graduate education, was founded in 1818 and is situated in a residential area of Halifax on the Atlantic coast of Canada.

Dalhousie began offering medical education 120 years ago. Today, Dalhousie's medical school is the central medical school of the Maritime provinces, graduating 84 M.D.s each year and providing medical care for the people of the region.

Halifax, one of Canada's most vital small cities, is known for its picturesque coastline, historic buildings, and modern entertainment, leisure, and shopping facilities. Medical students have easy access to many of the coastal region's major research centers and teaching hospitals.

Admissions

Of the 84 students admitted to each entering class, 76 are residents of the three Maritime provinces; eight seats are reserved for applicants from other parts of Canada and foreign countries. The decisions of the admissions committee are based on academic as well as nonacademic factors. Many of the school's students have had other careers and have decided to study medicine later in life.

Undergraduate Preparation

To be accepted for enrollment in the medical school, candidates must possess a bachelor's degree. The medical school faculty recognizes that preparation for medical school can be acquired through many academic avenues. The school seeks students who have had a broad education in the physical, life, and social sciences as well as the humanities.

All candidates for admission must take the MCAT.

Placement Records

Graduates of the medical school enter all areas of medicine—family practice, specialty medicine or surgery, laboratory medicine, and research.

Costs

All costs are in Canadian dollars.

Tuition for the 1990-91 academic year is $2,200 for residents of Canada. Non-Canadian students pay a differential fee of $1,700, for a total of $3,900. The student union fee is $92. Health insurance for foreign residents costs approximately $500 for single students (insurance costs for residents of Canada is minimal). The cost of books varies, but is estimated to total about $2,400 for all four years. Instruments for the first year cost approximately $650.

Financial Aid

All accepted students receive an application form for entrance scholarships and bursaries. Named scholarships, general entrance scholarships, and a number of bursaries are available. Financial aid is granted on the basis of need.

UNIVERSITY OF MANITOBA FACULTY OF MEDICINE

424 University Center
Winnipeg, Manitoba
Canada R3E 0WE
(204) 474-8815/8825

Accreditation	LCME, CACMS
Degrees Offered	M.D.
# Students Applied	191
Enrollment	82 / class
Mean GPA	3.84
% Men / % Women	64% / 36%
% Minorities	Not Available
Tuition	$2,581
Application Fee	$35
Application Deadline	November 15

The University

Set in the capital of Manitoba, the university enjoys its proximity to the beautiful Hudson Bay and Lakes Winnipeg and Manitoba. Winnipeg (pop. 584,842) is situated at the confluence of the Red and Assiniboine rivers. This great city is one of the largest wheat-marketing centers in the nation. The city is on the site of the French-built Fort Rouge (1738) and Fort Gibraltar, and grew as a center for prairie produce as a result of the opening of the railways. Outdoor winter and sporting activities, the parks, restaurants, and museums of this historic city offer ample opportunity for diversion and entertainment.

Admissions

The MCAT is required. Applicants seeking admissions for September of a given year must take the MCAT no later than the September of the year before. Preference is given to undergraduates and graduates of the Universities of Manitoba who are Canadian citizens. Applicants who are from the native populations of Canada, who are sponsored by faculty-approved agencies, who have completed the biomedical Ph.D., or who have an acceptable academic background are also given special consideration. In 1990, the mean GPA of those admitted was 3.84. The mean MCAT was 9.9, with a range of 8.2-13.8.

Undergraduate Preparation

Students must have graduated from a high school program that satisfies the department of education of the Province of Manitoba. If Canadian, students should have included 300-level mathematics, chemistry, physics, and English in their high school courses. In addition, students should have a bachelor's degree from a university recognized by the University of Manitoba. Applicants may be accepted who have completed their degrees in three regular academic sessions (30 semester hours each), with 24 hours minimum of credit in new courses in each session. Applicants with a regular B.A. or B.S. must complete six credit hours of English, plus one credit hour in the social sciences or humanities. In addition, the university expects six credit hours in the natural physical sciences. Students with honors degrees require fewer hours in social sciences, humanities, and natural and physical sciences.

Costs

All costs are in Canadian dollars.
Tuition for the 1990 year was $2,581. Student fees were $41.

Financial Aid

For information on financial aid, address all inquiries to Financial Aids & Awards, 422 University Centre (204) 474-9531.

Curriculum

During the first and second years there are 30 hours per week of formal instruction for 38 weeks. During the first year students will be introduced to normal human biology, integration of structure and function of organ systems, and disease. The second year is spent studying the clinical sciences and clinical skills. The third and fourth years are spent in clinical situations.

Facilities

Teaching hospitals includes the Health Sciences Centre, St. Boniface General Hospital, Deer Lodge Veterans Hospital, Grace Hospital, and Seven Oaks Hospital.

Grading Procedures

Students are graded on a pass/fail basis.

Application Procedures

The admissions office must receive applications no later than the end of the first week of January in the entry year. For the class of September 1992, the deadline is November 15, 1991. Applicants who qualify with GPAs and MCATs will be asked to submit an autobiographical essay of 800 words along with a recent photograph. The university then sends a standardized questionnaire to references named by the candidate. Each candidate is interviewed. A second interview may be requested. Applicants for advanced standing are considered only for entrance into the second year of medicine and must be in good academic standing at a medical school accredited by the LCME.

Contact
Admissions Office
The University of Manitoba
The Faculty of Medicine
424 University Centre
Winnipeg, Manitoba R3E 0WE
Canada
(204) 474-8815/8825

McGILL UNIVERSITY
FACULTY OF MEDICINE

3655 Drummond Street
Montreal, Quebec
Canada H3G 1Y6
(514) 398-3517

Accreditation	LCME
Degrees Offered	M.D.
# Students Applied	1,339
Enrollment	149 / class
Mean GPA	3.7
% Men / % Women	Not Available
% Minorities	Not Available
Tuition	$1,176 – Canadian residents
	$5,800 – Nonresidents
Application Fee	$25
Application Deadline	November 15 (Out-of-Province); February 1 (In-Province)

The University

The Faculty of Medicine was part of the original McGill University founded in 1829. Located in historic Montreal, students may enjoy the old city architecture, the parks (one of which was designed by Frederick Law Olmstead), and the charm of the historic colonial city.

Admissions

Applicants must take the MCAT. McGill selects students based upon achievement in the academic record, personal qualities (based on letters of references), interviews, and the MCAT. The mean GPA is 3.7.

Undergraduate Preparation

Students must be in the final year of undergraduate study or must have received their bachelor's degree. Students must be fluent in English, the language of instruction. Coursework should include six semester hours each (with lab) of general biology, general and organic chemistry, and physics. In addition, three hours each of cellular and molecular biology are required.

Student Body

The entering class for 1990 consisted of 149 students. Of these, 101 were from Quebec. Of the out-of-province students, 19 were U.S. citizens and seven from other foreign countries.

Costs

Tuition is $1,176 for Canadians and $5,800 for non-Canadians. Student fees amount to $650.

Financial Aid

Limited numbers of scholarships, bursaries, and loans are available to students in all years. Information is available from the student aid office.

Curriculum

The course of study lasts four years and consists of five academic periods. The first two periods (about two years) cover the basic biological and psychological sciences. Clinical work and electives begin in the third period, and clinical clerkships begin in the third year and carry over into the fourth. The fourth year includes study in ethics, sciences, professional development, and a number of electives.

Facilities

The university facilities include five teaching hospitals, seven affiliated teaching hospitals, and 13 special research centers.

Application Procedures

Applicants may apply starting on September 1. The deadline is November 15 for out-of-province and February 1 for Quebec residents. The application fee is $25. McGill does not have an early decision plan. The earliest acceptance notices are sent out on March 30. Applicants must accept offers for admission within two weeks. A $100 deposit is required to hold the applicant's place in class. Classes begin in August.

Contact

Admissions Office
McGill University
Faculty of Medicine
3655 Drummond Street
Montreal, Quebec H3G 1Y6
Canada
(514) 398-3517

McMASTER UNIVERSITY SCHOOL OF MEDICINE

1200 Main Street West
Hamilton, Ontario
Canada L8N 3Z5
(416) 525-9140

Accreditation	LCME, CACMS
Degrees Offered	M.D.
# Students Applied	2,068
Enrollment	400 / total school
Mean GPA	2.5 minimum
% Men / % Women	30% / 70%
% Minorities	Not Available
Tuition	$3,169 — Canadian residents
	$12,641— Nonresidents
Application Fee	$50
Application Deadline	November 1

The University

The School of Medicine at McMaster University was established in 1965, admitting its first students in 1969 and graduating its first class of physicians in 1972. The concept of health sciences education within the School of Medicine is based on the view that health is a broad subject encompassing not only the problems of ill health, but also the impact of biology, environment, and the way of life on health.

Admissions

Undergraduate academic standing with a B average (2.5) or better is required for applicants. A minimum of three years of undergraduate work must be completed at the time of application.

Undergraduate Preparation

There are no course prerequisites.

Student Body

Seventy percent of the students in the class of 1993 were female and 30 percent were male. Ninety-two were from the province of Ontario with the remainder of the class coming from other locations in Canada. Most of these medical students were between 21 and 24 years of age. Common undergraduate majors included arts and sciences, health care professions, and the natural/physical sciences.

Costs

Costs are in Canadian dollars.

For the 1989-90 academic year, tuition for Canadian residents was $3,169 annually during Years I and II and $2,175 during Year III. For foreign students, charges for Years I and II totaled $12,641 per year while Year III tuition was set at $8,491. Also, McMaster estimates that first-year medical students will have additional costs for books and diagnostic equipment that will total approximately $1,500.

Financial Aid

A variety of loan programs and scholarships are available through the university. Some are based on need and others on academic merit. The Ontario Hospital Services Commission offers a final-year clerkship stipend of approximately $4,000 to qualified students to aid in their educational development within a teaching hospital. The Canadian Department of National Defence administers the Canadian Forces Medical Officers Training Plan. Under this plan, the cost of a student's medical education is covered by the government in return for a commitment to military service upon graduation with an M.D. degree.

Curriculum

The medical program at McMaster is a three-year sequence of intensive study and training leading to an M.D. degree. The curriculum is divided into six units, each with a separate and distinct focus of study. Unit one provides an introduction to the medical program, in which students receive instruction in basic sciences and clinical skills. Units two through four focus on the systematic study of human structure, function, and behavior and are individually organized around different systems of the body. During Unit five students study health care problems from the community, including reproductive health, childhood and adolescent health, and occupational, environmental, and geriatric health. Unit six is devoted to clinical clerkships during which students participate in the direct care of patients and become clinically self-sufficient within the realm of contemporary medicine. Clerkship periods consist of rotations in medicine and surgery, family medicine, psychiatry, pediatrics, and obstetrics and gynecology, as well as an elective period.

Facilities

Affiliated teaching hospitals include Chedoke McMaster Hospitals, Hamilton General Hospital, Henderson General Hospital, St. Joseph's Hospital, Hamilton Psychiatric Hospital, and St. Peter's Hospital.

Grading Procedures

Much of the instruction in the medical school occurs within the tutorial setting so that students are continually being evaluated by other students as well as the tutor. Two problem-solving exercises are required in each of the six units. At the completion of the unit, the instructor prepares a written summary of observation of the student's performance in the tutorial and related activities.

Contact

Admissions and Records (HSC)
McMaster University
Room 1B7-Health Sciences Centre
1200 Main Street West
Hamilton, Ontario L8N 3Z5
Canada
(416) 525-9140, Ext. 2114

MEMORIAL UNIVERSITY OF NEWFOUNDLAND FACULTY OF MEDICINE

St. Johns, Newfoundland
Canada A1B 3V6
(709) 737-6615

Accreditation	LCME, CACMS
Degrees Offered	M.D., B.MS./M.D.
# Students Applied	576
Enrollment	56 / class
Mean GPA	Not Available
% Men / % Women	Not Available
% Minorities	Not Available
Tuition	$1,344
Application Fee	$25
Application Deadline	December 15

The University

Founded as Memorial College in 1925, Memorial University is today the sole university in the province of Newfoundland, Canada. The college attained university status in 1949. The university has a faculty of about 1,000 and enrolls about 12,000 undergraduate students. The medical school is one of the newest in Canada. It is part of the Health Sciences Centre, which also houses the university hospital.

Admissions

The school considers MCAT scores and academic record for admission. Priority is given to residents of Newfoundland and Labrador, with New Brunswick following. The school may then consider applicants from the rest of Canada and elsewhere.

Undergraduate Preparation

Applicants must have had at least two years of college-level education. Two semesters are required in each of the following subjects: general chemistry, organic chemistry, mathematics, and English.

Student Body

Each year, 56 students are admitted to the medical school. In 1990-91, the entering class consisted of 41 in-province students and 15 out-of-province students. All students took the MCAT, and 73 percent held bachelor's degrees.

Costs

For the 1990-91 entering class, tuition was $1,344, and student fees were $178.

Curriculum

An interim degree—the bachelor of medical science degree—is awarded after successful completion of the second year of the medical program. The M.D. degree is awarded after completion of four years of study.

The first year consists of basic medical studies in areas such as biochemistry, molecular genetics, microbiology, and nutrition/pharmacology. Students also study the behavioral sciences and community medicine, and will experience their first patient contact in one of a wide variety of clinical settings. During the following years, the basic sciences of anatomy, physiology, and pathology are integrated with the clinical aspects of the program. The first, third, and fourth years provide time for elective study, which may include research or courses in specialty areas.

Facilities

The Health Sciences Centre of the university consists of the medical school and General Hospital, a 320-bed facility. The Centre also houses a biomedical library. Internships and residencies may be taken at affiliated hospitals in St. John's and other medical facilities in Newfoundland, which represent a total of over 3,100 beds.

Application Procedures

Applications must be filed with the Faculty of Medicine between September 1 and December 15 of the year before the year of desired enrollment. The application fee is $25. The Faculty of Medicine does not have an early decision plan. Applicants will begin to be notified of acceptance the following April. Accepted students must submit a $100 deposit (applied toward tuition) to hold their place in the class.

Contact
Chairman, Committee on Admissions
Memorial University of Newfoundland
Faculty of Medicine
St. John's, Newfoundland A1B 3V6
Canada
(709) 737-6615

UNIVERSITY OF MONTREAL FACULTY OF MEDICINE

Montreal, Quebec
Canada H3C 3J7
(514) 737-6615

Accreditation	LCME, CACMS
Degrees Offered	M.D., M.D./M.S., J.D., M.D./Ph.D.
# Students Applied	1,974
Enrollment	170 / class
Mean GPA	Not Available
% Men / % Women	42% / 58%
% Minorities	Not Available
Tuition	$1,198 – Canadian residents
	$5,800 – Nonresidents
Application Fee	$15
Application Deadline	March 1

The University

The Faculty of Medicine of the University of Montreal was established in 1843. In 1891 the school merged with the Faculty of Medicine of the Montreal branch of Laval University. In 1920, an act of the Quebec Legislature granted the Montreal branch of Laval University its independence and became known by its present name. All instruction at the Faculty of Medicine is conducted in French.

Admissions

Students must be either Canadian citizens or landed immigrants; however, French-speaking candidates from other provinces and the United States are considered. Special consideration for admission is given to native American applicants.

Candidates are selected based on global scores from scholastic records, aptitude tests, and interviews.

Undergraduate Preparation

Entering students must have a thorough knowledge of the French language. Students must have a minimum of two years of college (health science program) and the diploma of collegial studies of the Department of Education Coursework (D.E.C.) which must include work in philosophy, behavioral and social sciences, French, English, mathematics, and sciences.

Student Body

The entering class of 1990 consisted of about 170 students, suggesting a student body of about 680 students. Ninety-one students had one to three years of college work. One hundred sixty-three were Quebec residents, and 99 were women.

Costs

Tuition for Canadians is $1,198; non-Canadians pay $5,800. Student fees amount to $204 per year.

Financial Aid

Sources of financial aid include the Kellogg Foundations Loan Fund, the Scholarships and Loan Committee of the University, and the Jean Frappier Fund. Some summer scholarships are available.

Curriculum

The course of study lasts four years. The first year is devoted to basic biological and behavioral sciences, with initial exposure to clinical work. Morphology and function, both normal and abnormal, take up the second year, and students must take 90 hours of elective learning. The third and fourth years consist of a clerkship that lasts for 80 weeks.

Facilities

All instruction is carried out in 14 affiliated teaching hospitals and research centers.

Special Programs

Combined M.D./M.S. and M.D./Ph.D. programs are available. Various courses and symposia may be taken in continuing education programs.

Application Procedures

The deadline for application is March 1. There is an application fee of $15. The Faculty of Medicine does not have an early decision program. Notification of acceptance begins on May 15. Candidates must accept the offer within two weeks of notification. No deposit is necessary for holding the applicant's place in class.

Contact
Committee on Admission
University of Montreal
Faculty of Medicine
P.O. Box 6128, Station A
Montreal, Quebec H3C 3J7
Canada
(514) 343-6265

UNIVERSITY OF OTTAWA
SCHOOL OF MEDICINE

451 Smyth Road
Ottawa, Ontario
Canada K1H 8M5
(613) 787-6463

Accreditation	LCME, CACMS
Degrees Offered	M.D.
# Students Applied	2,109
Enrollment	84 / class
Mean GPA	3.2
% Men / % Women	Not Available
% Minorities	Not Available
Tuition	$2,255 – Canadian residents
	$9,975 – Nonresidents
Application Fee	$50
Application Deadline	November 1

The University

Founded by the Missionary Oblates of Mary Immaculate, the University of Ottawa was chartered by the Province of Ontario in 1866. Since 1965, the university has been managed by a board of governors comprising various community members. It is an autonomously governed institution. The Faculty of Medicine, established in 1945, is part of the Faculty of Health Sciences, which, as of 1978, also includes the School of Nursing and the School of Human Kinetics.

Admissions

The major factor in the admissions decision is the applicant's level of academic achievement. To be competitive, students must have maintained a GPA of B+ or above in undergraduate coursework, and have achieved scores of 8 or above in each of the MCAT subtests. The difficulty of the undergraduate courses taken, and their relevance to the study of medicine, is considered. Personal qualities are also assessed as part of the admissions process, and no applicant can be accepted without having participated in an interview. The school accepts only Canadian citizens, landed immigrants, or children of alumni.

Undergraduate Preparation

The school seeks students who have had exposure to both the sciences and the humanities. Course requirements are one year each of general biology or zoology, general or inorganic chemistry, organic chemistry, and physics. Applicants should have completed at least two years of college or university work leading to the B.S. or B.A. degree. All candidates must take the MCAT.

Student Body

The 1990-91 class consisted of 84 students; 73 in-province students and 11 from outside Ontario.

Costs

For 1990-91, tuition was $2,255 for Canadian residents and $9,975 for non-Canadians. Student fees were $171.

Financial Aid

Financial aid is available on the basis of financial need as well as academic achievement. The school's financial aid office as well as the provincial governments of Canada offer loans and grants. Financial aid programs include the Ontario Medical Association Bursaries and Loan Fund, the Kellogg Foundation Loan Fund, and other special awards administered by the school's awards committee.

Curriculum

Training is intended to produce physicians for primary care/family medicine or for postgraduate study. The first two years consist of lectures and small-group instruction. Tutorials, seminars, and supervised study time are also available. The third year features a systems approach of study and 24 weeks of clerkships. Students may take a 52 week clerkship in the fourth year instead of the post-M.D. rotating internships.

Application Procedures

The Faculty of Medicine participates in OMSAS (Ontario Universities' Application Centre). The OMSAS application must be filed between July 1 and November 1 of the year preceding the year of desired enrollment. The OMSAS fee is $50. The school does not have an early decision policy. Accepted students must pay a $100 deposit (applied toward tuition) to hold their place in the class.

Contact

Admissions
University of Ottawa
Faculty of Medicine
451 Smyth Road
Ottawa, Ontario K1H 8M5
Canada
(613) 787-6463

QUEEN'S UNIVERSITY FACULTY OF MEDICINE

Kingston, Ontario
Canada K7L 3N6
(613) 545-2542

Accreditation	LCME
Degrees Offered	M.D.
# Students Applied	2,162
Enrollment	72 / class
Mean GPA	Not Available
% Men / % Women	Not Available
% Minorities	Not Available
Tuition	$2,083 – Canadian residents
	$9,157 – Nonresidents
Application Fee	$50
Application Deadline	November 1

The University

Queen's University enrolls over 10,000 full-time students. The Faculty of Medicine was founded in 1854. The campus is located in Kingston, Ontario, which is situated on Lake Ontario at the origin of the St. Lawrence river, and has a population of about 98,000. The overall aim of the M.D. curriculum is to provide a broad medical education and to prepare students for specialized postgraduate education.

Admissions

The faculty considers a wide range of academic and personal factors for admission, with about 60 percent of the evaluation based on scholastic record and 40 percent on the applicant's personal background. The committee examines the quality of the academic background and evidence of improvement during the course of undergraduate studies. Other factors, including personal extenuating circumstances that affect academic achievement, may be taken into account. The committee takes into account letters of recommendation and the candidate's personal essay. The school admits only Canadian citizens, Canadian permanent residents, or children of university alumni who reside outside Canada.

Undergraduate Preparation

The faculty requires students to have taken at least two full years of study at the university level. One undergraduate course (with lab) is required in each of the following areas: general chemistry, organic chemistry, general physics, and biology (or zoology). All applicants must take the MCAT. No specific major is required.

Student Body

The 1990-91 entering class had 72 students. Sixty-two were residents of the province of Ontario. All students in the class took the MCAT, and 30 percent held bachelor's degrees.

Costs

For the 1990-91 entering class, tuition was $2,083 for Canadian residents. Tuition for nonresidents was $9,157. Student's fees for the year totaled $296.

Curriculum

A new curriculum was established in 1991 that allows greater independent learning, and a new systems-based approach better integrates the basic sciences with the clinical sciences. The new program emphasizes elective choices and more time for independent study. It is designed to offer students a more flexible educational experience.

Phase I of the program focuses on principles of the basic medical sciences and their relation to clinical medicine. Phase II focuses on selected clinical topics and, again, is concerned with the integration of the basic sciences with the clinical aspects of medicine. Phase III introduces clinical clerkships.

Facilities

The campus houses all facilities for preclinical instruction. Students participate in clinical experiences in the Kingston General Hospital (located next to the campus), the Hotel Dieu Hospital, and a variety of other specialty hospitals.

Application Procedures

Queen's University Faculty of Medicine participates in OMSAS (Ontario Medical School Application Service). Candidates should file their applications between July 1 and November 1 of the year preceding the year of intended enrollment. The university does not participate in an early decision plan. The OMSAS fee is $50. The university's application fee and the deposit to hold a place in class are pending the admissions decision.

Contact

Admissions Office
Queen's University
Faculty of Medicine
Kingston, Ontario K7L 3N6
Canada
(613) 545-2542

UNIVERSITY OF SASKATCHEWAN COLLEGE OF MEDICINE

Saskatoon, Saskatchewan
Canada S7N 0W0
(306) 966-8664

Accreditation	LCME, CACMS
Degrees Offered	M.D., B.S.
# Students Applied	373
Enrollment	60 / class
Mean GPA	Not Available
% Men / % Women	Not Available
% Minorities	Not Available
Tuition	$2,247
Application Fee	$25 In-Province, $50 Out-of-Province
Application Deadline	January 15 In-Province; December 1 Out-of-Province

The University

Medical education at the University of Saskatchewan began in 1926. A four-year curriculum was implemented in 1953. In 1968 the curriculum changed to five years with a one-year premedical university requirement. The program is currently designed to educate physicians for family medicine, specialty practice, public health, research, and teaching.

Admissions

Academic achievement and personal qualities of the applicant are assessed for admission. The college also evaluates academic records, letters of recommendation, and the results of a personal interview.

Undergraduate Preparation

Candidates for admission must have had at least two years of undergraduate education. Required coursework includes six credit hours each of biology, general chemistry, and general physics, all with lab. Three hours of organic chemistry, six hours of English (literature and composition), and six hours of social sciences or humanities are also required. The college does not require applicants to take the MCAT. Only Canadian citizens or landed immigrants are considered for admission.

Student Body

Each year, the college admits up to 60 students. Of the 1990-91 first-year class, 58 students were from the province of Saskatchewan and two were from elsewhere in Canada. The average GPA of this class was 84.7 percent. About one-third held baccalaureate degrees.

Costs

Costs are in Canadian dollars.

For the 1990-91 entering class, tuition was $2,247 annually for both in-province and out-of-province students. Fees totaled $100 for the year.

Financial Aid

Both scholarships and loans are available. Bursaries may also be available to students who wish to pursue research during the time between academic years.

Curriculum

The clinical and basic sciences are organized by body system, and the general approach emphasizes problem solving. The four-year curriculum is divided into five phases. The first two phases provide an overview and also a more specific study of the basic medical sciences. Phase three introduces the connection between basic and clinical sciences and begins the student's training in clinical skills. Phase four provides a more intensive training in the clinical aspects of medicine. During phase five, students apply their skill and knowledge to actual patient care. Ample time is given throughout the curriculum for independent study and clinical electives.

Facilities

Students pursue their clinical experience at University Hospital, St. Paul's and Saskatoon City hospitals, and the Plains Health Centre and General Hospital in Regina.

Special Programs

The college offers students the opportunity to obtain a B.S. degree in basic medical sciences during the four-year M.D. program.

Application Procedures

Applications for in-province students must be filed with the college between September 1 and January 15. The deadline for out-of-province applicants is December 1. The application fee is $25 for in-province applicants and $50 for out-of-province applicants. The college does not participate in an early decision plan. Upon acceptance, students must submit a $100 deposit (applied toward tuition) to hold their place in class.

Contact

Administrative Assistant, Admissions
University of Saskatchewan
College of Medicine
Saskatoon, Saskatchewan S7N 0W0
Canada
(306) 966-8554

UNIVERSITY OF SHERBROOKE FACULTY OF MEDICINE

Sherbrooke, Quebec
Canada J1H 5N4
(819) 564-5208

Accreditation	LCME, CACMS
Degrees Offered	M.D., M.S., Ph.D.
# Students Applied	1,763
Enrollment	102 / class
Mean GPA	Not Available
% Men / % Women	65% / 35%
% Minorities	Not Available
Tuition	$2,355 – Canadian residents
	$8,700 – Nonresidents
Application Fee	$15
Application Deadline	March 1

The University

The Faculty of Medicine of the University of Sherbrooke enrolled its first class in 1966 and is today part of a modern health sciences center. Classes are conducted in French.

Admissions

The major factor considered in the admissions process is academic achievement in the preprofessional course of study. Preference is given to residents of Quebec (88 out of 100 spots in each entering class are reserved for those from Quebec). Two places may be available in the class for foreign applicants. All applicants must be fluent in French. Applicants are not required to take the MCAT.

Undergraduate Preparation

Applicants must have completed at least two years of college. Applicants are expected to possess a broad cultural background, with courses in the arts, humanities, and behavioral sciences as well as in premedical sciences. The following premedical courses are required as part of the undergraduate curriculum leading toward the bachelor's degree: two semesters each of biology, chemistry, and organic chemistry, all with lab, and three semesters of general physics with lab. Also required are three semesters of college math, including analytical geometry, algebra, trigonometry, and calculus. Candidates of the CEGEP (College D'enseignement General et Professionel) must have a college diploma (DEC) with a major in the sciences.

Student Body

Of the 1990-91 first-year class, 88 were from Quebec and 14 were out-of-province residents. Of the 102 new students, 13 percent held baccalaureate degrees.

Costs

All costs are in Canadian dollars.

In 1990-91, tuition was $2,355 for Canadian residents and $8,700 for nonresidents. Student fees totaled $1,000.

Financial Aid

Quebec residents can seek financial assistance through the Bursaries Division of the Provincial Ministry of Education, the university's Scholarships and Loans Committee, as well as from private foundations.

Curriculum

The four-year M.D. degree program features a problem-based approach to learning. Among the teaching methods used are seminars, small group discussion, field work, and audiovisual instruction. Formal lectures are minimal. Most teaching at the school is interdisciplinary in approach. Students gain exposure to the hospital setting from the start of the first year of study. The fourth year consists of 16 months of clerkships.

Facilities

The Health Sciences Center consists of a 400-bed teaching hospital as well as a Department of Nursing.

Special Programs

The school offers postgraduate programs leading to the M.S. and the Ph.D., as well as a diploma in community health.

Application Procedures

Applications must be filed with the school between November and March for entrance into the following year's first-year class. The application fee is $15. The school does not have an early decision plan. The school will send acceptance notifications between May 15 and August. Accepted students must submit a $75 deposit, which is applied toward tuition, to hold their place in the class.

Contact

Admissions Office
University of Sherbrooke
Faculty of Medicine
Sherbrooke, Quebec J1H 5N4
Canada
(819) 564-5208

UNIVERSITY OF TORONTO FACULTY OF MEDICINE

Toronto, Ontario
Canada M5S 1A8
(416) 978-2717

Accreditation	LCME, CACMS
Degrees Offered	M.D., M.D./Ph.D.
# Students Applied	2,300
Enrollment	250 / class
Mean GPA	3.4
% Men / % Women	67% / 33%
% Minorities	Not Available
Tuition	$2,367 – Canadian residents
	$10,072 – Nonresidents
Application Fee	$50
Application Deadline	November 1

The University

The University of Toronto was founded as King's College in 1843. The Faculty of Medicine at the university is Canada's largest medical school, where several major medical breakthroughs, including the discovery of insulin and the development of the cardiac pacemaker, have taken place through the years. The medical school is affiliated with 10 teaching hospitals in the surrounding Toronto area.

Metropolitan Toronto features countless attractions, such as concerts, museums, and major league sports. There are great opportunities for both winter and summer outdoor sports and activities. The southern Ontario region is filled with beautiful sights and scenes to explore. Spread out along the university campus are relaxing pubs, theaters, and special lectures.

Admissions

The admissions committee looks very closely at GPA and MCAT scores when evaluating the applicant pool. The average GPA ranges from 3.4 to 3.7. The average quantitative score from the Medical College Admission Test is 9.33. Students are advised to take the MCAT in the spring prior to applying. MCAT scores must reflect a test taken after 1990.

Undergraduate Preparation

Applicants are not required to major in any specific discipline. Students must obtain credit for one year each, with labs, in the following prerequisite courses: biology, physics, general chemistry, and organic chemistry, and are urged to acquire excellent oral and written English skills. In addition, familiarity with biostatistics and computer science would assist students in the medical program. Students belonging to a university outside of Canada must complete the equivalent of a Canadian bachelor's degree. Applicants should also have completed a standard first aid course in addition to a CPR basic rescuer course prior to enrollment in the medical curriculum. Before beginning the second year, students must have completed a course in biometrics or statistics. Fifty percent of the applicants who are admitted have had at least two years of university training. About 66 percent of the admitted applicants do not possess an undergraduate degree.

Student Body

A total of 252 students are accepted into the entering first-year class. The male/female ratio runs 67 percent to 33 percent. At least 89 percent of the students are Canadian residents. Close to 230 of the entering class come from Ontario.

Placement Records

During the fourth or final year of the medical program, students apply for postgraduate training through the Canadian Intern and Resident Matching Service (CIRMS). Most graduates find residency within Toronto or the affiliated hospital region.

Costs

All costs are in Canadian dollars.

The total annual tuition for Canadians is $2,367; students on a visa pay $10,072. Books and instruments for the first year cost $1,456. An additional $1,000 should be allocated each year for supplies. Room and board cost at least $126 per week.

Financial Aid

Scholarships, bursary, and loan funds are available under the Province of Ontario Student Assistance Program and the Canada Student Loan Program. Students are required to apply to the Ontario Student Assistance Program as soon as possible. Financial problems can be discussed with an awards officer or the assistant dean of student affairs.

Student Organizations

Medical students can be active on faculty committees or be student representatives through Arts and Letters, the Auricle (student newspaper), the Medical Journal, Medical Christian Fellowship, Men's Athletic Association, Medical Women's Association, and any other university organization.

Curriculum

The medical program is a four-year, systems-oriented curriculum. The first year is dedicated to the study of the normal structure and function of and basic medical sciences corresponding to the human body. Students study anatomy, embryology, histology, biochemistry, metabolism, and molecular genetics. The second and third years consist of the study of clinical medicine. Preclinical material is covered in the first term. For the clinical subjects each student is assigned to a "home base" hospital for training. A 48-week clerkship comprises the entire fourth year, during which, for varying periods of time, students concentrate on medicine, surgery, pediatrics, obstetrics and gynecology, psychiatry, otolaryngology, anesthesia, and family and community medicine.

Special Programs

A joint M.D./Ph.D. program is available primarily for students preparing for a career in biomedical research. There are four different routes offered for the combined degree. Many research opportunities are also available, such as the Undergraduate Programme in Medical Science, in which students are paired with supervisors involved in both clinical work and research. A stipend covers tuition and certain other expenses.

Application Procedures

The Faculty of Medicine participates in the Ontario Medical School Application Service (OMSAS). Students must apply no later than November 1 of the year prior to admission. There is a $50 OMSAS fee as well as a nonrefundable application fee of $50 for the university. Notices of acceptance will be sent out in the spring prior to the proposed date of admission. No more than 50 places will be offered to non-Ontario residents. An interview may be scheduled at the discretion of the admissions committee.

Contact

University of Toronto
Faculty of Medicine, Admissions
Toronto, Ontario M5S 1A8
Canada
(416) 978-2717

UNIVERSITY OF WESTERN ONTARIO FACULTY OF MEDICINE

London, Ontario
Canada N6A 5C1
(519) 661-3744

Accreditation	LCME, CACMS
Degrees Offered	M.D., M.D./Ph.D., M.D./M.S.
# Students Applied	2,211
Enrollment	105 / class
Mean GPA	Not Available
% Men / % Women	Not Available
% Minorities	Not Available
Tuition	$2,157
Application Fee	$50
Application Deadline	November 1

The University

The Faculty of Medicine started in 1882 and became a part of the University of Western Ontario in 1912. The university is a private school but receives some government grants.

Admissions

Each candidate for admission is evaluated according to his or her academic record, MCAT scores, interview, and essay. Particular attention is given to the last two undergraduate years (five full or equivalent courses in each year). An assessment is made of the level of difficulty of all courses and the student's achievement. Some credit is given to applicants with a graduate and/or professional degree, provided the candidate meets the minimum requirements.

Applicants must be Canadian citizens or permanent residents (landed immigrants) on the closing date for application. Two positions may be available for students supported by the Canadian International Development Agency or a similar agency. Candidates applying for admission with advanced standing or transferring from another medical school are considered only in very exceptional cases.

Undergraduate Preparation

Applicants for admission will be considered who are in, or have completed, a second-year program at a recognized university, provided that the program included a minimum of four honors courses (or the equivalent), or who have completed at least two years of a program at a recognized university. Applicants will also be considered who are in the final year of, or who have successfully completed, a graduate or undergraduate degree program at a recognized university, provided the program has included at least five full courses (of which three must have been senior/honors courses) in each of the last two undergraduate years. Graduate students will be expected to have completed all requirements for their graduate degree prior to registration.

Prerequisite areas of study include full laboratory courses in biology (university year I level), chemistry (university year I level), physics, and organic chemistry (university year II level). Grade 13/OAC English or the equivalent is required. Two full-year courses (university level) in arts or social science are also required. One of these courses must be literature (English) if the applicant does not have Grade 13/OAC or equivalent English.

Costs

Costs are in Canadian dollars.

Tuition costs $2,330 per year. Tuition fees are subject to change.

Financial Aid

Contact the student awards office, Somerville, at (519) 661-3775 for financial aid information.

Student Organizations

There is a branch of the medical honor society, Alpha Omega Alpha, on campus.

Faculty

There are more than 1,000 faculty members on the teaching staff.

Curriculum

The undergraduate medical program is a four-year program divided into five phases. The program is a blend of lectures, laboratory exercises, small group problem-based learning, and supervised clinical experiences. The first three phases are designed to provide the student with a solid grounding in the basic and clinical sciences. This method of teaching is structured around one problem-based learning day per week. Students take responsibility for their own learning, with the tutor assisting but not leading, allowing the student to develop skills in communication and in independent, self-directed learning.

Phase IV, the clinical clerkship, is a 52-week integrated learning experience. Phase V includes selected topics (six-week classroom block) and clinical selective and electives. Selectives are completed locally. Electives are subject to approval, and are completed by the individual at Western or in other centers.

Facilities

Western's Computer Based Learning Centre (CLBC), located in the medical sciences building, contains over 150 educational programs through which students can advance their understanding of the basic and clinical sciences, as well as gain practice in clinical decision-making while receiving feedback on the quality of their decisions.

Grading Procedures

An honors/pass/fail grading system is used. To progress to Phase IV, a preclinical comprehensive examination must be taken and passed. To progress to Phase V, the post-clinical comprehensive examination must be successfully completed.

Special Programs

The Faculties of Medicine and Graduate Studies have established combined M.D./Ph.D and M.D./M.S. programs. Candidates for these special programs must be enrolled in the undergraduate program of the Faculty of Medicine prior to entering the combined program and must be accepted by the relevant basic health science department and the Faculty of Graduate Studies. The minimum residence requirement for the Ph.D. program is six consecutive terms plus at least one additional summer term. The minimum residence requirement for the M.S. degree in the program is three consecutive terms.

Applications Procedures

The Medical College Admission Test (MCAT) is required. MCAT results before the spring of 1991 will not be acceptable for applications made on or after November 1991. No preference is given according to place of residence, age, or university attended.

Application to the Faculty of Medicine must be made upon the regular application form, which candidates may obtain from the Ontario Medical School Application Service (OMSAS). The completed application forms and additional information (the applicant statement/essay, and the confidential assessment form) must be mailed to OMSAS no later than November 1 for the class starting in the following September. All applicants must have an adequate knowledge of written and spoken English.

Contact

Admissions Office
University of Western Ontario
Faculty of Medicine
Health Sciences Centre
London, Ontario N6A 5C1
Canada
(519) 661-3744

A WORD ON FOREIGN MEDICAL STUDY

Some students choose to seek admission to medical school in a foreign country. There are many reasons why a student might seek admission to a foreign medical school: the student was unable to or thought he or she would be unable to gain admission to an American medical school; the student wishes to study in a different culture or with a different language which had previously been studied and enjoyed; or that parents or other relatives come from that country. There are many other reasons as well.

Whatever the case, foreign medical study is generally not recommended. It is very difficult to return to the United States as a practicing physician, because United States hospitals prefer American trained doctors, and that is where the residencies are. If you decide to study abroad, it should be with a clear understanding that you may not be able to come back with your degree and start a practice in the United States.

Another problem with foreign medical study is the obvious—the language barrier. The schools we contacted sent their admissions material in the native language, not in English. It was made quite clear to us that a student must have full and complete understanding of the country's language before considering study in their schools. Even if you have a fluent understanding of the language native to the country, it may be even more difficult to learn the concepts and curriculum using the native langauge. Do not assume that classes will be taught in English, or that textbooks will be in English. It seems that the majority of them are not.

If you are interested in studying abroad, the following is a list of some of the more popular countries and schools. If the school or country you are interested in is not listed, write to the consulate of that country.

Belgium
Contact:

University of Antwerp, Faculteit der Geneeskunde, Rijksuniversitair, Centrum Antwerpen, Goemaerelei, 52, 2000 Antwerpen, Belgium

University of Brussels, Faculté de Médecine, Université Libre de Bruxelles, Rectorat-Affaires Etudiantes, Avenue A. Buyl, 131, 1050 Bruxelles, Belgium

University of Ghent, Faculteit der Geneeskunde, Rijksuniversiteit to Gent, Voldersstraat, 13, 9000 Gent, Belgium

University of Liège, Faculté de Médecine, Université de Liège, Services des Étudiants, Place de XX Août, 4000 Liège, Belgium

University of Louvain, Faculté de Médecine, Université Catholique de Louvain, Secrétariat des Étudiants Etrangers, Avenue E . Mounier, 1200 Bruxelles, Belgium (French)

or contact:

Universiteit Katholik te Leuven, Studentensecretariat, Universiteithal Naamsestraat, 22 3000 Leuven, Belgium (Flemish)

Caribbean
Contact:

St. George's University, c/o Foreign Medical School Services Corporation, One East Main Street, Bay Shore, NY 11706

or contact:

American University of the Caribbean, School of Medicine, 100 N.W. 37th Avenue, Miami, FL 33125

Dominican Republic
Contact:

Admissions Office for Foreign Students, Universidad Central del Este, Tampico, Dominican Republic

Universidad Nacional Pedro Henriquez Urena, Director, Esceula de Medicina, Santo Domingo, Dominican Republic

England
Contact:

Universities Central Council on Admissions, PO Box 28, Cheltenham GL5O 1HY, England

France
Contact:

Théraplix, Secrétariat du Guide Théraplix des Études Médicales, 46-52 rue Albert, 75640 Paris Cedex 13, France

Germany
Contact:

Cultural Division, Consulate General of the Federal Republic of Germany, 460 Park Avenue, New York, NY 10022

Hungary
Contact:

University of Pecs, c/o Hungarian Consulate, 8 East 75th Street, New York, NY 10021

Ireland

Contact:

Royal College of Surgeons, 123 St. Stephen's Green, Dublin 2, Ireland

Israel

Contact:

Sackler School of Medicine of the University of Tel Aviv, Medical School Office of Admissions, 17 East 62nd Street, New York, NY 10021

Italy

For the following schools in Italy, please contact the school as Universita degli Studi, and the town in which it is located. For example, the University of Bologna can be reached at Universita degli Studi, Bologna, Italy.

University of Padua

University of Rome

University of Turin

University of Pisa

University of Pavia

University of Palermo

University of Florence

University of Genoa

University of Milan

University of Naples

or write to:

Italian Consulate, 690 Park Avenue, New York, NY 10021

Mexico

Contact:

Oficina de Informacion a Extranjeros, Universidad Autónoma de Guadalajara, Apartado Postal 1-440, Guadalajara, Jalisco, Mexico

Autonomous University of Ciudad Juarez, Instituto de Ciencias Biomedicas, Apartado Postal 1574, Sucursal "D", Ciudad Juarez, Chihuahua, Mexico

University of Monterrey, Direccion de Admisiones, Seccion de Extranjeros, Apartado Postal 4435, Sucursal "J", Ciudad Juarez, Chihuahua, Mexico

University Del Noreste (Tampico) Admissions Office, 120 East 41st Street, Suite 1000, New York, NY 10017

Philippines

Contact:

University of the Philippines, College of Medicine and Surgery, 547 Herren Street, Manila, Philippines

University of Santo Tomas, College of Medicine, España Street, Manila, Philippines

Manila Central University, College of Medicine, Samson Road, Caloocan City, Philippines

University of the East, Ramon Magsaysay Memorial Medical Center, College of Medicine, Aurora Boulevard, Quezon City, Philippines

Far Eastern University, Institute of Medicine, Science Building, Nicanor Reyes Sr. Street, Manila, Philippines

Southwestern University, College of Medicine and Surgery, Cebu City, Philippines

or write to the:

Consulate General of the Philippines, 556 Fifth Avenue, New York, NY 10009

Poland

Contact:

Embassy of the Polish People's Republic, 2640 16th Street, N.W., Washington, DC 20009

Spain

Contact:

Cultural Relations Department, Spanish Embassy, Columbia Road, N.W., Washington, DC 20001

## CHAPTER 3

Osteopathic Schools

OSTEOPATHIC MEDICINE

Osteopathic medicine has long been regarded as the "other" branch of medicine. Osteopathic medicine is, however, a special type of medicine which requires more training than "traditional" or allopathic medicine.

Philosophy

The philosophy of osteopathic medicine is what makes it different from any other type of medicine or treatment. The osteopathic physician (D.O.) recognizes that the musculoskeletal system (the muscle, bones, and joints) makes up over 60 percent of body mass. D.O.s also recognize that all body systems, including the musculoskeletal system, are interdependent, and a disturbance in one causes altered function in other systems of the body. This interrelationship of body systems is effected through the nervous and circulatory systems. The emphasis on the relationship between body structure and organic functioning gives a broader base for the treatment of the patient as a unit. These concepts require a thorough understanding of anatomy and the development of special skills in recognizing (diagnosing) and correcting (treating) structural problems through manipulative therapy. As physicians and surgeons, D.O.s use structural diagnosis and osteopathic manipulative therapy (a therapy in which the D.O. manipulates muscles, bones, and tendons to improve circulation and correct structural abnormalities) along with all of the other more traditional forms of diagnosis and treatment to care effectively for patients.

Training

Becoming an osteopathic physician is a challenging experience. Generally, a student must complete his or her undergraduate degree, while fulfilling requirements in the basic sciences. After completing the degree, the osteopathic medical student then goes on to one of 15 medical schools, where he or she embarks on a four year intensive training program. This program generally consists of two years of classroom instruction, followed by two years of clinical ("hands on") instruction. Required training during the second two years of education includes general medicine, pediatrics, obstetrics/gynecology, surgery, radiology, and preventive medicine. During this time, the student learns to recognize, diagnose, and treat a patient's symptoms. The student is also expected to attend lectures, clinical conferences, and seminars.

After the osteopathic medical student earns his or her degree, the internship begins. The new doctor spends 12 months in an approved internship in the primary care areas of internal medicine, surgery, general practice, obstetrics and gynecology, and pediatrics. The intern also will have an opportunity to sample other specialty and subspecialty areas of medicine. The osteopathic physician continues to receive additional training in more osteopathic principles and techniques.

After completing internship training, the osteopathic physician may choose to continue further education in order to specialize in a particular medical field, or a subspecialty of that field. If this is the case, two to six years of additional training are necessary.

Certification and Licensure

Osteopathic physicians can be board certified in anesthesiology, dermatology, emergency medicine, general practice, internal medicine, neurology and psychiatry, nuclear medicine, obstetrics and gynecology, ophthalmology and otorhinolaryngology, orthopedic surgery, osteopathic manipulation medicine, pathology, pediatrics, proctology, public health and preventive medicine, rehabilitative medicine, and surgery, and they can earn the Certificate of Competence for sports medicine.

An osteopathic physician must also pass required examinations in order to be allowed to practice medicine. There are three avenues to becoming licensed:

1. The National Board of Osteopathic Medical Examiners holds National Board Examinations in three parts. Students take the first two parts during school, and the third part is taken after six months of an approved internship.

2. FLEX, which stands for the Federal Licensing Examination, is administered twice a year over three days, and is given to both doctors of medicine and doctors of osteopathic medicine.

3. States give their own examinations throughout the year.

The Profession

Osteopathic medicine is one of the fastest growing health professions. D.O.s practice throughout the entire country, many in small communities of 50,000 or less, and many in communities of 500,000 or more. While D.O.s comprise only five percent of all physicians, they make up 15 percent of doctors practicing in areas of 10,000 people or less.

Approximately 60 percent of osteopathic physicians specialize in the combined areas of family practice, obstetrics/gynecology, general internal medicine, and general surgery—the traditional primary care fields. The remaining physicians practice in a specialty or subspecialty area.

There are fine osteopathic physicians all over the country. Most of these physicians can be found in Michigan, Ohio, New Jersey, Florida, Texas, and Missouri. Since there are osteopathic colleges in all these states, many graduates may have chosen to settle in the geographic area where they were trained. Keep in mind, however, that an osteopathic physician can practice in any state of the country.

Admission Requirements*

Admission to an osteopathic program requires a minimum of three years of undergraduate education. Virtually every entering student, however, holds at least a bachelor's degree.

Minimum requirements are as follows:

- Six semester credit hours of English

- Six semester credit hours of behavioral science

- One year of physics

- One year of biology

- One year of inorganic and organic chemistry elective courses

The MCAT exam should be taken before applying to an osteopathic program. Letters of recommendation to prove outstanding character, dependability, and maturity should also be sent with the student's application.

Further Contacts

For more information on osteopathic education, please contact:

American Association of Colleges of Osteopathic Medicine (AACOM)
6110 Executive Boulevard
Rockville, MD 20852
(301) 468-0990

or:

American Osteopathic Association
142 E. Ontario Street
Chicago, IL 60611
(312) 280-5800

For specific information on the 15 osteopathic colleges of medicine in the United States, please view the listings on the following pages.

---

*Admission requirements are as stated by the American Association of Colleges of Osteopathic Medicine. (AACOM)

OSTEOPATHIC SCHOOLS AT A GLANCE

School	Accreditation	Degrees Offered	# Students Applied	Enrollment
Chicago College of Osteopathic Medicine	AOA	D.O., D.O./Ph.D.	*	*
College of Osteopathic Medicine of the Pacific	AOA	M.S.H.P.E., D.O., B.S./D.O.	*	112 / class
University of Health Sciences College of Osteopathic Medicine	AOA	D.O.	*	130 / class
Kirksville College of Osteopathic Medicine	AOA	D.O.	1,000	140 / class
University of Medicine and Dentistry of New Jersey School of Osteopathic Medicine	AOA	D.O.	*	56 / class
Michigan State University College of Osteopathic Medicine	AOA	D.O., Ph.D., D.O./Ph.D.	*	104 / class
University of New England College of Osteopathic Medicine	AOA	D.O.	1,300	100 / class
New York Institute of Technology New York College of Osteopathic Medicine	AOA	D.O., B.S./D.O.	*	150 / class
Ohio University College of Osteopathic Medicine	AOA	D.O.	1,900	100 / class
Oklahoma State University School of Osteopathic Medicine	AOA	D.O.	691	88 / class
University of Osteopathic Medicine and Health Sciences College of Osteopathic Medicine and Surgery	AOA, CIHE	D.O.	1,400	190 / class
Philadelphia College of Osteopathic Medicine	AOA	D.O., M.Sc., D.O./M.B.A., D.O./M.P.H.	1,200	200 / class
Southeastern University of the Health Sciences College of Osteopathic Medicine	AOA	D.O., B.S./D.O.	1,000	100 / class
Texas College of Osteopathic Medicine	AOA	D.O.	1,200	100 / class
West Virginia School of Osteopathic Medicine	AOA	D.O.	800	237

* Not Available   ** Not Applicable   C/S – Contact School   I/S – In-State   O/S – Out-of-State

Mean GPA	% Male / % Female	% Minorities	In-State Tuition	Out-of-State Tuition	Application Fee	Application Deadline
*	*	*	$12,565	$16,115	C/S	C/S
3.3	66% / 34%	21%	$14,925	**	C/S	C/S
3.04	70% / 30%	*	$13,990	**	C/S	C/S
3.0	73% / 27%	11%	$17,850	**	$25	March 1
3.3	64% / 36%	18%	$10,457	$13,723	C/S	March 1
3.2	60% / 40%	15%	$7,086	$15,282	C/S	January 1
3.0	*	*	$16,690	**	$55	March 1
2.75	65% / 35%	24%	$13,500	**	$60	March 1
3.2	68% / 32%	17%	$5,593	$8,352	$25	January 15
3.2	75% / 25%	15%	$5,240	$12,710	C/S	April 1
3.19	62% / 38%	11%	$16,775	**	$45	February 1
3.1	63% / 37%	9.9%	$15,078	$15,467	$50	March 1
*	74% / 26%	*	$11,965	$15,965	$50	March 1
3.0	31% / 69%	4%	$5,463	$21,852	$50	December 1
3.17	75% / 25%	*	$6,152	$10,832	$20 I/S $40 O/S	March 1

* Not Available   ** Not Applicable   C/S – Contact School   I/S – In-State   O/S – Out-of-State

CHICAGO COLLEGE OF OSTEOPATHIC MEDICINE

555 Thirty-First Street
Downers Grove, Illinois 60515
(708) 747-4000

Accreditation	AOA
Degrees Offered	D.O., D.O./Ph.D.
# Students Applied	Not Available
Enrolled	Not Available
Mean GPA	Not Available
% Men / % Women	Not Available
% Minorities	Not Available
Tuition	$12,565 In-State
	$16,115 Out-of-State
Application Fee	Contact School
Application Deadline	Contact School

The University

The Chicago College of Osteopathic Medicine (CCOM) was founded by Dr. J. Martin Littlejohn in 1900 as the American College of Osteopathic Medicine and Surgery. Two years later, the college merged with another new osteopathic college that had opened in Chicago. The new institution was named Littlejohn College and Hospital, after Dr. Littlejohn.

The school changed its name to the Chicago College of Osteopathic Medicine in 1970. The college maintains the basic science facility at the 103-acre Downers Grove campus, in a western suburb of Chicago, where students take their first two years of study. Hospital affiliates are located in Olympia Fields and Hyde Park.

Admissions

The admissions committee evaluates the student's ability to successfully complete a rigorous medical program of study. Students must have earned a minimum 2.5 GPA in both general and science coursework. (Students should possess a bachelor's degree and a GPA of above 3.0 to be competitive.)

The committee evaluates MCAT scores, paying special attention to the reading and quantitative analysis scores. The committee also assesses factors such as motivation to study osteopathic medicine and personal, social, and work experiences. The student's personal statement and letters of recommendation are important factors in the admissions process.

Undergraduate Preparation

To qualify for admission, the student must have completed 90 semester hours of coursework at an accredited college with one academic year each in English, physics, biology, general chemistry, and organic chemistry.

Costs

For the 1990-91 academic year, tuition for Illinois residents was $12,565 and for nonresidents was $16,115, plus a $185 activity fee. Residence hall housing is $265 per month; apartment housing is $345 per month.

Financial Aid

A large majority of students receive at least one type of student loan. Some students receive fellowships and scholarships. The college's office of financial aid helps qualified students obtain aid from a variety of programs, most of which are need-based. These aid programs include Stafford Student Loans, Health Education Assistance Loans, Perkins Loans, American Osteopathic Association Scholarships, the CCOM Scholarship Fund, and CCOM Alumni Association Loans.

Student Organizations

The student council is the principal liaison between the student body and the administration. There are many other student organizations on campus, including the Student Osteopathic Medical Association, the Undergraduate American Academy of Osteopathy, the National Osteopathic Women Physicians Association/American Medical Women's Association, and the CCOM sports medicine club. The college also has a student newspaper, the *Osteon.*

Curriculum

CCOM supports the holistic philosophy of osteopathic practice, which regards the body as an integrated whole with structures and functions working interdependently. CCOM has therefore developed a four-year curriculum that educates students in the biopsychosocial nature of patient care, as well as the basic medical arts and sciences.

The first two years of the program emphasize a rigorous basic sciences curriculum and preparation for clinical training. Basic courses include gross anatomy, biochemistry, osteopathic manipulative medicine, introduction to clinical medicine, physiology, psychiatry, and microbiology.

During the third and fourth years, students rotate through a variety of clinics, accruing 105 weeks of direct health care experience.

Facilities

The Downers Grove campus includes science buildings, laboratories, a state-of-the-art outpatient clinic, student housing, and a recreational center. Also on the Downers Grove campus is the Osteopathic Medical Center of DuPage, offering a variety of outpatient services. In Hyde Park, the college maintains the Chicago Osteopathic Medical Center, a 300-bed hospital with primary medical-surgical facilities, 34 specialty clinics, and various special services. The medical center is staffed by 230 D.O.s and M.D.s.

The college also maintains the Olympia Fields Osteopathic Medical Center, which serves nearly one-half million residents in south suburban Chicago. Technologies here include a trauma center, a catheterization laboratory, a surgical suite, numerous specialty clinics, programs ranging from sports medicine to geriatric care, and comprehensive instructional facilities.

CCOM also has an ambulatory care network comprising 25 clinics. The college library is designated as a resource library by the National Library of Medicine.

Grading Procedures

Grades for courses and clerkships are either pass/fail or numerical grades in which 75 percent or above will represent satisfactory performance.

Special Programs

The D.O./Ph.D. program is open to sophomore students in good academic standing; they may begin their combined studies in the junior year. The program is for students who are interested in academic medicine. Students pursue the doctoral degree at a leading area university.

Application Procedures

The college participates in AACOMAS. After reviewing the AACOMAS application, the college will send a second application to its applicants, requesting additional information. The student must complete the form and return it with a letter of evaluation from two faculty members or a letter of evaluation from a premedical advisory committee. A letter of recommendation from an osteopathic physician is optional.

The college's admissions committee may invite candidates for personal interviews. An initial tuition deposit of $250 must be made upon acceptance.

Contact

Chicago College of Osteopathic Medicine
Office of Admissions
555 Thirty-first Street
Downers Grove, Illinois 60515
(708) 515-6472
(800) 458-6253

COLLEGE OF OSTEOPATHIC MEDICINE OF THE PACIFIC

Pomona, California 91766
(714) 623-6116

Accreditation	AOA
Degrees Offered	M.S.H.P.E., D.O., B.S./D.O.
# Students Applied	Not Available
Enrollment	112 / class
Mean GPA	3.3
% Men / % Women	66% / 34%
% Minorities	21%
Tuition	$14,925
Application Fee	Contact School
Application Deadline	Contact School

The University

The College of Osteopathic Medicine of the Pacific (COMP), the only osteopathic medical school in the far west, is a fully accredited, independent, nonprofit, four-year medical college. The college was founded in 1977 in Pomona, California, population 120,000. Many colleges and universities as well as hospitals and clinics are located near the college. Pomona offers various cultural activities in a multi-ethnic community setting, and in the immediate vicinity can be found parks, golf courses, and a lake. Skiers, backpackers, and campers enjoy the San Gabriel Mountains to the north, and the Pacific Ocean is less than an hour away to the south and west.

Admissions

Students are selected on the basis of grades, test scores, work experiences, letters of recommendation, and interest in and proclivity for osteopathic medicine. Most candidates have earned at least a four-year degree with a GPA of 3.3 and MCAT score of 9. The new MCAT is required.

Undergraduate Preparation

Qualified candidates will have completed 90 semester hours or three-fourths of the credits necessary to earn a baccalaureate degree, including one academic year of English, biology, physics, organic chemistry, inorganic chemistry, and behavioral sciences.

Student Body

Many students at COMP have had careers in the health care field. A large number enter medical school immediately after receiving an undergraduate degree, although a significant number have earned credit towards or obtained graduate degrees. Of the 425 students enrolled, 34 percent are women, 21 percent are minorities, 39 percent are married, and 22 percent have children.

Costs

Annual tuition is $14,925. Additional costs include a $300 curriculum fee covering all instructional materials, a $100 mandatory student health fee, $600 for health insurance, a $30 student body fee for the first and second years ($10 for the third and fourth years), and $1,000 for a microscope. Independent students studying for a D.O. degree can expect to pay a total of $44,915 for their education while dependent students can expect to pay $27,340.

Financial Aid

Students applying for financial aid should submit a Student Aid Application for California (SAAC) to the College Scholarship Service. Many forms of financial aid are available including California State Graduate Fellowships, Western Interstate Commission on Higher Education (WICHE), Guaranteed Student Loans, college work study programs, and Military Service Commitment Scholarships, plus various college loans and scholarships. A booklet describing financial aid is available from the COMP financial aid office.

Student Organizations

Student organizations include student council, American College of General Practitioners, American Medical Students Association, American Medical Women's Association, Chicano/Latino Medical Student Association, Christian Medical Society, COMP-Physicians for Social Responsibility, National Osteopathic Women Physicians Association, emergency medicine club, Journal Club, osteopathic sports medicine club, SANUS (the world's only osteopathic theater troupe), Sigma Sigma Phi, student associate auxiliary, surgery club, and wellness club.

Faculty

There are 42 full-time faculty members and over 1,000 adjunct faculty. The student/faculty ratio is low.

Curriculum

The curriculum is divided into three phases. During Phase I, which occurs during the first semester of the freshman year,

students study anatomy, biochemistry, microbiology, pathology, pharmacology, physiology, osteopathic principles and practices, emergency medicine, medical ethics, and substance abuse. In Phase II, from second semester freshman year to sophomore year, classes are designed to integrate basic sciences with clinical practice. Phase III involves 22 clinical clerkships.

Facilities

The medical library houses 400 journals and 10,000 bound volumes and offers services which include an interlibrary loan system, MEDLINE computer-based access to biomedical literature, Index Medicus, the Upjohn Media Learning Center, and a computer learning center. COMPNET consists of four medical centers which serve as training facilities for COMP students.

Grading Procedures

The College of Osteopathic Medicine of the Pacific uses a four-point letter grade scale ranging from A, signifying excellence and having a grade-point value of 4, to D, signifying deficient but passing and having a grade-point value of 1. As a graduation requirement, the college requires that students take the entire Part I of the National Board Examination.

Special Programs

Disadvantaged students are eligible for a grant from the Health Careers Opportunity Program. Other special programs include the tutorial program and summer anatomy program.

Application Procedures

Applicants should submit an application to AACOMAS. Students whose applications have been screened will receive a supplementary application. This application, along with three letters of recommendation or a preprofessional committee evaluation should be submitted to the director of admissions for evaluation by the admissions committee within 30 days of receipt. Invitations for interviews will be determined based upon this information. Official transcripts should be sent to COMP by June 1.

Contact

College of Osteopathic Medicine of the Pacific
College Plaza
Pomona, California 91766
(714) 623-6116 ext. 207 or
(800) 447-COMP

UNIVERSITY OF HEALTH SCIENCES COLLEGE OF OSTEOPATHIC MEDICINE

2105 Independence Boulevard
Kansas City, Missouri 64124
(816) 283-2000

Accreditation	AOA
Degrees Offered	D.O.
# Students Applied	Not Available
Enrollment	130 / class
Mean GPA	3.04
% Men / % Women	70% / 30%
% Minorities	Not Available
Tuition	$13,990
Application Fee	Contact School
Application Deadline	Contact School

The University

The University of Health Sciences-College of Osteopathic Medicine is the second oldest College of Osteopathic Medicine in the country. It is a four-year medical school that awards the doctor of osteopathy degree. The university was founded as the Kansas City College of Osteopathy and Surgery in 1916. The following year the school was relocated, and in 1921 the university acquired the site where it is currently located, one mile east of downtown Kansas City. More than 5,000 physicians have graduated from the second oldest College of Osteopathic Medicine since it was founded over 70 years ago. The university is on a 35-acre campus in an urban center with a population of 1.6 million. Kansas City's economy is considered one of the top 10 in the United States.

Admissions

Students who have a baccalaureate degree are given admissions preference. Applicants are evaluated on the basis of scores on the new Medical College Admissions Test, grades, and grade point average taking into account the difficulty of the classes.

Undergraduate Preparation

Students applying for entrance into the College of Osteopathic Medicine should have a baccalaureate degree or have completed at least three-fourths of the credits necessary to obtain the degree. In addition, the following courses with laboratory should be completed: eight semester hours of general chemistry, eight semester hours of organic chemistry (specifically aliphatic and aromatic compounds), 12 semester credits of general biology, and eight semester credits of physics. Also required are six semester hours of English composition and literature. Students are expected to be proficient in the biological and physical sciences including comparative vertebrate anatomy, genetics, bacteriology, and should also have mathematics skills. Courses in sociology, philosophy, and psychology are considered helpful.

Student Body

Approximately 550 students representing almost every state in the country and several foreign countries are enrolled in UHS-COM. Women comprise about 30 percent of the student body.

Costs

Tuition, fees and expenses for 1990-91 include a $500 acceptance fee and $500 matriculation fee, both credited toward the tuition; a $13,990 tuition fee, which includes library privileges and laboratory supplies; a $35 activities fee; $1,000 for a microscope; $410 for books the first year plus $215 for lecture supplements and lab manuals; and $770 for instruments the first year. Book fees increase annually.

Financial Aid

Students should apply for financial aid through the office of student financial aid. A GAPSFAS form should be submitted. Among the many forms of financial aid available are the Health Professions Student Loan, Stafford Loan, Health Education Assistance Loan, Perkins Loan, college work-study program, Exceptional Financial Need Scholarship, Financial Assistance for Disadvantaged Health Professions Students, Service Obligation Scholarships, and Military and National Health Service Programs.

Student Organizations

Student organizations on campus include Alpha Phi Omega, American Academy of Osteopathy, American College of General Practitioners, American Osteopathic Academy of Sports Medicine, Christian Medical Society, Delta Omega, Iota Tau Sigma, Phi Sigma Gamma, Psi Sigma Alpha, Sigma Sigma Phi, Society for the Advancement of Osteopathic Medicine, student council, student associate auxiliary, and Student Osteopathic Medical Association.

Curriculum

The academic program for the first term consists of biochemistry, gross anatomy, embryology, histology, osteopathic principle and practice, physiology, neuroanatomy, and basic life support (CPR). The second-year program includes microbiology, human sexuality, osteopathic diagnosis and technique, pathology, pharmacology, psychiatry, medical ethics, gynecology, obstetrics, pediatrics, physical diagnosis, and clinical radiology. Third-year classes include clinical osteopathic medicine and therapeutics, electrocardiography, obstetrics, medicine (including dermatology and nutrition), otorhinolaryngology, pediatrics, surgery, cardiovascular medicine, clinical radiology, gerontology, medical jurisprudence, neurology, anesthesiology, emergency medicine, oncology, ophthalmology, medical office management, and advanced life support. Clinical services during the third year involve four rotations. Fourth-year students have 12 rotations, a family medicine preceptorship in a rural area, and advanced life support.

Facilities

Teaching facilities include the university library which houses a collection of more than 50,000 volumes and 140 periodicals. Services also offered by the library are Apple IIe computer floppy disc with self-instruction, two interlibrary loan systems, and MEDLINE, CANCERLIT, BIOETHICS, HEALTH, and TOXLINE health science databases. Northeast Medical Clinic and University Towers Medical Pavilion are medical teaching facilities. Students receive training during the clinical year at 18 affiliated teaching hospitals and 14 rural clinics.

Grading Procedures

Students are evaluated with a letter grading system: A (excellent, four grade points), B (good performance, three grade points), C (passing, two grade points), F (failure, no grade points). A student whose GPA falls below 2.0 is put on probation. Students who have an incomplete or F may not be promoted. D.O. candidates must pass Part I of the osteopathic national board examination.

Application Procedures

Applications should be filed with AACOMAS by March 1. Transcripts should also be sent to AACOMAS, while MCAT scores should be sent directly to the university. The university requests a recommendation from the premedical committee, or one premedical advisor and two senior science faculty members, and a personal reference preferably from an osteopathic physician. Letters from an employer and supervisor are requested from students who have been employed off campus. After March 1, students should apply directly to the university by sending a completed application, a $50 application fee, transcripts, letters of recommendation, and MCAT scores. Invitations for interviews are based on evaluation of these materials.

Contact

Office of Admissions
The University of Health Sciences
College of Osteopathic Medicine
2105 Independence Boulevard
Kansas City, Missouri 64124
(816) 283-2100

KIRKSVILLE COLLEGE OF OSTEOPATHIC MEDICINE

800 West Jefferson Street
Kirksville, Missouri 63501
(816) 626-2354

Accreditation	AOA
Degrees Offered	D.O.
# Students Applied	1,000
Enrollment	140 / class
Mean GPA	3.0
% Men / % Women	73% / 27%
% Minorities	11%
Tuition	$17,850
Application Fee	$25
Application Deadline	March 1

The University

Kirksville College of Osteopathic Medicine (KCOM) celebrates its 100th anniversary in 1992. The college was established by Andrew Taylor Still, the founder of osteopathic medicine. The objectives of the college include research and service programs as well as a strong tradition in promoting manipulative medicine. The college has a special commitment to family practice, rural health care, and gerontology.

The college is situated on a 50-acre campus in Kirksville, Missouri, a community of approximately 20,000.

Admissions

The college evaluates students based on a range of factors that includes motivation for the practice of osteopathy, preprofessional academic record, letters of recommendation, MCAT scores, and the results of a personal interview. At the time of application, students must have completed most of the required undergraduate courses. A minimum of 2.5 in the overall GPA, as well as in the science GPA, must be maintained to be considered for admission. Of the Fall 1990 entering class, 98 percent held a bachelor's degree, and the mean overall GPA was over 3.0.

Undergraduate Preparation

Applicants must have taken at least 90 semester hours of undergraduate coursework at an accredited college or university. A broad scholarly background is important. The required coursework includes one academic year (or equivalent) of English, biology (with lab), physics (with lab), inorganic chemistry (with lab), and organic chemistry (with lab). Other recommended coursework includes biochemistry, human anatomy, and comparative anatomy.

Applicants are advised to take the MCAT at least one year before the date of anticipated admission.

Student Body

In the 1989-90 academic year, total enrollment at the college was 532. Each year, the college admits approximately 140 new students. The student body is diverse, representing almost every state and several foreign countries.

Women make up about 27 percent of the student body and minorities comprise about 11 percent. The majority of the students hold a baccalaureate degree.

Placement Records

The college has approximately 5,000 alumni, many of whom have returned to their home towns across the nation to establish a practice. Kirksville alumni comprise a strong national support network.

Costs

Tuition for the 1991-92 academic year is $17,850.

Financial Aid

Sources of financial aid include the Health Professions Scholarship Program, Exceptional Financial Need Scholarships, and KCOM scholarships. Over 20 percent of the student body receive scholarships. There are five government loans available: Health Education Assistance Loan, Stafford Loan, Health Professions Student Loan, Perkins Loan, and Supplemental Loans for Students. Special loans exist for women, minorities, and rural students, awarded by the Robert Wood Johnson Foundation.

Student Organizations

The college hosts a wide variety of student groups, including the Student Government Association, undergraduate chapters of professional organizations, service clubs, religious groups, and social fraternities.

Curriculum

The four-year curriculum leads to the D.O. degree, focusing on the preparation of osteopathic physicians for family practice or further training in medical specialties. Osteopathic theory and methods are taught throughout the curriculum together with basic sciences and clinical coursework.

The first two years consist of training in the basic sciences with some introduction to clinical education. Patient care begins in the second year. The third year highlights clinical education. In the last 17 months of the program, students must complete at least 58 weeks of clinical training. Students train in affiliated hospitals and in a general practice setting. Students also participate in psychiatry and emergency medicine rotations and take at least 20 weeks of electives.

Facilities

The Kirksville Osteopathic Medical Complex is comprised of the college, the KCOM Gutensohn Health and Wellness Clinic, the Kirksville Osteopathic Medical Center, and Laughlin Pavilion, a psychiatric hospital and substance abuse treatment center. The college also has nine rural clinics throughout Missouri, and provides a specialized gerontology program through the Twin Pines Adult Care Center near the main campus.

The Medical Center is a 119-bed acute care hospital with a new $8.2 million diagnostic and treatment facility. There is also a new cancer treatment center.

There are about 19 hospitals affiliated with KCOM that are located throughout the country.

The A. T. Still Memorial Library is the oldest established osteopathic library. The library subscribes to over 840 biomedical journals and has over 62,900 volumes of books, reference works, and bound journals. The library has about 5,000 audiovisual titles and provides interlibrary loan services as well as access to MEDLINE.

Grading Procedures

Students are evaluated using percentage grades, except for certain courses that are designated for pass/fail evaluation. A grade of 70 percent or more is a "pass" grade.

Special Programs

The college offers graduates the opportunity to participate in a number of postdoctoral and special fellowships offered by agencies such as the National Institutes of Health and the National Osteopathic Foundation.

Application Procedures

The college participates in AACOMAS. College transcripts and MCAT scores should be forwarded to AACOMAS. After the college receives the AACOMAS application, a supplementary application will be sent to applicants. A $25 fee is due along with the return of this application.

Applications should be submitted by March 1 of the year before the year of intended enrollment. The college participates in an early decision program.

Contact

Kirksville College of Osteopathic Medicine
Office of Admissions
800 West Jefferson Street
Kirksville, Missouri 63501
(816) 626-2237

UNIVERSITY OF MEDICINE AND DENTISTRY OF NEW JERSEY SCHOOL OF OSTEOPATHIC MEDICINE

301 South Central Plaza
Stratford, New Jersey 08084-1504
(609) 757-7706

Accreditation	AOA
Degrees Offered	D.O.
# Students Applied	Not Available
Enrollment	56 / class
Mean GPA	3.3
% Men / % Women	64% / 36%
% Minorities	18%
Tuition	$10,457 In-State
	$13,723 Out-of-State
Application Fee	Contact School
Application Deadline	March 1

The University

The School of Osteopathic Medicine, a division of the University of Medicine and Dentistry in New Jersey (UMDNJ) was established in 1976. UMDNJ-SOM is located in southern New Jersey, within convenient driving distance of New York City and Philadelphia. The area offers nearby culture, sports, and entertainment—and thousands of acres of farmlands, parklands, waterways, and wildlife sanctuaries. The shoreline of New Jersey offers fun for all seasons. South Jersey boasts 24 acute care and specialty hospitals. The medical research programs at the school are renowned by the international scientific community.

Admissions

In-state applicants should have a minimum GPA of 2.75 in both science and nonscience courses; out-of-state candidates must have an overall and science average of at least 3.0 to be considered. The average GPA of all currently enrolled students is 3.3. A baccalaureate degree is required, and MCAT scores must be submitted. The average MCAT score of last year's entering class was 7. Preference is given to New Jersey residents.

Undergraduate Preparation

All candidates must have earned an undergraduate degree, with a well-rounded curriculum. The minimum requirements include: one year of behavioral science (psychology, sociology, or cultural anthropology); two years of biology including introductions to natural history, evolution, genetics, embryology, structure and function of animals; eight semester hours each of organic and inorganic chemistry (or a one-year course in each) with lab, including quantitative concepts and techniques; a college course in physics with lab, covering modern concepts of the atom, nuclear structure, and isotopes; one year of English including one semester of composition; and one year of college-level math. The college strongly recommends one full year of English writing, as well as courses in biochemistry and calculus.

Student Body

Of the total 1989-90 enrollment of 209, 36 percent are women, 18 percent are minorities, and 90 percent are residents of New Jersey. About 14 percent hold graduate degrees. The average age of students is 26.

Costs

Tuition for the 1988-89 school year was $10,457 for residents, and $13,723 for nonresidents. A refundable $50 deposit is required for lab equipment. Book costs may exceed $500 per year.

Financial Aid

Financial aid is available in many forms, including student loans, scholarships, and grants. For those who demonstrate need, there are programs such as the Guaranteed Student Loan, the Perkins Loan, the Health Education Assistance Loan, the Health Professions Student Loan, and the college work-study program. Supplemental Loans to Students are available.

Minority Programs

The dean's minority research associates program assists local minority students. The minority admissions subcommittee reviews all minority applications, schedules and conducts interviews, and makes recommendations for action. There is a special teaching program for first-year minority students.

Student Organizations

Besides a student government, the school offers such organizations as the Student Osteopathic Medical Association, the Undergraduate Academy of Osteopathy, and the Eastern Regional Osteopathic Convention Organizational Committee.

Faculty

There are 307 full-time, part-time, and volunteer faculty members.

Curriculum

The first two years of basic science concentrate on the study of anatomy, biochemistry, physiology, histology, cell biology, pathology, pharmacology, and neurosciences. Introduction to clinical medicine is also begun, with history taking and physical diagnosis. Psychiatry, emergency principles, infectious diseases, human sexuality, and family medicine are introduced in the second year. Unique osteopathic principles and practices courses include history of the profession and medicine in general, in-depth study of the American Osteopathic Association, ethical principles in medicine, specific principles and practices of osteopathic diagnosis and therapeutics. Throughout the first two years, clinical correlations are offered in all the disciplines. In the third year, the first clinical training programs begin. Included are clinical rotations in ambulatory family practice, general internal medicine, osteopathic sciences, surgery, obstetrics and gynecology, and pediatrics. In the fourth year, students serve clinical clerkships in internal medicine, surgery, pediatrics, family practice, obstetrics and gynecology, emergency medicine, and psychiatry.

Facilities

In September 1991, Stratford became the site of a unified campus of the UMDNJ-School of Osteopathic Medicine. A new 60,000-square-foot ambulatory health care center houses the ambulatory practice sites of the clinical faculty, the UMDNJ Health Sciences Library/Learning Resource Center, the Center for Health Promotion and Wellness, classrooms, and the admissions office.

Grading Procedures

As of 1986, UMDNJ-SOM uses a five-point grading system: honors, high pass, pass, low pass, fail.

Application Procedures

UMDNJ-SOM participates in AACOMAS; deadline for applications is March 1. MCAT scores from tests taken no later than the spring of application must be submitted, as well as a letter of recommendation from the candidate's undergraduate preprofessional committee (or, if no such committee exists, from two members of the science faculty). Deadline for these materials is April 15. A $25 application fee is payable when a student is notified of further consideration. Selected applicants are invited for interviews starting in October. New Jersey residents interested in early admissions to the school are advised to contact the admissions office.

Contact

UMDNJ-School of Osteopathic Medicine
Admissions Office, Suite 1600
301 South Central Plaza
Stratford, New Jersey 08084-1504
(609) 346-7050

MICHIGAN STATE UNIVERSITY COLLEGE OF OSTEOPATHIC MEDICINE

East Lansing, Michigan 48824
(517) 355-1855

Accreditation	AOA
Degrees Offered	D.O., Ph.D., D.O./Ph.D.
# Students Applied	Not Available
Enrollment	104 / class
Mean GPA	3.2
% Men / % Women	60% / 40%
% Minorities	15%
Tuition	$7,086 In-State
	$15,282 Out-of-State
Application Fee	Contact School
Application Deadline	January 1

The University

Michigan State University (MSU) was founded in 1855 and is today one of the most extensive centers of higher education and research in the country. The 5,300-acre East Lansing campus hosts more than 42,500 students from all 50 states and 106 foreign countries. MSU is widely recognized as a leading public institution in many areas, hosting more Rhodes Scholars than any other public institution today and producing a competitive number of winners of National Science Foundation Graduate Fellowships.

The College of Osteopathic Medicine (MSU-COM) was the first state-assisted, university-based school of its kind. It was originally established as a private school, and later became part of the university by an act of the state legislature. The college enrolled its first class in 1971.

MSU-COM is part of the university's biomedical complex, which also comprises the colleges of veterinary medicine, human medicine, and nursing.

More osteopathic physicians are licensed in Michigan than in any other state, constituting about one-fifth of the state's practicing physicians.

Admissions

Candidates for admission are evaluated on the basis of undergraduate GPA, any graduate GPA available, and the MCAT score. Over the past five years, entering GPAs have averaged well above 3.0. For the 1990 entering class, the mean GPA was 3.2 and the mean MCAT was 7.0. Applicants are considered on the basis of their ability to meet the emotional, social, and physical needs of others through experience in human services activities, extracurricular activities, and any past involvement in research. Recommendations, commitment to the osteopathic profession, and the results of a personal interview are important factors in the admissions process.

A typical applicant pool consists of about 80 to 90 percent Michigan residents. Ultimately, about 20 out-of-state residents will be admitted.

Undergraduate Preparation

Applicants should have a background in the natural, social, and behavioral sciences and the humanities. While completion of at least 90 semester hours (three years) of college or university courses is mandatory, virtually all students admitted to the college will have earned their baccalaureate degree by the time of enrollment. Preference is given to students who have completed their preprofessional course of study by the time of application.

Preprofessional course requirements include completion of eight semester or 12 term credits including lecture and lab, with at least a 2.0 average, in biology, inorganic chemistry, organic chemistry, and physics. Requirements also include completion of six semester or nine term credits, with at least a 2.0 average, in English and in the psychosocial/behavioral sciences.

The MCAT must be taken by the fall of the year application is being made.

Student Body

The 1990 entering class had 79 men and 53 women. There were 18 Asian Americans, four Blacks, and two Hispanics. The average age was 25 years. The college has consistently maintained the highest ratios of both ethnic minority students (about 15 percent) and women (about 40 percent) of all osteopathic colleges.

Placement Records

More than two-thirds of those who have graduated from MSU-COM are currently practicing or training in primary care. The remainder of the graduates are working in specialties ranging from anesthesiology to public health and preventive medicine, from nephrology to neurosurgery.

Costs

In-state tuition and fees for the 1990 entering class are $7,086 for the first and fourth years, and $9,448 for the second and third years. Nonresident tuition is $15,282 for the first and fourth years and $21,376 for the second and third years. Costs can increase markedly, however, within a single year. Books and instruments range from $1,200 to $1,600 for the first two years. Rent (with utilities) ranges from $325 to $400 per month. Average total annual costs for four years for residents is $19,840; for nonresidents, $29,400. All students should anticipate the need for a car for clinical experiences in the second year, and should also plan for the possibility of relocating outside the Lansing area at the beginning of the third year.

Financial Aid

Most students who finance their education at MSU-COM use state, federal, and private financial aid programs. Few receive grants or scholarships. About one-tenth are on military or public health scholarships.

Faculty

In addition to full-time faculty, students receive clinical education from more than 600 volunteer physicians in community hospitals, ambulatory care sites, and physicians' offices throughout Michigan.

Curriculum

MSU-COM provides an academic program that assists students with the integration of basic science, behavioral science, and clinical science concepts related to the tenets of osteopathic philosophy. The curriculum provides students with comprehensive medical knowledge and skills, and prepares them to enter either general practice or to pursue further training related to a medical specialty.

The first year introduces the student to basic medical sciences along with basic osteopathic clinical skills. The student will study the basic body systems, including the musculoskeletal system, as well as the behavioral sciences, and will go on to participate in clinical preceptorships in the latter half of the curriculum.

The last 60 weeks of the program consists of required and elective clinical clerkships scheduled in college-affiliated hospitals, clinics, or family practitioners' offices.

Facilities

The Clinical Center was the first health care facility at MSU to offer complete outpatient services to the public. The center comprises ambulatory care facilities, a clinical laboratory, specialty diagnostic and treatment areas, a surgical suite, medical library, classrooms, and a lecture hall. Other campus medical units include the life sciences building, the veterinary clinical center, and the Olin health center for student health care. Faculty in the basic sciences are located in research facilities throughout campus.

Clinical training is conducted in communities across the state—in affiliated hospitals, in the offices of nearly 600 volunteer clinical faculty, and in a number of ambulatory care clinics administered and staffed by the college.

Other facilities on the MSU campus include a planetarium and observatory, botanical gardens, libraries, a museum, a daily newspaper, an art center gallery, theater, stadium, gymnasium, golf courses, swimming pools, baseball diamonds, tennis courts, an outdoor track, soccer fields, and an ice arena.

Special Programs

MSU-COM was the first among the nation's osteopathic schools to pilot a Medical Scientist Training Program, which grants the D.O./Ph.D. joint degree. Students in the program are highly motivated and have outstanding research and academic qualifications. Graduates are proficient in investigative research as well as clinical medicine. Students must be accepted separately to the medical school and graduate program.

Certain departments of the college offer either the M.S. or the Ph.D. independently in several of the science and health care fields.

MSU-COM also offers individualized programs in postdoctoral research training for students wishing to pursue careers in biomedical research.

Application Procedures

MSU-COM participates in AACOMAS. Applications must be filed with AACOMAS by January 1 of the year of entry; early application is strongly recommended. All official transcripts should be received by AACOMAS by January 15. Those who pass an initial screening will be sent a secondary application from the college, to be completed by the date specified.

Interviews are conducted in fall and early winter, and selection of admitted and alternate students is completed by mid-March. Approximately 250-300 candidates will be invited to interview for 125 seats.

Contact

MSU College of Osteopathic Medicine
Office of Admissions
C110 East Fee Hall
East Lansing, Michigan 48824-1316
(517) 353-7740

UNIVERSITY OF NEW ENGLAND COLLEGE OF OSTEOPATHIC MEDICINE

11 Hills Beach Road
Biddeford, Maine 04005
(207) 283-0171, ext. 212

Accreditation	AOA
Degrees Offered	D.O.
# Students Applied	1,300
Enrollment	100 / class
Mean GPA	3.0
% Men / % Women	Not Available
% Minorities	Not Available
Tuition	$16,690
Application Fee	$55
Application Deadline	March 1

The University

The University of New England was formed in 1978 when UNE's predecessor, St. Francis College, merged with New England's only College of Osteopathic Medicine. The 122-acre campus is located in Biddeford, Maine, on the Atlantic coastline.

The College of Osteopathic Medicine was established in the 1970s to serve the six New England states with osteopathic services. The school opened its doors in 1978 with its first class of 36 students.

Biddeford is a small city near Saco, Old Orchard Beach, and Kennebunk. The surrounding area is commercially undeveloped and is primarily a summer resort area. Portland, Maine's largest city, is a 20-minute drive from Biddeford.

Admissions

Factors considered in the admissions process include demonstrated scholastic ability and motivation to practice osteopathic medicine in New England. Personal qualities are also taken into account, including personality, emotional stability, maturity, breadth of background, work experience, extracurricular involvements, and sense of responsibility. All applicants must take the MCAT.

Undergraduate Preparation

The college seeks students who are broadly educated both in the humanities and sciences. Applicants must have had a minimum of 90 semester hours toward the bachelor's degree from an accredited college or university. The cumulative GPA must be 2.5 or better in both elective and required subjects.

Prerequisite courses for admission are one year of English composition and literature; eight semester hours of general chemistry; eight semester hours of organic chemistry; eight semester hours of physics; and eight semester hours of biology. Students should have taken labs with the science courses, and are encouraged to enroll in additional science and math courses.

Costs

1991-92 tuition is $8,345 per semester ($16,690 for the spring and fall semesters together). The microscope rental fee (first year only) is $125. The general services fee is $200. Students must have health insurance; the UNE medical plan costs $290 for 12 months of coverage.

Financial Aid

Financial assistance is available through a number of programs, including the Auxiliary to the American Osteopathic Association awards, Exceptional Financial Need Scholarships for Health Professions Students, Maine Osteopathic Association Scholarships, Health Education Assistance Loans, Stafford Student Loans, Maine Osteopathic Loan Fund, and Perkins Loans.

Detailed information can be obtained from the university's office of graduate financial aid.

Student Organizations

In addition to the student government association, the college has a number of professional clubs and organizations for students. These include the sports medicine club, the American Academic of Osteopathy, and the local chapter of the Student Osteopathic Medical Association. Sigma Sigma Phi, a national osteopathic honor society, maintains a chapter on campus.

Curriculum

Both the didactic curriculum and the clinical training programs of the curriculum emphasize the knowledge and skills basic to osteopathic general practice. The basic and clinical science foundation is augmented by a strong program in human behavior and community medicine.

The curriculum is divided into three sections: on-campus basic and clinical sciences curriculum, preceptee training curriculum, and clerkship training curriculum.

Students have the opportunity to participate in a first-year preceptorship, where they can experience the complexities of the patient/physician relationship in the office of a practicing physician.

Throughout the community medicine program, the student learns how to work as an integral part of the health care team, and becomes familiar with the wide range of community health needs and corresponding services.

Clinical clerkships are taken during the final one and one-half years of the curriculum. Required and elective clerkships are taken in a variety of affiliated hospitals, ambulatory care sites, and other clinical settings.

Facilities

Facilities include Stella Maris Hall, which houses laboratories and classrooms, and a multimillion dollar recreational facility.

The college maintains a variety of clinical affiliations for student training and practice. The college-operated university health service centers have been established as model family practice clinics. For ambulatory-based programs, the college uses the offices of clinical faculty members located throughout New England as well as a number of community health programs.

The Jack S. Ketchum Library houses over 86,000 volumes and subscribes to more than 600 journals. Literature searching, interlibrary loan, and MEDLINE are available.

Grading Procedures

The college uses numerical grades, letter grades, or pass/fail grades. Cumulative averages and class rank are determined using all numerical grades on the transcript.

Application Procedures

The college participates in AACOMAS, which collects materials and submits admissions information to the college. Official transcripts and MCAT scores should be submitted to AACOMAS (the MCAT must be taken no later than September of the calendar year prior to the desired year of enrollment).

The college will review the AACOMAS materials and ask qualified applicants to submit secondary information to the college along with a $55 application fee. This information should include recommendations from two faculty members and a recommendation from another professional person. A recommendation from one or more osteopathic physicians is strongly advised as well.

The college reviews and interviews students on a rolling basis beginning in the fall. Early application is strongly recommended.

Contact

University of New England
College of Osteopathic Medicine
11 Hills Beach Road
Biddeford, Maine 04005
(207) 283-0171

NEW YORK INSTITUTE OF TECHNOLOGY
NEW YORK COLLEGE OF OSTEOPATHIC MEDICINE

Old Westbury, New York 11568
(516) 626-6922

Accreditation	AOA
Degrees Offered	D.O., B.S./D.O.
# Students Applied	Not Available
Enrollment	150 / class
Mean GPA	2.75
% Men / % Women	65% / 35%
% Minorities	24%
Tuition	$13,500
Application Fee	$60
Application Deadline	March 1

The University

The New York College of Osteopathic Medicine (NYCOM) is the first school of osteopathic medicine in New York State. The school is located on the campus of the New York Institute of Technology, approximately 25 miles east of New York City. Located in a suburban Long Island community, it offers students the opportunity to serve in rural, suburban, and urban facilities.

Admissions

When considering an applicant for admission, academic records, MCAT scores, letters of references and extracurricular health-related activities are evaluated. The candidate must have earned a minimum overall GPA of 2.75 and a minimum science GPA of 2.5.

Undergraduate Preparation

Applicants must have completed a bachelors degree, or at least 90 semester hours (30 semester hours at the baccalaureate level) of college work at an accredited institution. At least one academic year sequence of the following courses must be completed: biology (including a basic course in general biology or zoology); English (composition is preferred); general chemistry; organic chemistry; and physics. Labs are required for the science courses. Applicants must have earned at least a C (2.0) in each required course. The study of physical chemistry, behavioral sciences, calculus, comparative anatomy, and English is encouraged.

Placement Records

Over 70 percent of graduating interns choose residency programs in the primary care specialties of family practice, pediatrics, internal medicine, and obstetrics/gynecology.

Costs

Tuition for first-year students amounts to $13,500. Student fees amount to $240.

Financial Aid

Financial aid is available from a variety of federal, state, and private offices. To receive aid, students must be in good standing with the college, have satisfactory academic progress, and have demonstrated financial need. Students must complete the Graduate and Professional School Financial Aid Service (GAPSFAS) form to begin the financial aid process.

Faculty

There are approximately 325 full- and part-time faculty members. Faculty members teach in the classroom and serve as instructors at affiliated and cooperating hospitals, and in the preceptorship program. All faculty members possess either the D.O., M.D., or Ph.D. degree.

Curriculum

Emphasis is placed on needs and opportunities in primary health care and community health services. The first two years of coursework consist of the study of basic and clinical sciences as well as osteopathic principles and practice. During the second year, the emphasis is more on the clinical sciences and the study of organ systems. Students rotate through the family health care center, located on campus, to learn how to perform patient history and physical examinations. Other courses include community medicine, dermatology, radiology, rehabilitation medicine, and surgery. The third year includes clinical rotations in medicine and surgery, obstetrics and gynecology, pediatrics, psychiatry, and family practice. Clinical rotations are offered at 24 training facilities in New York, New Jersey, Florida, and Pennsylvania. There is also an optional third-year rural clinical program. The fourth year consists of a series of four-week rotations and a six-week required rotation in emergency medicine. Students must choose three rotations in medicine from a list of 12 approved specialty fields, and one rotation in one of nine surgical areas. Two ambulatory rotations are offered. Students may also choose two elective rotations.

Facilities

The college is housed in two buildings, the Nelson A. Rockefeller Academic Center and the Academic Health Care Center. The Rockefeller Academic Center contains a multilevel library with an extensive collection of texts, journals, and audiovisual aids. The biomechanics laboratory uses the Vicon data analysis system to address the problems of musculoskeletal injuries in industry. The health care center contains a family health care center for research and evaluation in patient care. The W. Kenneth Ritand Institute of Neuro-Muscular Disorders is an anatomy laboratory for instruction, administrative, and faculty offices. Many hospitals are affiliated with the college, providing over 75 percent of the clinical rotations taken by students. On-campus housing is not available.

Special Programs

The college and the institute offer a combined seven-year B.S./D.O. degree. Allied health professionals (nurses, physician's assistants, and emergency medical technicians) may enroll in the college through the upward mobility plan.

Application Procedures

The college participates in the American Association of Colleges of Osteopathic Medicine Application Service (AACOMAS). Applications must be submitted by March 1 of the year of planned enrollment. Interviews are arranged with selected applicants, at which time a supplemental application must be completed, and a $60 application fee must be paid. Letters of reference are required and should include an osteopathic physician's recommendation. The MCAT is required. Acceptances are issued on a rolling basis.

Contact

Director of Admissions
New York College of Osteopathic Medicine
New York Institute of Technology
Old Westbury, New York 11568
(516) 626-6947

OHIO UNIVERSITY COLLEGE OF OSTEOPATHIC MEDICINE

102 Grosvenor Hall
Athens, Ohio 45701
(614) 593-1800

Accreditation	AOA
Degrees Offered	D.O.
# Students Applied	1,900
Enrollment	100 / class
Mean GPA	3.2
% Men / % Women	68% / 32%
% Minorities	17%
Tuition	$5,593 In-State
	$8,352 Out-of-State
Application Fee	$25
Application Deadline	January 15

The University

Founded in 1806, Ohio University is the oldest state-sponsored university west of the Allegheny Mountains. Total enrollment is about 23,000 with enrollment on the Athens campus at more than 16,000. Graduate enrollment is 2,700, including nearly 400 osteopathic students. There are over 700 full-time faculty members, more than 200 part-time faculty, and almost 900 graduate associates, graduate research associates, and graduate teaching associates.

Admissions

In order to be eligible for admission, applicants must meet the minimum requirements by June of the year of application. Possession of a bachelor's degree is preferred, although applicants with at least 90 semester hours of exceptional work at a regionally accredited college or university may be considered. U.S. citizenship or a permanent resident visa is required. According to state law, at least 80 percent of the entering class must be Ohio residents or agree to practice medicine in Ohio for five years after completing medical school. Other admissions criteria include superior academic performance, concern for human life, interest in osteopathic medicine, and ethics.

Undergraduate Preparation

Undergraduates are required to have completed six semester hours in English, eight semester hours in biology, eight semester hours in general chemistry, eight semester hours in physics, eight semester hours in organic chemistry (with one or two courses in biochemistry recommended), and six semester hours in behavioral sciences—all with a grade of C or above, by August of the year of application.

Student Body

For the entering class of 1990, 64 percent maintained residency in Ohio while 36 percent were out-of-state residents. Sixty-eight percent were males and 32 percent females. Minority students comprised 17 percent of the class with nine percent African Americans, two percent Hispanic, five percent Asians or Pacific Islanders, and one percent Native Americans. Eighty-five percent had undergraduate degrees in science and 13 percent had graduate degrees. Ages ranged between 21 and 44, with an average age of 25.

Placement Records

Sixty percent of OU-COM graduates practice family medicine while 69 percent provide primary care. Almost 50 percent have settled in communities with a population of less than 50,000.

Costs

Tuition for residents is $5,593 and $8,352 for nonresidents.

Financial Aid

More than 80 percent of the students attending the College of Osteopathic Medicine receive financial aid. Aid is available in the form of various scholarships and loans. Most of the scholarships require applicants to complete a GAPSFAS, submit information on their parents' financial status, complete an OU-COM application and apply by February 15. The scholarships are awarded by the College of Medicine largely based upon funding. Most loans also require applicants to submit a GAPSFAS form and an OU-COM application with half requesting information on the parents' financial status. The deadline for most is February 15. The College of Medicine awards at least half of the loans. The largest loan available is $20,000 maximum from the Health Education Assistance Loan.

Student Organizations

The student council serves as the representative organization for the American Medical Student Association, the American Medical Women's Association, the American Academy of Osteopathy, the American Osteopathic Association, the Atlas club, the Christian Medical Society, the emergency medicine club, the family practice club, the Ohio Osteopathic Association, Sigma Sigma Phi, the sports medicine club, the student associate auxiliary, the Student Osteopathic Medical Association, and the yearbook.

Faculty

The medical school faculty numbers more than 70 in Athens while 400 part-time faculty members teach in the Regional Teaching Centers all over Ohio. Specialties among the clinical staff include surgery, emergency medicine, radiology, ophthalmology, and obstetrics and gynecology.

Curriculum

The curriculum is divided into four phases. Phases I and II take place in Athens. During Phase I, students study medical biochemistry, gross anatomy, microanatomy, physiology, microbiology, immunology, pharmacology, metabolism, hematology, pathology, and the fundamentals of osteopathic medicine. Phase II begins during the first quarter of the second year and focuses on history and physical examination skills, osteopathic practices and principles, psychosocial awareness, public health and preventative medicine, professionalism and the history of medicine, medical jurisprudence, emergency medicine, and geriatrics. Phase III begins the clinical portion of study at one of seven regional teaching centers (RTCs). Phase IV, beginning in January and lasting 17 months, features rotations in internal medicine, pediatrics, obstetrics and gynecology, general surgery and anesthesiology, orthopedic surgery (hospital and ambulatory), otorhinolaryngology, emergency medicine, laboratory medicine and radiology, and geriatrics in a hospital setting. Students also choose electives and attend case conferences one half-day every week in an RTC as well as occasional clinical case conferences.

Facilities

Dayton, Columbus, Cleveland, Toledo, Massillon, and Youngstown are home to the six regional teaching centers, which have a combined capacity of almost 5,000 beds. The Osteopathic Medical Center, located on campus, served 87,746 patients in one year. Ohio University's recreational facilities include a gymnasium, an indoor ice skating ring, tennis courts, a new aquatic center that features a 50-meter indoor pool, and various other athletic fields.

Grading Procedures

The College of Medicine uses a four-letter scale of A, B, C, or F. Grades of I (incomplete) or PR (progress) are assigned for incomplete coursework. Pass or fail grades are given by the clinical instructor during Phase IV. To graduate, students must pass Part I of the national osteopathic boards and take Part II.

Application Procedures

Because the college participates in AACOMAS, applicants should obtain an application request card from the college or directly from AACOMAS. The application should be sent by January 15 and, once the application has been reviewed, the college may ask for supplemental information, which should be submitted along with a $25 application fee by February 15.

Contact
Admissions
102 Grosvenor Hall
College of Osteopathic Medicine
Ohio University
Athens, Ohio 45701
(800) 345-1440 (In-State)
(800) 345-1560 (Out-of-State)

OKLAHOMA STATE UNIVERSITY SCHOOL OF OSTEOPATHIC MEDICINE

1111 West 17th Street
Tulsa, Oklahoma 74107
(918) 582-1972

Accreditation	AOA
Degrees Offered	D.O.
# Students Applied	691
Enrollment	88 / class
Mean GPA	3.2
% Men / % Women	75% / 25%
% Minorities	15%
Tuition	$5,240 In-State
	$12,710 Out-of-State
Application Fee	Contact School
Application Deadline	April 1

The University

Oklahoma State University has four campuses and a total enrollment of about 26,000 students. As a large university, OSU offers a 1.5 million-volume library, modern research laboratories, excellent recreational facilities, and a wide variety of cultural events.

The College of Osteopathic Medicine was founded in 1972 and became part of Oklahoma State University in 1988. It serves the medical needs of residents of Oklahoma, Arkansas, Louisiana, New Mexico, Colorado, Kansas, and southwest Missouri. The 16-acre campus is located on the west bank of the Arkansas River, minutes from downtown Tulsa.

Admissions

Strong preference is given to residents of Oklahoma and the regional service area (Arkansas, Louisiana, New Mexico, Colorado, Kansas, and southwest Missouri). Applicants must have an overall GPA of at least 3.0, a preprofessional science GPA of at least 2.75, and a minimum score of 7.0 on the MCAT. Under special circumstances, the college may admit students who do not meet these minimum requirements. Those who have experienced unequal educational opportunities for social, cultural, or racial reasons are encouraged to apply. Applicants must be U.S. citizens or have obtained permanent resident status.

Undergraduate Preparation

Applicants must have completed at least three years (90 semester hours) and not less than 75 percent of the courses required for the bachelor's degree at a regionally accredited college or university at the time of enrollment. Completion of a full academic year sequence of the following courses (including necessary laboratory work in the science courses) is required: English, biology, general chemistry, organic chemistry, and physics. Applicants should have earned grades above a C (2.0) in all required courses, and must have completed at least one of the following undergraduate courses: biochemistry, comparative anatomy, embryology, microbiology, or histology.

Placement Records

The physician placement officer offers graduates assistance in setting up a practice following internship and residency training.

Costs

Tuition fees for Oklahoma residents amount to $5,240 per year. Tuition fees for nonresidents amount to $12,710 per year.

Financial Aid

Financial aid options include loans, scholarships, grants, work-study programs, and return service agreements.

Student Organizations

Student organizations on campus include the American College of General Practitioners-undergraduate chapter, the Christian Medical Society, Delta Omega, Osteopathic Sports Medicine Society, Sigma Phi, Society for the Advancement of Osteopathic Medicine, Student National Medical Association, Student Osteopathic Medical Association, and the Undergraduate American Academy of Osteopathy.

Curriculum

The curriculum emphasizes general practice. A coordinated spiraling systems approach is used, through which subject matter is continuously reintroduced in greater depth and complexity. The first year includes the basic sciences and preliminary clinical concepts. The next three semesters emphasize the interdisciplinary study of the structure and function of body systems. Students are also introduced to specialized clinical care and medical procedures related to each body system.

The final 16 months are devoted exclusively to clinical rotations. Students work under the supervision of faculty members, rotating through basic hospital services, and spend a few weeks at a small rural hospital, major urban hospital, primary care clinic, psychiatric facility, community health facility, office of a private physician, and one elective location.

Facilities

The college campus is a modern, three-building complex, located on the west bank of the Arkansas River, a short distance away from downtown Tulsa. The College Clinic is a health care resource for residents of the west Tulsa area as well as a teaching clinic for medical students. It is staffed by licensed osteopathic physicians who supervise students in the care of patients. Other institutions affiliated with the college include: Tulsa Regional Medical Center (533 beds); Dallas/Fort-Worth Medical Center (377 beds); Coffeyville Regional Medical Center, Enid Memorial Hospital; Riverside Hospital; and Paul Valley General Hospital.

Application Procedures

The college participates in the American Association of Colleges of Osteopathic Medicine Application Service (AACOMAS). The annual application deadline is April 1 of the year of entry. The MCAT is required, and should be taken in the spring prior to application. Fall scores are acceptable. All applicants from Oklahoma and the regional service area who meet the necessary requirements will be invited to an on-campus interview. Well-qualified applicants from outside the region will also be invited for an interview. The interview is required for admission.

Contact

College of Osteopathic Medicine
Oklahoma State University
1111 West 17th Street
Tulsa, Oklahoma 74107
(918) 582-1972
(800) 256-1972 (Toll-free in Oklahoma)

UNIVERSITY OF OSTEOPATHIC MEDICINE AND HEALTH SCIENCES COLLEGE OF OSTEOPATHIC MEDICINE AND SURGERY

3200 Grand Avenue
Des Moines, Iowa 50312
(515) 271-1400

Accreditation	AOA, CIHE
Degrees Offered	D.O.
# Students Applied	1,400
Enrollment	190 / class
Mean GPA	3.19
% Men / % Women	62% / 38%
% Minorities	11%
Tuition	$16,775
Application Fee	$45
Application Deadline	February 1

The University

The University of Osteopathic Medicine was founded in 1898 as the Dr. S. S. Still College of Osteopathy. The school's name has changed several times in its history, and the program of study has greatly expanded from the original two-year format. Since the college moved to its current 22-acre site in Des Moines, enrollment has more than doubled. Its current total enrollment makes it the second largest osteopathic medical college in America today. In 1987 the university opened an on-campus medical center, which operates as a regional referral center for osteopathic physicians. The university is accredited by the Commission of Institutions of Higher Education of the North Central Association of Colleges and Schools. The campus is centrally located in Des Moines near housing, restaurants, places of worship, and several cultural centers.

Admissions

The admissions committee of the College of Osteopathic Medicine and Surgery (COMS) bases its decisions on a candidate's academic achievements, activities, personality, motivation, and future promise. A diversified undergraduate academic background is helpful in developing the kinds of thinking and communications skills necessary for a successful osteopathic physician, and is viewed favorably by the admissions committee. Exceptional students may be admitted to COMS after completing 75 percent of the requirements toward an undergraduate degree; however, more than 95 percent of students admitted have attained a baccalaureate degree. A minimum overall GPA of 2.5 is required. Applicants must submit MCAT scores.

Undergraduate Preparation

Applicants must have attained a minimum grade of C in all required courses, which are: eight semester hours each of general biology, inorganic and organic chemistry, and physics—all with laboratory—and six semester hours in English composition, communication, or language arts. No more than four semester hours of biology/zoology may be taken in botany. Courses in biochemistry, genetics, comparative anatomy, mathematics, general psychology, and English literature are recommended.

Placement Records

Twelve-month internships at an osteopathic hospital can be secured only by participating in the intern match program (IMP) of the American Osteopathic Association.

Costs

Annual tuition for the College of Osteopathic Medicine and Surgery is $15,360. A first-year student should allot $2,500 for books, instruments, and supplies.

Facilities

An 82,000-square-foot academic center contains lecture halls, a library, a biomedical communications department, art museum, lounges, bookstore, and administrative offices. The Tower Medical Clinic on campus offers primary care, medical specialties, and ambulatory surgery facilities for complete diagnostic and therapeutic care of Iowa residents. The university medical library houses more than 28,000 books and bound periodicals and subscribes to more than 500 medical and scientific newsletters and journals. Students have access to six microcomputers; the library also provides access to MEDLINE and other on-line databases. The State Medical Library in Des Moines is open to university students. The university operates seven clinics within a 50-mile radius of Des Moines. The school maintains a minimal number of student housing units, but off-campus housing is readily available.

Grading Procedures

Courses are graded on a pass/fail basis.

Special Programs

For those with a doctoral degree in basic sciences or certain health professions, the university offers an accelerated, 36 month medical education program that leads to the D.O. degree. Applicants to this graduate professional education program (GREP) should have at least three years of postdoctoral experience through an internship, residency, fellowship, academic research, or employment.

Contact

Admissions Office
University of Osteopathic Medicine and Health Sciences
College of Osteopathic Medicine and Surgery
3200 Grand Avenue
Des Moines, Iowa 50312
(515) 271-1400

PHILADELPHIA COLLEGE OF OSTEOPATHIC MEDICINE

4150 City Avenue
Philadelphia, Pennsylvania 19131-1696
(215) 871-1000

Accreditation	AOA
Degrees Offered	D.O., M.Sc., D.O./M.B.A., D.O./M.P.H.
# Students Applied	1,200
Enrollment	200 / class
Mean GPA	3.1
% Men / % Women	63% / 37%
% Minorities	9.9%
Tuition	$15,078 In-State
	$15,467 Out-of-State
Application Fee	$50
Application Deadline	March 1

The University

The Philadelphia College of Osteopathic Medicine (PCOM) was chartered in 1899 and has graduated more than 7,600 physicians. It has grown steadily to become the hub of an educational/health care complex. PCOM today forms the heart of the Osteopathic Medical Center of Philadelphia.

The mission of the college is to provide programs of instruction and training in the art, science, and practice of osteopathic medicine in accordance with the osteopathic concept of etiology, diagnosis, prevention, and treatment. Emphasis is placed on training physicians for primary care practice.

PCOM is the second largest medical school in Pennsylvania, the largest of the 15 osteopathic colleges, and is accredited by the American Osteopathic Association.

Admissions

Admission is competitive and selective. MCAT scores and the GPA are reviewed. Admission is also based on fulfillment of undergraduate course requirements. PCOM seeks well-rounded, achievement-oriented students, and students demonstrating breadth of education, quality of character, and dedication to service.

Undergraduate Preparation

The school seeks students with a strong liberal arts background that will complement an education in the sciences. A bachelor's degree is required for admission. The following courses are prerequisites for admission: at least eight semester hours each of biology, inorganic chemistry, organic chemistry, and physics, and at least six semester hours of English. A minimum of two hours of the required eight semester hours of each of the science courses must be laboratory work.

Student Body

PCOM is the largest of the osteopathic colleges, with a student enrollment of 826. Seventy percent of the student body is composed of Pennsylvania residents, and the remainder represent 20 states of the union. Women comprise about 37 percent of the most recent entering class. More than 200 undergraduate colleges are represented in the student body.

Placement Records

About 80 percent of PCOM's graduates enter primary care practice.

Costs

For the 1990-91 academic year, Pennsylvania residents pay tuition of $15,078 and nonresidents pay $15,467. The annual equipment usage fee for first- and second-year students is $100.

Financial Aid

PCOM helps students assemble a financial aid package and offers financial planning seminars. Upon acceptance to the college, students are advised to contact the office of financial aid as soon as possible, where information and application forms are available. The college offers loans, scholarships, and student employment opportunities. These include Auxiliary to the American Osteopathic Association awards (open to sophomores), American Osteopathic Association/National Osteopathic Foundation Loans (available to third and fourth year students), PCOM Alumni Loans, Stafford Loans, and Health Education Assistance Loans.

Minority Programs

The college organizes an annual conference for minority undergraduate students and an annual awards dinner honoring the contributions of minority physicians. The college's Summer Start program is offered to minority students accepted for admission, and two Ethel Allen memorial scholarships are given annually to first-year minority women students.

Student Organizations

In addition to the student council, the college has numerous professional and social societies for students. These include the Student Osteopathic Medical Association, a chapter of the Academy of Applied Osteopathy, the Pennsylvania Osteopathic Medical Association, the surgery club, the neuropsychiatry club, the Student National Medical Society, and Physicians for Social Responsibility. Also represented are Phi Sigma Gamma and Lambda Omicron Gamma fraternities.

Faculty

The faculty comprises a highly qualified body of certified or board-eligible osteopathic physicians and scientists. PCOM has a faculty of 233 based at its Philadelphia campuses, among whom are 206 D.O.s and 27 Ph.D.s. In addition, the academic program is served by hundreds of practicing physicians across the country who provide clinical instruction at various affiliated sites as volunteers.

Curriculum

PCOM emphasizes the basics to prepare students for the practice of medicine in the next century, and is supported by the best modern technology. Students are trained to treat the whole person and to understand the importance of the neuro-musculoskeletal system to health and well-being. The curriculum also provides extensive opportunities for students to explore the specialty disciplines.

The first two years focus on basic sciences complemented by courses in bioethics, human sexuality, medical law, and medical economics. Early clinical courses are also introduced at this time, as well as the opportunity to provide care to geriatric patients as a special ongoing experience beginning in the first year of study.

The last two years of study consist of clinical rotations throughout Pennsylvania and neighboring states. This phase of study is designed to afford progressive student responsibility for all phases of patient care under the direction of experienced physicians. The clinical curriculum includes history-taking, physical examination, daily patient rounds, lectures, conferences, and case presentations.

Facilities

Educational facilities include the seven-story Evans Hall, which houses amphitheaters, sophisticated instructional media, and the college library. The college has an anatomy museum and an electron microscopy laboratory.

The Hospital of PCOM is a 424-bed acute care general hospital devoted to patient care, teaching, and research. Available technologies include CAT scan, MRI, full imaging and invasive radiological procedures, and complete ultrasound. Month-long rotations in the hospital and other affiliated hospitals begin during the third year. PCOM sponsors one rural and four urban health care centers where students deliver hands-on primary care under supervision. Twenty-eight other affiliated hospitals and numerous outpatient units and physician's offices serve as clinical teaching sites.

The O.J. Snyder Memorial Library houses about 63,000 volumes and subscribes to 785 medical periodicals, 109 of which are osteopathic publications. Other resources include the PALINET/OCLC Network, MEDLINE, and audio- and videocassettes. The library is a member of the Health Sciences Libraries Consortium, along with a group of other medical libraries located throughout Pennsylvania.

Special Programs

The college offers a clinical master of science degree (M.S.) based on a proposed thesis. The applicant must be in full-time residency to be accepted into this program.

Together with Saint Joseph's University, the college offers a combined D.O./M.B.A. degree. The five-year course of study was created in 1989 as the nation's first D.O./M.B.A. program.

Students who have successfully completed their first year of study at PCOM may enter the D.O./M.P.H. program, offered in conjunction with Temple University. This newly created five-year program specializes in community health education.

Application Procedures

Application packets are available from the director of admissions beginning June 1. Each applicant must submit a completed application along with a $50 nonrefundable fee, MCAT scores, certified academic transcripts, and a letter of recommendation from the premedical committee or advisor. A letter of recommendation from an osteopathic physician is strongly advised but not required.

The application must be postmarked no later than March 1 preceding the opening of the next academic year. The college also has an early admission program. Upon acceptance of admission, students must pay a $500 tuition deposit to hold a place in class.

Contact

Director of Admissions
Philadelphia College of Osteopathic Medicine
4150 City Avenue
Philadelphia, Pennsylvania 19131-1696
(215) 871-1000

SOUTHEASTERN UNIVERSITY OF THE HEALTH SCIENCES COLLEGE OF OSTEOPATHIC MEDICINE

1750 N.E. 168th Street
North Miami Beach, Florida 33162-3097
(305) 949-4000

Accreditation	AOA
Degrees Offered	D.O., B.S./D.O.
# Students Applied	1,000
Enrollment	100 / class
Mean GPA	Not Available
% Men / % Women	74% / 26%
% Minorities	Not Available
Tuition	$11,965 In-State
	$15,965 Out-of-State
Application Fee	$50
Application Deadline	March 1

The University

The Southeastern University of the Health Sciences (SECOM) is the only private, not-for-profit institution of higher learning in Florida entirely given to health care education. The college was first chartered by Florida in 1979 and was accredited by the American Osteopathic Association. In 1987, SECOM added the College of Pharmacy and in 1989, opened the College of Optometry. Located in a quiet suburb in the heart of North Miami Beach, the campus is close to transportation, recreation, and housing. Two international airports close by afford ready access to long distance travel. SECOM is also licensed by the State Board of Independent College and Universities in Florida.

Admissions

Students must take the MCAT in the spring of the junior undergraduate year and no later than the fall of the senior year. SECOM seeks students with "superior" GPAs and "creditable" MCATs.

Undergraduate Preparation

Applicants must have a bachelor's degree from an accredited college or university. They must complete one year (usually six semesters) each, including lab, of the following courses: general biology, inorganic and organic chemistry, and physics.

One year of English composition and literature is also required.

Student Body

Out of 1,000 applications received annually, 100 are chosen for each entering class. The average age of the entering class is 25, and more than 25 percent are female. Some students come from careers in pharmacy, surgery, and engineering.

Costs

Tuition is $11,965 for Florida residents and $15,965 for nonresidents. Living expenses and other costs total about $4,100 per year.

Financial Aid

SECOM encourages students to investigate independent sources of funds. Some college work-study programs and short-term loans are available. About 15 federal programs, loan and scholarship funds are available, including a full-tuition SECOM minority scholarship.

Student Organizations

Delta Omega, a female student professional organization has a chapter on campus. Other special organizations include the Sports Medicine Club, Student Osteopathic Medical Association (representing over 90 percent of SECOM's student body), the Undergraduate American Academy of Osteopathy (UAAO), the ACGP in Osteopathic Medicine and Surgery, and the undergraduate chapter of the American College of Osteopathic Pediatricians.

Faculty

The faculty for all of SECOM consists of about 290 professors from all parts of the nation and from all major disciplines, suggesting a student/faculty ratio of about 4:3.

Curriculum

The course of study lasts four years. The first two-and-one-half years develop a foundation in the basic sciences, including anatomy, microbiology, pathology, biochemistry, physiology, and pharmacology. Special attention is given to community medicine, geriatrics, rural medicine, minority medicine, and the humanities. Hands-on training, including clinical teaching rotations, begin in the sixth semester. After 17 months of clinical work, students return for an eighth semester of basic clinical science and personal preparation for internship, residency, and practices.

Facilities

SECOM consists of a central three-level education building. The Student Activities Building, along with the usual student recreational and eating facilities, houses the 12,000-square-foot library with a vast collection of medical books and journals. SECOM works in close affiliation with a number of area hospitals and clinics.

Grading Procedures

While no specific grading procedures are indicated, in order to graduate, students must pass all prescribed examinations and complete the program of study required for the degree including all assignments. Successful candidates will take and pass Parts I and II of the National Board Examination.

Special Programs

In addition to its programs in pharmacy and optometry, SECOM provides programs of training out of the state's Area Health Education Center (AHEC). Students work to develop skills in remote and underserved areas. Florida International University participates in nursing, social work, and allied health; Palm Beach Junior College offers dental hygiene and Broward Community College offers continuing education and health professions programs. The University of Miami's Dade County AHEC program works closely with SECOM. A Rural Medicine Program is a particular specialty of SECOM, and the college also offers a combined degree program (B.S./D.O.) in affiliation with Florida International University, a program covering seven years.

Application Procedures

Students must apply through AACOMAS. Applications may be obtained from SECOM or by writing to AACOMAS. AACOMAS must receive the following by March 1: AACOMAS application, official transcripts, and MCAT scores. SECOM must receive the following by April 15: supplemental application, $50 application fee, letter(s) of recommendation, and one letter of recommendation from an osteopathic physician. An interview may follow.

Contact

Admissions Office
Southeastern University of the Health Sciences
College of Osteopathic Medicine
1750 Northeast 168th Street
North Miami Beach, Florida 33162-3097
(305) 949-4000

TEXAS COLLEGE OF OSTEOPATHIC MEDICINE

3500 Camp Bowie Boulevard
Fort Worth, Texas 76107-2690
(817) 735-2000

Accreditation	AOA
Degrees Offered	D.O.
# Students Applied	1,200
Enrollment	100 / class
Mean GPA	3.0
% Men / % Women	31% / 69%
% Minorities	4%
Tuition	$5,463 In-State
	$21,852 Out-of-State
Application Fee	$50
Application Deadline	December 1

The University

The Texas College of Osteopathic Medicine (TCOM) was founded in 1970 and became a state-supported college in 1975.

Admissions

Factors considered for admission to the medical school include MCAT scores, overall GPA, and GPA in preprofessional science courses. The MCAT must have been taken within three years prior to application. Both overall and science GPA should be at least a 3.0. An applicant with weaknesses in one academic area may be compensated for by strength in other areas, but no applicant with either an overall or a science GPA of less than 2.5 will be considered.

Undergraduate Preparation

Applicants must have completed at least 90 semester hours at an accredited college or university. Undergraduate academic requirements include one academic year of biology with lab, one academic year of physics with lab, two academic years of chemistry with lab, and one academic year of expository writing.

Student Body

Of the 400 students enrolled at TCOM, 90 percent are Texas residents.

Placement Records

About 70 percent of TCOM's graduates practice in Texas. Almost 75 percent become family or primary care physicians, and about 40 percent serve rural and small-town areas. Specializations include anesthesiology, surgery, sports medicine, and pediatrics, among other fields.

Costs

Annual tuition is $5,463 for Texas residents and $21,852 for nonresidents. Additional expenses for fees, books, supplies, room and board, transportation, and personal expenses are about $12,447. A disadvantaged financial position may warrant waivering the application fee.

Financial Aid

Financial aid may be obtained from federal programs; state, institutional, and private scholarship/loan programs; and private foundation scholarships and loans. Federal programs include the college work-study program, Disadvantaged Health Professions Program, Exceptional Financial Need Scholarship program, Health Education Assistance Loan program (HEAL), Health Professions Student Loan program (HPSL), Perkins Loan program, Stafford Student Loan program, Supplemental Loans for Students (SLS), and armed forces programs. All those applying for financial aid must first file the Financial Aid Form (FAF) with the College Scholarship Service.

Faculty

TCOM students are taught by 150 full-time faculty members in classrooms and labs, and more than 300 community physicians in clinics, hospitals, and private offices.

Curriculum

The first two years of the medical curriculum consist of the following coursework: developing dimensions in health care, osteopathic clinical practices, biochemistry, embryology, gross anatomy, medical histology and cell biology, basic and clinical immunology, medical physiology, neuro-biology, medical microbiology, pathology, pharmacology, psychiatry, and computer literacy. Second year students are assigned to the office of an osteopathic physician to experience general practice. The third-and fourth-year consists of courses in dermatology, obstetrics, pediatrics, radiology, and surgery. The last year and a half of medical school consists of clinical rotations in ambulatory care, emergency medicine, general practice, medicine, mental health, obstetrics and gynecology, pediatrics, subspecialty internal medicine, surgery, and various electives. The final semester also includes preparation for comprehensive examinations.

Facilities

Medical students gain clinical experience in the college's six general and family practice clinics, 13 specialty clinics, and

12 affiliated hospitals. TCOM's library boasts computer search systems and a communications network that allows access to virtually all of the world's current medical information.

Application Procedures

Applications must be processed through the American Association of Colleges of Osteopathic Medicine Application Service (AACOMAS) beginning July 1 and no later than December 1. The Texas College of Osteopathic Medicine Office of admissions must receive all application material from early decision plan applicants by September 1. College or university transcripts must be submitted to AACOMAS by December 15. Early applications receive first consideration. Candidates are advised to take the MCAT in the spring prior to the year of intended matriculation. The necessity of an interview will be determined by the admissions committee upon reviewing the applicant's academic record, the AACOMAS application, supplemental application, and letters of evaluation. One letter must be from a premedical/health professions advisory committee, one from a faculty member, and one from a recent employer or another person other than a relative who knows the candidate well. Faculty letters may take the place of an advisory committee letter, and letters from employers or supervisors may take the place of faculty letters for those applicants who have worked extensively during college or have worked for several years after college. Admissions decisions on EDP applicants are made by November 1. Applicants who wish to defer matriculation for one academic year must submit a request before June 1.

Contact

Office of Medical Student Admissions
Texas College of Osteopathic Medicine
3500 Camp Bowie Boulevard
Fort Worth, Texas 76107-2690
(817) 735-2204
(800) 535-TCOM

WEST VIRGINIA SCHOOL OF OSTEOPATHIC MEDICINE

Lewisburg, West Virginia 24901
(304) 645-6270

Accreditation	AOA
Degrees Offered	D.O.
# Students Applied	800
Enrollment	237
Mean GPA	3.17
% Men / % Women	75% / 25%
% Minorities	Not Available
Tuition	$6,152 In-State
	$10,832 Out-of-State
Application Fee	$20 In-State; $40 Out-of-State
Application Deadline	March 1

The University

The West Virginia School of Osteopathic Medicine (WVSOM) is a state-supported professional college emphasizing rural primary health care for West Virginia and Appalachia. The school is located in Lewisburg, the nation's most rural medical college community.

WVSOM also serves nine other states throughout the Appalachian region and has added gerontological studies to its curriculum to enhance health care for the elderly in these rural states. Since the college's establishment in 1974, the state's osteopathic profession has grown by nearly 500 percent.

Admissions

Factors considered in the admissions process include scholarship, health-related experience, level of maturity, motivation for osteopathic medicine, outside activities, and letters of recommendation. The results of a personal interview are also considered. Applicants must take the MCAT.

Preference is given to West Virginia residents and to residents of the Southern Regional Education Board (SREB) contract states of Georgia, Mississippi, and Alabama. Second preference is given to applicants from the southern Appalachian states of Virginia, Maryland, Kentucky, Tennessee, North Carolina, and South Carolina.

Undergraduate Preparation

The majority of candidates selected for admission will have completed four or more years of preprofessional study; the minimum acceptable is 90 semester hours from an accredited college or university. Minimum course requirements are six hours of English, eight hours each of biology (general biology or zoology), physics, inorganic chemistry, organic chemistry (including aliphatic and aromatic compounds), and 52 hours of electives.

Applicants are expected to have earned a minimum GPA of 2.5.

Student Body

Total enrollment is 237. Of these, 146 are West Virginia residents, 54 are SREB state residents, and 37 come from other states in the Appalachian region. About 59 are women.

The average age of the student body is 30. Almost 200 hold bachelor's degrees, and 27 hold other graduate or professional degrees.

Placement Records

WVSOM is the state leader in providing rural physicians in West Virginia. The majority (95 percent) of WVSOM graduates now in West Virginia are practicing in primary care medical fields.

Costs

Tuition for West Virginia residents is $6,152. Nonresidents pay $10,832. Books and supplies (including microscope rental) are estimated to cost $3,200 for first-year students.

Financial Aid

WVSOM participates in a variety of federal, state, and institutional financial aid programs. Financial aid packages are determined on the basis of need, and all applicants must file a GAPSFAS form. All necessary documentation for first-year students requesting financial aid must be in the financial aid office by June 1.

Federal programs include College Work-Study, Perkins Loans, Stafford Loans, and Health Education Assistance Loans. Other financial aid programs include Armed Forces Scholarships, Veterans Administration, University of West Virginia Board of Trustees Medical Student Loan Program, and WVSOM Tuition Fee Waiver Scholarships.

Other financial aid options are available, including awards and loans from the National Osteopathic Association Foundation, the West Virginia Federation of Women's Club, and the West Virginia Attorney General's Office.

Faculty

The full-time clinical and basic science faculty comprise 20

Ph.D.s, 12 D.O.s, and one M.D. More than 60 guest lecturers visit campus each year.

Curriculum

The curriculum is designed to prepare students for practice in small towns and rural areas, with an osteopathic emphasis on the integrity of the body, the interrelationship of structure and function, and the role of the musculoskeletal system in health and disease. Preventive medicine, nutrition, and behavioral medicine are all taught as part of the osteopathic concept of health maintenance. Occupational medicine, rural medicine, geriatric health care, physical diagnosis, and family practice help prepare students for practice in West Virginia.

Phase I of the four-year curriculum comprises the majority of the first year and includes courses in basic and clinical sciences. During Phase II, preclinical and clinical instruction are arranged to study one organ system at a time. Phase III, the third and fourth years, consists of concentrated clinical training conducted at public health sites, rural clinics, nursing homes, hospitals, and other instructional settings.

Facilities

Affiliated hospitals, clinics, and physicians' offices used as training sites for WVSOM student physicians range from the nation's largest osteopathic teaching hospitals to a growing network of small community and rural clinical sites throughout Appalachia.

Application Procedures

The college participates in AACOMAS. Undergraduate transcripts and MCAT scores should be mailed directly to AACOMAS. The WVSOM application, letters of recommendation, and an application fee ($20 for residents, $40 for nonresidents) should be mailed directly to the college. Applicants may be invited for personal interviews. The AACOMAS application deadline is March 1 of the year of desired matriculation. The deadline for submission of the WVSOM supplemental materials is April 15 of that year.

Contact

West Virginia School of Osteopathic Medicine
Office of Admissions
400 North Lee Street
Lewisburg, West Virginia 24901
(304) 647-6251
(800) 356-7836 (In-State)
(800) 537-7077 (Out-of-State)

CHAPTER 4

Podiatric Schools

THE PODIATRIC PROFESSION

Dancing, walking, and jogging can be enjoyable and healthy activities, but if your feet hurt, even the thought of standing can make you miserable. Being unable to stand or move about easily is an inconvenience at the very least, but if the disability is permanent, it can be a crushing blow. Podiatrists, also known as doctors of podiatric medicine (DPMs), diagnose and treat disorders and diseases of the foot and lower leg.

Podiatrists treat the major foot conditions: corns and calluses, ingrown toenails, and bunions. Other conditions treated by podiatrists include hammertoes, ankle and foot injuries, and foot complaints associated with diseases such as diabetes. For example, diabetics are prone to ulcers and infections due to their poor circulation.

Some practitioners specialize in surgery. Other specialties are orthopedics and public health. Besides these three recognized specialties, podiatrists may choose subspecialty areas such as elderly care, sports medicine, and diabetic foot care. One of the biggest subspecialty areas is primary podiatric medicine, which is considered the family medicine of foot care.

Going to a podiatrist for treatment of a foot problem may be the entry point into the health care system for some patients since clinical signs of diseases such as arthritis, diabetes, and heart disease may first appear in the foot. Podiatrists are trained to spot these and other systemic diseases and to refer patients to other medical specialties when appropriate.

Podiatrists usually work independently in their own offices. They work over 48 hours a week, on average. Podiatrists with solo practices set their own hours. Podiatrists who are employed in hospitals, health maintenance organizations (HMOs), or clinics may work nights and weekends and be on call.

The vast majority of podiatrists, however, are in private practice. Traditionally, podiatrists have been solo practitioners and most still are. Recently, other practice arrangements such as partnerships and group practices have begun to emerge.

All 50 states and the District of Columbia require a license for the practice of podiatric medicine. Each state and jurisdiction defines its own licensing requirements. Generally, however, the applicant must be a graduate of an accredited college of podiatric medicine and pass written and oral examinations. Many states also require applicants to have completed an accredited residency program. Some states permit applicants to substitute the examination of the National Board of Podiatric Examiners, given in the second and fourth years of podiatric medical college, for part or all of the written

state examination. Certain states grant reciprocity to podiatrists who are licensed in another state.

The six colleges of podiatric medicine are located in California, Illinois, New York, Ohio, Pennsylvania, and Iowa. There are no colleges of Podiatric Medicine in Canada. If you are Canadian and interested in becoming a podiatrist, you may attend an American school. Prerequisites for admission include the completion of at least 90 semester hours of undergraduate study, a certain grade point average, and certain scores on the Medical College Admission Test (MCAT). Usually, eight semester hours each of biology, inorganic chemistry, organic chemistry, and physics and six hours of English are required. Please see the individual profiles on the following pages for more specific requirements for each school.

Colleges of podiatric medicine offer a four-year program whose core curriculum is similar to that in other schools of medicine. Classroom instruction in the basic sciences, including anatomy, chemistry, pathology, and pharmacology, given during the first two years. Third and fourth year students have clinical rotations in different practice settings, including private practice, hospitals, and clinics. During these rotations, they acquire clinical skills—learning how to take general and podiatric histories, to perform routine physical examinations, to interpret tests and findings, to make diagnoses, and to perform therapeutic procedures. Graduates are awarded the degree of doctor of podiatric medicine (DPM).

Most graduates complete a 1–3 year residency after receiving the DPM degree. Residency programs are hospital based. The first-year resident receives advanced training in podiatric medicine and surgery and serves clinical rotations in anesthesiology, internal medicine, pathology, radiology, emergency medicine, and orthopedic and general surgery. Second and third year residencies provide more extensive training in one of the three specialty areas.

There are three recognized certifying boards for the specialty areas: the American Board of Podiatric Surgery, the American Board of Podiatric Orthopedics, and the American Board of Podiatric Public Health.

Certification means that the DPM meets higher standards than those required for licensure. Each board has specific requirements, including advanced training, successful completion of oral and written examinations, and experience as a practicing podiatrist.

Those considering a career in podiatry should have scientific aptitude, manual dexterity, and interpersonal skills. They must be able to acquire scientific knowledge and stay abreast of new developments in the field of medicine; develop the motor functions and professional skills needed for clinical practice; and develop personal rapport and empathy with patients. A good business sense and congeniality are assets, as in any medical profession.

For further information, call

American Podiatric Medical Association
9312 Old Georgetown Road
Bethesda, MD 20814-1621

or:

American Association of Colleges of Podiatric Medicine
1350 Piccard Drive, Suite 322
Rockville, MD 20850-4307
(800) 922-9266
(301) 990-7400
FAX (301) 990-2807

PODIATRIC SCHOOLS AT A GLANCE

School	Accreditation	Degrees Offered	# Students Applied	Enrollment
California College of Podiatric Medicine	CPME, WASC, APA	D.P.M.	326	100 / class
New York College of Podiatric Medicine	CPME	D.P.M.	500	132 / class
Ohio College of Podiatric Medicine	CPME, APMA, NCA	D.P.M.	*	125
University of Osteopathic Medicine and Health Science College of Podiatric Medicine and Surgery	CPME	D.P.M.	*	70 / class
Pennsylvania College of Podiatric Medicine	MSACS, CPME	D.P.M., D.P.M./Ph.D.	*	*
Dr. William M. Scholl College of Podiatric Medicine	CPME, AACPM	D.P.M.	457	119 / class

* Not Available   ** Not Applicable   C/S – Contact School

Mean GPA	% Male / % Female	% Minorities	In-State Tuition	Out-of-State Tuition	Application Fee	Application Deadline
*	70% / 30%	*	$17,000	C/S	$50	August 1
2.91	68% / 32%	*	$17,595	C/S	C/S	C/S
2.7	65% / 35%	*	$14,000	C/S	C/S	August 15
3.1	67% / 33%	20%	$13,461	C/S	C/S	C/S
*	*	*	C/S	C/S	C/S	C/S
3.0	68% / 32%	26.8 %	$15,000	$15,300	C/S	August 1

* Not Available   ** Not Applicable   C/S – Contact School

CALIFORNIA COLLEGE OF PODIATRIC MEDICINE

1210 Scott Street
San Francisco, California 94115
(800) 334-2276

Accreditation	WASC, APA
Degrees Offered	D.P.M.
# Students Applied	326
Enrollment	100 / class
Mean GPA	Not Available
% Men / % Women	70% / 30%
% Minorities	Not Available
Tuition	$17,000
Application Fee	$50
Application Deadline	August 1

The University

Founded in 1914, the California College of Podiatric Medicine (CCPM) is a private, independent, four-year health professional school. Facilities at the college include the Pacific Coast Hospital (a hospital designed and equipped for foot surgery), outpatient clinics, and the Primary Care Center, which provides medical care for residents of the community.

San Francisco is a cosmopolitan urban area which offers a wide variety of cultural activities, including the San Francisco Symphony and Opera, theaters, and museums. The Golden Gate National Recreation Area offers jogging, biking, and hiking trails. Skiing, camping, and hiking facilities are available within a half-day drive at Gold Rush Country, Lake Tahoe, and Yosemite National Park.

Admissions

The admissions and standards committee chooses candidates on the basis of scholarship, motivation, character, ability, and achievement. Applicants are first screened on the basis of undergraduate academic credentials and the results of the MCAT. Interviews are offered to applicants who have passed the preliminary screening of the admissions process. Most of the students admitted to the college have completed the baccalaureate degree.

Undergraduate Preparation

Applicants must have completed at least three years of undergraduate preprofessional education at an accredited institution. Completion of the following courses is required:

biological sciences (16 semester hours); organic chemistry (eight semester hours); inorganic chemistry (eight semester hours); physics (eight semester hours); English/communication skills (six semester hours). Laboratories are required for all science courses. A course in biochemistry can be substituted for one organic chemistry course. At least 12 semester hours of other liberal arts courses are also required. Most students enrolled at the college have taken at least three of the following courses: anatomy, biochemistry, embryology, histology, microbiology, and physiology.

Placement Records

Every CCPM student is guaranteed a residency upon graduation through a program of speciality rotations in affiliated teaching hospitals, VA hospitals, private institutions, and district hospitals.

Costs

Tuition for the 1992-93 academic year is estimated to be $17,000. Additional fees are estimated to be $920.

Financial Aid

The college attempts to provide as much financial assistance as possible to students with demonstrated need. Financial assistance is limited by the amount of funding provided to the college by government sources. Financial aid is available through the college and from a variety of federal, state, and private offices.

Student Organizations

Student organizations on campus include Alpha Gamma Kappa, Pi Delta (a national podiatric medical student honor society), the American Podiatric Medical Students Association, the Student National Podiatric Medical Association, Women in Podiatry, and student chapters of the American College of Foot Surgeons, the American Academy of Podiatric Sports Medicine, and the California Podiatric Medical Association. All students are members of the California Podiatric Medical Students Association, a student government organization.

Faculty

The faculty consists of 524 full-time members, 89 part-time faculty members, and 2,071 volunteer faculty members.

Curriculum

The basic science courses stress the study of the lower extremities. The first year concentrates primarily on the basic sciences, including lower extremity anatomy and histology. The second year includes courses in medical microbiology, pathology, and pharmacology. Clinical rotations begin during the summer following the second year, although academic coursework continues into the third year. The fourth year consists entirely of clinical rotations, which are completed at the college, the Pacific Coast Hospital, and at affiliated medical centers in San Francisco, the University of Southern California, and other locations in the United States. Research opportunities are available.

Facilities

The Pacific Coast Hospital is the only acute-care hospital specializing in podiatric medicine located on a college campus. At the hospital and adjoining outpatient clinics, students are exposed to more than 1,400 surgical cases and 22,000 outpatient visits each year. The outpatient clinics at the college offer 64 private treatment rooms, a physical therapy department, a clinical laboratory, and pharmacy, radiology, and biomechanical laboratories for the creation of orthopedic devices. The medical library contains approximately 22,000 books and bound journal volumes, and annually receives over 450 serial titles. Index Medicus, a system which allows patrons to run their own literature searches, is also available.

Housing is available for single students through an arrangement with the University of San Francisco. Graduate dorms are located less than a quarter mile from CCPM.

Grading Procedures

A letter grading system is used. Part I of the National Board of Podiatric Medicine Examination is given upon completion of the second year of study. Part II is given during the spring term of the fourth year.

Application Procedures

Applications should be received between September 1 and April 1 to receive priority consideration. August 1 is the regular application deadline. The college participates in the American Association of College of Podiatric Medicine Application Service (AACPMAS). The MCAT is required. CCPM will accept scores no more than three years old. Recommendations are required from a preprofessional advisory committee or from two science faculty members. One recommendation from a podiatric physician is also required (applicants are encouraged to contact the college admissions office for an alumni directory). Applications are considered on a rolling basis. The admission, evaluation, and notification process usually takes four to eight weeks. Interviews are arranged by invitation of the admissions and standards committee. There is an application fee of $50.

International candidates are encouraged to apply by April 1 to have time to obtain a student visa. Some international students must take the Test of English as a Foreign Language (TOEFL). A minimum score of 600 is required. All applicants are responsible for obtaining certified translations of all original documents that are not in English. Financial certification showing that educational expenses will be provided is needed if an offer of admission is made.

Applicants for advanced standing must have completed one or two years of professional school at an accredited institution and must be in good academic standing at their original college.

Applicants for advanced standing may be admitted to the second and third years.

Contact

Admissions Office
California College of Podiatric Medicine
1210 Scott Street
San Francisco, California 94115
(800) 334-2276 (Out-of-State)
(800) 443-2276 (In-State)

NEW YORK COLLEGE OF PODIATRIC MEDICINE

1800 Park Avenue
New York, New York 10035
(212) 410-8000

Accreditation	CPME
Degrees Offered	D.P.M.
# Students Applied	500
Enrollment	132 / class
Mean GPA	2.91
% Men / % Women	68% / 32%
% Minorities	Not Available
Tuition	$17,595
Application Fee	Contact School
Application Deadline	Contact School

The University

The New York College of Podiatric Medicine is the oldest and largest college of podiatric medicine in the United States. It was founded in 1911, and has since graduated more than 3,000 podiatric physicians, accounting for approximately 25 percent of the practicing foot specialists in the nation. The college is located in upper Manhattan, near many other medical training facilities, including Columbia Presbyterian Medical Center, Mount Sinai Medical Center, the Hospital for Joint Diseases, and North General Hospital.

New York City offers a wide variety of cultural attractions, from traditional to avant-garde, including museums, concert halls, art galleries, and theaters. Every professional sport is represented, many by two teams. The Adirondack Mountains and the beaches of New Jersey and Long Island are a short ride away.

Admissions

The admissions committee selects candidates who have demonstrated not only high academic performance, but who give promise of becoming ethical, capable, and responsible physicians.

Undergraduate Preparation

Mature, well-qualified students may be admitted after completing 90 semester hours of undergraduate coursework, but the college recommends the completion of a bachelor's degree from an accredited college of arts and sciences. Completion of at least one year (or eight semester hours) of general biology, inorganic chemistry, organic chemistry, and physics is required for admission. A minimum of one year (or six semester hours) of English is also required. The admissions committee has no preference as to a student's major.

Student Body

The student population represents most American states and several countries throughout the world.

Placement Records

More than 90 percent of NYCPM graduates pass the state license exam on their first attempt, and 97 percent of NYCPM students pass the final national board exam the first time. Eighty-five percent of graduating seniors are placed in fully credentialed, full-time residency programs.

Costs

Tuition and fees for first-year residents and nonresidents amount to approximately $17,595 (tuition and fees are subject to change). The cost of books, instruments, and supplies for a first-year student is approximately $3,075. Students with a modest standard of living would spend about $9,340 per year on room and board and personal expenses if living alone, or about $6,280 if living with parents or relatives.

Financial Aid

The college offers aid in the form of scholarships, grants, loans, and work-study programs from institutional, federal, and state sources. Students who demonstrate high need may also be offered scholarship awards from the Exceptional Financial Need program. Candidates for admission will receive debt management materials discussing loan programs and sample repayment schedules. Applicants are not required to complete and submit a loan application before being accepted to the college.

Student Organizations

The student council's social activities committee organizes a number of recreational activities for the student body.

Faculty

The college has a student/faculty ratio of 4:1, allowing students to receive individual attention and special assistance when needed.

Curriculum

The college believes that the "hands on" approach is the best way to train physicians. Therefore, the basic science credit hours are condensed, allowing students to begin clinical training after one and one-half years. After completing 78 credit hours of basic sciences, students take a transition semester that serves as a bridge between classroom training and clinical training. In addition to the clinical training they receive in the foot clinics, students rotate for up to five months at various hospitals, clinics, or private practices throughout the country. Over 100 such externship programs are available to NYCPM students.

The need for individual initiative is stressed throughout the four years of training. The entire program revolves around a specific number of objectives that each student is required to master. Weekly examinations enable faculty members to detect any problems a student may be having. Clinical training is based on a systematic rotational block approach. Each student must master each area before moving on to the next. To prepare students for private practice, courses in ethics, practice management, legal issues, and regulations regarding third-party participation are offered.

NYCPM maintains an active Division of Institutional Research, supporting projects on AIDS, arthritis, tinea pedis, neoplasms, orthotic materials, anti-inflammatory and dermatological pharmaceuticals, and pulse electromagnetism.

Facilities

The New York College of Podiatric Medicine is a part of the Foot Clinics of New York, the largest foot care center in the world. The clinics treat an average of 60,000 patients per year, mostly underprivileged area residents, with a wide variety of podiatric pathologies. The clinics comprise seven clinical divisions: podiatric medicine, surgery, general podiatry, orthopedics, pediatrics, radiology, and sports medicine.

The college offers a print library of approximately 10,000 bound texts, an audiovisual department that videotapes all lectures, note-taking services, and a faculty and student tutor network.

The student affairs office maintains affiliation with several dormitory and apartment-type residences that cater to medical students, including the 92nd Street Clara De Hirsch Residence, a dormitory-style facility.

Application Procedures

The college participates in the American Association of Colleges of Podiatric Medicine Application Service (AACPMAS). Although applications to the college are reviewed on a rolling basis, applicants are strongly urged to apply before

May 1. The MCAT is required. Candidates must also submit three letters of recommendation (one of which must be written by a practicing podiatrist). Interviews are required for admission and are arranged only by invitation of the admissions committee.

Contact

New York College of Podiatric Medicine
Office of Admissions
1800 Park Avenue
New York, New York 10035
(212) 410-8053
or (800) 526-6966

OHIO COLLEGE OF PODIATRIC MEDICINE

10515 Carnegie Avenue
Cleveland, Ohio 44106-3082
(216) 231-3300

Accreditation	CPME, APMA, NCA
Degrees Offered	D.P.M.
# Students Applied	Not Available
Enrollment	125/ class
Mean GPA	2.7
% Men / % Women	65% / 35%
% Minorities	Not Available
Tuition	$14,000
Application Fee	Contact School
Application Deadline	August 15

The University

The Ohio College of Podiatric Medicine was founded in 1916 as the Ohio College of Chiropody. In 1976, the college moved to its current location at the center of University Circle. Also located within University Circle are Case Western Reserve University, Mt. Sinai Medical Center, Veteran's Administration Hospital, the Cleveland Museum of Art, Western Reserve Historical Society, the Museum of Natural History, and Severance Hall (home of the Cleveland Orchestra and site of OCPM's graduation ceremonies).

Many cultural attractions are available throughout the city,

including a selection of theaters, music centers, and art museums. Recreational activities are abundant in the "Emerald Necklace," Cleveland's popular park system.

Admissions

Applicants are evaluated by their academic records, commitment to the profession and its advancement, and demonstrated moral and professional character. The admissions committee places great emphasis on its appraisal of the character, personality, and general background of the applicant through the interview process.

Students who attended a foreign college or university must have completed undergraduate coursework equivalent to standard requirements for the entering class, and must present evidence that they have command of written and spoken English by achieving a satisfactory score on the Test of English as a Foreign Language (TOEFL).

Undergraduate Preparation

Completion of at least 90 semester hours (or 135 quarter hours) of credit at an accredited college or university is required to apply for admission to OCPM. Approximately 90 percent of OCPM students have completed a bachelor's degree. The following are prerequisite courses: eight semester hours of biology or zoology, inorganic chemistry, organic chemistry, and physics; and six semester hours of English. All science courses must include laboratory work.

Placement Records

The Ohio College of Podiatric Medicine has a full-time graduate placement office, which has consistently placed more than 90 percent of graduates in residency programs. In 1990, the total placement in residencies, preceptorships, and private practice was 95 percent. Many OCPM graduates open their second practices within five years of opening their first.

Costs

Tuition costs $14,000 per year. The cost of books, instruments, and supplies for first-year students is $949. Additional fees, including insurance, for first-year students total $595.

Financial Aid

About 90 percent of OCPM students receive some form of financial assistance. Financial aid workshops are offered for continuing students at the beginning of the application process to review details about the types of aid available, including government loans, scholarships, and work-study programs. Similar assistance is offered to prospective students during the Day on Campus program.

Student Organizations

Student organizations on campus include the Ohio Podiatric Medical Students Association, the Student National Podiatric Medical Association, the Ohio Chapter of the Canadian Association of Podiatry Students, the American Association of Women in Podiatry, and the Sports Medicine Club. There are also three professional fraternities on campus.

Curriculum

Classes are taught within five major departments: basic sciences, general medicine, orthopedics/biomechanics, podiatric medicine, and podiatric surgery. The first two years of the study of podiatric medicine is much like the first two years of medical and dental school, including instruction in the basic biological sciences. The third and fourth years focus on the specifics about the foot and lower extremity, while concentrating on courses in the clinical sciences and offering experiences in community clinics, accredited hospitals, and offices of podiatric physicians. The interrelation of the lower extremity with the entire human body is investigated. General diagnostic and therapeutic procedures for all systems of the body are examined as well. At the end of the fourth year, students must take a comprehensive clinical examination.

Facilities

Students receive most of their clinical training at the Cleveland Foot Clinic, which has been in operation for over 40 years. It includes a clinical out-patient treatment center, clinical staff offices, clinical support areas for radiology medical records, and a pharmacy. Students also receive training at several affiliated hospitals; in addition, more than 300 private practitioners and 45 hospitals provide externship and clerkship training to OCPM students.

The Locomotion Laboratory and intricate research equipment enables professors and students to research diseases of the lower anatomy. The biomedical communications department is a multimedia facility that contains videotape equipment, a television studio, photography equipment, and illustration materials. Lectures and surgical procedures may be videotaped so students may view the tapes at home.

The OCPM Library contains more than 12,000 volumes and 225 medical and podiatric journals. Medical information is also available through the Cleveland Health Sciences Library and Case Western Reserve University.

Some graduate and professional students reside on the campus of Case Western Reserve University, while the majority live off campus.

Grading Procedures

During the first three years of the program, a letter grading system is used. Grading for the clinical evaluation is based on an honors/pass/fail system. The academic standards and promotions committee makes a recommendation for promotion after each semester upon consideration of a student's grade records. Part I of the National Board exams is taken after successful completion of the second year, and Part II is taken toward the end of the fourth year. The comprehensive clinical examination is given to fourth-year students.

Special Programs

Preprofessional internships are offered to highly-qualified undergraduates. This program is designed to provide insight into the education and scope of practice involved with podiatric medicine. A binary degree program allows qualified undergraduate students at participating institutions to enter OCPM after three years of academic study. Upon completion of the first and/or second years at OCPM, students will receive the B.S. or B.A. degree from their undergraduate institution. The five-year program allows specified students to complete the first two years of the curriculum in three years.

Application Procedures

The college participates in the American Association of Colleges of Podiatric Medicine Application Service (AACPMAS). The college should receive the application by April 1 of the year of planned enrollment for primary consideration, although the official application deadline is August 1. Interviews are arranged by invitation of the admissions committee. The MCAT is required and should be taken in April or September of the year prior to planned enrollment. Applicants must furnish at least two letters of recommendation, one from a premedical advisor or committee and one from a health professional (preferably a podiatrist).

Transfer students and applicants for admission with advanced standing will be considered for admission.

Contact

The Ohio College of Podiatric Medicine
University Circle
10515 Carnegie Avenue
Cleveland, Ohio 44106-3082
(216) 231-3300
(800) 821-6562 (In-State)
(800) 238-7903 (Out-of-State)

UNIVERSITY OF OSTEOPATHIC MEDICINE AND HEALTH SCIENCE COLLEGE OF PODIATRIC MEDICINE AND SURGERY

300 Grand Avenue
Des Moines, Iowa 50312
(515) 271-1469

Accreditation	CPME
Degrees Offered	DPM
# Students Applied	Not Available
Enrollment	70 / class
Mean GPA	3.1
% Men / % Women	67% / 33%
% Minorities	20%
Tuition	$13,461
Application Fee	Contact School
Application Deadline	Contact School

The University

The University of Osteopathic Medicine and Health Sciences was founded in 1898. The College of Osteopathic Medicine and Surgery is the second oldest and second largest osteopathic and medical school in the nation. In 1980, it received university status through the addition of the College of Podiatric Medicine and Surgery (CPMS) and the College of Biological Sciences. The College of Podiatric Medicine and Surgery is the only podiatric medical college within a health sciences university that offers students the benefit of concentrating on the specialty of podiatric medicine while interacting with students of other health professions.

With a population of approximately 250,000, Des Moines is large enough to offer a variety of cultural attractions, but is close enough to several lakes and rivers to offer recreational activities, such as fishing, boating, camping, and picnicking. There are several colleges and universities in the area, including Drake University and Iowa State University in nearby Ames.

Admissions

Qualified students usually have a cumulative GPA of 2.5 or higher. The mean GPA of the applicants accepted in 1991 was 3.1. Most applicants have completed a baccalaureate degree by the time of registration.

Undergraduate Preparation

Candidates for admission must have completed a minimum of 90 semester hours of undergraduate work, although most applicants have completed an undergraduate degree by the time of registration. Applicants must have completed at least eight semester hours of the following prerequisite courses (including necessary laboratory work): biology, general chemistry (college chemistry, qualitative and/or quantitative analysis, or physical chemistry), organic chemistry (four credit hours of biochemistry can substitute for four semester hours of organic chemistry), and physics. Six semester hours of English or the language arts are also required. Additional recommended coursework includes English literature, biochemistry, genetics, comparative anatomy, mathematics, and psychology. All work must be completed at a regionally accredited institution.

Student Body

Sixty-one percent of the class of 1995 are from the north-central region of the country. About 25 states throughout the nation are represented in this class. The students' academic backgrounds range from the traditional premedical major to a practicing attorney. About one third of the entering class are female and between 15 and 20 percent represent ethnic and racial minorities.

Of the class of 1994, approximately 83 percent possessed a bachelor's degree or higher at the time of enrollment. The majority of students reside in Kansas, Minnesota, Iowa, and Illinois. However, 28 states and Puerto Rico are represented.

Placement Records

Graduating students often enter residency programs where they receive clinical training. Virtually 100 percent of the 1990 CPMS graduates obtained a postgraduate program (residency and/or preceptorship).

Costs

Tuition for residents and nonresidents amounts to $13,461 and is adjusted annually by the board of trustees. Additional fees and supplies amount to $2,480 for first-year students.

Financial Aid

Upon acceptance, students receive a financial aid packet that includes application and need-analysis forms. Financial aid is available from federal, state, and private sources, and is granted on the basis of need and/or ability. The college participates in many federal and campus-based loan programs. A limited number of partial scholarships are available to academically superior students.

Student Organizations

Student medical organizations and clubs include the American Podiatric Medical Student Association, the Iowa Podiatric Medical Student Association, the Student National Podiatric Medical Association, the American Association of

Women Podiatrists, the Pi Delta Honor Society, the surgery club, the emergency medicine club, the podogeriatrics club, the podopediatrics club, the podiatric sports medicine club, and others.

Faculty

The college has a full-time, campus-based faculty and staff.

Curriculum

The first year of study includes basic medical sciences, nutrition, and behavioral science/medicine. The second year consists of the integration of the study of basic sciences, clinical medicine, and podiatric medicine with the study of various organ systems. In each of the system courses, the interrelationship and interdependence of body systems is emphasized. The basic sciences that apply to a certain body system are studied in tandem with the clinical problems of that system.

During the third year, the curriculum is self-directed and problem based. Groups of approximately seven students meet with a faculty member for six- to eight-week blocks of time, during which they actively learn by solving patient problems and becoming involved with all diagnostic and therapeutic modalities. Students see each patient through all phases of care. Afterwards, they are then assigned to five or six other faculty members for similar blocks of time.

During the last 18 months of study, students receive clinical training in four medical environments: the ambulatory clinic, the hospital, long-term care facility, and community practice. Students apply classroom learning to the clinical setting while working with other members of the health care team. Four-to six-week rotations are often completed at major medical centers throughout the nation, including Yale, Loma Linda, University of Texas Health Science Center at San Antonio, University of Washington, and the University of Missouri.

Facilities

The Tower Medical Clinic offers primary care and many medical specialties. Students receive part of their clinical training in the Tower's podiatric medicine department and ambulatory surgery center.

The university also operates seven family practice clinics, some of which are in rural locations and in underserved areas. Rotations at these clinics provide a variety of learning experiences in both urban and rural settings.

Application Procedures

The college participates in the American Association of Colleges of Podiatric Medicine Application Service (AACPMAS). The MCAT is required and should be taken in April of the year preceding planned enrollment. A letter of recommendation from the applicant's preprofessional advisory committee, or three letters of reference from professors (at least two from science faculty) must be sent to the admissions office. Official transcripts of all college courses are also required. Interviews are arranged by invitation of the admissions committee and are required for admission.

Contact

University of Osteopathic Medicine and Health Sciences
Recruiting Office
College of Podiatric Medicine and Surgery
3200 Grand Avenue
Des Moines, Iowa 50312
(515) 243-4830

PENNSYLVANIA COLLEGE OF PODIATRIC MEDICINE

8th at Race Street
Philadelphia, Pennsylvania 19107
(215) 629-0300

Accreditation	MSACS, CPME
Degrees Offered	D.P.M., D.P.M./Ph.D.
# Students Applied	Not Available
Enrollment	Not Available
Mean GPA	Not Available
% Men / % Women	Not Available
% Minorities	Not Available
Tuition	Not Available
Application Fee	Contact School
Application Deadline	Contact School

The University

The Pennsylvania College of Podiatric Medicine (PCPM) was established in 1963. By 1973, it found a permanent home on a one-and-one-half-acre site at Race Street in Philadelphia. PCPM is fully accredited by the MSAC and the Council of Podiatric Medical Education of the American Podiatric Medical Association.

Located in historic Philadelphia, the college sits in the midst of American history, architecture, and urban life. Independence Hall, the Liberty Bell, Penn's Landing, the Philadelphia Museum of Art, and numerous parks, restaurants, and shopping areas in the city make PCPM an attractive locale, serving many cultural and social needs.

Admissions

Applicants should plan to complete or have completed four years of undergraduate education. PCPM requires at least 90 semester hours at an accredited college or university. The college does participate in an accelerated admissions program with various colleges. The new MCAT is required. Transfer students need to take a proficiency exam to be admitted.

Undergraduate Preparation

Required courses include one year each (with lab) of inorganic and organic chemistry, biology or zoology, and physics. Six semester hours in English are also required. Courses in embryology, histology, evolution, cell biology, genetics, and physiology are highly recommended, along with at least 52 semester hours (combined) in a foreign language, philosophy, history, and political science.

Costs

Students live on and off campus at competitive rates. Please call the school for tuition information.

Curriculum

The course of study for the D.P.M. lasts four years. Students take part in clinical observation starting in the first year. Courses in the basic sciences are covered early. The entire fourth year concentrates on clinical training at the college and at hospital externships throughout the country.

Facilities

The recently renovated Foot and Ankle Institute handles 30,000 patient visits a year. Most of the student's clinical work in the third and fourth years is done here. The Annenberg Communications Center has state-of-the-art audiovisual equipment with hookups in all clinical laboratories and conference rooms. There are 16 individual basic science laboratories on two floors of the college, as well as 10 well-equipped research labs. The Gait Study Center, where patients with biomechanical abnormalities are diagnosed and treated, is among the most sophisticated in the country. PCPM has the largest, most complete podiatric medical library in the world. The Charles E. Krauz Library houses about 21,000 volumes and more than 375 current journal subscriptions in related sciences. A computer laboratory is also located here.

Special Programs

In addition to the D.P.M., PCPM offers the joint D.P.M./Ph.D. program in biomedical engineering, in conjunction with the University of Pennsylvania, and in biomedical engineering or biomedical sciences with Drexel University.

Application Procedures

Students must apply through AACPMAS (American Association of Colleges of Podiatric Medicine Application Service), 6110 Executive Boulevard, Suite 204, Rockville, Maryland 20852. Students must submit scores from the new MCAT; the test is offered in April and September. All relevant transcripts are required, and applicants should forward them directly to the college. PCPM requires recommendations from a prehealth professions advisory committee or two letters from science faculty or health professionals. Selected candidates are invited for an interview.

Contact

Recruitment Officer
Pennsylvania College of Podiatric Medicine
Eighth at Race Street
Philadelphia, Pennsylvania 19107
(215) 629-0300 or (800) 220-FEET

DR. WILLIAM M. SCHOLL COLLEGE OF PODIATRIC MEDICINE

1001 North Dearborn Street
Chicago, Illinois 60610
(312) 280-2880

Accreditation	CPME, AACPM
Degrees Offered	D.P.M.
# Students Applied	457
Enrollment	119 / class
Mean GPA	3.0
% Men / % Women	68% / 32%
% Minorities	26.8 %
Tuition	$15,000 In-State
	$15,300 Out-of-State
Application Fee	Contact School
Application Deadline	August 1

The University

Located in Chicago's stylish Gold Coast neighborhood, the Dr. William M. Scholl College of Podiatric Medicine opened in 1912 as the Illinois College of Chiropody and Orthopedics. In 1981, officials renamed the college to honor the late Dr. Scholl. Scholl College is the first podiatric college to enter into a joint venture with a major teaching hospital, the renowned Illinois Masonic Medical Center. This arrangement offers students educational experiences within a multidisciplinary medical setting. The Dr. William M. Scholl College of Podiatric Medicine is accredited by the Council on Podiatric Medical Education of the American Podiatric Medical Association and the Commission on Institutions of Higher Education of the North Central Association of Colleges and Schools. The college is also a member of the AACPM, the ACE, the AGBUC, and the NAICU.

Chicago is a cosmopolitan urban center with small-town appeal. Professional sports, movies, theaters, museums, and a multitude of recreational, social, and cultural opportunities abound in this historic city.

Admissions

Scholl College has a nondiscriminatory policy and encourages all academically-qualified students to apply. Candidates for admission may come from any academic discipline and should have completed at least three years of undergraduate study in an accredited college or university. All candidates must take the MCAT before enrollment. Transfer students are considered and should inquire about special conditions. Students who need to apply for financial aid must have a GPA of 3.4 or higher.

Undergraduate Preparation

Applicants must have completed at least 90 semester credit hours (135 quarter hours) from an accredited college or university. Required courses include 12 semester hours of biology (with lab), and eight semester hours each (with lab) of inorganic and organic chemistry and physics. In addition, the college requires six semester hours of English. Also valuable are skills gained in classes such as anatomy, physiology, biochemistry, microbiology, histology, embryology, algebra, trigonometry, and computer science.

Student Body

About 85 percent of the entering students have earned a baccalaureate or advanced degree. The total college enrollment is about 428, ranging in age from 21 to 41. Students come from 44 states and three foreign countries, and all ethnic and racial minority groups are represented.

Placement Records

One of every three podiatrists in the nation is a graduate of Scholl. Ninety percent of Illinois' podiatrists are alumni of the college. In 1990, over 905 (90 percent) of Scholl College graduates were placed in hospital-based residencies.

Costs

In-state tuition is $15,000; out-of-state tuition is $15,300. Fees amount to $412 for the first year. Room and board, personal costs, and transportation are estimated at $1,385 per month; the total cost for the first year is estimated at $28,930.

Financial Aid

About 96 percent of all Scholl students receive some form of financial aid. Students who show documented financial need are supported through endowed scholarships, 50 half-tuition scholarships, and the Exceptional Financial Need Scholarship program, which provides scholarships to students who have extremely limited financial resources. Grants and loans for residents of Arkansas, Louisiana, and Massachusetts, federal educational loan programs, educational loans from private sources, and student employment are all available to help support the student during the course of study at Scholl.

Student Organizations

Students take part in the campus life through the Illinois Podiatric Medical Students Association (IPMSA) and the American Podiatric Medical Students Association (APMSA). Three active podiatric medical fraternities (Kappa Tau Epsilon, Phi Alpha Pi, and Alpha Gamma Kappa) sponsor a variety of professional and social events every year. Other organizations of interest to Scholl students are the Podiatric Sports Medicine Club, the Podiatry Student Hillel Association, and student chapters of the American College of Foot Surgeons, the American Society of Podiatric Dermatology, and several others. The office of student services offers a number of sporting and recreational activities to round out student life.

Faculty

The faculty consists of about 45 full-time and 23 part-time members in all relevant disciplines. One hundred percent of the basic science staff are Ph.Ds, while all professors at the clinical level are either D.P.Ms or M.Ds.

Curriculum

The course of study for the D.P.M. lasts four years. The first year covers the basic sciences, including biochemistry, gross anatomy, histology, lower extremity anatomy, neuroscience, and physiology. The second year covers microbiology, pathology, and pharmacology. The clinical science courses are offered in the semester format and begin in the second year with a variety of workshops, labs, and rotations, and this continues into the third year. Fourth-year students take part in SCPM clinical rotations in affiliated hospitals for 52 weeks. Fourth-year students are also assigned to podopediatrics, sports medicine, blood flow laboratory, and diabetic foot clinic rotations.

Facilities

Scholl has a new bilingual Hispano Clinic serving Chicago's rapidly growing Hispanic community. Most of the laboratories and classrooms are housed in the 12-story Scholl complex, which also contains outpatient surgery suites and diagnostic areas, a medical library, a fitness center and swimming pool, and a historical museum. A newly renovated Basic Science Research Laboratory and the Scholl College Center for Gait and Locomotion Study offer ample opportunity for research.

Special Programs

The college offers a number of outreach programs to work in the community, including the Hispano Foot Center, Help for the Homeless, and a community foot screening program. Students with appropriate prior experience can participate in advance research training through Scholl's summer research fellowship program, which provides a summer of research training at a number of prestigious Chicago-area medical schools and hospitals.

Application Procedures

Students must apply through AACPMAS. Applications must be received by August 1. The school prefers a composite evaluation from the preprofessional advisory committee, but three letters of evaluation may be substituted. A personal interview may follow. All students must submit a complete health inventory.

Contact

Office of Admission
Scholl College of Podiatric Medicine
1001 North Dearborn Street
Chicago, Illinois 60610
(312) 280-2940 or
(800) 572-2367 (In-State)
(800) 843-3059 (Out-of-State)

## CHAPTER 5

Chiropractic Schools

THE PROFESSION OF CHIROPRACTIC MEDICINE

Chiropractors are health practitioners who primarily treat patients whose health problems are associated with the body's structural and neurological systems, especially the spine. Interference with these systems is believed to impair normal functions and cause lower resistance to disease. Chiropractors believe that malalignment or compression of the spinal nerves, for example, can alter many important body functions by affecting the neurological system.

The chiropractic approach to health care reflects a holistic view, which stresses the patient's overall well-being. It recognizes that many factors affect health, including exercise, diet, rest, environment, and heredity. In keeping with holistic tradition, chiropractors encourage the use of natural, non-drug, nonsurgical health treatments. In cases where chiropractic is inappropriate, chiropractors refer patients to other health practitioners. Like other health practitioners, chiropractors follow a standard routine to secure the information needed for diagnosis and treatment. They take the patient's medical history, conduct physical, neurological, and orthopedic examinations, order laboratory tests, and take X-rays, if needed. They also employ a postural and spinal analysis unique to chiropractic diagnosis.

Some chiropractors specialize in areas related to athletic injuries, diseases and disorders of children, or mental and nervous disorders. Others specialize in taking or interpreting X-rays in orthopedics.

Chiropractors, like other health professionals, are subject to state laws and regulations that specify the types of services they may or may not provide. All states, for example, prohibit chiropractors from prescribing drugs and performing surgery.

In 1988, an estimated 36,000 persons practiced chiropractic. About 70 percent of active chiropractors are in solo practice. The remainder are in group practice or work for other chiropractors. A small number teach and conduct research at chiropractic colleges.

All 50 states and the District of Columbia regulate the practice of chiropractic and grant licenses to chiropractors who meet educational requirements and pass a state board examination. Many states have reciprocity agreements that permit chiropractors already licensed in another state to obtain a license without taking an examination.

The scope of the practice permitted and the educational requirements for a license vary considerably from one state to another, but, in general, state licensing boards require successful completion of a four-year chiropractic college course following two years, equal to 60 semester hours, of undergraduate education. Most state boards recognize only academic training in chiropractic colleges accredited by the Council of Chiropractic Education. Several states require that chiropractors pass a basic science examination, similar to that required for other health practitioners.

All states require a licensure exam. Most state boards recognize either all or part of the three-part test administered by the National Board of Chiropractic Examiners. State examinations may supplement the National Board tests, depending on individual state requirements.

To maintain licensure, 44 states require completion of a specified number of hours of continuing education each year to remain current in the field. Continuing education programs are offered by the American Chiropractic Association (ACA), International Chiropractors Associations, and state chiropractic associations. Special councils within the ACA also offer programs leading to certification, called "diplomatic status," in the areas of orthopedics, nutrition, and radiology and internal disorders.

Chiropractic colleges emphasize classroom and laboratory work in basic science subjects, such as anatomy, public health, microbiology, pathology, physiology, and biochemistry. The last two years stress physical and laboratory diagnosis, neurology, orthopedics, geriatrics, physiotherapy, nutrition, in addition to adjustment techniques and clinical experience. Students completing chiropractic education earn the Doctor of Chiropractic degree (D.C.).

Newly licensed chiropractors have a number of options upon graduation. They can apply for a residency program, set up a new practice, purchase an established one, enter into partnership with an established practitioner, or take a salaried position with an established chiropractor to acquire the experience and the funds needed to open and equip an office.

For more information on chiropractic, contact:

American Chiropractic Association
1701 Clarendon Boulevard
Arlington, VA 22209

or:

Council on Chiropractic Education
4401 Westown Parkway Suite 120
West Des Moines, IA 50265

CHIROPRACTIC SCHOOLS AT A GLANCE

School	Accreditation	Degrees Offered	# Students Applied	Enrollment
Canadian Memorial Chiropractic College	CCE	D.C.	*	*
Cleveland Chiropractic College of Kansas City	CCE	D.C.	*	*
Cleveland Chiropractic College of Los Angeles	CCE	D.C.	137	58 / class
Life Chiropractic College West of Los Angeles	CCE	D.C.	*	100 / class
Life College	CCE, SACS	D.C., B.S., M.S.	500	200
Logan College of Chiropractic	CCE	B.S., D.C.	*	75 / class
Los Angeles College of Chiropractic	CCE	D.C., B.S.	265	100 / class
National College of Chiropractic	CCE	B.S., D.C.	300	101 / class
New York Chiropractic College	CCE	D.C.	*	*
Northwestern College of Chiropractic	CCE	D.C., B.S.	225	116 / class
Palmer College of Chiropractic	CCE, NCACS	D.C., B.S., M.S.	376	221
Palmer College of Chiropractic-West	CCE	DC	*	125 / class
Parker College of Chiropractic	CCE, SACS	D.C., B.S.	*	250
Texas Chiropractic College	CCE, CCSACS	D.C., B.S.	*	*
Western States Chiropractic College	CCE, NWASC	D.C., B.S.	*	*

* Not Available   ** Not Applicable   C/S – Contact School

Mean GPA	% Male / % Female	% Minorities	In-State Tuition	Out-of-State Tuition	Application Fee	Application Deadline
*	*	*	$7,365	$9,245	$75	January 31
*	*	*	$3,774 / trimester	$2,862 / trimester	$50	C/S
2.50	65% / 35%	*	$3,760	C/S	$50	No deadline, rolling admissions
2.25	*	*	$2,750 / quarter	C/S	$35	C/S
2.8	74% / 26%	5%	$2,425 / quarter	C/S	$50	Two weeks prior to start of class
2.25	71% / 29%	6.6%	$3,605 / trimester	C/S	$35	C/S
3.0	70% / 30%	25%	$3,891 / trimester	C/S	$25	C/S
2.75	75% / 25%	10%	$155 / credit hour	C/S	$50	No deadline, rolling admissions
2.25	*	*	$3,150	C/S	$50	C/S
3.0	68% / 32%	4%	$3,585 / trimester	C/S	$35	C/S
2.90	60% / 40%	5%	$10,170	C/S	$50	No deadline
3.0	70% / 30%	*	$2,890 / quarter	C/S	$40	C/S
*	75% / 25%	*	$3,600 / trimester	C/S	$35	C/S
*	*	*	$9,900	C/S	$50	C/S
2.25	*	*	$10,000 / year	C/S	C/S	C/S

* Not Available   ** Not Applicable   C/S – Contact School

CANADIAN MEMORIAL CHIROPRACTIC COLLEGE

1900 Bayview Avenue
Toronto, Ontario, Canada M4G 3E6
(416) 482-2340

Accreditation	CCE
Degrees Offered	D.C.
# Students Applied	Not Available
Enrollment	Not Available
Mean GPA	Not Available
% Men / % Women	Not Available
% Minorities	Not Available
Tuition	$7,365 Canadian Residents (except Quebec)
	$9,245 Canadian Residents (including Quebec)
Application Fee	$75
Application Deadline	January 31

The University

Canadian Memorial Chiropractic College is the only chiropractic educational institution in Canada. It is a charitable, nonprofit organization. Members of the chiropractic profession have accepted complete financial responsibility and pay an annual fee to the college. CMCC is accredited by the Councils on Chiropractic Education of the United States and Canada, which allows graduates to apply for licensure in most states in the U.S. as well as Canada. The college has a no-smoking policy.

Admissions

Applicants must have achieved at least a C average in the required courses and must have a cumulative GPA of 2.25 or above. Non-Canadian applicants will be considered for admission. All students for whom English is a second language must submit evidence of their proficiency in English with their application. Applications for advanced standing may be obtained from the registrar's office. Transfer students from other chiropractic colleges will also be considered for admission.

Undergraduate Preparation

Candidates must have completed at least two years (or the equivalent) of study at a university in Canada. Applicants from Quebec must have completed at least two years in the

Colleges of General and Professional Education Health Sciences (CEGEP), supplemented with a minimum of one year at a university. The following prerequisite courses (including necessary laboratory work) must be successfully completed by the university's spring final examination session: one credit (or six units) each of biology, general or inorganic chemistry, organic chemistry, and physics; psychology, one-half credit (three units); English or communication skills, one credit (six units); and two and one-half credits (15 units) of social science or the humanities.

No more than 20 semester hours of a candidate's preprofessional education (in courses other than the required natural, biological, or physical sciences) can be acquired through the College Level Examination Program (CLEP) or other college proficiency exams. These credits must be certified by an institution accredited at the college level.

Costs

All costs are in Canadian dollars.

Tuition for residents of all provinces except Quebec amounts to $7,365. Tuition for residents of Quebec and all other nonresident students is $9,245. Additional expenses for first-year students, including a flexible vertebral column model for chiropractic courses and laboratory, and library fees, amount to $295. Textbooks and classroom supplies cost approximately $850 per year.

Financial Aid

Under the Canada Student Loan Program, bank loans are available to full-time students in financial need. Only Canadian citizens or those with landed immigrant status are eligible. Financial aid is also available from various provincial student awards programs. Additional aid is available through the college and is awarded on the basis of need and/or achievement. For more information, contact the CMCC student affairs office. It is important to apply early for financial aid.

Outside employment is available, but students must ensure that employment or outside activities will not interfere with the requirements of the curriculum.

Student Organizations

The student's administrative council supervises the direction of extracurricular activities and services, represents student interests on various college governing bodies and committees, and refers problems to the appropriate college authorities. Professional organizations on campus include the Canadian Student Council of Women Chiropractors, the Chiropractic Christian Fellowship, the Student Canadian Chiropractic Association, and the Canadian Chiropractic Toastmaster Club.

Curriculum

The first three years of study are divided into two semesters each. The fourth year has three semesters. The first two years are devoted to the basic sciences, with an introduction to chiropractic and clinical diagnostic studies. The third year includes the study of chiropractic science with an emphasis on clinical diagnostic studies and methodology in clinical investigations. During the fourth year of study, the presentation of chiropractic and clinical studies is continued in specialized areas and clinical training is intensified.

The fourth-year student must complete an investigative project in order to graduate. Before beginning the project, students are given instruction in research methodology and biometrics. Groups of students, under the supervision of a faculty member, then select a research problem. Upon approval, students either develop an independent investigation or assist in a faculty research study.

Facilities

Most clinical education is given at the college's two outpatient clinics. The outpatient clinic on the Bayview Avenue campus contains consultation treatment rooms, administrative offices, a clinical laboratory, and radiology departments. The satellite clinic is located in west Toronto on the lower level of the Crossways Mall. It contains a reception/waiting area, consultation and treatment rooms, and a radiology department. The Midtown Chiropractic Clinic is a faculty-based teaching clinic offering treatment and assessment facilities.

Laboratory facilities include the human gross anatomy laboratory, the biochemistry, microbiology and laboratory diagnosis facility, and the physiology laboratory. The C.C. Clemmer Health Sciences Library provides materials and resources necessary to supplement the teaching and learning process and to support scientific investigation and research. The library has on-line access to the MEDLARS, CAN/OLE, BRS, and DIALOG information retrieval systems.

CMCC has no facilities for student housing.

Grading Procedures

A letter grading system is used. Evaluation for promotion takes place at the end of each year of study.

Application Procedures

Applications for admission can be obtained by contacting the registrar's office. The deadline for application is January 31. Applications should include a nonrefundable application fee of $75, reference letters from two individuals (mailed directly from those individuals to the registrar's office), and official transcripts of academic records. When all supporting documents are received by the registrar's office, a letter of acknowledgment will be mailed to the applicant. If all academic requirements are fulfilled, an applicant may be scheduled for a private interview. At this time, the applicant must provide a recent photograph and pay an interview fee of $50.

Contact

The Registrar
Canadian Memorial Chiropractic College
1900 Bayview Avenue
Toronto, Ontario
Canada M4G 3E6
(416) 482-2340

CLEVELAND CHIROPRACTIC COLLEGE OF KANSAS CITY

6401 Rockhill Road
Kansas City, Missouri 64131
(816) 333-8230

Accreditation	CCE
Degrees Offered	D.C.
# Students Applied	Not Available
Enrollment	Not Available
Mean GPA	Not Available
% Men / % Women	Not Available
% Minorities	Not Available
Tuition	$3,774 / trimester (9-trimester program);
	$2,862 / trimester (12-trimester program)
Application Fee	$50
Application Deadline	Contact School

The University

Established in 1922, Cleveland Chiropractic College of Kansas City is recognized as a major institution for chiropractic education and research. The college seeks to educate practitioners as primary health care providers.

The college is located in Kansas City, Missouri, a major midwestern city with a population of more than 1.5 million (including surrounding areas).

Admissions

The college considers undergraduate grades, letters of recommendation, and the candidate's personal statement. In general, the cumulative GPA and the cumulative GPA in science and mathematics must be at least 2.5. The student must demonstrate certain physical capabilities such as strength and coordination for the performance of chiropractic procedures and techniques, the necessary tactile senses, and an appropriate level of manual dexterity.

Undergraduate Preparation

Candidates must have completed at least two years (90 semester hours) of undergraduate work at an accredited institution. Undergraduate coursework must include one year each of biology, inorganic chemistry, organic chemistry, and physics, all with lab; six semester hours of English; three semester hours of psychology; three semester hours in the social sciences; and 12 hours of humanities or other social sciences courses.

Costs

The college has a nine-trimester and a 12-trimester program. The current cost for the first trimester of the nine-trimester program is $3,774 per trimester. The current cost for the first trimester of the extended twelve-trimester program is $2,862 per trimester. Tuition costs, which are normally adjusted each September, include malpractice insurance coverage, student council dues, and a university activity card. At present, the cost of textbooks and lecture notes range from $400 to $500 per trimester. Expenditures for diagnostic instruments vary. In addition, an $86-per-trimester student activity fee is charged. Dormitory rooms on the university campus, including a meal plan, cost between $2,500 and $3,000.

Financial Aid

A wide variety of financial aid plans are available. Federal assistance includes Pell Grants, Supplemental Educational Opportunity Grant, Perkins Student Loans, college work-study programs, and Stafford Loans. Private scholarships are usually available to students who have a record of good academic standing. Veterans benefits are also available.

Student Organizations

Student organizations at Cleveland College provide students with a chance for leadership, extracurricular activity, and interaction with faculty, alumni, and other students. There are more than a dozen organizations, including Activator Methods Club, Baha'i Association, Beta Chi Rho Fraternity, Radiology Club, Student American Chiropractic Association, and student council. In addition, students have the opportunity to participate in intramural sports, such as basketball and softball. Students can also attend the educational program of the Cleveland Chiropractic College Alumni Association.

Curriculum

The standard chiropractic program consists of nine trimesters (four months per trimester for a total of 36 months). The school also has an extended 12-month course of study (48 months).

The program encompasses the content and methodology necessary for the development of expertise in chiropractic health care. The curriculum is designed to qualify graduates for the state licensure examination and to prepare graduates to be primary health care providers. The curriculum provides training in the relationship of the structural and neurological aspects of the body, and how this relationship relates to health.

The curriculum consists of basic science and clinical skills courses as well as clinical and laboratory experiences.

Facilities

The college comprises three interconnecting buildings representing 46,000 square feet of floor area. The college clinic has consultation rooms, conference rooms, examination and treatment rooms, clinical laboratories, radiological laboratories, and other facilities. The college laboratories have facilities for instruction in anatomy, chemistry, microbiology, physiology, radiology, diagnosis, and technique. Facilities also include a student center and a bookstore.

The Ruth R. Cleveland Memorial Library houses a collection that supports the chiropractic and health sciences. The library subscribes to over 200 national and international journals. Computer search facilities include MEDLINE and BIOSIS, and standard indexes are available. The library contains a radiologic learning laboratory, a collection of over 4,000 films of bone, chest, neurological, gastrointestinal, and other anatomical areas. Video and audiocassettes and slides are also available. Students have access to interlibrary loan service with 30 member libraries in the Kansas City library network and other libraries both nationwide and abroad.

Grading Procedures

The college uses a letter grading system of A, B, C, D, and F.

Special Programs

Special programs include a postdoctoral research fellowship program for those already holding doctoral degrees in a health field. The college offers continuing education courses for practicing doctors in various areas of specialty or particular need.

Application Procedures

Candidates must submit a completed application form (available from the college's office of admissions) along with a $50 nonrefundable application fee. High school and undergraduate college transcripts must be submitted directly to the office, as well as two letters of recommendation—one from a professor and one from a health care professional. Students must submit a personal statement of motivation along with the application.

Candidates can begin study in any of three terms—fall, winter, or summer. Within two weeks of acceptance, students must submit a $150 reservation deposit.

Contact

Office of Admissions
Cleveland Chiropractic College of Kansas City
6401 Rockhill Road
Kansas City, Missouri 64131
(816) 333-8230
(800) 274-0617

CLEVELAND CHIROPRACTIC COLLEGE OF LOS ANGELES

590 North Vermont Avenue
Los Angeles, California 90004-2196
(213) 660-6166

Accreditation	CCE
Degrees Offered	D.C.
# Students Applied	137
Enrollment	58 / class
Mean GPA	2.50
% Men / % Women	65% / 35%
% Minorities	Not Available
Tuition	$3,760
Application Fee	$50
Application Deadline	No deadline, rolling admissions

The University

Dr. C.S. Cleveland, Sr., founder of the Cleveland Chiropractic College in Kansas City, Missouri, proposed in the 1940s that the college acquire Ratledge Chiropractic College in Los Angeles. The board of trustees acted on his advice, and after Ratledge was purchased in 1950, it was renamed the Cleveland Chiropractic College of Los Angeles. In 1976, the college acquired its current three-acre campus, a few miles from the original site, in metropolitan Los Angeles near Hollywood, downtown Los Angeles, and Southland beaches. Los Angeles, the largest city in California in terms of population and size, is ranked second nationally in population. The Los Angeles area offers a variety of cultural, ethnic, and social opportunities. Entertainment in the form of theater, ballet, opera, classical concerts, and celebrity appearances is easily accessible. Outdoor sports and activities from skiing to surfing are popular throughout the year.

Admissions

A candidate must have completed 60 semester units of prechiropractic courses with a GPA of at least 2.50. Applicants who have a bachelor's degree in liberal arts are preferred. Each candidate must meet physical requirements needed to perform the duties of a chiropractor.

Undergraduate Preparation

Required courses for the doctor of chiropractic program include six semester hours (with lab) of general biology, anatomy, physiology, microbiology, or zoology; six semester hours (with lab) of general or inorganic chemistry and organic chemistry; six semester hours of English/communications (including composition/writing/rhetoric). Also required are 12 additional semester hours of social sciences or humanities; three semester hours of general psychology; and 24 semester hours of electives.

Costs

Tuition is $3,760 per term. In addition, there are clinic fees for chiropractic health care that cover a complete physical neurological examination, initial X-ray study, treatment including adjustments, and physiological therapeutics laboratory testing. Books and supplies cost $1,000 per year.

Financial Aid

Students may apply for financial aid in the form of scholarships, grants, work study, and loans. Most students receive aid primarily from loan sources. Federal student financial aid programs include Pell Grant, college work-study program, Perkins Loan, Supplemental Education Opportunity Grants, Stafford Student Loans, Supplemental Loans for Students, Health Education Assistance Loans, Parent Loan for Undergraduate Students, and Professional Educational Program. California residents may apply for CAL GRANT A and B. Veterans should contact the V.A. representative in the student affairs office for information about Veterans Administration benefits. Private grants and scholarships are awarded on the basis of both need and qualifications.

Student Organizations

Students may participate in a variety of organizations and activities including the student body association, Sigma Chi Psi, Delta Tau Alpha, International Chiropractors Association, American Chiropractic Association, California Chiropractic Association, technique clubs including Gonstead, Thompson, applied kinesiology, motion palpation, pediatrics, sports injuries, club chiropractic, Christian Chiropractors Association, Korean club, and Asian club.

Faculty

In addition to the three department chairs, there are nine associate professors, six full professors, 17 assistant professors, two instructors, one clinician, and one radiologist on staff at the college. The continuing education faculty consists of 30 members, most of whom are Doctors of Chiropractic.

Curriculum

The chiropractic degree program is composed of courses in basics sciences, including anatomy, physiology, chemistry, pathology, microbiology, and public health; diagnostic sciences, including diagnosis and X-ray; and chiropractic sciences, including orientation, philosophy, technique, physiotherapy, clinic, management, research, and office procedures. In order to graduate, a student must fulfill the following requirements: the last three full-time trimesters must be completed at Cleveland Chiropractic College of Los Angeles; passing grades should be earned in all courses with a minimum 2.0 GPA in basic, diagnostic, and chiropractic sciences; satisfactory performance of clinical requirements; and fulfillment of all requirements within six years.

Facilities

The main building contains classrooms, laboratories, clinics, student lounges, a cafeteria, and administrative offices. Laboratories are designed for the study of bacteriology, chemistry, pathology, histology, human dissection, palpation, and clinical laboratory analysis. The library, adjacent to the main building, houses approximately 14,000 books, journals, and pamphlets. Visual and non-print materials are kept in the learning resource center. In addition to the collection, the library offers interlibrary loan services and the computerized services of interdisciplinary library networks, the Medical Library Association, and various university, public, and hospital libraries.

Grading Procedures

Grades are based on exams, attendance, and class participation. A letter grading system of A, B, C, D, and F is used.

Special Programs

The senior intern program gives 10th-trimester students the opportunity to explore a specialty in the areas of administration, insurance, diagnosis, adjustive skills, physical therapy, X-ray, faculty, and referral clinic. The preceptorship program, also available to 10th-trimester students, enables participants to apprentice with a practicing chiropractor in a clinic. Other special programs include the sports medicine program, the research program, and continuing education studies in which relicensing seminars are conducted.

Application Procedures

An application, along with a $50 application fee, official transcripts, two personal recommendations, a cover letter specifying prerequisite courses currently being taken, and a recent photograph, should be submitted to the office of admissions. Trimesters begin in January, May, and September.

Contact

Office of Admissions
Cleveland Chiropractic College
590 North Vermont Avenue
Los Angeles, California 90004-2196
(213) 660-6166

LIFE CHIROPRACTIC COLLEGE WEST

2005 Via Barrett
San Lorenzo, California 94580
(415) 276-9013

Accreditation	CCE
Degrees Offered	D.C.
# Students Applied	Not Available
Enrollment	100 / class
Mean GPA	2.25
% Men / % Women	Not Available
% Minorities	Not Available
Tuition	$2,750 / quarter
Application Fee	$35
Application Deadline	Contact School

The University

Life Chiropractic College West was founded and incorporated in 1976 as Pacific States Chiropractic College. In March 1981, Dr. Sid E. Williams made possible the merger between Pacific and Life Colleges to produce the college with its current name. Life Chiropractic College West is accredited by the CCE. Located in San Lorenzo, a suburban community in the San Francisco Bay area, the campus allows for quick and easy access to all the amenities of San Francisco, San Jose, Oakland, and Berkeley, but still keeps the friendly small-town atmosphere of San Lorenzo itself.

Admissions

Life Chiropractic College West offers equal education and employment opportunities to all without regard to race, sex, creed, age, color, ethnic origin, or physical handicap. Entering students must have a minimum of 60 college semester credits with a GPA of at least 2.25. Up to 20 semester hours of CLEP credit is acceptable.

Undergraduate Preparation

Required courses include six semester hours each (with lab) of biology and/or zoology, inorganic and organic chemistry, and physics. At least six hours of English composition or communication skills are also required, along with three hours of psychology, and three hours in the social sciences and humanities. Beginning in 1991, 24 of the total 60 hours required must be in the humanities. Students must pass all science courses with a C or better.

Student Body

The college enrolls 400 students, suggesting an entering class of about 100.

Costs

Tuition is $2,750 per quarter. Other fees come to about $700. The college provides assistance in locating housing. Reasonably priced accommodations are available nearby.

Financial Aid

Students may apply for a full range of grants, loans, employment programs, scholarships, and Veterans Educational Benefits. Grants include the Pell Grant, SEOG, CAL Grant A, and the Bureau of Indian Affairs Grant. Loans include the Stafford and HEAL loan funds.

Student Organizations

Numerous technique clubs and a wide variety of athletic and social programs complement Life's academic program.

Faculty

The college enjoys a faculty and staff of 130 members. The student/faculty ratio is 8.5:1.

Curriculum

The curriculum consists of 12 quarters of full-time study. A 14-quarter option is available. In the 12-quarter program, students cover the basic sciences in the first six quarters and must pass Part I of the National Boards at the end of the fifth quarter. The study of the clinical sciences begins in the seventh quarter, and internships begin as early as the eighth quarter. In the 11th quarter students must take and pass Part II of the National Boards.

Facilities

The college operates a 12,000-square-foot state-of-the-art clinic in downtown Hayward. The latest equipment, experienced faculty, and spacious areas for study and clinical work offer the student a comprehensive venue for study. The 9,000-square-foot library complex is centrally located and consists of circulating and reference collections, historic archives, audio-visual facilities, and a roentgenology lab. Ten well-equipped laboratories support the curriculum with up-to-date technology.

Grading Procedures

Life College uses a letter grading system, A-D (4-1 points), with A for superior work, and D for poor but passing work. An F indicates failure, and students must repeat the course and pass. An F and/or a WF will remain on the student's permanent record, though he or she may repeat and complete the course. Honors, cum laude, and other such recognitions are offered to those who qualify.

Application Procedures

Applications for admission may be obtained from and submitted to the admissions office. The nonrefundable application fee is $35. Applicants should also send high school transcripts, college transcripts, and a personal photo. Call admissions to arrange an interview. International students may apply but should write to admissions for their special academic requirements. Upon acceptance all students must reserve a place in class by submitting a $500 acceptance fee, which will be applied to the first-quarter tuition. Students may be considered for advanced standing and transfer.

Contact

Life Chiropractic College West
2005 Via Barrett
San Lorenzo, California 94580
(415) 276-9013

LIFE COLLEGE

1269 Barclay Circle
Marietta, Georgia 30060
(404) 424-0554

Accreditation	CCE, SACS
Degrees Offered	D.C., B.S., M.S.
# Students Applied	500
Enrollment	200
Mean GPA	2.8
% Men / % Women	74% / 26%
% Minorities	5%
Tuition	$2,425 / quarter
Application Fee	$50
Application Deadline	Two weeks prior to start of class

The University

Life College was founded in 1974 by Dr. Sid E. Williams. The college is a private nonprofit institution dedicated to helping people discover their own natural abilities to heal. With an enrollment of more than 2,000, it is the largest chiropractic college in the world. In addition to its chiropractic program, the college has both undergraduate programs and professional graduate programs.

The college is located on a 100-acre campus in Marietta, Georgia, a suburb of Atlanta with about 43,000 residents. It is situated near the Chattahoochee River and near the lakes and mountains of northern Georgia. The Appalachian Mountains are a perfect setting for many kinds of outdoor recreation; the city of Atlanta provides many cultural opportunities: theaters, art museums, the Atlanta Symphony, Zoo Atlanta, the Martin Luther King Center, the Jimmy Carter Presidential Library, and the Fernbank Science Center, to name but a few.

Admissions

The admissions committee carefully examines many factors to determine what the applicant can bring to the chiropractic profession. The undergraduate GPA must be 2.25 in order to be considered for admission. Each required undergraduate science course must be passed with a C grade or better.

Undergraduate Preparation

Applicants must have taken at least 60 semester hours or 90 quarter hours in the arts and sciences toward the bachelor's degree. Students from a community college or junior college must be working toward an associate's degree. Undergraduate coursework must include six semester hours of English; three semester hours of psychology; three semester hours of social sciences or humanities; six semester hours of biology (with lab); 12 semester hours of chemistry with lab (including six semester hours each of inorganic and organic chemistry); and six semester hours of physics (with lab). Other courses in mathematics are recommended.

Student Body

The average age of the Life College student is 24 years. Eighteen percent of the students are Georgia residents and 26 percent are women. More than 25 percent hold the baccalaureate degree at time of matriculation. Life College students are from 42 states and 27 foreign countries.

Costs

Tuition for 1991-92 is $2,425 per quarter for the D.C. program (quarter-hour tuition rate is $115.48 per credit hour). Most other fees are minimal. Off-campus one-bedroom apartments typically rent for about $300 per month.

Financial Aid

Financial aid programs available to Life College students include Pell Grants, Supplemental Educational Opportunity Grants, college work-study programs, Perkins Loans, and Life College Foreign Student Loans. State grants are also available.

Minority Programs

Life College has a special minority student scholarship.

Student Organizations

The college has over 50 service, social, and fraternal organizations for students. These include a nationally chartered chiropractic fraternity and a national sorority. There is a wide variety of intramural sports for students, including a prize-winning rugby team, and basketball, ice hockey, and tennis teams.

Faculty

The college has more than 125 faculty members.

Curriculum

The curriculum includes studies in biological and health sciences, chiropractic philosophy, and practice management. Students have extensive clinical experience in the college's outpatient clinics. The special focus of Life's program is on the relationship between structural and neurological aspects of the body in health and disease. Upon graduation, students are eligible for licensure as chiropractors in 49 states and in many foreign countries. Students may also participate in research along with faculty members.

Facilities

Life College has comprehensive facilities, which include a recent multimillion-dollar expansion and improvement project. The expansion has provided for a new functional cadaver laboratory, biochemistry and bacteriological laboratories, and equipment for standard hematological and urinalysis procedures. There is also a new wellness center for students and the public.

There are both tutorial rooms and large lecture rooms for teaching. The Neil K. Williams Learning Resource Center houses 50,000 books, periodicals, and audiovisual materials. The center is a member of the chiropractic library consortium, the National Library of Medicine Regional Program, and the Medical Library Association.

Special Programs

The college offers a B.S. in nutrition for the chiropractic sciences, which focuses on nutrition for the prevention of disease. The college also offers the master of sports health science degree and a four-quarter program for chiropractic technicians. For those who have not taken the preprofessional courses necessary for admission, the college offers undergraduate courses to satisfy these requirements.

Application Procedures

Life College has its own application for admission, which

should be completed and submitted to the school's director of admission services. High school and college transcripts must be submitted along with two letters of recommendation from practicing chiropractors and a $50 nonrefundable application fee. Candidates can apply for the winter, spring, summer, or fall quarters.

Foreign students must apply through the World Education Services, Inc., P.O. Box 745, Old Chelsea Station, New York, NY 10011.

Contact

Life College
Director of Admission Services
1269 Barclay Circle
Marietta, Georgia 30060
(404) 424-0554, ext. 231

LOGAN COLLEGE OF CHIROPRACTIC

1851 Schoettler Road
Chesterfield, Missouri 63006-1065
(314) 227-2100

Accreditation	CCE
Degrees Offered	B.S., D.C.
# Students Applied	Not Available
Enrollment	75 / class
Mean GPA	2.25
% Men / % Women	71% / 29%
% Minorities	6.6%
Tuition	$3,605 / trimester
Application Fee	$35
Application Deadline	Contact School

The University

Dr. Hugh B. Logan founded the Logan College of Chiropractic in 1935. The first class consisted of seven men and women; classes were held in a converted residence in St. Louis. By the following fall the school had outgrown the original site, and a 17-acre site in Normandy was chosen as Logan's permanent location. Enrollment increased steadily even during the Second World War. In 1958 Logan College merged

with the Carver Chiropractic College, Oklahoma, and in 1964 merged with Missouri Chiropractic College. To meet the needs of increasing numbers of students interested in studying chiropractic, in 1973 Logan moved to a 103-acre wooded hilltop in the city of Chesterfield, a suburb of St. Louis. Its proximity to St. Louis affords all the advantages of city life while providing the amenities of a small town. Dances, outings, and sporting events are organized on the Logan campus, and recreational and cultural activities are available in the St. Louis area.

Admissions

Students are admitted in either the fall trimester in September, the spring trimester in January, or the summer trimester in May. In order to be selected, a candidate must have finished at least two years of undergraduate work and have an overall GPA of at least 2.25 and a GPA of 2.0 in biology, chemistry, and physics. Additionally, candidates for admission must have participated in a personal interview, received a recommendation from a Doctor of Chiropractic plus three additional personal references, and submitted an essay describing professional goals.

Undergraduate Preparation

Undergraduate requirements include six semester hours of language and/or communication skills; three semester hours of psychology; 15 semester hours of social sciences or humanities; one year of biological sciences (specifically general biology, anatomy, physiology, microbiology, or zoology); one year of general or inorganic chemistry; one year of organic chemistry; and one year of physics. All science courses must be taken with a lab and a grade of C or better must be earned. Electives enough to complete 60 semester hours or two years of study should be taken, preferably in the humanities, social sciences, language or communication skills, or general sciences.

Student Body

Students are enrolled from all over the United States as well as Canada, South America, Europe, Asia, Africa, and Australia. About 96 percent of the students who enroll at Logan earn the D.C. degree.

Costs

Tuition costs $3,605 each trimester, and students must pay an $85 clinic entrance fee during the fifth and eighth trimesters. Additional annual costs include $8,616 for room and board for a single student living off campus, approximately $860 for books, and $3,300 for personal expenses.

Financial Aid

Scholarships, grants, loans, and employment are among the forms of financial aid programs available to Logan students. These programs include the Pell Grant, Supplemental Educational Opportunity Grant, college work-study program, Perkins

Loan, Stafford Student Loan, PLUS/Supplemental Loan, Health Education Assistance Loan, and the Missouri Grant Program. Department fellowships and research grants are given to students demonstrating academic excellence and experience. Disabled students may be eligible for benefits from their state vocational rehabilitation service. In order to qualify for financial aid, a student must be enrolled in the D.C. program full time, have satisfactory grades, have no outstanding loans or grant refunds, and be a U.S. citizen or permanent resident.

Student Organizations

Campus organizations include Student Doctor's Council, four national professional chiropractic societies, student chapters of the ACA and ICA, student state clubs, Women's Club, and various technique clubs.

Faculty

There are 76 faculty members on staff. Seventy percent have D.C. degrees and many also have masters or doctoral degrees in medicine, pharmacy, radiology, humanities, law, and business.

Curriculum

The 10-trimester or five-year program incorporates courses from five divisions including basic science, chiropractic science, clinical science, the health center, and research. In the area of basic science, students study gross anatomy, cell biology, physiology, and biochemistry. Chiropractic science courses include chiropractic philosophy, office management, the Logan system of body mechanics, and other adjusting techniques. The study of clinical science follows human biology with coursework in clinical diagnosis. Actual clinical work, lectures, and case studies are the focus of the health center division. Methods of research leading to the completion of a senior research project are part of the academic experiences designed by the research division.

Facilities

Facilities on campus include technique, science, research, and ergonomic laboratories, the learning resources center, the health center, and a science, research, and ergonomics center. The learning resources center contains the library, library media room, and media production studio. Located in the main building, the library's collection includes about 10,000 volumes, 200 serials, and anatomical models, as well as chiropractic newsletters, statutes, newspaper clippings, articles and reprints, and the DYNIX computerized interlibrary loan system. The library media room houses 700 audiovisual titles. Media production provides equipment and services for instruction. The Logan health center is a teaching clinic equipped with offices, a radiology and clinical laboratory, and private adjusting rooms. The ergonomics center, located in the science, research, and ergonomics building, contains a human performance laboratory. Off-campus facilities include the Community Health Center, the Dellwood Health Center, and the Harbor Light Clinic, all in St. Louis.

Grading Procedures

The college uses a letter grading system of A-F and AF (failure due to absences).

Special Programs

Logan College of Chiropractic offers various postdoctoral programs including diplomate programs, certification programs, paraprofessional programs, residency programs, continuing education seminars, and adult continuing education courses.

Application Procedures

Students may apply for entrance into the D.C. program by applying six months in advance of the trimester (September, January, or May) they wish to begin. An application and a $35 application fee should be sent to the admissions office along with transcripts from all colleges attended, a letter of recommendation from a D.C., and three personal references. An interview is required and should be arranged through the admissions office.

Contact

Logan College of Chiropractic
Admissions Office
1851 Schoettler Road
PO Box 1065
Chesterfield, Missouri 63006-1065
(314) 227-2100
(800) 782-3344

LOS ANGELES COLLEGE OF CHIROPRACTIC

16200 East Amber Valley Drive
Whittier, California 90609-1166
(213) 947-8755

Accreditation	CCE
Degrees Offered	D.C., B.S.
# Students Applied	265
Enrollment	100 / class
Mean GPA	3.0
% Men / % Women	70% / 30%
% Minorities	25%
Tuition	$3,891 / trimester
Application Fee	$25
Application Deadline	No deadline

The University

A nonprofit institution founded in 1911, Los Angeles College of Chiropractic (LACC) received its CCE accreditation in 1966. Today, the college enrolls 1,000 students and occupies a 39-acre campus.

The college is located in Whittier, California, a quiet residential community near the Pacific beaches and the southern ridges of the Sierra Nevada Mountains. With a population of about 71,000, Whittier offers sports, cultural, and commercial attractions.

Admissions

Candidates for admission are evaluated based on high school and college transcripts, personal references attesting to good moral character, and the results of an interview. Factors considered include professional character, aptitude, scholarship, and good health. Applicants must have at least a 2.5 overall GPA to be admitted; the average GPA of the accepted candidate is 3.0.

Physical qualifications must also be met to ensure students have the necessary strength and coordination to stand alone and use the limbs in chiropractic techniques. A level of manual dexterity is needed in addition to oral communication skills.

Undergraduate Preparation

Minimum requirements for admission include undergraduate coursework in the following: one year of biological sciences with lab (biology preferred, zoology, anatomy, or physiology accepted); one year of general chemistry (with lab); one year of organic chemistry (with lab); one year of physics (with lab); six semester units in English or communication skills (including one English composition course); three semester units of psychology; and three units in social sciences or humanities, with a minimum grades of C in each. Preadmission counseling is recommended before starting the preprofessional course of study.

Student Body

LACC admits a new class of 150 students twice a year. The student body comprises about 70 percent men and 30 percent women.

Placement Records

LACC graduates rank above the national average in the National and the State Board examinations. The college assists its students in preparing for a career through its preceptor program, in which students take internships in a licensed chiropractor's office. Three-year residency programs in radiology and clinical chiropractic are offered for graduates, as are careers in teaching and research.

Costs

For September 1991 through August 1992, tuition is $3,891 per trimester. The cost of books is estimated to be $300 per trimester. Equipment costs are estimated to be $700 per trimester.

Financial Aid

Most LACC students receive some form of financial aid, from scholarships to loans to work-study for pay or academic credit. Institutional awards include the Mindlin Award, the Scholars Program Awards, and the James W. Fitches Endowment Fund. There are a variety of federal and state grants, including Pell Grants; and about two dozen scholarships are available from various chiropractic associations and organizations. Other types of aid include Stafford Loans, Health Education Assistance Loans, and work-study program opportunities.

Minority Programs

LACC has special tuition grants and special scholarships for ethnic minorities, women, and foreign students.

Student Organizations

The college has a variety of service clubs and student organizations. These include the Student American Chiropractic Association, the Women's Health Council, the World Congress of Chiropractic Students, the Sports Injury Council, Toastmasters, Student International Chiropractic Association, Delta Tau Alpha, Sigma Chi Psi, and a range of clubs based on various chiropractic concerns, among them the Motion Palpation Club, Nutrition Council, and the Applied Kinesiology Club.

Faculty

The LACC faculty and staff number about 200 full-time members. All members of the basic sciences faculty have either a Ph.D. or M.D. related to their field of teaching. All clinical sciences faculty hold a first professional degree and California license.

Curriculum

The academic program is built on trimesters of 15 weeks each. The regular program of 10 trimesters can be completed in three and one-half years. Recently revised, the new Doctor of Chiropractic curriculum—called the "Advantage" Program—is based on teaching chiropractic competencies rather than academic subjects.

Basic science courses are taught as they relate to clinical diagnosis and treatment. Students begin clinical training from the start of the program, and all instruction is integrated with clinical experience. Chiropractic and diagnostic skills are emphasized. Students take their internships in one of five modern clinical facilities, where they care for patients under faculty supervision.

Facilities

The five clinics of the college are located in Whittier (on campus) and in Anaheim, El Monte, Glendale, and La Habra. Other public clinics in Los Angeles and Pasadena are used by the college.

The recently remodeled Learning Resource Center provides comprehensive facilities for LACC students, including an up-to-date collection of books and access to over 500 scientific journal titles. The center has audio and video study aids as well as radiological films for study. The center provides access to the MEDLARS bibliography and is connected to hundreds of other databases through the DIALOG Information System. The center serves as the west coast depository for the Chiropractic Research Archives Collection.

Grading Procedures

The college uses a letter grading system, A through F.

Special Programs

The college offers a bachelor of science degree in biology. The college also has a division of postgraduate education for those who seek membership or certification in a specialty area. These postgraduate specialities include chiropractic consulting in the workplace, chiropractic neurology, and sports and recreational injuries. There are residency programs and a program to educate chiropractic assistants.

Application Procedures

Candidates for admission must submit an application, official transcripts from all high schools and colleges attended, a $25 application fee, and three recommendations (at least one must be from a D.C.). Candidates will also be asked to participate in a personal interview.

Early application is strongly recommended. Applications should be submitted not less than 12 months before the date of desired enrollment. LACC admits foreign students and transfer students.

Contact

Los Angeles College of Chiropractic
Admission Department
16200 East Amber Valley Drive
PO Box 1166-P
Whittier, California 90609-1166
(213) 947-8755
(800) 221-LACC

NATIONAL COLLEGE OF CHIROPRACTIC

200 East Roosevelt Road
Lombard, Illinois 60148-4583
(708) 629-2000

Accreditation	CCE
Degrees Offered	B.S., D.C.
# Students Applied	300
Enrollment	101 / class
Mean GPA	2.75
% Men / % Women	75% / 25%
% Minorities	10%
Tuition	$155 / credit hour
Application Fee	$50
Application Deadline	No deadline, rolling admissions

The University

In 1906 the college was established as the National School of Chiropractic. The school was moved to Chicago in 1908, and in 1912 was chartered and incorporated under Illinois state laws. In 1920 the name of the school was officially changed to the National College of Chiropractic. The college became a nonprofit institution in 1942. In 1963, the school was moved to its current location, a 30-acre site in Lombard and in 1981 it received accreditation by the North Central Association of Colleges and Secondary Schools.

The college publishes the only referenced, internationally indexed, chiropractic journal, the Journal of Manipulative and Physiological Therapeutics. As a five-year, co-educational, private college, NCC enrolls about 800 students. Lombard, a suburban town 25 miles west of Chicago, affords easy access to many outdoor sports activities. Employment is available and cost of living is moderate.

Admissions

In order to be eligible for admission into the doctor of chiropractic program, candidates must have a high school diploma, two years consisting of 60 semester hours at a junior college, college, or university, a grade of C or higher in each course taken, and a GPA of no less than 2.25.

Undergraduate Preparation

Undergraduate admissions requires 24 to 32 semester hours of coursework in the sciences, including general or inorganic chemistry, organic chemistry, physics, and biology; six semester hours of English; 18 semester hours of humanities and social sciences with three of those hours in basic psychology; and four to 12 semester hours of electives. Each science course sequence must have a value of no less than six semester hours of credit completed in two or more academic terms and must include a lab.

Costs

Tuition is $155 per credit hour. The base education fee, including tuition and fees, is $3,670.

Financial Aid

Most financial aid is received in the form of federal and state loans, grants, and scholarships. Students may also apply for work-study programs and fellowships. Among the aid available are Pell Grants, Supplemental Educational Opportunity Grants, state grants and scholarships, Illinois Student Assistance Commission, Veterans' Administration Education Benefits, Grant-In-Aid Program for Citizens of the United States, Scholarship Program for Foreign Students, and Grant-In-Aid for Canadian Students. Students may apply for Perkins Loans, the Stafford program, Parent Loans for Undergraduate Students, Supplemental Loan for Students, and the Health Education Assistance Loan. College work-study is awarded on the basis of need and skill for available positions.

Minority Programs

The Grant-In-Aid Program is available to minority students who are Illinois residents.

Student Organizations

The student council coordinates the activities of many groups on campus including the aerobic club, applied kinesiology, Chi Rho Sigma international professional fraternity, cycling club, Delta Tau Alpha honorary society, fellowship of Christian chiropractors, hockey club, Jewish chiropractic organization, yearbook, motion palpation club, performing arts club, rugby team, Sigma Phi Kappa fraternity, ski club, soccer team, soft-style martial arts club, soft tissue club, specific adjusting club, and sports injury council, among others.

Faculty

Eighteen assistant professors, 18 lecturers, 13 associate professors, 19 full professors, 20 instructors, four residents, eight fellows, and one adjunct faculty member comprise the teaching staff.

Curriculum

The doctor of chiropractic program takes at least five years to complete. Subject areas include human embryology, gross anatomy, human histology, chiropractic awareness, biochemistry, normal radiographic anatomy, human neuroanatomy, cells and body fluids, genetics, biomechanics, palpation, clinical psychology, emergency care, and first-aid procedures. In order to graduate with a doctor of chiropractic degree a student must have spent at least five years studying chiropractic education with a minimum of the last two years as a resident at the National College of Chiropractic, fulfilled all course requirements within eight years, have the support of the faculty and clinic staff, have no financial debt to the college, be 21 years of age and of good moral character, and attend the graduation ceremony.

Facilities

The National College of Chiropractic has six teaching clinics including the student clinic, Chicago General Health Service, Brookfield Chiropractic Clinic, National College Chiropractic Center, two Salvation Army clinics and 21 laboratories. The Sordoni-Burich Library, the audio-visual library, and the audiovisual department are all part of the learning resource center. The Sordoni-Burich Library houses approximately 25,000 volumes and 500 serial subscriptions, provides access to on-line databases, and is part of an interlibrary loan system. The audiovisual library provides computer programs, X-rays, and microcomputers for student use. The audio-visual department has audio, graphics, photography, video, and television production services in its collection. Additionally, the college operates a 56,000-square-foot patient and research center on campus.

Grading Procedures

First trimester grades are based on a comprehensive final examination, a midterm, tests, quizzes, performance on assignments in the laboratory and class participation, attendance and overall attitude. Letter grades of A-F are given as evaluations of academic achievement.

Application Procedures

Students may apply for admission in September, January, and April. In order to apply, students should submit an application for matriculation available from the office of admissions, a $50 application fee, college transcripts, a recent photograph, and two letters of recommendation (one preferably from a chiropractor). Applicants are accepted on a rolling admissions basis. Interviews may be conducted in person or by phone.

Contact

The National College of Chiropractic
Office of Admissions
200 East Roosevelt Road
Lombard, Illinois 60148-4583
(708) 629-2000
(800) 222-0274 or (800) 826-NATL
(800) 826-2957 in Illinois

NEW YORK CHIROPRACTIC COLLEGE

Glen Head, New York 11545
(516) 626-2700

Accreditation	CCE
Degrees Offered	D.C.
# Students Applied	Not Available
Enrollment	Not Available
Mean GPA	2.25
% Men / % Women	Not Available
% Minorities	Not Available
Tuition	$3,150
Application Fee	$50
Application Deadline	Contact School

The University

New York Chiropractic College, a nonprofit, co-educational school, offers a Doctor of Chiropractic degree program. The college, founded in 1919, is the oldest chiropractic college in the northeast. The college comprises two campuses, one in Old Brookville and one in Seneca Falls. The Seneca Falls campus, opening in fall 1991, occupies 283 acres in the scenic Finger Lakes region of New York. The town of Seneca Falls is about 45 minutes from Syracuse, Ithaca, and Rochester, where

many cultural and recreational activities are available. Opportunities for recreation are also abundant all year in Seneca Falls and surrounding areas.

Admissions

An applicant must have a high school diploma or equivalency certificate, two years of study toward a bachelor's degree, and a minimum GPA of 2.25. Students accepted into the D.C. program usually have surpassed the minimum requirements for undergraduate work and grades. Most have earned a baccalaureate degree. Candidates are selected on the basis of oral and written communication skills, familiarity with the responsibilities of a chiropractic health care worker, desire to enter the chiropractic profession, and grades.

Undergraduate Preparation

Applicants should have completed one year of science courses with laboratories in general or inorganic chemistry, organic chemistry, general physics, and general biology or zoology. All science courses should be designed for science majors and be passed with a grade of at least a C. In addition, six semester hours of English composition, three semester hours of general psychology, and three semester hours of other social sciences or humanities are prerequisite to admission. The last 12 credits should be earned in social sciences or humanities.

Costs

Tuition per trimester is $3,150. Student housing costs $950 for a shared room and $1,400 for a single room.

Financial Aid

Funds are available from federal, state, institutional, and private sources. A financial aid form should be filed with the college scholarship service. Applicants must also file signed copies of their federal and state income tax returns as well as their parents' returns if they are dependents, and a copy of their social security card and birth certificate or passport. Federal aid or Title IV, tuition assistance program, veteran benefits, and state vocational rehabilitation programs are available. Loan programs include the Stafford Student Loan Program, Supplementary Loans for Students, Health Education Assistance Loans, and Perkins Loans. Scholarships include SEEK, available to New York State residents, and institutional scholarships. New York Chiropractic College and the federal government fund a college work-study program.

Minority Programs

The Regents Professional Opportunity Scholarship, in the amounts of $1,000 to $5,000 per year, is awarded to an economically disadvantaged student who is a member of a minority group.

Student Organizations

Students may participate in various clubs and societies on

campus including A.C.A. and I.C.A., student chapters of several state associations, Christian Chiropractic Association, Clinic Colloquium, Garden Club, Gonstead Club, Karate Club, Applied Kinesiology Club, Lay Lecture Club, Motion Palpation Club, Nutrition & Homeopathy Club, Photography Club, and Sports Injury Club, among others.

Faculty

There are 18 faculty members in the clinical studies department, 17 in the preclinical studies department, 18 in chiropractic studies, two at the Syracuse Health Center, 17 at the Levittown Health Center, and 76 in the postgraduate and continuing education department.

Curriculum

In order to graduate, a student must complete at least four years of study (the last four trimesters in residence at NYCC), fulfill all academic requirements with a 2.50 GPA, and have taken Parts I, II, and III of the National Board of Chiropractic Examiners examination. Students are expected to complete 1,440 hours in preclinical studies including courses in anatomy, biochemistry, physiopathology, microbiology, and public health. Clinical studies comprise 990 hours of study in diagnosis, roentgenology, clinical laboratory, and associated studies. Chiropractic studies (990 hours) include chiropractic principles, chiropractic procedures, and ancillary therapeutic procedures. A total of 1,765 hours is spent participating in clinical conferences and seminars, and providing clinical services.

Facilities

The 15 classrooms and laboratories and the student chiropractic clinic are located in the academic center. The library/anatomical center contains the human anatomy laboratory as well as books, periodicals, microform, rare and out-of-print chiropractic materials, and multimedia study aids, and offers interlibrary loan services and computer databases in the health sciences. There is a gymnasium, pool, fitness center, two handball/racquetball courts, a student lounge, and student activities offices in the student center. Students may be able to find housing in one of 10 residence halls on campus.

Grading Procedures

Letter grades are assigned for coursework. Students may earn an A (superior performance), H (superior performance in practical courses), B+ (substantial performance), B (above-average performance), S (above-average performance in practical courses), C+ (average), C (below average), D (minimally acceptable), and F (unsatisfactory performance).

Special Programs

Postgraduate and continuing education programs leading to diplomate status include neurology, nutrition, and orthopedics. Certification programs are available in sports injury, thermography, nutrition, Meridian therapy, industrial relations,

and rehabilitation procedures. A certificate can be earned in chiropractic assistant training, skeletal and soft tissue radiology, and nutrition. Technique programs are offered in soft tissue technique, extremity adjusting, micro-manipulation, and flexion distraction technique.

Application Procedures

Applicants should submit an application, a $50 application fee, a recent photograph, high school transcripts and SAT scores, college transcripts, and three reference letters or letters of recommendation to the office of admissions.

Contact

Office of Admissions
New York Chiropractic College
PO Box 167
Glen Head, New York 11545
(800) 228-6922

NORTHWESTERN COLLEGE OF CHIROPRACTIC

2501 West 84th Street
Bloomington, Minnesota 55431
(612) 888-4777

Accreditation	CCE
Degrees Offered	D.C., B.S.
# Students Applied	225
Enrollment	116 / class
Mean GPA	3.0
% Men / % Women	68% / 32%
% Minorities	4%
Tuition	$3,585 / trimester
Application Fee	$35
Application Deadline	April

The University

Northwestern College of Chiropractic (NWCC) was founded in Minneapolis in 1941. In 1949, with an enrollment of 280, NWCC was reorganized under a nonprofit corporate structure and was moved from Nicollet Avenue to Park

Avenue. Northwestern was among the first colleges to adopt the six-year academic program. The Commission on Accreditation of the Council on Chiropractic Education accredited Northwestern in 1971. A new campus is located on 25 acres in nearby Bloomington. The Twin Cities of Minnesota offer camping, boating, and recreation in dozens of parks. Over 15,000 lakes offer almost unlimited opportunity for outdoor activity. Theaters, professional team sports, and a vast range of indoor cultural events stand ready to amuse, educate, and delight.

Admissions

The mean GPA for a class of entering students is usually about 3.0. Students typically have three and one-half years of preprofessional college experience, but they must have completed two academic years (60 semester or 90 quarter hours) of college credit. No more than 20 CLEP hours are allowed.

Undergraduate Preparation

Students must have six semester hours each (with lab) of biology and/or zoology, general and inorganic chemistry, and physics. Also required are six semester hours of English or communication skills; three hours of psychology; and at least 15 hours in the humanities or social sciences. All courses must be passed with a grade of C or better. Applicants should have a cumulative GPA of at least 2.5 and a science GPA of 2.0.

Student Body

Students come from 30 states. The typical fall class averages 25 years of age. Thirty-two percent are women, and about one-fifth of the students are married.

Placement Records

Most graduates go directly into practice in the areas of their choice.

Costs

Tuition is $3,585 per trimester. General fees, books, and supplies amount to approximately $3,458; most of this expense is incurred in the first two years. All housing is off campus.

Financial Aid

Students are awarded aid based on the information submitted in the needs analysis forms. Northwestern also accepts the FAF and the FFS forms. Besides Stafford and Perkins Loans, two other loan funds are available. Students may apply for three grant programs and the college work-study program. Some 41 scholarships are available at Northwestern.

Student Organizations

NWCC has one of the most active chapters of the Student American Chiropractic Association (S.A.C.A.). Other student groups include the World Congress of Chiropractic Students (WCCS) and the Chi Omega Phi fraternity, which admits both men and women.

Faculty

Sixty-four full-time faculty members and about 78 postdoctoral faculty in all disciplines deliver the course of study.

Curriculum

The course of study lasts five years. Each year consists of two 15-week trimesters. In the first two trimesters, students take courses in basic sciences and introductory chiropractic principles and methods. In the third through fifth trimesters, the basic sciences are completed, and progress is made in the clinical sciences, including diagnosis and radiology. In trimesters six and seven, students complete the core curriculum in radiological science and chiropractic science. Finally, in trimesters eight through ten, students serve in the college clinics for 12 months, complete the clinical sciences, and select an elective opportunity in private practice as a physicians' associate.

Facilities

The Bloomington campus includes a full library, fitness center, and other facilities for recreation and study. The five public teaching clinics as well as the student health service offer ample room for research and practice. The clinics include the St. Paul Clinic, the Minneapolis Clinic, the Robbinsdale Clinic, the Burnsville Clinic, and the Student Health Service. The library on the main floor of the college has over 9,000 volumes covering the basic sciences and chiropractic and 250 journal titles. NWCC students may also use several area libraries.

Grading Procedures

NWCC uses a letter grading system, each letter having a point assignment from 4-1, respectively: A (excellent), B (above average), C (average), and D (minimal achievement). Students must pass every course. Students with a GPA of less than 2.0 are placed on probation. Failure to bring up the average within two trimesters results in dismissal.

Special Programs

NWCC conducts continuing postdoctoral education programs. In addition to the D.C., NWCC offers the B.S. in human biology.

Application Procedures

Applications may be obtained from the associate director of admissions. The nonrefundable application fee is $35. Students must send official transcripts from both high school and colleges directly to NWCC and three completed character reference forms or letters of recommendation. At least one must be from a college science professor or teaching assistant. New students are admitted for the trimesters beginning in January and September. Transfer students may be admitted in January, April, or September. Upon acceptance, students must pay a tuition deposit of $200.

Contact

Associate Director of Admissions
Northwestern College of Chiropractic
2501 West 84th Street
Bloomington, Minnesota 55431
(800) 888-4777 or (612) 888-4777

PALMER COLLEGE OF CHIROPRACTIC

1000 Brady Street
Davenport, Iowa 52803
(319) 326-9600

Accreditation	CCE, NCACS
Degrees Offered	D.C., B.S., M.S.
# Students Applied	376
Enrollment	221
Mean GPA	2.90
% Men / % Women	60% / 40%
% Minorities	5%
Tuition	$10,170
Application Fee	$50
Application Deadline	No deadline

The University

D.D. Palmer, the father of chiropractic, founded Palmer College of Chiropractic nearly 100 years ago in 1895. The five cities that comprise the Quad Cities region have a combined population of 390,000. Unlike most of the Midwest, the area is hilly, forested, and bucolic, offering a number of excellent outdoor activities. The region has art galleries, planetariums, a symphony, parks (more than 80), music festivals, ski resorts, golf courses (18 in the area), theaters, and the Mississippi Paddle Steamer for recreation and diversion. The campus itself offers a number of extra curricular activities and social groups. Palmer is fully accredited by the CCE and the North Central Association of Colleges and Schools.

Admissions

The average entering student has a GPA of 2.90 and 100 hours of undergraduate credit. Applicants must have at least a 2.50 GPA to be competitive. No applicant is eligible to matriculate with less than a 2.25 GPA and less than 60 total semester hours of undergraduate credit.

Undergraduate Preparation

Required courses include six semester hours each (with lab) in biology, inorganic and organic chemistry, and physics. In addition, six semester hours of English or English communication skills are required, along with three hours each of psychology and social sciences. Students must have passed their courses with a grade of C or better.

Student Body

Enrollment consists of 1,650 students representing all 50 states and 18 foreign countries.

Placement Records

One out of every three chiropractors in the world is a Palmer College graduate. Palmer graduates have successful practices in cities across the U.S. and throughout the world. The college has more alumni than any other chiropractic college. About 30,000 doctors of chiropractic graduated from Palmer since its founding.

Costs

Tuition, books, and supplies for 12 months amount to $10,170. Palmer estimates that housing costs an average of $250 per month for a one-bedroom apartment.

Financial Aid

Primary sources of assistance to students who qualify include Stafford, HEAL, and SLS loans. Students may apply to three grant funds, a number of scholarships, graduate assistantships, and college work-study programs.

Student Organizations

The college has over 90 student organizations. Three active fraternities and a sorority sponsor both social and professionally-oriented activities. The International Chiropractors Association and the American Chiropractors Association have student chapters on campus.

Faculty

Palmer employs 129 full-time faculty. The average professor has been teaching 12-and-a-half years. The student/faculty ratio is 13:1.

Curriculum

The curriculum is divided into four basic areas, and the course of study lasts 10 trimesters. Basic science courses include anatomy, physiology, and chemistry. Preclinical subjects cover

X-ray diagnosis and chiropractic technique. Clinical training takes place in a practical real-life setting. The first trimester consists of courses in philosophic principles, neuroanatomy, fundamental anatomy, gross anatomy, embryology, biochemistry, and cellular physiology.

Facilities

Palmer has the largest chiropractic library in the world, some 48,000 volumes. The school's four clinical facilities see more than 500 patients a day. The home campus consists of 12 buildings used for research, lectures, and clinical practice.

Special Programs

Palmer offers the B.S., the M.S. in chiropractic, the M.S. in anatomy, the chiropractic technologist certificate (offered at Palmer's School of Chiropractic Technology), and the associate of applied science.

Application Procedures

Students should apply one year in advance so they may enter during the trimester of choice, either July, October, or February and complete the doctor of chiropractic application for admission. The nonrefundable application fee is $50. Applicants should also submit transcripts from all relevant colleges, three letters of recommendation mailed directly to admissions from a doctor of chiropractic, a college professor, and a personal reference. An interview may then be required of the selected candidate. International students may apply under special conditions.

Contact

Admissions Department
Palmer College of Chiropractic
1000 Brady Street
Davenport, Iowa 52803
(319) 326-9882 or (800) 722-2586

PALMER COLLEGE OF CHIROPRACTIC-WEST

1095 Dunford Way
Sunnyvale, California 94087
(408) 244-8907

Accreditation	CCE
Degrees Offered	D.C.
# Students Applied	Not Available
Enrollment	125 / class
Mean GPA	3.0
% Men / % Women	70% / 30%
% Minorities	Not Available
Tuition	$2,890 / quarter
Application Fee	$40
Application Deadline	Contact School

The University

The tradition of Palmer College of Chiropractic-West dates back to the late 1800s, when the original Palmer College of Chiropractic (the profession's oldest and largest college) was founded in Davenport, Iowa. The western college, incorporated in 1980, shares a common background and philosophy with its Iowa counterpart. One of the newest chiropractic colleges in the country, Palmer-West seeks to educate high-caliber students of chiropractic who will graduate to serve as primary care providers.

The college is situated at the southern end of the San Francisco Bay area in California on two large campuses—the original 23-acre Sunnyvale campus and the newly acquired Santa Clara campus less than a mile south. The Bay Area, with a population of about 1.4 million, is a growing region rich in educational, cultural, and recreational attractions, and provides an ideal opportunity to build a thriving career in chiropractic.

Admissions

The college considers a variety of academic and personal factors in its admissions decisions. The college seeks students who have demonstrated academic achievement, especially in the sciences. Communication skills and knowledge of chiropractic are evaluated. The candidate's personal statement is also important—it should explain motivation and describe the applicant's personal background and life experience. Letters of recommendation and results of an interview are also reviewed in the admissions process. The average GPA of Palmer-West students is 3.0.

Undergraduate Preparation

Applicants must have completed at least 60 semester units (90 quarter units) of college or university coursework leading to the bachelor's or associate's degree. The following courses comprise the required preprofessional studies: two semesters of biology (with lab); two semesters of general chemistry (with lab); two semesters of organic chemistry (with lab); two semesters of physics (with lab); two semesters of English; 15 semester units of humanities and/or social sciences; and one semester of psychology. It is highly recommended that at least three to four human biology courses (anatomy, cell biology, microbiology, physiology, and zoology, for example) be completed.

Student Body

Total student enrollment at Palmer-West is 500, with 50 to 70 students admitted each quarter. Most students come from California and the other western states, but a growing contingent come from the northeast and other areas of the country. About 70 percent are men and 30 percent are women. There are also many foreign students. The average age is 27 years old.

Costs

Tuition for 1990-91 is $2,890 per quarter. Books are estimated to cost $275 per quarter, and equipment for the entire program is estimated to cost about $500. Assuming housing is shared, single students can expect to pay $350 per month for off-campus housing, and $225 monthly for board.

Financial Aid

The college helps students obtain financial aid as needed through federal, state, and private sources. CAL Grants are for California residents only. A limited number of students may be eligible for Pell Grants and Supplemental Educational Opportunity Grants. Available loans include Perkin Loans, Stafford Loans, Health Education Assistance Loans, and Supplemental Loans for Students. There are also work-study opportunities. The college will assist students in obtaining veterans' benefits and assistance from state and private sources.

Student Organizations

Students can participate in student council. The college also has branches of the International Chiropractors Association, American Chiropractic Association, and the California Chiropractic Association. There are a wide variety of clubs and intramural sports organizations to suit individual interests.

Faculty

The student/faculty ratio is 12:1.

Curriculum

The program consists of 13 quarters of lecture, laboratory, and clinical experience. Students can choose to complete the program in four years, or shorten their course of study to three-and-a-third calendar years. The program of study is characterized by a strong emphasis on chiropractic technique, which is taught during every term of the program. Basic sciences in the first half of the curriculum are followed by clinical sciences in the second half.

At the end of the third year, students take a clinic entrance exam. After passing the exam, students move on to the final year of the program in the on-campus public clinic. The clinical experience stresses the relationship of the structural and neurological aspects of the body in health and disease.

Students are required to complete two research courses. An elective program is offered in the senior year.

Facilities

The 23-acre campus comprises seven buildings, which include a public clinic, laboratories, the library, and a cafeteria. Recreational facilities for students include a 15-acre playing field, and the surrounding area offers swimming facilities, golf courses, and parks.

The campus clinic is where students participate in patient care. Here, students gain experience in epidemiological investigations, clinical outcome research, and evaluations of physician-practice-based disciplines, such as radiography, thermography, spinal manipulation, and health education. The college has several research laboratories for biomechanics, physiology, and biochemistry. Students have access to modern computer facilities, including a large variety of information databases.

Grading Procedures

Students must complete Parts I and II of the National Board exams prior to graduation.

Application Procedures

The college accepts students four times a year—January, March, July, and October. Students are encouraged to apply at least six months in advance of their desired date of entry (for October entry, at least nine months).

Students should submit an application form with a $40 application fee, two letters of recommendation, a personal essay of one or two pages in length, a passport-type photo, and all high school and college transcripts. The college will schedule a personal interview once all materials have been submitted.

Contact

Palmer College of Chiropractic-West
Admissions Office
1095 Dunford Way
Sunnyvale, California 94087
(408) 983-4024
(800) 44-CHIRO

PARKER COLLEGE OF CHIROPRACTIC

2500 Walnut Hill Lane
Dallas, Texas 75229-5612
(214) 438-6932

Accreditation	CCE, SACS
Degrees Offered	D.C., B.S.
# Students Applied	Not Available
Enrollment	250
Mean GPA	Not Available
% Men / % Women	75% / 25%
% Minorities	Not Available
Tuition	$3,600 / trimester
Application Fee	$35
Application Deadline	Contact School

The University

Parker College of Chiropractic is a private, nonprofit institution created to educate doctors of chiropractic as primary health care providers. Parker College of Chiropractic (PCC), founded by Dr. James W. Parker, was chartered by the state of Texas in early 1978; later that same year, it received non-profit status. The school officially opened with 27 students in 1982. Five years later PCC was accredited by the Southern Association of Colleges and Schools; and in 1988, by the CCE. Ten years after it enrolled its first class, the college anticipates a 1992 enrollment of 1,000—making it the third largest school of chiropractic in the world. The first Parker College public clinic was opened in 1984 on the original Irvine campus, which now also houses a research and rehabilitation department, an auditorium, and a student lounge. In 1989 the school moved to its 11.3-acre Dallas campus in the mainstream Dallas-Ft. Worth Metroplex, close to every conceivable convenience and the finest living, entertainment, shopping, recreational, and cultural opportunities in the vicinity.

Admissions

The college seeks students who demonstrate concern for mankind and have a strong desire to serve. The college considers high school and college transcripts and letters of recommendation. The college requires a minimum of 60 semester hours of credit at an accredited college. The courses must be part of a program leading toward a degree (bachelor at a four-year college or associate at a junior college). Certain physical criteria must be met, including demonstration of coordination of upper limbs and manual dexterity.

Grades in undergraduate science courses must be at least a C to be considered for admission; the overall GPA must be 2.25.

Undergraduate Preparation

Required undergraduate courses include one year each of biology, general chemistry, organic chemistry, and physics (all with lab), and English. The sciences courses should be two subsequent or sequential courses, each with a lab. Psychology and humanities or social sciences courses are also required. Anatomy and physiology are not prerequisite to enrollment, but are highly recommended.

Student Body

By September 1992, the college anticipates enrolling about 1,000 students. The college has students from every state, from Canada, and from about 22 overseas countries.

Costs

Tuition (fall 1991) is $3,600 per trimester. Students must pay a laboratory fee of $30 per class. Books and equipment average $250 to $300 per trimester. Most other fees are minimal.

Financial Aid

Eligibility for financial aid is determined by needs analysis. Students who have been accepted will be sent a complete financial aid packet. Students are required to file a FAF with the necessary documentation in order to be considered for financial aid.

Available forms of financial aid include Pell Grants, Texas Equalization Grants, state and national chiropractic organization scholarships, Stafford Loans, Health Education Assistance Loans, and Supplemental Loans for Students. There is also a campus-based college work-study program.

Student Organizations

The college has well over a dozen student organizations. In addition to the student government, the college has an affinity group called chiropractic adventures into research and education. Other student groups include the bicycling club, the international students club, the motion palpation club, the student American Chiropractic Association, and the World Congress of Women Chiropractors. There are also chapters of Delta Sigma Chi and Delta Sigma Chi Sisters.

Faculty

The college has about 61 faculty members.

Curriculum

The curriculum consists of nine trimesters of 15 weeks each. The first five trimesters consist of courses in basic medical sciences and chiropractic, such as palpation, public health, normal radiographic anatomy, and spinal biomechanics. The last four trimesters include courses such as bone pathology, emergency care, extra-spinal manipulation, Leander/Cox technique, radiology, subluxation, obstetrics/gynecology, diagnostic imaging interpretation, clinical applied kinesiology, and three internships.

Facilities

The student clinic includes care facilities and state-of-the-art facilities for ultrasound, diathermy, and other techniques. The college also has a public clinic that averages about 200 patient visits per day. Other facilities include the anatomy laboratory, histology and neurology laboratories, X-ray physics laboratories, diagnostic and physiological therapeutics laboratory, and a host of other lab facilities.

The library and resource center is equipped with spacious and modern facilities for study. In addition to books, videos, and other training materials, the center has nationwide borrowing and computer research capabilities. Students can borrow from other chiropractic colleges, and interlibrary loan service is available.

Grading Procedures

The college normally uses letter grades A through F. In some circumstances, students may be evaluated using P (pass), I (incomplete), or F (fail). Students must take Parts I and II of the National Board of Chiropractic Examiners test to graduate.

Special Programs

In addition to the D.C. degree, the college also offers a B.S. in anatomy and several postgraduate programs leading to diplomate status. These include the Diplomate American Board of Chiropractic Orthopedists (D.A.B.C.O.) and the Diplomate American Chiropractic Academy of Neurology (D.A.C.A.N.). The college also offers the 100-hour certification in sports injuries.

Application Procedures

Students can be admitted to the January, May, or September trimester. The college has its own application form, which must be submitted along with a $35 application fee. High school and college transcripts must be sent directly to the admissions office, and three letters of recommendation must accompany the application. Upon acceptance, students have a specified period of time to submit a matriculation fee of $250, which is applied toward tuition.

Contact

Parker College of Chiropractic
Admissions Office
2500 Walnut Hill Lane
Dallas, Texas 75229-5668
(800) 438-6932

TEXAS CHIROPRACTIC COLLEGE

5912 Spencer Highway
Pasadena, Texas 77505
(713) 487-1170

Accreditation	CCE, CCSACS
Degrees Offered	D.C., B.S.
# Students Applied	Not Available
Enrollment	Not Available
Mean GPA	Not Available
% Men / % Women	Not Available
% Minorities	Not Available
Tuition	$9,900
Application Fee	$50
Application Deadline	Contact School

The University

Texas Chiropractic College was founded in 1908 as a state-chartered college for chiropractors. Originally located in San Antonio, it became a private college and moved to its present location in Pasadena in 1965. The college offers modern laboratory and clinic facilities, education and learning centers, and specialty rotations within the Texas Medical Center in Houston.

Pasadena is a city of over 120,000 inhabitants. It is located near Houston, Clear Lake, the beaches of Galveston Island, and Johnson Space Center (NASA). Houston offers a wide variety of cultural activities, including musical concerts, live theater, opera, and museums. Many colleges and universities are located in the city, including the University of Houston, Rice University, and Houston Baptist University.

Admissions

A minimum GPA of 2.25 is required. International applicants, are welcome. The college has a long history of attracting students from throughout the world, from countries such as Chile, Colombia, Nigeria, France, Japan, Pakistan, and Vietnam.

Undergraduate Preparation

Applicants must have completed at least 60 semester hours (90 quarter hours) of prechiropractic study at an accredited college or university by the time of enrollment. Only 20 hours of general preprofessional credit may be earned through credit by examination. Credit by examination will not be accepted for required science courses. Completion of six semester hours of the following courses is required (including at least two semesters of laboratory work): biological sciences (biology, zoology, anatomy, and physiology are acceptable); general inorganic chemistry courses for preprofessional majors; organic chemistry for preprofessional majors; general physics at a preprofessional or trigonometry level. Six semester hours of English or communication skills are also required, including two semesters in composition, literature, speech, or approved substitutes. Three semester hours are required in general psychology, and 12 semester hours are required in the social sciences or humanities.

Costs

Tuition is currently $9,900 per year. Additional fees are approximately $100 per year.

Financial Aid

Financial aid is available from a variety of federal, state, and private offices. Information about applying for scholarships, grants, loans, and other forms of assistance is available from the financial aid office. Additional information about scholarships may be available from state chiropractic associations. Information about veteran's benefits is available from state rehabilitation agencies. International students should contact the chiropractic association or society in their country for scholarship and other aid information, as financial aid for international students is not available from the college.

Applicants should begin the financial aid process at least six months prior to enrollment.

Student Organizations

Student organizations on campus include the student body association, student chapters of the American Chiropractic Association and the Texas Chiropractic Association, the International Student Association, fraternity and sorority groups, and numerous professional clubs.

Curriculum

The program includes classroom instruction and hands-on training in the basic and clinical sciences and in the science and practice of chiropractic. Five academic years (10 trimesters in three and one-third calendar years) of prescribed study are required.

The first six trimesters are devoted to the basic sciences and an introduction to chiropractic clinical diagnostic studies. The last four trimesters include the study of chiropractic science with an emphasis on clinical studies. Also included are courses in ethics and jurisprudence, insurance procedures, and office procedures. During the last trimester, there is a clinical preceptorship.

The college sponsors the chiropractic and hospital orientation in clinical experience (CHOICE) program, a group of observational rotation programs. These include rotations in orthopedic surgery and neurosurgery. These rotation programs encourage a continuing dialogue between the chiropractic and medical communities.

Facilities

The 18-acre campus includes classroom, laboratory, research, and clinic facilities. Laboratories are fully supplied and equipped for instruction in the basic sciences. The college operates an outpatient clinic and research laboratory where students receive clinical training. The neurodiagnostic center houses a CAT scan and offers students the opportunity to learn diagnostic imaging procedures. Specialty rotations are offered within the Texas Medical Center in Houston, the world's largest health sciences complex. The Mae Hilty Memorial Library provides learning resources to supplement classroom instruction and laboratory experience.

On-campus housing is not available.

Grading Procedures

In order to graduate, students must have completed all course and clinic requirements within seven calendar years with a minimum overall GPA of 2.0. Of the five academic years of study, the last must have been in residence at Texas Chiropractic College.

Application Procedures

Applications are available from the admissions office. Applications, transcripts, two recommendation forms (one form from a doctor of chiropractic and another from a health professions advisor or natural sciences professor) and the nonrefundable application fee of $50 must be submitted to the admissions office. A campus visit is not required, but is encouraged. Appointments can be scheduled by contacting the admissions office.

International students are urged to begin the application process at least six months before anticipated enrollment. In addition to following the regular application procedures, international students must also submit a minimum score of 500 on the Test of English as a Foreign Language (TOEFL), and evidence of financial resources to complete a minimum of one year of study. Foreign college and university transcripts must be submitted through an approved evaluation service such as Spantran Educational Services, P.O. Box 35404, Houston, TX 77235; or World Education Services, P.O. Box 745, Old Chelsea Station, New York, NY 10113-0745.

Contact

Admissions Office
Texas Chiropractic College
5912 Spencer Highway
Pasadena, Texas 77505
(800) 468-6839
(713) 487-1170

WESTERN STATES CHIROPRACTIC COLLEGE

2900 N.E. 132nd Avenue
Portland, Oregon 97230-3099
(503) 256-3180

Accreditation	CCE, NWASC
Degrees Offered	D.C., B.S.
# Students Applied	Not Available
Enrollment	Not Available
Mean GPA	2.25
% Men / % Women	Not Available
% Minorities	Not Available
Tuition	$10,000 / year
Application Fee	Contact School
Application Deadline	Contact School

The University

Dr. D.D. Palmer, the father of modern chiropractic, founded Western States Chiropractic College (WSCC) in 1907. The college is fully accredited by the Northwest Association of Schools and Colleges and the Council on Chiropractic Education. The college is a member of the Oregon Independent Colleges Association and the American Public Health Association. WSCC's campus offers a wonderful view of Mt. Hood and Mt. St. Helens. The 22-acre campus lies nestled among expansive green lawns and the Northwest's flowering and evergreen woods. The Portland area has an almost unlimited variety of recreational, cultural, and entertainment possibilities. The city's new $100 million performing arts center hosts a wide variety of world-class artists, and Oregon's famed coast is only 90 minutes from the campus.

Admissions

All CCE requirements are in effect at Western States Chiropractic College. Entering students must have completed two years of prechiropractic credits (60 semester or 90 quarter credits) at an accredited junior or community college, college, or university. Students must also have at least a C+ (2.25) GPA, as well as a C+ GPA in chemistry and biology combined. WSCC accepts up to 20 semester or 30 quarter hours of nontraditional credit (CLEP). Some international students are accepted.

Undergraduate Preparation

Required courses include one academic sequence (two or more academic terms—i.e., quarters, semesters, or trimesters) with lab in general and organic chemistry and physics, and one academic year in biological science, regardless of the number of credits earned. Entering students must have completed at least 24 semester hours of social sciences and humanities, including three in psychology and six in English composition or communication skills.

Costs

Tuition, fees, books, and equipment for the four-year program amount to about $40,000. Student housing is safe, affordable, and close to campus.

Financial Aid

Grants, loans, and employment are available to students in need. WSCC administers all U.S. Title IV programs and the Health Education Assistance Loan program, as well as a scholarship program. The Veterans Administration approves the course of study. Some special scholarships include the Honors at Entrance Scholarships, Service to Minority Communities, and International Scholarships.

Minority Programs

WSCC is committed to equal opportunity. African-American students are encouraged to apply for the Harvey Lillard scholarship, awarded annually to an outstanding student. The college's minority scholarship assists Native Americans, Hispanic Americans, and Asian Americans in meeting the costs of study at WSCC.

Student Organizations

Students can take part in study clubs and student chapters of the American Chiropractic Association and the International Chiropractors Association.

Faculty

All of the basic science faculty have at least a master's degree and 60 percent hold a Ph.D. The faculty numbers some 70 full-time members from all relevant disciplines.

Curriculum

The course of study lasts four years, or about 4,500 classroom hours. All students must be enrolled full time. During the first and second years, students cover a combination of chiropractic and basic sciences. The third year emphasizes the clinical and chiropractic sciences and includes an internship at the student health center. The fourth year provides practical clinical experience through internship at the outpatient clinic.

Facilities

The clinic program is housed in two campus facilities and provides an efficient professional atmosphere. The student health center serves as a first step into practice and houses the Raymond W. Klier Diagnostic Laboratory with state-of-the-art equipment. Senior students work in the campus outpatient clinic, specifically built to serve for patient care and chiropractic teaching.

Special Programs

Students may pursue the B.S. along with their D.C. WSCC also offers a 10-weekend certificate program in nutrition.

Application Procedures

Students enter in the fall only and should apply nine months to one year ahead of their anticipated entry date. Application forms may be obtained directly from the admissions office.

Contact

Admissions Office
Western States Chiropractic College
2900 NE 132nd Avenue
Portland, Oregon 97230
(503) 256-3180
(800) 641-5641

CHAPTER 6

Dental Schools

TRENDS IN DENTAL SCHOOL APPLICANTS

There are approximately 158,000 dentists in the United States. Ideally, this figure would average approximately one dentist for every 1,773 people. Certain places, however, such as rural and inner-city areas, are severely in need of dentists. There is also a need for dentists in government, dental societies, national scientific organizations, and educational institutions. The field of dentistry has been experiencing significant changes in the past ten years, both in dental education and professional dental practice.

Ironically, the number of dental school enrollments has been on the decline. In the school year 1977-78, there were 5,945 first-year enrollments. In the school year 1988-89, there were only 4,196 first-year enrollments. The number has risen slightly between 1990 and 1991 from 3,979 to 4,001. There is no significant increase, however, predicted for dental school enrollments at present.

The significant changes dental schools have seen in their applications have been in the number of women and minority applicants. The number of women submitting dental school applications increased from 7,154 in the school year 1989-90 to 8,377 in the school year 1990-91. Women made up 38 percent of the total first-year enrollments in dental school for 1990-1991.

The number of minority applicants increased as well. The number of first-year enrollments for minority students has risen by 13.8 percent. Despite a total attrition rate of 2.8 percent, the number of minority graduates has also increased by 14 percent in the past ten years.

Another important trend seen in today's dental school graduates is the interest in developing a specialty practice. Eight specialty practices are recognized by the American Dental Association: Dental Public Health, Endodontics, Oral Pathology, Oral Surgery, Orthodontics, Pediatric Dentistry, Periodontics, and Prosthodontics. In 1987, 20 percent of active dentists specialized in one of these fields. Part of the reason for this trend could be the increasing number of elderly people needing specialized dental care, such as dentures and dental implants. Although elderly people do not have the opportunity to benefit from the new preventive techniques, there is now a growing awareness of preventive dental care among younger people. The growing trend of preventive care may lead to more pediatric dentists, helping children to preserve and maintain their natural teeth.

Dentists are also becoming more active in research and dental education. This is evident in the new drugs, dental equipment, and restorative materials. Continued dentist involvement will result in even more discoveries in the future.

Dentists are also offered incentives for careers in the armed forces, serving the military personnel, and advising the government on such issues as public health policy. Dentists are commissioned as captains in the Army and Air Force, and as lieutenants in the Navy. There are also over 2,000 civilian dentists serving the Federal Government in the Veterans Administration and the U.S. Public Health Service.

Before you begin your career in dentistry, however, you must choose where you will obtain your dental education. Our book will provide you with complete and specific school profiles and guide you through the individual admissions processes. You should select a school based on how you think their programs will fit your personal and professional needs, goals, and objectives. Once this task has been accomplished, you have made the most important choice in becoming a dentist.

EXPERIENCES WITH DENTAL SCHOOL

by Adam B. Stern, D.M.D., Temple University

Congratulations on your decision to become a dentist! You have chosen a profession that combines interest in the sciences, interaction with people, and the use of manual dexterity skills.

In addition to being an academic science, dentistry is an art. You will be learning how to restore lost or deteriorating teeth, and how to maintain the dental health of your patients over a lifetime.

Now that you have aspired to become a dentist, the next important step is choosing the dental school which is best for you. The first thing that you should take into consideration when choosing a dental school is the location. I suggest that you look into schools which are close to your home. This is because family support is very important. Also, I have found that parents and relatives make very good, reliable patients for your clinical requirements in the third and fourth years.

There are some advantages to choosing a dental school in a large city, because these schools are more likely to have large patient pools for the school clinic. Lower and middle income patients tend to live in large cities and may choose the dental services of a university rather than the work of a private dentist in the same local area, since the service is less expensive.

Another consideration to make when choosing a dental school is the cost factor. Since the curriculum will be the same at virtually every school, you would be receiving the same education at an Ivy League dental school as you would at a state university. Therefore, I find it is wise to choose a dental school with the least tuition combined with other considerations such as location, clinical facilities, and academic reputation of the school.

Keep in mind that dental school in general is expensive, and most students leave school with debts ranging from $10,000 to $120,000—the average debt is $60,000. You should realize now that you will be paying back all your potential loans after dental school. Because of this, and the fact that you will probably open your own practice, keep your loans to a minimum. If you are sensible about your financial situation, you will be able to make your life easier after graduation.

One of the most important considerations in choosing your school is the quality of the clinical facilities. I recommend that you arrange a tour with the admissions office at the dental schools you are considering. During the tour, you will want to ascertain whether the school provides modern dental equipment. If you compare the equipment you see in the school to that of your own dentist, you may be able to make a fair assessment of the equipment's condition. Other clues in assessing the equipment's condition would be to find

out when the clinic was last renovated and the age of the chairs in the clinic. Be sure to ask your tour guide these kinds of questions.

Approach dental school as a consumer, and expect the most for your money. Another consideration in dental schools is the status of the faculty members. I suggest that you ask what percentage of the faculty are part-time and what percentage are full-time. A 50-50 ratio of full-time to part-time faculty is ideal. Full-time professors do not practice outside the dental school, and although they are very good academic instructors, they may lack practical experience. Part-time instructors, on the other hand, have a good working knowledge of practical treatment planning and patient management. Keep in mind, however, that the instructors with practical experience can make dental school a little confusing. While the full time instructors tend to standardize their teaching techniques, practicing dentists don't.

Another consideration is what type of students will be attending your classes. Your first two years of dental school consist mostly of science text courses such as histology, gross anatomy, dental anatomy and occlusion, biochemistry, and microbiology. Some of these courses are also given to medical students and other health care professional students. At some universities, anatomy courses are taught to dental and medical students together. This is not advantageous for the dental student, since dental students begin working "hands-on" much earlier in their schooling. Medical students are in the classsroom almost completely in the first two years of medical school, and thus have more time and energy to devote to classwork than dental students, who are focusing not only on their classwork, but also on their pre-clinicals.

My general feeling is that dental students have less time to devote to textbook courses than medical students since the emphasis of learning is on practical experience. Therefore, I recommend that you choose a dental school which offers few classes with medical students. You will want the slant of your dental courses to concentrate on the practical experience of dentistry rather than on the scientific data of the field.

Many people think that a "predental advisor" will help them to find the right dental schools to apply to, as well as explain prerequisites, and so forth. If you are lucky enough to have a predental advisor, congratulations. Hopefully, this person will be well-informed and will help you to make intelligent and informed choices.

I was not so lucky as to have a "predental advisor," and I have the feeling that there are many others just like me. I had what my school called a "pre-health advisor" who was not at all helpful. He did not know which tests were required to enter dental school, or even if my GPA qualified for the dental schools to which I wanted to apply.

I became my own advisor. I called the ADA in Chicago. They sent me the listing of every dental school in the United States and Canada. The listing included such valuable information as GPA means, DAT scores, tuition, fees, and a brief description of the dental school facilities. (You will find all that information in this publication also!)

Becoming my own advisor paid off for me. In the course of my research, I discovered that one does not need a bachelor's degree to enter dental school. As a result of this finding, I applied to dental school in October of my junior year in college and was accepted in March of that same academic year. I entered dental school a whole year earlier, but without my bachelor's degree. If you are absolutely intent on going to dental school and would not miss getting your bachelor's degree, I highly recommend that you apply a year early. If you are accepted a year early, you will save a year of your life, and a year's tuition of undergraduate school.

I would like to make one suggestion about the DATs: either take them as soon as you complete your organic chemistry course, or in the middle of the second semester of organic chemistry. This way everything from that difficult course will be fresh in your mind, and you will be confident when you take your DAT.

As an undergraduate, you will need to choose a major. If you are intent on going to dental school, biology is the best major to pursue. You do not have to be a biology major to get into dental school, though. You can choose any other major that interests you, and take only the necessary prerequisite courses to get in. For dental school, this includes a course in general biology. I also suggest that you take a comparative vertebrae anatomy course, histology, embryology, biochemistry, physiology, and microbiology. If you are a biology major, you will be taking most or all of these courses anyway. If you are not, choose some of these electives that you are interested in, but don't feel that you have to take all of them. I didn't. I think that two of these courses are sufficient.

Another good place to get "predental" information is your own dentist. A good idea is to become employed as a dental assistant during your summer break or part-time after school. In addition to earning a salary, you will gain practical knowledge by observing a dentist treat his or her patients. This opportunity will help you decide if dentistry is the right profession for you.

A friend of mine in undergraduate school decided to work for his uncle, a dentist, during one summer break to get a feel for dentistry. He discovered after working in a dental office for several months that dentistry was not right for him. Ultimately, he changed his major and pursued a different career. Because he did this during his undergraduate years, he was able to change his course easily and without wreaking too much havoc on his life. If he had waited until dental school, he would have wasted valuable time and money making this discovery.

People often assume that dentistry is similar to medical practice, and so when they fail to get into medical school, they assume that dental school is an excellent alternative. Wrong! There is more to dentistry than diagnosing an illness and writing a prescription. There is a lot of manual dexterity involved, among other things. When you interview at dental schools, do not tell the interviewer that you originally wanted to go to medical school. You will most certainly be rejected.

Now that you are sure that you want to be a dentist, and you have been accepted to the school of your choice, you will start to get mentally prepared for that big first day. What can you expect?

On day one of dental school you will be sitting in a new classroom surrounded by strangers who have all gone through the stress of applying to dental school. And just like you, they have all been accepted.

You can expect that the deans and some select faculty and upperclass students will talk to you and welcome you to the school. After the introduction, you will be issued dental instruments. This is an exciting experience, as you will be holding the first dental tools which will be with you as you receive your dental education. You will notice that there will be mass confusion as each student tries to figure out which instrument is which. Other events which take place are the issuing of locker keys and book lists. While all this is going on, you will be meeting your peers and making friendships that may last a life time.

Besides everything else that will happen on your first day of dental school, you will be given a book list, with which you will head down to the university bookstore. I'd like to give you some hints for handling that list economically.

First of all, if you were to buy all the required and recommended books on your list, you would spend approximately $500 to $600 in one semester. I suggest that you only buy the required books first. Buy the recommended reference books only as you need them. Talk to second-year students and find out which books to buy; many upperclass students will not only give you good suggestions on what to buy, but they will often agree to sell or give you their old science textbooks. If you will be purchasing your science textbooks from the bookstore, try to find used ones to help defray costs a little. You will want to buy your dental books new, as these books will stay with you in your personal dental library long after you finish your education.

The first real pressures in dental school arrive when the first exam is a week or two away. You then realize how far behind you are in your reading, and how incomplete your notes seem to be. Everyone feels the same way, and everyone panics. This is when the class begins to buckle down.

Throughout the educational process, pre-professional students strive to make the grade. In high school, students struggle to acquire high GPAs and SAT scores in order to get into the best college possible. In college the focus is on GPAs and class rank, along with DATs in order to get into dental school. The competition is always stiff, since there are always more students than seats available in any given program. Now that you have finally arrived in dental school, plan to work together with your classmates so that you can see each other through. There is no reason to foster competition, since from here you will all graduate and become dentists. It is no longer necessary to have high GPAs. Don't be discouraged if the GPA you are accustomed to achieving suddenly drops. Most people find themselves in the same situation. The only dental students who need to obtain GPAs of at least 3.0 are the 20 percent which will go into specialties such as orthodontics, oral surgery, etc.

My point is that you should take a lot of pressure off yourself and expect that you will work harder than ever while receiving worse grades than ever. Grades are really not important—just get through the program. The person who finishes first in the class and the person who finishes last will both get to be called "doctor."

Dental school is unique from other graduate health professions because there are preclinical laboratory courses. Dental anatomy lab, for example, involves carving anatomically correct teeth out of wax. For most, this is a significant challenge, since so few students have any formal training or experience in carving sculpture. Another lab course includes dental materials, where you take impressions on classmates and make plaster models. There is an operative dentistry lab where you prepare (drill) cavities on mannequin models. These lab courses are extremely time-consuming as you strive to meet deadlines for projects. This cuts into your studying time for the basic science courses which you will be required to take at the same time.

Time management will become very important to you as you try to meet your responsibilities. Work out a schedule on paper. Include a reading schedule which consists of a number of pages or chapters that must be read by the next class. Always be sure to include meal time, recreation, and relaxation time. Try to take time to exercise or find some other relaxing activity. Even with the best time organization, it is possible to fall behind. Use the weekend to catch up, or even to get ahead.

Low moments may occur. You may fail an exam or come close to failing. Lab projects on which you spent hours may get poor grades or be rejected completely. Don't get discouraged—chances are you are not the only one this is happening

to. If you have trouble on an exam, get help. Find a competent classmate to tutor you, or seek help from the instructor. Most instructors will bend over backwards to help you learn the material. Don't be embarrassed to ask someone for help.

You or a classmate may consider dropping out when you are going through this rough time. A student who considers dropping out is usually failing more than one course. His or her lab projects are sloppy and also receive poor grades. Some students have trouble meeting the manual dexterity requirement. Don't be surprised if, at the beginning of the second semester, you notice that there are fewer students than there were in the first. It takes a lot of energy and stamina to get through the program, but it is well worth it.

Although dental school has its share of tough times, there are a lot of great things that go on there, too. After major exams, you will always find a party where you can relax and get to know your classmates better. You will form many close and lasting relationships. In addition, many students find spouses during dental school. I was one of them.

As you sit in the library studying histology or some other basic science course, you will wonder what this has to do with the practice of dentistry. Your thoughts are, to some extent, fairly accurate. These basic science courses have little or no value when you get to the clinic. Basic knowledge of the sciences is necessary to understand concepts in other clinically related courses. The National Board Exam Part I is the other time when you will need a command of the basic sciences. My personal feeling about the study of the basic science courses is that they make you into a doctor as opposed to a "mouth mechanic."

Good luck as you move forward into the profession of dentistry. Now that I have completed my program at Temple University, I feel the four years went swiftly. They will for you too, if you just persevere.

—*Adam Brandon Stern, D.M.D., graduated in May 1991 from Temple University School of Dentistry. Dr. Stern is a practicing dentist in Somerset, N.J.*

U.S. DENTAL SCHOOLS AT A GLANCE

School	Accreditation	Degrees Offered	# Students Applied	Enrollment
University of Alabama School of Dentistry	CDA	D.M.D.	155	56 / class
Baylor College of Dentistry	CDA, SACS	D.D.S.	233	95 / class
Boston University Medical Center Henry M. Goldman School of Graduate Dentistry	CDA	D.M.D., M.S., D.M.D./M.Sc., D.M.D./D.Sc.	729	79 / class
University of California–Los Angeles School of Dentistry	CDA	D.D.S., M.S.	495	93 / class
University of California-San Francisco School of Dentistry	ADA	D.D.S., M.S., Ph.D., B.S.	307	88 / class
Case Western Reserve University School of Dentistry	CDA	D.D.S.	432	51 / class
University of Colorado School of Dentistry	CDA	D.D.S.	318	35 / class
Columbia University School of Dental and Oral Surgery	CDA	D.D.S., M.P.H./D.D.S.	680	58 / class
University of Connecticut School of Dental Medicine	ADA	D.M.D., D.M.D./M.D., D.M.D./Ph.D., D.M.D./M.P.H.	403	44 / class
Creighton University School of Dentistry	ADA	D.D.S.	700	75 / class
University of Detroit School of Dentistry	ADA, AADS	D.D.S., B.S., M.S.	358	55 / class
University of Florida College of Dentistry	ADA	D.M.D.	303	77 / class
Harvard School of Dental Medicine	CDA	D.M.D., D.M.S., M.M.S., M.D.	256	24 / class
Howard University College of Dentistry	CDA	D.D.S., B.S./D.D.S.	438	63 / class
University of Illinois at Chicago, Health Sciences Center College of Dentistry	CDA	D.D.S., D.D.S./M.S.	334	68 / class
Indiana University School of Dentistry	CDA	M.S.D., D.D.S., D.M.D.	404	80 / class
The University of Iowa College of Dentistry	CDA	D.D.S.	314	68 / class
University of Kentucky College of Dentistry	ADA	D.M.D.	*	40 / class
Loma Linda University School of Dentistry	CDA	D.D.S., B.S., M.S.	426	78 / class

* Not Available   ** Not Applicable   C/S – Contact School   I/S – In-State   O/S – Out-of-State

Mean GPA	% Male / % Female	% Minorities	In-State Tuition	Out-of-State Tuition	Application Fee	Application Deadline
3.34	89% / 11%	4%	$3,057	$6,102	$25	April 1
3.02	64% / 36%	27%	$4,511	$18,044	$15	Flexible
2.6	76% / 24%	28%	$21,400	**	$40	April 1
3.25	59% / 41%	11%	$1,590	$7,506	$40	January 1
3.12	52% / 48%	29%	None	$5,916	$40	January 1
2.75	70% / 30%	15%	$18,500	**	$35	March 1
3.08	86% / 14%	30%	$5,729	$17,112	$35	March 1
2.92	80% / 20%	47%	$16,950	**	$45	March 1
3.1	62% / 38%	*	$5,800 In-State $7,250 N. Eng.	$13,300	$50	April 1
2.90	92% / 8%	3%	$13,824	**	$25	March 1
2.86	61% / 39%	9%	$12,500	**	$25	Flexible
3.0	65% / 35%	36%	$5,618	$13,576	$15	October 15
3.43	59% / 41%	41%	$18,030	**	$60	January 1
2.63	50% / 50%	*	$8,200	**	$25	March 1
3.85	61% / 39%	13%	$1,553	$3,893	$20	April 1
3.05	63% / 37%	4%	$5,750	$11,930	$20	April 1
2.5	63% / 37%	20%	$4,264	$11,994	$20	November 30
3.17	50% / 50%	*	$4,320	$15,900	None I/S $10 O/S	April 1
3.1	69% / 31%	48%	$15,669	**	$25	February 1

* Not Available   ** Not Applicable   C/S – Contact School   I/S – In-State   O/S – Out-of-State

School	Accreditation	Degrees Offered	# Students Applied	Enrollment
Louisiana State University School of Dentistry	CDA	D.D.S.	127	53 / class
University of Louisville School of Dentistry	ADA, AADS	D.M.D., B.S./D.M.D.	308	61 / class
Loyola University of Chicago School of Dentistry	CDA	D.D.S.	841	94 / class
Marquette University School of Dentistry	CDA	D.D.S., M.S., B.S./D.D.S., D.D.S./M.S., M.S.	753	64 / class
University of Maryland at Baltimore Dental School, Baltimore College of Dental Surgery	CDA	D.D.S., Ph.D., D.D.S./Ph.D., B.S., M.S., B.S./D.D.S.	677	95 / class
Medical College of Georgia School of Dentistry	ADA	D.M.D., M.S./D.M.D.	176	53 / class
Medical University of South Carolina College of Dental Medicine	CDE, ADA	D.M.D.	310	46 / class
University of Medicine and Dentistry of New Jersey, New Jersey Dental School	CDA	D.M.D.	470	90 / class
Meharry Medical College School of Dentistry	CDA	D.D.S.	353	46 / class
University of Michigan School of Dentistry	ADA	D.D.S., M.S., Ph.D., B.S., D.D.S./B.S., D.D.S./B.A., D.D.S./B.G.S.	545	96 / class
University of Minnesota School of Dentistry	CDA	D.D.S., B.S., M.S., Ph.D. in Oral Biology	349	76 / class
University of Mississippi School of Dentistry	ADA	D.M.D.	68	30 / class
University of Missouri-Kansas City School of Dentistry	ADA	D.D.S., B.S., M.S., B.A./D.D.S.	444	69 / class
University of Nebraska, Medical Center–Lincoln College of Dentistry	ADA	D.D.S., Ph.D., M.S.	192	42 / class
New York University College of Dentistry	MSACS	D.D.S., B.A./D.D.S.	716	158 / class
University of North Carolina School of Dentistry	CDA	D.D.S., B.S., D.D.S./Ph.D., D.D.S./M.P.H.	380	66 / class
Northwestern University Dental School	ADA	D.D.S., B.A./D.D.S., M.S.	646	64 / class
The Ohio State University College of Dentistry	CDA	D.D.S., Ph.D., M.S.	536	101 / class

* Not Available   ** Not Applicable   C/S – Contact School   I/S – In-State   O/S – Out-of-State

Mean GPA	% Male / % Female	% Minorities	In-State Tuition	Out-of-State Tuition	Application Fee	Application Deadline
3.06	63% / 37%	11%	$3,647	$8,247	$30	March 31
3.03	74% / 26%	5%	$4,110	$15,798	$10	April 1
2.7	63% / 28%	32%	$14,100	**	$30	March 31
2.74	72% / 28%	50%	$19,310	**	$25	April 1
3.05	62% / 38%	26%	$6,778	$15,550	$25	March 1
3.25	65% / 35%	9%	$3,942	$7,884	None	November 1
2.91	65% / 35%	27%	$3,500	$9,800	$25	December 30
2.95	56% / 44%	22%	$10,457	$13,723	$25	March 1
2.59	60% / 40%	95%	$12,000	**	$25	March 15
3.11	67% / 33%	24%	$9,086	$16,814	$30	April 1
3.02	71% / 29%	14%	$6,278	$9,416	$30	April 1
3.3	83% / 17%	10%	$4,050	$10,038	$25 I/S $50 O/S	March 1
3.23	68% / 32%	16%	$6,378	$10,119	None	April 1
3.19	75% / 25%	9%	$6,231	$14,418	$25	March 1
2.87	61% / 39%	41%	$22,282	**	$35	June 1
3.1	65% / 35%	5%	$3,011	$17,034	$35	December 1
2.99	65% / 35%	11%	$20,283	**	$35	March 1
2.93	71% / 29%	12%	$4,849	$14,497	$20	March 1

* Not Available   ** Not Applicable   C/S – Contact School   I/S – In-State   O/S – Out-of-State

School	Accreditation	Degrees Offered	# Students Applied	Enrollment
University of Oklahoma College of Dentistry	ADA, CDA	D.D.S.	203	50 / class
Oregon Health Sciences University School of Dentistry	CDA	D.M.D.	325	67 / class
University of the Pacific School of Dentistry	CDA	D.D.S.	549	120 / class
University of Pennsylvania School of Dental Medicine	CDA	D.M.D., D.M.D./M.B.A., D.M.D./M.D., D.M.D./Ph.D.	495	80 / class
University of Pittsburgh School of Dental Medicine	AADS, CDE, CDA	D.D.S.	335	75 / class
University of Puerto Rico School of Dentistry	ADA	D.M.D., M.S.D.	97	250
University of Southern California School of Dentistry	ADA, CDA	D.D.S., B.S., M.S., Ph.D.	792	109 / class
Southern Illinois University School of Dental Medicine	ADA	D.M.D., B.S./D.M.D.	206	49 / class
State University of New York at Buffalo School of Dentristry	ADA	D.D.S., M.S., Ph.D., B.S./D.D.S., D.D.S./Ph.D., M.S./Ph.D.	451	80 / class
State University of New York at Stony Brook School of Dental Medicine	ADA	D.D.S., M.S., Ph.D.	302	28 / class
Temple University School of Dentistry	CDA	D.D.S., D.M.D., D.M.D./M.B.A.	800	100 / class
University of Tennessee College of Dentistry	CDA	D.D.S., M.S.	187	90 / class
University of Texas Health Science Center at Houston, Dental Branch	ADA	D.D.S., M.S.	332	95 / class
University of Texas Health Science Center at San Antonio, Dental School	CDA	D.D.S., D.D.S./M.S., D.D.S./Ph.D.	435	96 / class
Tufts University School of Dental Medicine	ADA	D.M.D., M.S., B.S./D.M.D.	749	129 / class
Virginia Commonwealth University, Medical College of Virginia School of Dentistry	CDA	D.D.S., D.D.S./M.S., D.D.S./Ph.D.	531	35 / class
University of Washington School of Dentistry	CDA	D.D.S.	450	200 / class
West Virginia University School of Dentistry	CDA	D.D.S., M.S., B.S., Ph.D.	217	250

* Not Available   ** Not Applicable   C/S – Contact School   I/S – In-State   O/S – Out-of-State

Mean GPA	% Male / % Female	% Minorities	In-State Tuition	Out-of-State Tuition	Application Fee	Application Deadline
3.18	64% / 36%	20%	$4,860	$12,060	$10 I/S $15 O/S	March 1
3.3	82% / 18%	13%	$3,510	$8,610	$40	November 15
2.77	70% / 30%	30%	$29,100	**	$35	March 1
3.07	65% / 35%	25%	$21,210	**	$35	February 1
2.96	73% / 27%	*	$13,940	$19,700	$25	March 1
3.25	50% / 50%	*	$2,500	**	$15	December 15
3.07	57% / 43%	41%	$22,380	**	$40	April 1
2.93	70% / 30%	25%	$3,100	$9,300	$20	April 1
3.01	80% / 20%	*	$5,670	$13,070	$50	March 1
3.24	57% / 43%	18%	$5,550	$12,950	$50	March 31
*	65% / 35%	17%	$12,482	$18,950	$30	March 1
2.99	81% / 19%	10%	$4,264	$8,230	$25	February 28
2.94	61% / 39%	48%	$4,511	$18,044	$35 I/S $70 O/S	November 1
3.05	62% / 38%	38%	$4,511	$18,044	$35 I/S $70 O/S	November 1
2.86	57% / 43%	23%	$19,285	**	$35	April 1
3.02	78% / 22%	23%	$5,770	$10,800	$35	April 1
3.19	75% / 25%	25%	$4,926	$12,513	$35	December 1
*	70% / 30%	*	$3,839	$8,413	$30	November 1

* Not Available   ** Not Applicable   C/S – Contact School   I/S – In-State   O/S – Out-of-State

UNIVERSITY OF ALABAMA SCHOOL OF DENTISTRY

Birmingham, Alabama 35294
(205) 934-4720

Accreditation	CDA
Degrees Offered	D.M.D.
# Students Applied	155
Enrollment	56 / class
Mean GPA	3.34
% Men / % Women	89% / 11%
% Minorities	4%
Tuition	$3,057 In-State
	$6,102 Out-of-State
Application Fee	$25
Application Deadline	April 1

The University

The University of Alabama was founded in 1831 at Tuscaloosa. Federal cavalrymen burned the campus on April 4, 1865; only the observatory was left standing. After rebuilding, instruction began again in April 1869. In 1966, the University of Alabama at Birmingham became one of the three main university campuses. The campus in Birmingham consists of the Medical Center, University College, and the Graduate School. It is now the major urban university in the state. The University of Alabama School of Dentistry, a unit of the Medical Center, was created by an act of the state legislature in 1945.

Admissions

Preference is given to residents of Alabama. Selection is based on criteria which includes academic performance, recommendations from the predental advisory committee and/or science instructors, DAT scores, and personal characteristics.

Undergraduate Preparation

Applicants must have completed 90 semester hours of undergraduate coursework with a maximum of 60 semester hours earned at a junior college. Required courses include 12 semester hours of biology or zoology, eight semester hours of inorganic chemistry with lab, eight semester hours each of inorganic and organic chemistry with lab, eight semester hours of physics with lab, six semester hours of mathematics, and 30 semester hours of nonscience coursework. Highly recommended areas of study include biochemistry, analytic geometry, differential and integral calculus, and English.

Costs

Tuition per year is $3,057 for Alabama residents and $6,102 for nonresidents. Other expenses over the four years, including books, supplies, equipment, and laboratory and clinic fees, are about $10,668.

Financial Aid

Students must file financial aid forms each year. Available loan programs include the Stafford Student Loan, the Health Professions Student Loan Program (HPL), the Perkins Loan, the Supplemental Loan for Students (SLS), and Health Education Assistance Loan Program (HEAL). The State of Alabama Scholarship/Loan program provides funds for Alabama residents. Other forms of aid include college work-study programs as well as various loan and scholarship funds.

Minority Programs

Advice and special counseling is available to minority students during the application procedure. Tutorial assistance is available if necessary.

Student Organizations

Every dental student automatically becomes a member of the Student Government Association of the University of Alabama School of Dentistry at UAB. The dental fraternities, Psi Omega and Delta Sigma Delta, provide social functions.

Curriculum

The first two years of dental studies include the basic sciences; a PCD (Preclinical/Clinical Dentistry) Program in which teams of instructors teach preclinical technique courses; clinical sessions on screening for oral diseases, preventive techniques, and prophylaxis; and a multi-disciplinary patient management core course in data collection and analysis, diagnosis, treatment planning, and therapeutic modalities. The third and fourth years involve providing dental care to patients in the school clinics, participating in extramural rotations, completing programs in physical diagnosis, medicine, and life support, acquiring medical histories, and performing a complete physical examination. All students must pass Parts I and II of the examination of the National Board of Dental Examiners before graduating.

Facilities

The Lister Hill Library contains more than 210,000 volumes and receives about 2,900 biomedical journals. Reference services include the computerized bibliographical systems of MEDLINE and LISTER. The Hammonds Reading Room, located in the School of Dentistry Building, contains current issues of journals dealing with clinical dentistry.

Grading Procedures

Depending on the course, either the A through F grading system or the pass/fail grading system is used.

Special Programs

Qualified high school students may enroll in a seven-year combined Bachelor of Science/Doctor of Dental Medicine program. Those who are judged eligible during the first two years of dental study may join the Honors Program and pursue independent study. Each year a limited number of students may do summer research under the preceptorship of a senior faculty member. Students with special needs may be eligible for individualized curricula. Postgraduate certificate programs, one to four years long, are offered in the specialties of general dentistry, dental public health, dental radiology, endodontics, maxillofacial surgery, orthodontics, pediatric dentistry, periodontics, and prosthodontics. The combined D.M.D./Ph.D. degree may be earned in about seven years with a major in the departments of anatomy, biochemistry, microbiology, pharmacology, physiology, and biophysics. Administration-health services and nutrition, taught at the School of Health-Related Professions, are also possible majors.

Application Procedures

Applicants must file an application with the American Association of Dental Schools Application Service (AADSAS) by April 1 preceding the matriculation date. All Alabama residents and those nonresidents who are seriously being considered will be requested to file a supplemental application that includes either a recommendation from a predental advisory committee or two letters of recommendation from professors in the candidate's academic major. The application, transcripts, and letters must be received by the admissions office before the spring DAT testing date preceding matriculation.

Contact

University of Alabama School of Dentistry
Admissions Office
P.O. Box 16-SDB
University Station
Birmingham, Alabama 35294
(205) 934-3387

BAYLOR COLLEGE OF DENTISTRY

3302 Gaston Avenue
Dallas, Texas 75246-2097
(214) 828-8100

Accreditation	CDA, SACS
Degrees Offered	D.D.S.
# Students Applied	233
Enrollment	95 / class
Mean GPA	3.02
% Men / % Women	64% / 36%
% Minorities	27%
Tuition	$4,511 In-State
	$18,044 Out-of-State
Application Fee	$15
Application Deadline	Flexible—No set deadline

The University

Baylor College of Dentistry is located in the Dallas metropolitan area, about one mile from the downtown business district. It is within the Baylor University Medical Center complex, although it is a distinct corporate entity. The Dallas-Fort Worth metropolitan area offers many cultural, educational, and religious organizations. There are more than 40 colleges and universities within a 100-mile radius of Dallas. In addition, there is a professional theater, opera, symphony, and many museums and galleries.

Admissions

Preference is given to residents of the state of Texas and residents of the surrounding states which do not have a college of dentistry. The committee on admissions first evaluates GPA scores and the results of the DAT. The committee also evaluates an applicant's personal interview, biographical sketch, and recommendations, as well as the care taken in filling out the application form. Preference is not given to any major. Applicants who have attended a college offering an active predental advisory committee are preferred.

Undergraduate Preparation

Applicants must have completed 60 semester hours of coursework at an accredited college or university to be considered for admission. At least eight semester hours (including laboratory work) of inorganic chemistry, organic chemistry, physics, and biology are required for admission. Most students accepted to the college have completed 12-24 semester hours of biology or zoology. Six semester hours of English are also required. Recommended electives include physiology, embryology, anatomy, psychology, sociology, small business management, bookkeeping, reading improvement, mechanical drawing, and speech.

Student Body

Most students are residents of Texas, although students from many other states attend the College.

Placement Records

Most graduates work in private practice after graduation. Other graduates pursue their profession by working in hospital clinics, industrial clinics, public health agencies, commercial companies, or working as dental educators and consultants.

Costs

Tuition and fees are subject to change. Tuition (per quarter) for a Texas resident amounts to $1,128. For a nonresident student, tuition is $4,511. The cost of individual courses, per quarter hour, is $50. The summer clinic fee is $100. The cost of books, instruments, and supplies for the complete curriculum is estimated to be $4,243 for the first year, $7,350 for the second year, $424 for the third year, and $160 for the fourth year.

Financial Aid

Financial aid is available from federal, state, and private sources. The college provides scholarship funds each year for first-year students who are Texas residents and who are either members of a minority group or who will commit to practice in rural areas of Texas. Financial need is the primary criteria for these scholarships. Academic performance will also be considered. The College Scholarship Service is used by the college to evaluate an applicant's need for financial aid. Application for aid should be submitted to the office of financial aid. The college discourages students from holding outside employment which may interfere with their education.

Student Organizations

Student organizations of special interest to dental students include Omicron Kappa Upsilon, a dental honor society, the Baylor Odontological Honor Society, the Student Council, the Lambda Chapter of Delta Sigma Delta, Delta Psi Chapter of Psi Omega, Alpha Phi Chapter of Xi Psi Phi, and the Alpha Chi Chapter of Alpha Omega.

Faculty

There is a favorable student-faculty ratio, offering opportunity for interaction and individual instruction. Many faculty members are internationally prominent in their areas of specialization.

Curriculum

The curriculum is designed to correlate the basic biological sciences with the science and art of dentistry. The first two years consist of the study of the basic biological and dental sciences. Students must develop their psychomotor abilities on laboratory models before beginning patient care. The third and fourth years consist of clinical practice supported by didactic instruction. An electives program is offered, allowing students to study areas of special interest. Each fourth-year student must complete a minimum of two quarter hours of electives to fulfill graduation requirements. Dental students are encouraged to work with faculty members on research projects.

Facilities

Facilities include the main building, a seminar building for small groups, and the dental clinics, whose modern operatories provide a semi-closed cubicle of unique design, with all the advantages of a private dental office. The College of Dentistry serves nearly 21,000 patients per year. There is also a stomatology clinic, which has received an award from the American Dental Association and is the only one of its kind in the southwest.

The Baylor Health Sciences Library contains approximately 36,000 volumes and 600 current journal titles. In addition, approximately 2,000 volumes comprise the Sellars' Collection of rare books in medicine, religion, and art. Students also have access to materials in all major college and university libraries in the area. On-line access is available to databases, such as MEDLARS from the National Library of Medicine, DIALOG Information Services, and NIDR ONLINE at the National Institute of Dental Research.

The College also has arrangements with private dental offices in the North Texas area and various community agencies through which students are offered specialized experience in short-term, extramural rotations.

Application Procedures

In-state applicants must request application materials from the office of the registrar. Out-of-state applicants must apply through the American Association of Dental Schools Application Service. A list of courses in progress, a list of future courses, a biographical sketch, the application fee, and a photograph must be included with the application. Transcripts must be sent from each academic institution the applicant has attended. Recommendations are required from the applicant's preprofessional advisory committee, a dentist, and an individual who knows the applicant well.

The DAT is required and should be taken by April of the year prior to planned enrollment. DAT scores must be sent directly to the college. Residency information and forms are provided by the office of the registrar and must be submitted by August 1. Applicants should check periodically with the office of the registrar to be sure that all application materials are being received. Failure to supply transcripts or recommendations is perceived as an indication that the applicant is no longer interested in admission. Selected students are invited to the college for a personal interview. Personal interviews are required for admission.

Contact

Office of the Registrar
Baylor College of Dentistry
3302 Gaston Avenue
Dallas, Texas 75246-2097
(214) 828-8230

BOSTON UNIVERSITY MEDICAL CENTER, HENRY M. GOLDMAN, SCHOOL OF GRADUATE DENTISTRY

100 East Newton Street
Boston, Massachusetts 02118
(617) 638-4780

Accreditation	CDA
Degrees Offered	D.M.D., M.S., M.S.D., C.A.G.S., D.Sc.
# Students Applied	729
Enrollment	79 / class
Mean GPA	2.6
% Men / % Women	76% / 24%
% Minorities	28%
Tuition	$21,400
Application Fee	$40
Application Deadline	April 1

The University

The Goldman School of Graduate Dentistry, founded in 1963, is part of Boston University and is located in BU's Medical Center in the South End of Boston along the Charles River. The Medical Center is comprised of the School of Medicine, The University Hospital, the Humphrey Cancer Research Center, and the Cardiovascular Institute, and claims more than 20 New England health care affiliates. Attending school in Boston gives students the opportunity to enjoy history, theatre, sports events, and many other forms of recreation.

Admissions

Applicants are judged on their undergraduate record, Dental Admission Test (DAT) scores, letters of recommendation, quality and difficulty of courses taken, improvement in grades, leadership ability, motivation to study dentistry, and outstanding nonacademic achievement.

Undergraduate Preparation

Undergraduate requirements include 12 semester hours of biology, 16 semester hours of both inorganic and organic chemistry, eight semester hours of physics, two years of English, 18 semester hours of social sciences, and six semester hours of math, including calculus. Courses in genetics, embryology, molecular biology, psychology, humanities, sociology, anthropology, and economics are also recommended.

Placement Records

The Goldman School's Career Resource Center has a computerized list of job opportunities nationwide.

Costs

Accepted applicants who plan to attend the Goldman School have four weeks from the acceptance date to submit a nonrefundable initial tuition deposit of $500. A second deposit of $1,000 is required within 30 to 45 days after the first deposit. Both the postdoctoral and graduate programs require a $1,000 deposit. Annual tuition is $21,400 for the Doctor of Dental Medicine (D.M.D.) program, $19,850 for the postdoctoral programs, and $14,950 for the graduate programs in dental public health and nutritional sciences. Monthly payment plans are available through academic management services. Preclinical and clinical fees for the D.M.D. program over four years are about $3,325. Two required instrument kits cost about $5,896.

Financial Aid

Available loans include the Stafford Student Loan, the Spencer N. Frankl Student Revolving Loan, the Health Professions Student Loan, the Perkins Loan, the Health Education Assistance Loan (HEAL), Supplemental Loans for Students (SLS), and other loans through such lending agencies as TERI and MELA. Other sources of aid include college work-study, summer work-study, partial Exceptional Financial Need Scholarships, Financial Assistance for Disadvantaged Health Professions Students (FADHPS), state assistance, and state and local dental society loans and scholarships. Four Smith-Holden Scholarships of $300 each are awarded yearly to qualified applicants from Connecticut, Rhode Island, New Hampshire, or Massachusetts.

Minority Programs

Dental Scholarships for Undergraduate Disadvantaged Minority Students are available. Information and applications are processed through the American Fund for Dental Education.

Student Organizations

Students may get involved in community dental education programs, The Yankee Dental Congress, the student government, and various other extracurricular activities.

Faculty

All staff dentists at The University Hospital, as well as those dentists with admitting privileges, teach at the Goldman School.

Curriculum

In 1989 a new facet was added to the dental school's curriculum in the form of the APEX (Applied Professional Experience) Program. Through this program, students work as paid interns in a dental office during all four years of dental school. Students also participate in simulated practice in comprehensive care teams, which are made up of clinical faculty and students from each class. In a six-week extramural program, fourth-year students work in a new clinical setting located at any one of more than 20 affiliated sites from coast to coast. Settings include military installations, Veteran's Administration Hospitals, public health clinics, and major medical centers. First-year courses concentrate on basic sciences and a preparatory program in oral radiology, dental assisting techniques, and preventive dentistry. Second-year students study the basic, preclinical, and clinical sciences. Clinical study increases in the third and fourth years. Clinical rotations include oral surgery, pediatric dentistry/orthodontics, preventive dentistry, dental emergency care, and oral diagnosis/radiology.

Facilities

The University Hospital, a 379-bed, private, nonprofit facility, is a major teaching hospital of the Goldman School. The Institute for the Correction of Facial Deformities operates within the Goldman School and is also a teaching resource. The library, located in the Instructional Building of the Medical Center, contains over 101,790 medical and dental volumes and receives current serial publications and periodicals.

Grading Procedures

Work is graded on an A through F letter scale.

Special Programs

Qualified high school seniors may earn both the baccalaureate degree and the D.M.D. degree in the seven-year Liberal Arts/Dental Education Program. With the exception of the graduate programs in dental public health and nutritional sciences, all postdoctoral programs require the applicant to have completed a D.M.D. or D.D.S. degree. The Certificate of Advanced Graduate Study (CAGS) may be earned in advanced general dentistry, dental public health, endodontics, advanced operative dentistry, oral and maxillofacial surgery, orthodontics, pediatric dentistry, periodontics, and prosthodontics. Students interested in teaching or research may acquire a Master of Science in dentistry and a CAGS in three years. The Doctor of Science may be earned in dentistry or oral biology.

Application Procedures

All applications are processed through the American Association of Dental Schools Application Service (AADSAS) while a $40 application fee is sent to the Office of Predoctoral Admissions at Boston University. An official transcript and letters of recommendation are required. If a premedical or predental advisory committee is not available to evaluate a candidate, three letters of recommendation, including two from science professors, must be sent. Applicants will be notified of acceptance on or after December 1. Interviews at the dental school are arranged by invitation. Regional interviews are arranged by appointment. Transfer students and students with a dental degree from other countries may apply for admission to the D.M.D program with advanced standing. Complete applications to any postdoctoral program must include the application form, a $50 nonrefundable application fee, National Board scores, final official transcripts from dental and undergraduate schools, one letter from the dean of the dental school where the degree was earned, and two letters of recommendation from the dental school faculty. Interviews are required by most departments.

Contact

Boston University School of Dentistry
Office of Predoctoral Admissions
100 East Newton Street, Room 708
Boston, Massachusetts 02118
(617) 638-4787

UNIVERSITY OF CALIFORNIA LOS ANGELES SCHOOL OF DENTISTRY

Los Angeles, California 90024-1762
(213) 825-4321

Accreditation	CDA
Degrees Offered	D.D.S., M.S.
# Students Applied	495
Enrollment	93 / class
Mean GPA	3.25
% Men / % Women	59% / 41%
% Minorities	11%
Tuition	$1,590 In-State
	$7,506 Out-of-State
Application Fee	$40
Application Deadline	January 1

The University

The UCLA School of Dentistry was established in 1960. In 1964, 28 students attended the first class. In the spring of 1966, the school was dedicated. With program expansion came diversification, and the school established a research institute, started postdoctoral programs, organized a satellite clinic in the Venice community, and began to collaborate with adjacent colleges for the training of dental hygienists and dental assistants. Located on 419 acres, UCLA is a large urban university about five miles from the Pacific Ocean at the foot of the Santa Monica Mountains on the west side of Los Angeles. Situated in sunny California and in the home of Hollywood, a wide variety of cultural, social, and recreational entertainment is available to local students.

Admissions

Applicants must take the DAT within three-years prior to the year of anticipated enrollment. Students in a recent entering class achieved mean DAT scores (both academic and PAT) of 6. UCLA urges students to take the exam in April, and they require letters of recommendation. The student scholastic record (including class standing, course load, breadth of study, extracurricular activities, and work experience) is all taken seriously into account. The mean overall and science GPA of the 1989 entering class was 3.25.

Undergraduate Preparation

The school encourages students with undergraduate de-grees from accredited four-year universities or colleges. Applicants must have completed a minimum of 135 quarter hours (90 semester hours) of instruction. A maximum of 105 quarter hours (70 semester hours) of junior college work may be applied in calculating this total. Required predental courses include six semester units each of English and organic chemistry (with lab), eight semester units each (with lab) of inorganic chemistry, physics, and biology. In addition, three semester hours each of biological chemistry and introductory psychology are required.

Student Body

Ninety-three students were admitted in 1989. Thirty-eight were women and 10 were of minority background. Sixty-nine had completed baccalaureate degrees, and all but 11 were residents of California.

Costs

California residents pay tuition of $1,590 for the first and fourth years and $1,958 for the middle two years. Nonresidents pay an additional $5,916. Equipment and supplies amount to $6,800 for the first year, and room and board are about $5,230 to $8,306 annually for singles. Married couples, however, may pay up to $12,614 for room and board. In addition, a $25 microscope fee is required.

Financial Aid

Loan applications must be submitted by March 2 for the following year. Students are awarded loans and scholarships based on financial need and academic excellence. About 15 loan and scholarship funds support student study. Some private funds, donor scholarships and loans, and a National Health Service Corps Scholarship are also available.

Student Organizations

Recreational clubs bring students together for activities in amateur radio, dance, fishing, snow skiing, and martial arts, among many others. Two huge recreation centers support a wide range of sporting and recreational activities. The Epsilon Zeta chapter of the Omicron Kappa Upsilon (OKU) national dental honor society resides on campus.

Faculty

In a recent nationwide survey, UCLA faculty was judged second in the nation among public universities. About 400 faculty members from all related disciplines teach at the UCLA School of Dentistry.

Curriculum

The course of study lasts four years. In the first year, over half of the time is devoted to the basic sciences, including anatomy, biological chemistry, microbiology and immunology, oral biology and radiology, periodontics, physiology, public health dentistry, and restorative dentistry. In the second year, 87 percent of the time is given to didactic dental coursework. Courses include fixed prosthodontics, operative dentistry, oral diagnosis, removable prosthodontics, orthodontics, pediatric dentistry, and endodontics. In the third year, 61 percent of the coursework is devoted to clinical experience, and 34 percent to didactic dental courses. Students learn hospital dentistry, oral and maxillofacial surgery, or facial pain and occlusion, and special patient care. The fourth year includes 92 percent clinical experience and eight percent didactic dental coursework.

Facilities

UCLA has one college, 13 professional schools, and 24 research institutes and centers situated on the campus. The university research library, the college library, 18 specialized libraries contain nearly 6 million volumes and over 95,000 serial publications. The Louise Darling Biomedical Library contains 485,000 volumes and 6,000 serial publications, and features computer databases such as MEDLINE, MELVYL, and CANCERLIT.

Grading Procedures

UCLA uses a pass/not pass grading system. The pass (P) grade is given for satisfactory performance. The marginal (M) grade is a passing grade at the lower end of the criteria for passing. The not pass (NP) grade must be made up within a period of time stipulated by the course chairperson.

Special Programs

The School of Dentistry now offers postdoctoral programs in endodontics, oral and maxillofacial surgery, orthodontics, pediatric chemistry, periodontics, prosthodontics, implant prosthodontics, and maxillofacial prosthodontics. A combined orthodontic-pediatric dentistry program, two general dentistry postdoctoral programs, and a graduate training program in oral biology which leads to the M.S. degree are available.

Application Procedures

Students must apply through AADSAS, and materials are available from May 1 to November 1. The deadline for completed applications is January 1 of the year in which students wish to enroll. Applicants must submit substantive letters of recommendation from persons who have known the applicant well in the past four years. A comprehensive bibliography and personal history form are required as substitutes for a personal interview. The majority of notifications of acceptance come between December and March. Accepted students must send a $50 deposit within 45 days to reserve a place in class.

Contact

Office of Admissions, Recruitment
UCLA School of Dentistry
Student and Alumni Affairs, Room A3-042
Center for Health Sciences
Los Angeles, California 90024-1762
(213) 825-6141

UNIVERSITY OF CALIFORNIA SAN FRANCISCO SCHOOL OF DENTISTRY

San Francisco, California
94143-0988 (415) 476-1323

Accreditation	ADA
Degrees Offered	D.D.S., M.S., Ph.D., B.S.
# Students Applied	307
Enrollment	88 / class
Mean GPA	3.12
% Men / % Women	52% / 48%
% Minorities	29%
Tuition	None In-State
	$5,916 Out-of-State
Application Fee	$40
Application Deadline	January 1

The University

One of nine campuses of the University of California system, the San Francisco campus (UCSF) is totally devoted to education in the health sciences. The history of the campus dates back to 1873, and the School of Dentistry dates back to 1881.

UCSF is state supported. The campus comprises the schools of dentistry, medicine, nursing, and pharmacy; a major health center complex with three hospitals; and one of the largest ambulatory care programs in the state. Its professional schools are highly ranked in their respective fields.

Admissions

For its D.D.S. program, the school seeks students who share its educational goals and have the ability to handle the difficult curriculum. The school reviews academic transcripts and the DAT score to evaluate the potential for success in dentistry. Other important factors are many personal qualities, including sense of commitment to the community, open-mindedness, evidence of discipline, and leadership capabilities. The school assembles a student body that represents the diversity of the people of California; state residents are favored in the admissions process. Students with a GPA of less than 3.0 are not likely to be accepted for admission. The mean total GPA of a recent class was 3.12; the mean science GPA was 3.0. Applicants must submit DAT scores; those with scores below four are rarely admitted. Mean DAT scores for a recent entering class were six for both academic and PAT sections.

Note: the school also has a program in dental hygiene, which has a different set of admissions criteria.

Undergraduate Preparation

Students must complete 135 quarter units (90 semester units) at an accredited undergraduate institution in order to be considered for admission to the D.D.S. program.

Minimum undergraduate coursework required includes six semesters of English; eight semesters of inorganic chemistry with laboratory; four semesters of organic chemistry with laboratory; eight semesters of physics with laboratory; and eight semesters of biology (or zoology) with laboratory. Other requirements include courses in social sciences, psychology, and the humanities.

Student Body

Forty-one of the 88 students in a recent class were women, and 52 were of various minority backgrounds. All but 20 had bachelors degrees. All but seven were from California. The mean age was 23.

Placement Records

Virtually all the graduates of 1989 who sought employment found placement upon graduation. The school has a placement office, which assists students in career guidance and keeps student records for prospective employers.

Costs

There is no tuition or fees for California residents. Tuition for the 1991-92 school year is estimated at $5,916 for non-residents. The annual university registration fee is $642. There are other fees, including the $903 education fee and the $213 student health service fee.

Equipment, books, and supplies for the first year of the D.D.S. program are estimated to be $5,000, and $6,800 for the second year; thereafter, these costs decrease significantly.

Financial Aid

Financial aid is available to students on the basis of demonstrated need. The types of financial aid available include loans, scholarships, grants, and work-study programs. Scholarships awarded by the financial aid office include Regents Scholarships and University Scholarships. A limited number of awards are available from the Health Professional Exceptional Financial Need Scholarships for First-Year Students.

Numerous University of California loan funds exist for UCSF students, in addition to the Health Professional Student Loans, Stafford Student Loans, and emergency funds from the Associated Dental Students Loan Fund. Work-study and veterans benefits are also available.

Incoming students should apply for aid immediately after acceptance.

Minority Programs

The school has a special services program to recruit socio-economically disadvantaged health sciences students and assist them throughout their dental education. Services include financial aid assistance, tutoring, and an orientation program.

Student Organizations

Student organizations include Associated Dental Students and the Associated Students of the University of California, San Francisco. All dental students become members of the UCSF School of Dentistry Alumni Association.

Curriculum

The school seeks to train students not only in the traditional skills of dentistry but also to acquaint students with a strong biomedical approach to dentistry. Many diseases and conditions that have not been emphasized in the past—such as periodontal diseases, herpes infections, oral cancer, temporomandibular joint disorder, and geriatric problems—will need more attention by dentists who are well-trained in their diagnosis and treatment.

The first year consists of lectures, seminars, and laboratory sessions in the basic sciences. Students engage in an intensive study of topics such as biochemistry, head and neck anatomy, and neurobiology; and are introduced to preventive dentistry, periodontology, and AIDS treatment and research.

The second year emphasizes the clinical experience. Students are exposed to areas such as oral pathology, dental radiology, local anesthesia, fixed and removable prosthodontics, and behavioral science. In the third year, students master their clinical skills under supervision. In the fourth year, students gain experience in total patient care.

Students choose elective courses throughout the four-year program.

Facilities

In 1980, a new School of Dentistry building was constructed. The school, with its two community clinics, is one of the most modern and well-equipped dental institutions in the country. These teaching clinics provide comprehensive services in general and specialized dental and oral health care to more than 100,000 patients per year.

UCSF's medical center comprises the Moffitt/Long Hospital (including the Children's Medical Center) and Langley Porter Psychiatric Hospital. The school sponsors affiliated dental and dental auxiliary programs in hospitals and community colleges and offers continuing education courses via the Center for Continuing Dental Education.

Known as one of the finest health sciences libraries in the world, UCSF's library houses about 680,000 volumes, which include more than 200,000 foreign medical dissertations and almost 10,000 journal titles. The library has a media center, a rare collection in the history of the health sciences, and an oriental medical collection. The library has the MELVYL on-line catalog (the computer-assisted, on-line public union catalog for the entire UC system). Students also have access to MEDLINE.

The student union provides a wide range of facilities and services for students, including an automated teller machine, lockers, video games, ping pong and billiard tables, music practice rooms, and an athletic fitness center with a swimming pool, gymnasium, exercise room, massage service, and saunas.

Grading Procedures

The school uses the letter grading system of student evaluation, A through F.

Special Programs

The school has programs that lead to either the M.S. or Ph.D. in oral biology. Other postgraduate programs include those in dental clinical epidemiology, oral medicine, orthodontics, geriatric dentistry, and oral and maxillofacial surgery.

Application Procedures

The school participates in the AADSAS. The deadline for submission of applications to AADSAS is January 1 of the year of intended enrollment. Qualified applicants are sent a secondary application from the school. Candidates must return this application along with a $40 application fee and other materials, such as transcripts and pertinent personal information. The UCSF application should be returned to the school by November 1.

Contact

Dental Admission Office
University of California—San Francisco
School of Dentistry
619 Medical Sciences Building
San Francisco, California 94143
(415) 476-2737

CASE WESTERN RESERVE UNIVERSITY SCHOOL OF DENTISTRY

2123 Abington Road
Cleveland, Ohio 44106
(216) 368-3266

Accreditation	CDA
Degrees Offered	D.D.S.
# Students Applied	432
Enrollment	51 / class
Mean GPA	2.75
% Men / % Women	70% / 30%
% Minorities	15%
Tuition	$18,500
Application Fee	$35
Application Deadline	March 1

The University

Founded in 1892, the School of Dentistry has developed a "centennial plan" for dentistry—a program of dental education to prepare students for the changing role of dentistry (caring for an aging population, keeping abreast of new advances in technology, etc.). The school also hopes to continue its tradition of focusing on the needs and goals of its students.

Cleveland is experiencing a renaissance of business expansion and cultural activity. Cultural attractions include the Museum of Art, NASA Lewis Research Center, the Cleveland Playhouse, the world-renowned Cleveland Orchestra, and the International Film Festival. The "emerald necklace," an 185,000-acre system of parks surrounding Cleveland, offers many recreational activities. There are also three ski resorts in the area.

Admissions

Applicants are required to take the DAT. Primary consideration is given to applicants with a superior overall and science GPA. The mean DAT scores for a recent entering class were 4.36 (academic) and 4.52 (PAT). The mean overall GPA was 2.75; mean science GPA was 2.55.

An applicant for admission with advanced standing will be considered for admission if he or she is: a student formerly enrolled in another U.S. accredited dental institution, a foreign dental school graduate of an accredited dental institution who has satisfactorily completed a postgraduate program in a dental specialty recognized in the United States, or a foreign dental school graduate who has completed Part I of the National Board exam with a minimum average of 80.

Undergraduate Preparation

Applicants must have completed at least 60 semester hours of college courses, not including physical education and military training, by the time of enrollment. At least six semester hours each of general chemistry, organic chemistry, physics, biology, and English must have been completed; science courses must include laboratory work. Electives should include comparative anatomy, cell biology, genetics, biochemistry, microbiology, and physiology. Applicants are encouraged to take courses in the humanities, social sciences, and business. All applicants are considered, regardless of major.

Student Body

Students range in age from under 20 to over 50. About 15 percent of dental school students are members of minority groups, and 30 percent are women. Some students hold professional degrees, some are entering dental school many years after graduating from college, and some are beginning a second career. About 50 percent earned undergraduate degrees prior to matriculating at CWRUSD.

Costs

Tuition costs for a first-year student amount to $18,500. Other expenses, including laboratory fees, instruments, health insurance and books, amount to approximately $4,424. Living expenses are not included in this estimate.

Financial Aid

Financial aid is available from a variety of federal, state, and private offices. The university offers financial aid programs, including merit scholarships, available to minorities, Ohio residents, and exceptional students. Through the Tuition Stabilization Plan, tuition money can be borrowed from the university and repaid in equal monthly installments.

Minority Programs

The School of Dentistry has a minority coordinator who assists in the recruitment of minority students, monitors their progress through the dental program, provides academic or other assistance, and investigates sources of financial aid. The office of international student services offers nonacademic assistance to foreign students.

Student Organizations

Student organizations of special interest to dental students include Psi Omega, Alpha Omega, Delta Sigma Delta, the National Dental Association, and the Cleveland Association for Women Dentists.

Faculty

There are 33 full-time faculty members and more than 200 other instructors, specialists, and scientists.

Curriculum

The School of Dentistry offers a broad-based dental education and a demanding training program. The first year consists of the study of normal human biology, with an emphasis on the oral region. The fundamentals of dental health and the principles of preventive dentistry are taught. Students also participate in the dental clinic. The second year includes the study of abnormal human biology and oral pathology, symptoms and diagnosis of oral disease, and technical skills in restorative and prosthetic dentistry (students construct a complete denture prosthesis). Students continue to participate in the clinic. The third year consists of the study of advanced procedures in surgery, prosthetics, and restorative dentistry. Students spend time learning about the therapeutic needs of dental patients and provide clinical service under the supervision of faculty members. The fourth year includes training in comprehensive dental care in the clinic under the supervision of a preceptor, with consultation services provided by specialists. Students are encouraged to become involved in community health.

The school plans to add to the curriculum the study of health care delivery systems, ethical principles and jurisprudence, and interdisciplinary professional studies.

Facilities

The dental clinic offers fully-equipped private operating areas and five specialty clinics, as well as the Bolton-Brush Growth Study Center which has a unique collection of radiographs, dental casts, and comprehensive health data, offering opportunities for research in cranio-facial growth and development. The School of Dentistry is affiliated with several local hospitals and health clinics in Greater Cleveland.

The Cleveland Health Science Library has a collection of more than 320,000 volumes and over 2,000 journals. Facilities at the Andrew Jennings Computing Center are available to students, as well. Student housing is available on campus.

Special Programs

Under the six-year dental program, selected undergraduate applicants spend their first two years in an undergraduate program at CWRU or elsewhere, then enter the School of Dentistry. Students in this program earn a B.A. or B.S. and the D.D.S. in six years.

Application Procedures

The school participates in the American Association of Dental Schools Application Service. Applications should be received by March 1 of the year of planned enrollment. Those who wish to apply after March 1 should contact the admissions office for information concerning late admission procedures. The office reviews applications and interviews applicants throughout the year. Letters of recommendation from the predental advisory committee or from two instructors in basic sciences must be sent to the admissions office. A personal interview, arranged by invitation of the admissions committee, is required.

Transfer students must submit a written request for an application to the admissions office. There is an application fee of $55. Applications should be received by April 1. A "bench test" is given to test hand skills.

Contact

Office of Admissions
School of Dentistry
Case Western Reserve University
2123 Abington Road
Cleveland, Ohio 44106
(216) 368-2460 or (800) 362-8600 (In-state)
(800) 321-6984, ext. 2460 (Out-of-state)

UNIVERSITY OF COLORADO SCHOOL OF DENTISTRY

Denver, Colorado 80262
(303) 394-8282

Accreditation	CDA
Degrees Offered	D.D.S.
# Students Applied	318
Enrollment	35 / class
Mean GPA	3.08
% Men / % Women	86% / 14%
% Minorities	30%
Tuition	$5,729 In-State
	$17,112 Out-of-State
Application Fee	$35
Application Deadline	March 1

The University

The School of Medicine was established on the Boulder campus in 1893. In 1911, the university moved the School of Medicine to Denver, where it was merged with the Denver and Gross College of Medicine. The School of Dentistry was established in 1957. In 1967, capital and construction funds for the School of Dentistry were authorized by the Colorado Legislature. The first dental students graduated in May 1977.

Denver is a large city which offers a wide variety of cultural activities, including a symphony orchestra and excellent natural and fine arts museums. Many recreational activities are available, including skiing, hiking, and camping.

Admissions

Strong preference is given to residents of Colorado. The admissions committee evaluates an applicant's GPA (general and science), DAT scores, evaluations made by college predental committees and other faculty, personal letter and personal interview. Average entrance exam scores for students admitted to the program were: a DAT score of 15 and a mean GPA 3.08. Applications from women and minorities are encouraged.

Undergraduate Preparation

Completion of at least 90 semester hours of college coursework is required for admission. Most students accepted to the School of Dentistry have completed at least four years of undergraduate work and have received a Bachelor's degree. Completion of at least one year of the following courses (including lab) is required for admission: biology, general chemistry, organic chemistry, physics, and English literature or the humanities. One semester of English composition is also required. Recommended electives include the humanities and the social, biological, and behavioral sciences.

Student Body

The average age of students enrolled in the School of Dentistry is 25.

Costs

For the 1990-91 entering class, tuition was $5,729 for residents and $17,112 for nonresidents. Other expenses averaged $6,400 for first-year students.

Financial Aid

Financial aid usually consists of a combination of part-time work and long-term low interest loans and grants. All applicants for financial aid must be working towards a degree. Foreign students who have an immigrant or permanent visa are eligible. Preference is given to full-time students. Applicants who have not been officially accepted to a program at the Health Center or placed on an alternate list cannot obtain applications for financial aid.

Students must apply for financial aid by March 15 preceding the academic year for which assistance is desired (or 30 days after the date of the letter of acceptance for entering students). Students must reapply for financial aid each year.

Minority Programs

The Center for Multicultural Enrichment (CME) attempts to recruit students from groups underrepresented on the university campus. It also seeks to retain those students by providing support services that help to ensure their success.

Faculty

There are nearly 1,100 faculty members at the campus. The professional schools enroll approximately 1,500 students, with an additional 700 interns, residents, and fellows (all graduate physicians).

Curriculum

Class size is small, offering extensive faculty-student interaction. Dental students are provided with practice-oriented training through a clinic with a patient population selected for educational purposes. The first and second years consist of basic science instruction, reinforced by clinical faculty. Patient care experience takes place mainly in the third and fourth years. Electives are available during the latter two years. The Advanced Clinical Training and Service Program is available during a student's final eight months, enabling the student to spend time outside the school in extramural clinical rotations.

Facilities

The Health Sciences Center houses the University Hospital and the Colorado Psychiatric Hospital, as well as the School of Dentistry, the School of Medicine, the School of Nursing, the Graduate School, programs in the allied health professions, and eight affiliated institutes.

Grading Procedures

Evaluation is on a letter-grade basis.

Application Procedures

The School of Dentistry participates in AADSAS. Applications may be filed after June 1 of the year preceding planned enrollment, and all requested material must be received by AADSAS on or before March 1 of the year of planned enrollment. Late applications will not be considered for the following year. DAT results must be sent directly to the school. After the school has received the AADSAS packet, the following materials will be requested: an application fee of $35, verification of Colorado residency, college transcripts, letters of recommendation, and a recent photograph. Additional items may be requested. Interviews are arranged by invitation of the admissions committee.

Contact

School of Dentistry Recruitment Office
University of Colorado Health Sciences Center
4200 East Ninth Avenue, Box C284
Denver, Colorado 80262
(303) 270-7259

COLUMBIA UNIVERSITY SCHOOL OF DENTAL AND ORAL SURGERY

630 West 168th Street
New York, New York 10032
(212) 305-4171

Accreditation	CDA
Degrees Offered	D.D.S., M.P.H./D.D.S.
# Students Applied	680
Enrollment	58 / class
Mean GPA	2.92
% Men / % Women	80% / 20%
% Minorities	47%
Tuition	$16,950
Application Fee	$45
Application Deadline	March 1

The University

The School of Dental and Oral Surgery was founded in 1852, when the New York state legislature chartered the New York College of Dentistry. In 1923, it was joined with the dental school at Columbia University, the New York Postgraduate School of Dentistry, and the New York School of Dental Hygiene. The School has been a leading force in dental education and research since its establishment. In 1926, Professor William J. Gies of the Biochemistry Department prepared the report Dental Education in the United States and Canada, after which dental schools throughout the country adopted the basic educational policies and objectives developed at Columbia University.

New York City offers dental students exposure to leading authorities in every field of dentistry. There are many opportunities for extracurricular learning and recreation. New York City is an important cultural center, offering innumerable museums, galleries, concert halls, and cinemas, to name but a few places of interest.

Admissions

The admissions committee primarily considers an applicant's preparation and intellectual capacity. An applicant's personal character is also considered. All applicants must take the Dental Admission Tests (DAT). Mean scores from a recent entering class were 18 on the academic portion and 18 on the PAT portion. The mean total GPA is 2.92 and the mean science GPA is 3.0.

Undergraduate Preparation

Three years of undergraduate education at an accredited U.S. institution is required for admission. Eight semester hours each (including laboratory work in the science courses) of the following courses must be completed before registration: English composition and literature, physics, biology, inorganic chemistry, and organic chemistry. Additional courses in chemistry, advanced courses in biology, courses in mathematics, foreign languages, sociology, history, and the fine and industrial arts are also recommended.

Student Body

Twelve of the 58 students in a recent class were women and 27 were minorities. Thirty-five students were state residents, and all had earned baccalaureate degrees prior to matriculation.

Costs

Tuition and fees are subject to change. Tuition for a full-time D.D.S. student amounts to $16,950 per year. Health service and hospital insurance fees amount to approximately $888. Each student must purchase a package of instruments, necessary for preclinical and clinical dental instruction, from the university. The estimated costs of these instruments for students entering in September 1989 was approximately $6,000, which can be paid over a four-year period. Microscopes and certain clinical instruments can be rented. Books cost approximately $500 in the first year, $600 in the second, $300 in the third, and $100 in the fourth.

Financial Aid

Students may apply for financial aid through the financial aid office. The School uses the Graduate and Professional School Financial Aid Service (GAPSFAS) to determine each student's need. Summer work-study positions are available, but the School does not encourage outside employment during the academic year.

Student Organizations

Organizations of interest to dental students include the Columbia University student council, The William Jarvie Society (a dental honor society), and the Student Dental Association.

Curriculum

First-year dental students study the basic science "core program" with medical and graduate students. Included in the dental studies are courses offering an introduction to dentistry, as well as preclinical courses. The second year includes basic science courses, which are correlated with oral and dental problems that will be faced later in clinical practice. "Areas of Concentration," a comprehensive program that offers in-depth educational experiences in areas not ordinarily covered in the regular curriculum, is required during the second year. The student selects one of four general categories: advanced clinical dentistry, research, comprehensive general dentistry or oral medicine/oral pathology/hospital dentistry, and later chooses from more than 15 specialized elective "tracks" that include radiology, research, pediatric dentistry, and geriatric dentistry.

The third year is primarily clinical, with training in all phases of dentistry. Students begin to practice clinical dentistry under close preceptor supervision. A modular system of clinical training allows a student to work at his/her own pace, taking the time to master a technique before moving on. There is also a one-month rotation that all students spend off-campus at an affiliated hospital. The fourth year is the major clinical dentistry year, with students assuming the responsibility for giving comprehensive dental care to a practice panel of patients assigned to them while completing studies in their chosen area of concentration.

Voluntary participation in a research project of the student's own choice and in programs under the guidance of members of the faculty is encouraged. A limited number of student research fellowships are available.

Facilities

The school is located in the Columbia-Presbyterian Medical Center, where the student learns firsthand to provide dental care for hospitalized patients, gaining experience in the diagnosis and care of those cases where a relationship exists between oral and general systemic disease. In addition, the school has a modern dental teaching center with facilities for group practice by faculty members, general practice residents, and students.

The Health Sciences Library contains more than 400,000 volumes and receives almost 4,000 periodical titles. The media center is equipped with microcomputers and a variety of audiovisual materials. Literature searching is offered on many computerized databases, including MEDLARS. Other Columbia libraries on the Morningside campus are also available to dental students.

Limited student housing is available.

Grading Procedures

A letter grading system is used. A faculty committee meets annually to review each student's performance. Students are informed in writing of the academic decisions of each class committee.

Special Programs

The School of Dental and Oral Surgery and the School of Public Health offer a joint program leading to the Master of Public Health/Doctor of Dental Science degree. Applicants to the programs must be accepted first to the School of Dental and Oral Surgery, then to the School of Public Health. Students can enter the program during the first two-and-a-half years and can complete the program in up to two years after dental school graduation.

Application Procedures

The school participates in the American Association of Dental Schools Application Service (AADSAS). Applications should be received between July 1 of the year preceding planned enrollment and March 1 of the year of planned enrollment. A $45 application fee is required upon submission of the AADSAS application. The DAT is required. A personal interview is arranged with selected candidates upon invitation from the committee on admissions. Applicants living on the West Coast will have the option of being interviewed in California.

Applicants for advanced standing will be considered for placement into the second or third year. Applications for admission are accepted until April 1 for May enrollment. Graduates of dental schools may also be considered for placement into the second or third year of the program. A minimum score of 600 on the Test of English as a Foreign Language (TOEFL) is required.

Contact

Associate Dean for Academic Affairs
School of Dental and Oral Surgery
Columbia University
630 West 168th Street
New York, New York 10032
(212) 305-4174

UNIVERSITY OF CONNECTICUT SCHOOL OF DENTAL MEDICINE

Farmington, Connecticut 06030
(203) 679-2808

Accreditation	ADA
Degrees Offered	D.M.D., D.M.D./M.D., D.M.D./Ph.D., D.M.D./M.P.H.
# Students Applied	403
Enrollment	44 / class
Mean GPA	3.1
% Men / % Women	62% / 38%
% Minorities	Not Available
Tuition	$5,800 In-State,
	$7,250 New England
	$13,300 Out-of-State
Application Fee	$50
Application Deadline	April 1

The University

The University of Connecticut (UConn) traces its roots to the establishment of the Storrs Agricultural School in 1881. Its main campus is in Storrs, Connecticut, where the university enrolls 20,000 graduate and undergraduate students.

The university's health center, formed in the early 1960s, enrolled its first class in 1968. In addition to the School of Dental Medicine, the center comprises the School of Medicine and the John Dempsey Hospital. The health center is situated on a wooded, suburban campus near I-84 in Farmington, part of the Greater Hartford area.

The School of Dental Medicine is the only public dental school in New England. The school has consistently ranked among the top three dental schools in regard to the amount of funding received from the National Institute of Dental Research.

Farmington is close to the Berkshire Mountains and Long Island Sound beaches. Hartford affords students a wide variety of cultural, recreational, and sports events.

Admissions

The school seeks a student body that represents the groups found in society at large. While preference is given to residents of Connecticut and other New England states, many students come from other areas of the country. The school admits students based on their academic background as well as their personality and sense of motivation. The mean total GPA of the class that entered in fall 1989 was 3.1; the mean science GPA of this class was 3.0. The mean score for the academic part of the DAT was 5.41/17; for the PAT section, 5.46/16.85.

Undergraduate Preparation

Students are expected to have earned a bachelor's degree by the time of enrollment. Required undergraduate coursework includes one year (two semesters) each of general chemistry, organic chemistry, biology, and physics. English skills are highly valued, and students are encouraged to take courses in biochemistry or cell biology. All candidates for admission are required to take the DAT.

Student Body

Each entering class numbers about 40 students. They represent a diversity of backgrounds and a variety of undergraduate institutions. Many have had full-time career experience before applying to dental school. Of the 44 students who enrolled in 1989, 38 had bachelor degrees, and 17 were women. Ages of the students ranged from 21 to 29, the mean age being 23.

Placement Records

Generally, about 70 percent of the school's graduates set up practice in Connecticut. The school has a placement service that assists students in finding employment in Connecticut and nationwide.

Costs

For 1991-92, tuition for Connecticut residents is $5,800. Other New England residents pay $7,250. All others pay $13,300. Fees for all students total $2,450 per year. For first- and second-year students, books, supplies, and instruments cost approximately $3,000 to $3,300.

Financial Aid

More than 90 percent of the student body receives some form of financial aid. The award of aid is based on need as determined by information supplied on the GAPSFAS form. Scholarships include both need- and merit-based awards. Awards specific to the University of Connecticut include scholarships from the UConn Health Center Auxiliary, the Parents Association, and the Alumni Association. Other scholarships include the Health Professions Extreme Financial Need scholarships and Financial Assistance for Disadvantaged Health Professionals scholarships.

A wide variety of loans are available in addition to the Stafford, Perkins, and Health Professions Student Loans.

The school has a financial aid office and a minority student affairs office, which assist students in obtaining financial aid and with budget planning and debt and expense management.

Minority Programs

The office of minority student affairs supports minority students enrolled in the dental and medical schools, and administers special programs such as the Minority Scholars Institute, the Scholars Training Academy, and a research apprentice program for minority high school students.

Student Organizations

Students can become active on numerous committees of the Dental Council, the governing body of the dental school. Students can also become members of the Dental Student Association or the dental student research group, or join special interest groups formed around a variety of issues important to students.

The school also has chapters of Alpha Omega and Delta Sigma Delta.

Curriculum

The basic science curriculum is the same as that of the medical school. The school emphasizes an "organ-system" approach and the education of practitioners who can provide care to the whole person. Electives are an important part of the curriculum, and they include summer research opportunities as well as internships and externships in all the clinical specialties. Faculty members actively promote research opportunities for dental students.

First- and second-year courses foster an understanding of normal human biology and pathophysiology. Basic medical science courses are taught by committees. Students are also introduced to the basic clinical sciences in these years, which include oral, physical, and laboratory evaluation. This part of the program prepares the student for the major part of the clinical program in the last two years.

In the third and fourth years, students provide care to actual patients under the guidance of faculty members. The clinical part of the curriculum is considered a continuum through these last two years. During these years, students participate in about 2,500 hours of clinical work in all disciplines and over 700 hours of didactic education. Students take clinical rotations in many specialty areas and are also introduced to practice management during this part of the program.

Facilities

The school has 10 dental clinics consisting of 14 to 16 individual dental stations or operatories in each clinic. Students develop a comprehensive treatment approach using modern equipment that includes computer-assisted dispensing of sterilized instrument packages. During the 1989-90 academic year, the undergraduate clinics accommodated 20,000 patient visits. Extensive laboratory facilities are also available to dental students.

The library houses about 163,000 volumes, including 105,225 bound journals, and subscribes to approximately 2,770 journal titles. The audiovisual collection is considered one of the best in the country. The library also has a computer education center. Additional support facilities include a seven-floor center for laboratory animal care and a computer education center, which contains 28 Macintosh SEs, four laser printers, and 270 microcomputer programs for student use.

Grading Procedures

Students are evaluated on a pass/fail basis.

Special Programs

The school sponsors a joint D.M.D./Ph.D. program, which is designed for a small number of outstanding students who have specific goals in research and teaching and who are highly motivated. Other joint degree programs include the D.M.D./M.D. and the D.M.D./M.P.H.

Application Procedures

UConn School of Dental Medicine participates in AADSAS. Applications can be submitted to AADSAS between July and April 1. The student should, at the same time, send supplementary materials to the school's admissions office. These include the application fee of $50, letters of recommendation from predental advisory committee members (or letters from three faculty members, if no such advisory committee exists), and DAT scores. (The DAT should be taken in the spring of the undergraduate junior year or the fall of the senior year.) An interview is required prior to acceptance. The student, when notified of acceptance, must submit a $400 deposit, which is applied toward tuition.

Contact

Admissions Office
Office of Dental Student Affairs
University of Connecticut
School of Dental Medicine
Farmington, Connecticut 06030
(203) 679-2175

CREIGHTON UNIVERSITY SCHOOL OF DENTISTRY

California at 24th Street
Omaha, Nebraska 68178
(402) 280-2862

Accreditation	ADA
Degrees Offered	D.D.S.
# Students Applied	700
Enrollment	75 / class
Mean GPA	2.90
% Men / % Women	92% / 8%
% Minorities	3%
Tuition	$13,824
Application Fee	$25
Application Deadline	March 1

The University

The history of Creighton University dates back over a century. Its first division, the College of Arts and Sciences, was founded in 1878. Today, the university is a privately endowed, independent institution affiliated with the Jesuit tradition and enrolling nearly 6,000 students.

In addition to the School of Dentistry, Creighton has schools of medicine, nursing, pharmacy, and allied health professions. Almost one-quarter of its student body is enrolled in one of the health sciences programs. Creighton is the smallest university in the nation that has a full complement of health science schools. The School of Dentistry was founded in 1905.

The campus is situated in northwest downtown Omaha, Nebraska. Omaha is a major midwestern city with a population of well over 600,000, including its surrounding area. Omaha has 17 hospitals, the largest pediatric hospital between Denver and Chicago, and two university-based medical and research centers. The city has many opportunities for cultural and recreational diversions.

Admissions

The school seeks students judged to be the highest qualified to study and practice dentistry. Factors considered in the admissions decision include evidence of superior scholarship, DAT scores, and letters of recommendation. Of the 1989 entering class, the mean DAT (academic) score was 15.47; the mean GPA was 2.90.

Undergraduate Preparation

Candidates for admission must have had at least 64 semester hours (96 quarter hours) from an accredited college of arts and sciences. The preprofessional course of study must include six semester hours of biology (or zoology) with lab, eight semester hours of inorganic chemistry (lab recommended), six semester hours of organic chemistry with lab, six semester hours of English, and six semester hours of physics. These courses must be completed by the end of the spring term preceding the fall of intended enrollment. Students are expected to have at least a 3.0 overall GPA in undergraduate coursework.

Students should take the DAT preferably in October of their last preprofessional year in college, or in April preceding their last academic year.

Student Body

The school's entering class numbers about 75. Creighton's overall student body represents all geographical areas of the United States as well as numerous foreign countries. Of the 1989 entering class, eight percent were women and three percent were minorities. The ages of students ranged from 19 to 38, with a mean age of 25.

Costs

Effective August 1990, tuition per semester is $6,912. Books cost about $225 in the first and third years, about $700 in the second year, and about $145 in the fourth year. Instruments cost anywhere from about $2,500 to $3,600 for years one and two. All fees and costs are subject to change without notice.

Financial Aid

To apply for financial aid, students must submit a FAF and provide to Creighton all financial aid transcripts from all previous institutions attended. Application should be made between January 1 and April 1 preceding the fall semester of intended enrollment.

Types of loans available include the Health Professions Loan, Perkins Loan, Health Education Assistance Loan, Dental Alumni Loan, and the Frederick W. Schaefer Scholarship Loan (based on merit as well as need). Government grants and scholarships include Exceptional Need Scholarships for Dental Sciences, the Indian Fellowship Program, and the National Health Service Corps Scholarship. Several university dental school scholarships are also available.

A limited number of qualified students can receive partial tuition remission from Idaho, New Mexico, Utah, and Wyoming ("compact" states).

Student Organizations

Dental students are automatically members of the Creighton American Dental Association, a chartered chapter of the American Student Dental Association. Other student groups are organized around social, dramatic, literary, debating, and religious interests.

Fraternities and honor societies on campus include Delta Sigma Delta, Alpha Sigma Nu, and Omicron Kappa Upsilon.

Curriculum

The curriculum is geared toward educating dentists who will specialize in diseases of the oral cavity. Students are educated to possess the ability to provide comprehensive dental health care with little or no dependence on other specialists.

The four-year program is designed to take the student from basic science to mastery of basic clinical skills and total patient care.

First- and second-year courses include community dentistry field experiences, biochemistry, microbiology, general gross anatomy, general pathology, radiology, pulp biology, endodontics lecture, and dental anatomy lecture.

Typical courses of the third and fourth years include community dentistry field experience, geriatric dentistry, oral hygiene clinic, operative dentistry clinic, oral medicine and diagnosis, oral surgery clinic, removable prosthodontics clinic, and ethics in the practice of dentistry.

The program is based on a semester system. Elective courses are optional and carry no credit.

Facilities

Facilities include the Bio-Information Center, Saint Joseph Hospital (the university teaching hospital), the Omaha Health Professions Center, and the Boys Town National Research Hospital. The dental school building was completed in 1973.

The school, which has a total of 150,000 square feet, contains classrooms and preclinical laboratories, adult clinical facilities, children's clinics, basic science laboratories, and other facilities. Students have access to a surgical suite and X-ray equipment. On-campus housing is available for full-time students, and the nearby Creighton Child Care Center has reasonable rates—of interest to students with children.

Grading Procedures

Letter grades are used to evaluate students in all courses and as interim grades for academic and technical courses. Interim grades are also issued for clinical courses based on the A-F letter grading system.

Application Procedures

Creighton University School of Dentistry participates in AADSAS. Applications must be filed with AADSAS between May 1 and March 1 of the preceding academic year before year of enrollment. Early application is strongly recommended.

The dental admissions office will request supplemental information from the applicant, including a $25 application fee, DAT scores, official college transcripts, three letters of recommendation (two from science instructors and one from a nonscience instructor), and a supplementary application form.

Contact

Creighton University
Dental Admissions Office
California at 24th Street
Omaha, Nebraska 68178
(402) 280-2700

UNIVERSITY OF DETROIT SCHOOL OF DENTISTRY

2985 East Jefferson Avenue
Detroit, Michigan 48207-4282
(313) 446-1806

Accreditation	ADA, AADS
Degrees Offered	D.D.S., B.S., M.S.
# Students Applied	358
Enrollment	55 / class
Mean GPA	2.86
% Men / % Women	61% / 39%
% Minorities	9%
Tuition	$12,500
Application Fee	$25
Application Deadline	Flexible, will accept applicants until class is filled

The University

The University of Detroit was originally established as Detroit College in 1877. It is the oldest independent university in Michigan.

The dental school began in 1932. Its first class enrolled 47 students. Today, the school admits 62 students per year. In 1981, the school opened the university's dental service at Detroit Receiving Hospital, part of the Detroit Medical Center complex. This service provides an educational and training environment that closely simulates working conditions in private dental practice.

The dental school is located one mile east of downtown Detroit. Detroit offers a full range of intellectual, artistic, and recreational activities. As the birthplace of Motown, Detroit offers rock, soul, jazz, symphonic, and various ethnic kinds of music. For performing arts, there's the Fox Theatre. The Institute of Arts, containing 101 galleries, is the largest municipally owned museum in the U.S. Its excellent and varied restaurants have earned the city the honor of being named the third best culinary city in the nation. Lakes, ski trails, and camping and hiking areas can be found beyond the metropolitan area, in outlying Michigan and Canada.

Admissions

The admissions committee considers a variety of factors. These include academic performance in undergraduate studies, DAT scores, personal characteristics, and potential for success as determined by letters of recommendation and personal interviews.

It is strongly recommended that the DAT be taken no later than October of the year preceding anticipated enrollment. Students are also advised to take the DAT only after basic requirements in chemistry and biology have been completed.

Undergraduate Preparation

Students considering applying to the School of Dentistry should enroll in a four-year undergraduate program leading to a bachelor's degree. Most applicants who are accepted for admission have completed at least three years (90 semester hours) of undergraduate education. The choice of major is not critical as long as course requirements are fulfilled. They are as follows: eight semester hours each of inorganic or general chemistry (with lab), organic chemistry (with lab), general biology or zoology (with lab), and physics (with lab); and six semester hours of English. In addition, biochemistry is highly recommended. Also useful are courses in comparative anatomy, histology, embryology, and mathematics.

Student Body

Of the 55 students enrolled in 1989, 39 percent were women and ninepercent were minorities. About 55 percent had undergraduate degrees. Seventy-one percent were state residents. The mean age was 24.

Costs

Tuition for both residents and nonresidents is $12,500. Instruments cost $6,000 the first year, $3,800 the second year, $725 the third year, and $100 the last year. Annual expenses are a $120 lab fee, a $200 general fee, a $35 student activity fee, and $48 for personal insurance.

Financial Aid

Need-based aid is distributed on a first-come, first-served basis, so the school encourages students to apply early—as soon as possible after January 1 preceding the date they expect to enroll. Application for non-need-based aid can be submitted as early as the April preceding enrollment.

Several types of need-based aid are available, including Michigan Tuition Grants, Perkins Loans, Health Professions Loans, and Exceptional Need Scholarships. Programs not based on need include Dental Merit Grants (based on academic achievement) and Supplemental Loans to Students.

The school requires that financial aid applicants file a FAF and submit supplemental information to the university's financial aid office.

Student Organizations

Students play a major role on academic committees. There are a variety of professional and social organizations, including Delta Sigma Delta, Alpha Omega, and Psi Omega, and students are involved in student government, American Dental Student Association activity, and the school newspaper.

Faculty

The faculty at the School of Dentistry numbers approximately 190.

Curriculum

During the four-year D.D.S. curriculum, students are guided through the development and attainment of professional knowledge and skills in a program that begins with extensive faculty supervision and ends with the relative independence that will be carried into private practice.

Students are taught patient care with an emphasis on skills of evaluation, diagnosis, and prevention. A structured, systematic approach in the basic sciences provides the foundation for clinical work. The comprehensive curriculum includes studies in the behavioral sciences and fosters self-reliance and sensitivity to the needs of the community as a whole, especially urban and other underserved areas.

First- and second-year courses include basic pathology, biochemistry, dental anatomy and occlusion, oral pathology, clinical experience, orthodontics, oral diagnosis, operative dentistry, and pain and anxiety control.

Third- and fourth-year courses include oral surgery, therapeutics, community dentistry, practice management, and implant dentistry.

Facilities

Clinical facilities at the school include 147 stations, each accommodating chairside teaching and assistance. Students also rotate on assignment through satellite clinics and programs in local hospitals.

The dental service at Detroit Receiving Hospital provides a complete range of patient care, from general dental maintenance to periodontics, maxillofacial prosthetics, and oral and maxillofacial surgery.

The dental library is centrally located on the school's campus. The library houses an extensive collection of books and journals in the dental, biomedical, and behavioral sciences, as well as a media collection. On-line bibliographic services are provided by computer interaction with the National Library of Medicine.

Special Programs

The School of Dentistry has a 22-month postdoctoral program in endodontics and a 24-month postdoctoral program in orthodontics. These programs lead to an M.S. degree and a certificate of clinical competence.

The school also offers a three-year program leading to the certificate in dental hygiene and a four-year baccalaureate degree program leading to a B.S. in dental hygiene.

Application Procedures

The School of Dentistry participates in the AADSAS. Candidates should submit AADSAS applications between July 1 of the year preceding anticipated entry and March 1 of the year of entry (early application is encouraged).

An application fee of $25 should be sent directly to the school. Letters of recommendation from a preprofessional advisory committee or from science faculty are required, and should be submitted directly to the school. A personal statement is optional.

Students should try to achieve at least average scores on the academic and perceptual ability tests of the DAT.

Contact

Admissions Office
University of Detroit
School of Dentistry
2985 East Jefferson Avenue
Detroit, Michigan 48207
(313) 446-1858

UNIVERSITY OF FLORIDA COLLEGE OF DENTISTRY

Gainesville, Florida 32610-0445
(904) 372-2946

Accreditation	ADA
Degrees Offered	D.M.D.
# Students Applied	303
Enrollment	77 / class
Mean GPA	3.0
% Men / % Women	65% / 35%
% Minorities	36%
Tuition	$5,618 In-State
	$13,576 Out-of-State
Application Fee	$15
Application Deadline	October 15

The University

The University of Florida Health Science Center opened its first units in 1956—the College of Medicine and the College of Nursing. Today, the Health Science Center is among the most modern and advanced centers for health education in the country. The Center complex also comprises the College of Dentistry, College of Health Related Professions, College of Pharmacy, College of Veterinary Medicine, Shands Hospital, and the University of Florida clinics.

The College of Dentistry is the only dental school in the state of Florida. All the units of the Health Science Center work closely with each other—physicians, nurses, pharmacists, and others—to foster an approach that considers the total health of the individual.

The College of Dentistry admitted its first class in 1972. Currently, about 80 students are admitted each year.

Admissions

In general, the college looks closely at scholastic achievement, moral character, and motivation. Students with at least a B (3.0) average are given preference. Other factors considered in the admission process are DAT scores, breadth of undergraduate education, extracurricular activities, personal statement, knowledge of the profession, and personality factors. The DAT academic average for the 1990 entering class was 16.66; the PAT average was also 16.66. In recent years, the average total GPA of the entering class has ranged between 3.09 and 3.27. The average science GPA has been between 3.01 and 3.20. Florida residents are given preference.

Undergraduate Preparation

A baccalaureate degree is preferred; applicants must have had at least 90 semester hours of undergraduate coursework. The quality of the preprofessional program is an important factor in considering candidates for admission. The following courses are required: eight semester hours each of biology, general chemistry, organic chemistry, and physics—all with lab; and basic math as a prerequisite to physics and chemistry.

Student Body

About 80 students are accepted to each first-year class.

About 90 percent of the entering class are Florida residents. Generally, 30 to 40 percent of the class are women. The 1990 entering class comprises about 36 percent minorities. Fifty-nine of the 77 students in this class hold baccalaureate degrees.

Placement Records

Most College of Dentistry graduates find meaningful employment, with the majority remaining in the state of Florida. Many work in clinics or become associates in private practice. About 30 to 40 percent of UF dental graduates go on for more education, whether it be residency experience or two- or four-year graduate programs.

Costs

Tuition and fees for Florida residents is $5,618. Nonresidents pay $13,576. Textbooks and instruments for the total program are estimated to cost $10,800, about $6,500 of which is for the instrument package purchased for the second semester of the first year.

Financial Aid

Scholarship funding is very limited. Federal scholarships include the Exceptional Financial Need Program and the Federal Assistance for Disadvantaged Health Professions Students Program. Other scholarships include those provided by Florida dental centers, the American Association of Women Dentists, and the University of Florida Dental Guild.

A wide range of loan funds is available from federal, state, and private organizations and individuals, and from other sources. These include the Florida Dental Association fund, the Guaranteed Student Loan fund, the Health Education Assistance Loan Program, and the Auxiliary Loans for Students Program.

Funds are awarded according to need and availability of funds. Financial needs analysis forms are sent to students upon acceptance to the college.

Curriculum

The first two years focus on the basic sciences education. Dental students take many courses with medical and graduate students; these classes are taught by faculty teams. The core curriculum for dental students consists of dental science courses, preclinical technique programs, and clinical courses. Extramural rotations and hospital dentistry are part of the clinical curriculum. The elective portion of the curriculum allows students to tailor the program to their individual interests.

Clinical experience allows students to develop applied knowledge and skills. The clinical portion of the program teaches prevention, etiology, diagnosis, treatment planning, and treatment of disease and disease processes. During this phase, students have responsibility for total patient care.

Curricula format is a combination of self-paced study, self-instruction, seminar, conference, and lecture. Students are encouraged to participate in research through the Student Research Training Program.

Facilities

The Health Science Center underwent expansion in 1975. The Center's Communicore is a four-level multipurpose building that houses labs, classrooms, a learning resources center, the library, and other facilities. The Veterans Administration Medical Center in Gainesville operates as an integral unit of the Health Science Center.

The twelve-story Dental Sciences Building includes dental outpatient clinics, postgraduate and specialty clinics, faculty offices, seminar rooms, and teaching and research laboratories. On-campus housing is available; accepted students should apply early.

Grading Procedures

Most courses are graded by letter—A, B+, B, C+, C, D+, D, and E (failure). Elective courses may be graded S (Satisfactory) or U (Unsatisfactory). To graduate, students must pass Parts I and II of the National Board exam.

Special Programs

A wide variety of advanced programs in dentistry are offered. These include one-year certificate programs in areas such as pediatric dentistry, orthodontics, and geriatric dentistry. The college offers a general practice residency program and an oral and maxillofacial surgery residency program.

The college also offers graduate degree programs in dental biomaterials, oral biology, speech pathology, and behavioral sciences in dentistry.

Application Procedures

The college participates in AADSAS. The deadline for submission of AADSAS applications is October 15 of the year prior to anticipated enrollment. After the admissions committee reviews the AADSAS application, it will send a secondary application to promising applicants. This secondary application must be submitted to the college along with supplementary materials (letters of recommendation) by November 15 along with an application fee of $15. Selected candidates will be invited for interviews.

It is preferable that applicants take the DAT in the spring preceding the submission of the application to AADSAS.

Contact

Office of Admissions
University of Florida
College of Dentistry
Box J 445
J. Hillis Miller Health Science Center
Gainesville, Florida 32610
(904) 392-4866

HARVARD SCHOOL OF DENTAL MEDICINE

Cambridge, Massachusetts 02138
(617) 262-1401

Accreditation	CDA
Degrees Offered	D.M.D., D.M.S., M.M.S., M.D.
# Students Applied	256
Enrollment	24 / class
Mean GPA	3.43
% Men / % Women	59% / 41%
% Minorities	41%
Tuition	$18,030
Application Fee	$60
Application Deadline	January 1

The University

Harvard College first opened its doors in Cambridge, Massachusetts in 1636 for the newly settled New England colonies. During the 19th century the school added graduate and professional schools, of which there are now 10. These world-renowned professional institutions include the Business School, the School of Dental Medicine, the Medical School, and the School of Public Health. Now one of the world's most outstanding universities, Harvard has a total graduate and undergraduate enrollment of approximately 17,000 degree candidates. Since its foundation in 1867, the School of Dental Medicine has attracted the world's most gifted students from all around the United States and over 100 countries.

Admissions

All applicants are required to take the Dental Admission Test (DAT). It is strongly recommended that the DAT be taken by April of the junior year. The mean academic DAT score for a recent class was 19/6; the mean score for the PAT portion of the DAT was 19/5. The same class had a mean science GPA of 3.33 and a mean total GPA of 3.43.

Undergraduate Preparation

All applicants must have completed one full year of biology (with lab), chemistry (eight semester hours each of inorganic and organic), physics, English (including composition) and mathematics. It is also highly recommended that students have two or three advanced science courses, such as biochemistry, physiology, comparative anatomy, and genetics. To enhance the student's awareness of the world in which he or she lives the study of social and behavioral sciences, arts and humanities, and a foreign language is recommended.

Student Body

The Harvard professional school has a very competitive pool of applicants. Students from all sections of the world compose a gathering of truly gifted medical students. Twenty-four students enrolled in the 1989 entering class. Of these, 10 were women, 10 were minorities, and three were foreign nationals. The age range was 22 to 32; the mean age was 25.8 years. All had undergraduate degrees.

Placement Records

The Harvard professional graduate schools have some of the finest reputations for scholarly achievement and placement in the world.

Costs

Tuition is $18,030. Student health fees and room and board will run close to $10,000. An average of $350 should be allotted for books and supplies each year. There is a $250 microscope rental fee. Students should allow anywhere from $30,000 to $38,000 for total expenses each year.

Financial Aid

Financial aid is available in the form of loans, scholarships, and work-study programs for qualified candidates. Qualification is determined by the Graduate and Professional Schools Financial Aid Service (GAPSFAS). The School of Dental Medicine participates in the Title IV Student Assistance Programs and the Federal Health Professions Educational Assistance Programs. The loans available include the Stafford Guaranteed Student Loan, SLS Loan, Perkins Loan, and college work-study. Students are asked to contact the office of student affairs for further information.

Minority Programs

Several organizations cater to minority students, including the National Chicano Health Organization, Black Health Organization, Boricua Health Organization, and the Native American Health Organization.

Student Organizations

Dental students can participate in organizations such as the American Association of Dental Schools, the American Student Dental Association, the Student National Dental Association, and the HSDM student council. Issues of registration, financial aid management, academic and personal counseling, and curriculum can be discussed through the HSDM office of student affairs.

Faculty

Dental students can look forward to benefiting from the over 300 professional instructors and administrators.

Curriculum

The four major areas of the five-year predoctoral curriculum are divided into 20 months of basic science/preclinical core, 13 months of major clinical dentistry, 11 months of externship/ electives, and 11 months of biomedical research/health care research tracks. During the well-balanced introduction to medicine, students will study the human body, genetics, reproduction and development, pharmacology, and pathophysiology. Six additional courses are part of the introduction; these include oral biology, gerontology, oral radiology, oral pathology, dental anatomy, and occlusion. Dental students are required to participate in research experiences that result in a research proposal in the third year and a paper and defense at the end of the fourth year. Fifth-year students can choose to focus on either biomedical studies or health care issues. Both choices are "research tracks" that require students to develop and present a thesis in both written and oral forms and defend it before a thesis committee.

Facilities

The Francis A. Countway Library of Medicine combines the resources and services of the Harvard Medical Library and the Boston Medical Library. Countway is one of the largest libraries serving health professional schools in the country, with recorded holdings of nearly 500,000 volumes and more than 5,000 current periodicals. The library possesses some of the most important writings of medical interest published in the United States and Europe. These writings include documents that span throughout the previous four centuries and an additional 800 books published prior to 1501. Teaching and learning sessions take place in many affiliated hospitals.

Grading Procedures

The school uses a grading system of honors/pass/fail.

Special Programs

Students may earn a Master of Public Health or Master of Science degree and receive both the D.M.D. and the M.P.H. or M.S. degrees at the end of year five. Students may choose to spend up to five months of the fifth year performing research and/or patient care services in a developing country. The Peace

Corps and Project Hope may help cover some travel and living expenses. Opportunities for research and patient care exist on Indian reservations, as well.

Application Procedures

The Harvard School of Dental Medicine participates in the American Association of Dental Schools Application Service (AADSAS). Students are urged to apply between June and September of the year prior to matriculation. Applicants are to send along with the standard form a $60 application fee, official high school and college transcripts, letters of recommendation from the undergraduate school's predental advisory committee, and the scores from the Dental Admissions Test.

Contact

Admissions Office
Harvard School of Dental Medicine
188 Longwood Avenue
Boston, Massachusetts 02115
(617) 432-1443

HOWARD UNIVERSITY COLLEGE OF DENTISTRY

Washington, D.C. 20059
(202) 797-4440

Accreditation	CDA
Degrees Offered	D.D.S., B.S./D.D.S.
# Students Applied	438
Enrollment	63 / class
Mean GPA	2.63
% Men / % Women	50% / 50%
% Minorities	Not Available
Tuition	$8,200
Application Fee	$25
Application Deadline	March 1

The University

Howard University was founded in 1867 as an educational institution for liberal arts and sciences. Today it is a major university complex operating from four campuses and comprising 18 schools and colleges. The 89-acre main campus is located within five minutes of downtown Washington, D.C. Howard University is accredited by the Middle States Association of Secondary Schools and Colleges.

The College of Dentistry was founded in 1881. It is the fifth oldest dental school in the country. The college is part of the university's Center for the Health Sciences, which also includes the colleges of medicine, pharmacy and pharmaceutical sciences, allied health sciences, nursing; Howard University Hospital; and the Health Sciences Library.

Admissions

Applicants are evaluated on the basis of their academic records, DAT scores, and recommendations from preprofessional advisers and teachers. It is preferred that the DAT be taken in the spring preceding the submission of their application. Mean DAT scores from the 1989 entering class are 14 and 13, for the academic and PAT sections of the test, respectively. The minimum course requirements for admission are two full years of credit from an accredited college or university, or 60 credits as evaluated by Howard University. The quality of courses taken and the individual performance of the student is an important factor in the evaluation process. The mean overall GPA of a recent class was 2.63; the mean science GPA for the same class was 2.54.

Undergraduate Preparation

The following coursework is required for admission: eight semester hours of inorganic chemistry, with lab; eight semester hours of organic chemistry, with lab; eight semester hours of physics; eight semester hours of general biology or zoology; six semester hours of English composition and literature; and 22 semester hours of liberal arts electives, preferably in languages, social sciences, humanities, and behavioral sciences.

Student Body

In a recent entering class of 63 students, 32 were women, 20 were foreigners, 39 were from out of state, and 35 had an undergraduate degree. The age range was from 21 to 39, with 35 being the mean age.

Costs

As of April 1991, tuition was $8,200 per year. The university fee is $250 per year and the student activity fee is $75 per year. Books and instruments cost almost $6,000 the first year, about $3,400 the second year, and $460 the third year. There is a health fee of approximately $300 per year.

Financial Aid

Priority in receiving financial aid is given to those demonstrating the greatest need. Some scholarships are given on the basis of academic achievement. Most students applying for financial aid will receive loans, grants, scholarships, or work-study employment, or a combination of these resources. University-administered programs include the Howard University

Trustee Tuition Scholarship program, the Health Professions Student Loan program, Supplemental Loans for Students, and the Health Education Assistance Loan program.

To apply for financial assistance, students must submit the college's financial aid application, the FAF, parents' and students' 1040 and W2 forms, the financial aid transcript form, and the selective service compliance form.

Student Organizations

The academic reinforcement program (ARP) helps train disadvantaged but competent dental students. Phase I is an intensive eight-week summer program that evaluates a participant's intellectual and practical potential for a career in dentistry, and introduces him or her to basic sciences and to all phases of the dental profession. Phase II grants continuing assistance throughout the matriculated dental student's education.

Faculty

The college has a faculty of more than 160.

Curriculum

The basic four-year program leads to the D.D.S. degree. Courses in the first two years include anatomy, histology, restorative dentistry, dental hygiene, community dentistry, oral dentistry, and prosthodontics. The last two years include clinical dentistry, oral surgery, endodontics, dental research, and a variety of other advanced courses.

Activities that enhance the student's clinical skills include extramural rotations, table clinics, and summer externships.

Facilities

The college has a modern, five-story building with classrooms, clinics, laboratories, offices, and research facilities. There is also a new learning resources area, which helps students keep abreast of local and national activities in the field of dentistry and provides access to dental information services.

The college developed the world's first convertible clinic-laboratories for teaching preclinical techniques and clinical skills. The college's central research facility hosts a histological laboratory, tissue culture area, operating room, and electron microscope laboratory. Community-based learning experiences are provided at the 500-bed Howard University Hospital as well as other health-care sites.

The Health Sciences Library houses 300,000 volumes and receives 4,000 current serial publications. It subscribes to 180 dental journals from all over the world. Dental students have access to the world's most complete collections of dental books in the National Library of Medicine, the National Institutes of Health Library, the Library of Congress, and other area libraries.

Grading Procedures

A letter grading system is used: A (90-100), B (80-89), C (70-79), F (below 70), I (incomplete) and W (withdraw).

Special Programs

The B.S./D.D.S. program is a special curriculum spanning the predental and dental curricula. The program allows students to complete the requirements for both the B.S. and D.D.S. degrees in six years instead of the traditional eight years.

The university also offers a two-year dental hygiene program and postgraduate programs in oral and maxillofacial surgery, orthodontics, pediatric dentistry, general practice residency, and advanced general dentistry.

Application Procedures

The college participates in AADSAS. Application materials are mailed to applicants after June 1. DAT scores and transcripts from each post-secondary institution attended should be submitted directly to AADSAS.

The application must be returned to AADSAS by March 1 of the year of anticipated enrollment. Three letters of recommendation are required from all applicants.

Contact

Howard University College of Dentistry
Office of Admissions
M. W. Johnson Administration Building
Room 110
Washington, D.C. 20059
(202) 806-2700

UNIVERSITY OF ILLINOIS AT CHICAGO, HEALTH SCIENCES CENTER, COLLEGE OF DENTISTRY

Chicago, Illinois 60680
(312) 996-1040

Accreditation	CDA
Degrees Offered	D.D.S., D.D.S./M.S.
# Students Applied	334
Enrollment	68 / class
Mean GPA	3.85
% Men / % Women	61% / 39%
% Minorities	13%
Tuition	$1,553 In-State
	$3,893 Out-of-State
Application Fee	$20
Application Deadline	April 1

The University

The College of Dentistry was established in 1898 and became part of the University of Illinois in 1913. Originally known as the Columbian Dental College, it is now one of several health care institutions affiliated with the university, including the College of Medicine, the College of Pharmacy, and the College of Nursing.

Admissions

The school's criteria for admission include the undergraduate school attended and the academic record of the applicant, as well as letters of recommendation, DAT scores, and the health of the applicant. The college encourages applications from minorities and from those with a particular desire to practice dentistry in rural areas.

Undergraduate Preparation

Candidates are expected to have completed a minimum of 60 semester hours (or 90 quarter hours) or undergraduate school in order to be considered for admission. Required undergraduate courses included 14 semester hours of chemistry, six semester hours each of biology, physics, and English. It is recommended that students take a variety of courses in social and behavioral sciences, business, humanities, and accounting. The minimum GPA considered for admission is 3.25.

Student Body

There were 68 students in the 1991-92 entering class. Most students are residents of the state of Illinois. The entering class of 1989-90 had a mean GPA of 3.85 and a mean science GPA of 3.61.

Costs

For the 1989-90 year, tuition was $1,553 for residents and $3,893 for nonresidents. There is a laboratory fee of $300 per year. The purchase of instruments is estimated to be about $3,500 for the first year and $2,800 for the second year. Books cost about $500 for the first year.

Financial Aid

About 60 percent of students receive scholarships and/or loans. A limited number of scholarships and nonrepayable grants are available to entering students. Guaranteed student loans are available.

Minority Programs

The college has a Minority Recruitment and Admissions Program which provides counseling on the preprofessional curriculum and assists students academically while in dental school. The office also assists with the application procedure and with financial assistance.

Curriculum

The four-year curriculum includes basic medical sciences, preclinical skills, behavioral sciences, and clinical experience. The basic sciences are taught within the first two years. Clinical practice begins in the second semester of the first year, and exposure to clinical skills training increases with each semester after that. The fourth year consists primarily of clinical experience. Attendance at summer clinics is recommended between the second and third and third and fourth years.

The main methods of instruction are lectures, seminars, laboratory work, and supervised clinical practice. Students must maintain a GPA of at least 3.0 in order to graduate.

Grading Procedures

The college uses a letter grading system for student evaluation, A, B, C, D, and F.

Special Programs

Students enrolling in the program without a baccalaureate degree may earn their degree while in dental school. The college also offers a joint D.D.S./M.S. degree.

Application Procedures

The college participates in AADSAS. These applications must be filed between July 1 and April 1 of the year preceding the year of intended enrollment. There is a $20 application fee. Applicants are notified of acceptance between December 1 and June 15. The college does not have an early decision plan. Accepted students must pay a $100 deposit to hold their place in the class; this deposit will be applied toward tuition.

Contact
> University of Illinois at Chicago
> Director of Admissions
> P.O. Box 6998
> Chicago, Illinois 60612
> (312) 996-7755

INDIANA UNIVERSITY SCHOOL OF DENTISTRY

1121 West Michigan Street
Indianapolis, Indiana 46202
(317) 274-7461

Accreditation	CDA
Degrees Offered	M.S.D., D.D.S., D.M.D.
# Students Applied	404
Enrollment	80 / class
Mean GPA	3.05
% Men / % Women	63% / 37%
% Minorities	4%
Tuition	$5,750 In-State
	$11,930 Out-of-State
Application Fee	$20
Application Deadline	April 1

The University

A four-year, public university for men and women, Indiana University attracts students from all 50 states and around the world. The school has 882 degree programs and 39 certificate programs. Founded in 1820 in Bloomington, it is one of the oldest and largest institutions of higher education in the midwest. Over 80,000 students are enrolled at the eight campuses at Gary, Fort Wayne, Kokomo, New Albany, Richmond, South Bend, Bloomington, and Indianapolis. The School of Dentistry is located on the campus of Indiana University-Purdue University at Indianapolis (IUPUI). The IU Medical Center is also located here. It contains the schools of medicine, nursing, several major hospitals, outpatient clinics, laboratories, libraries, and special research facilities. The study of dentistry dates back to 1879 at the Indiana Dental College, which became affiliated with Indiana University in 1925.

Admissions

Preference is given to Indiana residents and students whose overall and science GPA exceeds 3.0. Students should have an overall and science GPA of at least 2.5. All applicants must take the Dental Admission Test (DAT), as provided by the American Dental Association. Applicants are advised to complete the test no later than October preceding the year of enrollment. Of the 1989 entering class, mean DAT scores were 15.72 and 16.76 for the academic and PAT portions, respectively. The overall average GPA was 3.05; the average science GPA was 2.9.

Undergraduate Preparation

High school students should take courses in biology, chemistry, physics, mathematics, shop work, art, and a foreign language. Most accepted students have earned a baccalaureate degree, however, some exceptional students may be accepted into dental school after 90 college credit hours. The more diverse the background, the better. Students are encouraged to take courses in social sciences, humanities, and mathematics. All applicants must have taken one year (two semesters) of biology or zoology, inorganic chemistry, and physics, all with laboratory. One semester of organic chemistry with a laboratory is required. In addition, students must have taken one semester of introductory psychology, English composition, and interpersonal communication (or public speaking). Strongly recommended (but not required) are courses in genetics, solid art, business administration or personal finance, histology, biochemistry, medical terminology, anthropology, and human anatomy.

Student Body

Of the 80 students entering in 1990, 50 were men and 30 were women. Most of the undergraduates majored in biology or chemistry. The average age is 24. The majority of students hold baccalaureate degrees. Sixty-eight are residents, 12 are nonresidents.

Placement Records

Approximately 15 to 20 percent of the dental school's alumni are self employed (with or without a partner), 10 to 15 percent are employed by group practice (salary, commission, or percentage), 30 to 40 percent are employed in other types of practice, 15 to 20 percent pursue advanced dental education, and 15 to 20 percent enter government service.

Costs

The tuition for Indiana residents for the 1990-91 year was $5,750. Nonresidents paid $11,930. Microscope rental amounts to $50, and instruments cost about $2,100. The estimated cost of books is $825. The total estimated living expenses for 12 months is about $12,312.

Financial Aid

Several loans and scholarships are available to qualified candidates. Such scholarships include Robert J. Alber, Milo V. Smith Dental, Indiana University Dental Alumni Association, Louise Kutka Memorial, and Michael T. Wilson. Other sources of aid include the Stafford Loan, Health Professions Student Loan, Perkins Loan, and the IDA Student Loan.

Minority Programs

Educational and moral support is offered to Blacks, Hispanic Americans, American Indians, and Eskimos by the IU School of Dentistry office of minority students, which offers predental counseling, assistance in acquiring financial aid, supplemental services, and one-on-one support assistance.

Student Organizations

"Hoosier hospitality" is actively demonstrated through groups like the student affairs council. Student counselor systems have been created to support the school's faculty counselor program. Student representatives have a say in the meetings of the faculty council and its committees. Membership to the local chapter of the American Dental Students Association is open to IUSD students; the national dental honorary fraternity, Omicron Kappa Upsilon, also has a chapter on campus.

Faculty

Many faculty members have made scientific and scholarly contributions to the world's professional dental literature. Many full-time members keep a hand in clinical dentistry by maintaining private practices. There are over 660 teaching professionals.

Curriculum

The first three years encompass the core curriculum, when the basic and preclinical sciences are studied. Courses consist of oral diagnosis, biochemistry, operative dentistry, periodontics, human physiology, endodontics, oral surgery, complete denture lab and clinic, periodontics, and pharmacology. During the fourth year students are exposed to cardiopulmonary resuscitation, family practice program, and electives. The fifth year consists of 25 credits of continuation of the fourth-year program. An average of six students per year apply to the two-year operative dentistry program.

Facilities

The school is proud to be one of the first to establish a special care clinic where difficult patient cases are treated. The in-house library contains some 48,000 volumes and subscriptions to more than 640 journals. The IU dental library has a comprehensive collection of dental literature that dates back to the early 1800s. The library contains an on-line computer that searches for fast references, as well as state-of-the-art audiovisual materials and microcomputers and software for student use. The IUPUI campus has a new, multimillion dollar natatorium and track and field stadium. On-campus housing is available, but competitive.

Grading Procedures

The School of Dentistry utilizes a letter grading system (A, B, C, D, S, and F).

Special Programs

The Bloomington campus of Illinois University, along with several IU regional campuses, offers a combined degree program in biology and chemistry with three years of predental study and the first year of dental school to fulfill the undergraduate degree requirements (B.A. or B.S.). Besides the D.D.S. degree, IUSD offers five programs each in dental hygiene and dental assisting, and one in dental laboratory technology. Students are open to participate in the many investigations that are conducted by the Oral Health Research Institute.

Application Procedures

Applications should be sent a full year prior to the beginning of the academic year. However, the deadline for having a completed application on file is February 1. All students must include with their application a $20 application fee, a current photo, official transcripts from all colleges attended, official DAT scores, and three academic letters of recommendation.

Contact

Office of Records and Admissions
Indiana University School of Dentistry
1121 West Michigan Street
Indianapolis, Indiana 46202
(317) 274-7461

THE UNIVERSITY OF IOWA COLLEGE OF DENTISTRY

Iowa City, Iowa 52242
(319) 335-3500

Accreditation	CDA
Degrees Offered	D.D.S.
# Students Applied	314
Enrollment	68 / class
Mean GPA	2.5
% Men / % Women	63% / 37%
% Minorities	20%
Tuition	$4,264 In-State
	$11,994 Out-of-State
Application Fee	$20
Application Deadline	November 30

The University

The University of Iowa established a Department of Dentistry in 1882 with 14 students enrolled. In 1900, it became a college of The University of Iowa. Located in a community of 50,500, the full university campus consists of 1,900 acres. The Iowa River flows through the middle of the campus. Iowa City is a comfortable place to live, free of big city complications. Students may take advantage of the Center for the Arts, The Museum of Art, and movie theaters. Fishing, sailing, and hunting are also available.

Admissions

Preference is given to residents of Iowa who meet certain academic requirements. The college prefers students who have completed a standard baccalaureate degree or who are pursing a combined program in which they earn a baccalaureate while completing their freshman year in dentistry. Applicants should have at least a 2.5 GPA. Students must take the DAT. DEAP is available to qualified students. Foreign applicants have additional requirements and should inquire at the office of admissions.

Undergraduate Preparation

Students should have at least three academic years of accredited work totaling at least 94 semester hours. Specific course requirements include eight semester hours each (with lab) of physics, organic and inorganic chemistry, and biology. In addition, college credit in English composition is required.

The balance of coursework should reflect a well-rounded pursuit of knowledge through electives.

Student Body

The total university enrollment is about 24,000 undergraduates and 6,000 graduates. Students come from all 50 states and 94 foreign countries. The College of Dentistry enrollment is 288.

Costs

Resident tuition is $4,264; nonresident tuition is $11,994. First-year fees amount to $3,785, and books and supplies cost $370 per year. University family housing costs $161-$307 per month, and fraternity housing is $290 per month.

Financial Aid

Major sources of support include scholarships, loans, and research and teaching assistantships. Students are asked to look for their own resources first before applying for financial aid. Eligibility for aid is based on need as determined by the applicant's FAF. Students may receive Health Professions Loans, Perkins Loans, and Stafford Loans. Some short-term loans are available through the ADA, the Iowa Dental Association, and the Kellogg Foundation. Inquire at the Office of Student Aid, 208 Calvin Hall.

Minority Programs

Financial assistance and counseling services are available to minority students who qualify under the University of Iowa's EOP and the Opportunity at Iowa program. For further information write or call the College of Dentistry Academic Affairs Office.

Student Organizations

Student organizations include chapters of the AADA, AADR, AAWD, ASDC, and SNDA. Many students belong to the two dental fraternities on campus, Delta Sigma Delta or Psi Omega. Students at Iowa can participate in many intramural sports groups, including wrestling, basketball, and volleyball.

Faculty

The student/faculty ratio is 3:1, suggesting a faculty of about 100. Faculty include generalists and specialists in every discipline as well as many faculty who hold Ph.D.'s in disciplines other than dentistry.

Curriculum

The course of study lasts for four years. During of the first two years students take courses in the biomedical sciences, including anatomy, biochemistry, embryology, histology, microbiology, pathology, pharmacology, and physiology. Some pre-clinical technical courses are also taught. Students are introduced to clinical patient situations during the first year, and during the second year they treat patients in restorative and preventive dentistry. Third-year students rotate through clinical clerkships in eight disciplines. Seniors deliver comprehensive dental care.

Facilities

The College of Dentistry works closely with other area colleges in the health sciences center. The Dental Science Building houses one complete wing devoted to clinical teaching and facilities. The Hardin Library for the Health Services has more than 18,000 volumes on dental subjects and 283 dental journals.

Special Programs

Iowa's College of Dentistry is one of only two in the nation that offers graduate programs in all dental specialties. Residencies in advanced general dental education and in general practice are also available.

Application Procedures

Apply through AADSAS. Students may submit applications beginning June 1 of the year before the year for which entry is sought. At the same time, send directly to the UI Office of Admissions three letters of recommendation and transcripts from each institution attended. The deadline for AADSAS applications is November 30. After this, UI asks applicants to send a final application to the college and to schedule a personal interview. Students should submit DAT scores and plan to complete the DAT no later than the fall of the year before the year for which they seek admission. Notification of acceptance starts after December 1.

Contact

Office of Admissions
116 Calvin Hall
The University of Iowa
Iowa City, Iowa 52242
(319) 335-1521 or 1-800-553-IOWA

UNIVERSITY OF KENTUCKY COLLEGE OF DENTISTRY

Lexington, Kentucky 40536-0084
(606) 233-5786

Accreditation	ADA
Degrees Offered	D.M.D.
# Students Applied	Not Available
Enrollment	40 / class
Mean GPA	3.17
% Men / % Women	50% / 50%
% Minorities	Not Available
Tuition	$4,320 In-State
	$15,900 Out-of-State
Application Fee	None for residents, $10 for nonresidents
Application Deadline	April 1

The University

The College of Dentistry was activated in the fall of 1962 with 26 students. The University of Kentucky College of Dentistry is fully accredited by the ADA. Located in Lexington (pop. 230,000), the heart of the Bluegrass region of Kentucky, the college sits on 716 acres. Lexington is the major center for raising thoroughbred horses in the United States. It has a huge tobacco and bluegrass seed market. In the midst of a historic geography, the homes of Henry Clay ("Ashland") and Mary Todd Lincoln are notable attractions. The Daniel Boone National Forest and other sites for outdoor sports and recreation are within easy drives of the campus.

Admissions

The college prefers applicants with a GPA of 3.0 or better and a DAT of 15 or better. Graduates of an accredited college or university are given preference, but students with less than four years of undergraduate coursework will receive serious consideration. In addition, the admissions committee considers the applicant's quality of educational experience, record of academic improvement, knowledge of dentistry, interviews, letters of recommendation, and involvement in leadership activities.

Undergraduate Preparation

Although the College of Dentistry has no specific course requirements for admission, qualified students will usually have two semesters of English composition. In addition, they will have completed one year each (with lab) of general and organic chemistry, biology, and physics. Courses in algebra and calculus are highly recommended.

Student Body

The University fo Kentucky enrollment is about 23,000. The College of Dentistry admits 40 Kentucky residents in each entering class. There is no limit to nonresident enrollment; however, there were only six nonresidents accepted for the class of 1994. Twenty-three of the students were men, and 23 were women. The youngest was 19 and the oldest was 41. The GPA for 1994 was 3.17, and the DAT academic average was 14.89, and the science average was 13.87. The D.M.D. program has a total enrollment of 170 students. Seventeen colleges are represented in the entering class.

Costs

Resident tuition for 1990-91 was $4,320; nonresident tuition was $15,900. The average total cost of living, tuition, plus fees and supplies amounts to $16,310 for residents and $27,890 for nonresidents.

Financial Aid

Nine scholarships, six loan fund programs, a few fellowships, and college work-study programs are available on the basis of academic merit and/or financial need. For further information apply to the office of financial aid.

Faculty

The college has a full-time faculty of 66 with a student/faculty ratio in the D.M.D. program of 3:1.

Curriculum

The college offers a four-year D.M.D. program. The program is composed of a diagonal curriculum in which basic sciences and clinical courses are taught throughout the four years. Clinical coursework intensifies in the third and fourth years. "Hands-on" experience begins, however, with the first year and involves matching patients' needs with students' skill levels.

Facilities

The college includes the Dental Sciences Building, a wing of the A.B. Chandler Medical Center, and has two floors of clinical facilities, two floors for special clinics, and 120 operatories in the general clinical areas. There are 53 chairs for specialized dental care and teaching. Students have access to additional clinical and research experiences in the Warren Wright University Medical Plaza.

Special Programs

Seven advanced education programs are offered at the college: oral and maxillofacial surgery, orthodontics, periodontics, pediatric dentistry, and general practice residency, as well as fellowships in orofacial pain and geriatric dentistry.

Application Procedures

Apply through AADSAS. Applicants will not receive packages before June 1, but apply early. The admissions committee will invite qualified students for an interview who have satisfactorily completed and submitted the AADSAS application.

Contact

Office of Student Affairs
College of Dentistry
University of Kentucky
D-155 Chandler Medical Center
Lexington, Kentucky 40536-0084
(606) 233-6071

LOMA LINDA UNIVERSITY SCHOOL OF DENTISTRY

Loma Linda, California 92350
(714) 824-4683

Accreditation	CDA
Degrees Offered	D.D.S., B.S., M.S.
# Students Applied	426
Enrollment	78 / class
Mean GPA	3.1
% Men / % Women	69% / 31%
% Minorities	48%
Tuition	$15,669
Application Fee	$25
Application Deadline	February 1

The University

Loma Linda University was founded in 1905 by Seventh-day Adventist church leaders. Its motto is "Make Man Whole." The School of Dentistry was opened in 1953 and is located about 60 miles east of Los Angeles. Loma Linda University School of Dentistry is nestled in a valley facing the San Bernadino Mountain Range to the north and east. Loma Linda itself has small-town appeal, with the cultural attractions of large cities like Los Angeles nearby. The desert, beaches, mountains, snow ski resorts, and Disneyland can be reached by car or bus within an hour.

Admissions

Preference is given to students who have taken the DAT no later than October of the academic year before the desired year of entry. Students will have completed a baccalaureate degree before entrance. However, a B.S. in human biology may be obtained concurrently with a D.D.S., if a broad base of general education coursework is completed before entrance.

Undergraduate Preparation

A minimum of 96 semester hours or 144 quarter units of coursework from an accredited college is required. Applicants must have a "superior" GPA, with particular strength in predental coursework. Courses should include one year each (with lab) of biology/zoology, general and organic chemistry, and physics. One year of English composition and literature are also required.

Student Body

The enrollment at Loma Linda University is 4,000. The School of Dentistry accepts about 70 students into the dental program and 35 students into the dental hygiene program, suggesting a student body of about 420.

Placement Records

Each year, the School of Dentistry has more opportunities than their dental graduates can fill—students can practice, enter partnerships, or become associates in an established practice. About half of the graduating students do work in other countries, including Mexico, Bangladesh, Malawi and others. The School of Dentistry is the main source for candidates to staff Seventh-day Adventist mission dental clinics all over the world. About 60 to 75 percent of these clinicians come from LLU School of Dentistry.

Costs

Tuition for residents and nonresidents is $15,669.

Financial Aid

Loma Linda offers financial aid to eligible students with documented needs.

Faculty

Faculty members number well over 1,800 from all relevant fields and disciplines, suggesting an overall student/faculty ratio of about 3:1.

Curriculum

The program lasts for four years. Students begin with classes in the basic and clinical sciences and then begin treating patients in the clinic.

Special Programs

The School of Dentistry offers an 18-month curriculum for the D.D.S. for graduates of dental schools outside the United States. Students may obtain the B.S. in dental hygiene. Graduate study leading to a certificate and/or M.S. degree is offered in the following clinical areas: endodontics, orthodontics, periodontics, oral and maxillofacial surgery.

Application Procedures

Apply through AADSAS before February 1. After a review, applicants submit a supplementary application, DAT scores, transcripts, and recommendations. A personal interview may follow. Applications are accepted from June 1 to February 1. The first letters of acceptance are mailed December 1.

Contact

School of Dentistry
Loma Linda University
Loma Linda, California 92350
(714) 824-4621 or (800) 422-4558

LOUISIANA STATE UNIVERSITY SCHOOL OF DENTISTRY

1100 Florida Avenue
New Orleans, Louisiana 70119
(504) 948-5400

Accreditation	CDA
Degrees Offered	D.D.S.
# Students Applied	127
Enrollment	53 / class
Mean GPA	3.06
% Men / % Women	63% / 37%
% Minorities	11%
Tuition	$3,647 In-State
	$8,247 Out-of-State
Application Fee	$30
Application Deadline	March 31

The University

Louisiana State University School of Dentistry is a state-supported institution that provides oral health care services, research, and education for the people of Louisiana. The school enrolled its first class in 1968 and built a $16-million complex of buildings in 1972. It is part of the LSU Medical Center.

Admissions

The main factors considered in the admissions process are academic records, DAT scores, preprofessional faculty recommendations, and the personal interview. The school seeks evidence that students can successfully complete the dental program. Residents of Louisiana and Arkansas are given preference in the admissions process.

Undergraduate Preparation

Applicants should have a minimum of three years (90 semester hours) of preprofessional college education. Required courses are eight hours of inorganic chemistry, eight hours of organic chemistry, eight hours of physics, 12 hours of biology, and nine hours of English. The school recommends that students take additional courses in the biological sciences, such as histology and anatomy, as well as psychology, sociology, and art courses such as sculpture that develop the student's manual skills.

The mean GPA of the 1989-90 entering class was 3.06. The mean science GPA was 2.96. The mean DAT score (academic) was 16. The mean DAT (PAT) score was 15.8.

Student Body

The 1989-90 entering class was comprised of 53 students. Twenty were women, four were black, and two were Hispanic. Most students were residents of Louisiana. The mean age of the student body was 21 years old.

Costs

For 1990-91, resident tuition was $3,647. Nonresidents paid $8,247 per year. Instrument purchase/rental is about $3,600 for the first year (these costs decrease for the subsequent years of dental school). Hospital insurance costs $450 per year, and books cost about $1,300 for the first two years.

Financial Aid

Students who are Louisiana residents may be eligible for assistance from the Louisiana State Guaranteed Loan Fund (maximum amount of loan, $5,000). A limited amount of scholarship and loan funds are available from dental organizations and private sources. The LSU Medical Center has an office of financial aid that assists students obtain funds.

Curriculum

The major goal of the curriculum is to educate practitioners to be highly skilled in diagnosis and to perform advanced dental procedures. Students are also thoroughly educated in the biological sciences, behavioral sciences, and practice management. Students have the option of pursuing careers as specialists, or in research or teaching.

The program consists of basic sciences combined with clinical skills and courses in behavioral science. Students are introduced to clinical experience early in the program. The basic science component is integrated into the clinical component. Total patient care is the major focus of the clinical part of the program. In addition to delivering patient care, the student will also supervise a team of other students in the clinical setting.

Special Programs

Students can earn a baccalaureate degree while in the dental program. Arrangements must be made with the student's undergraduate college.

Application Procedures

The school participates in AADSAS. Applications must be filed with AADSAS between July 15 and March 31 for entry the following fall. The school does not have an early decision plan. There is a $30 application fee. Students are notified of acceptance between December 1 and June 15. Upon acceptance, students must pay a nonrefundable $200 deposit, which is applied toward tuition.

Contact

Louisiana State University
School of Dentistry
Admissions Committee
1100 Florida Avenue
New Orleans, Louisiana 70119
(504) 948-8947

UNIVERSITY OF LOUISVILLE SCHOOL OF DENTISTRY

Louisville, Kentucky 40292
(502) 588-5295

Accreditation	ADA, AADS
Degrees Offered	D.M.D., B.S./D.M.D.
# Students Applied	308
Enrollment	61 / class
Mean GPA	3.03
% Men / % Women	74% / 26%
% Minorities	5%
Tuition	$4,110 In-State
	$15,798 Out-of-State
Application Fee	$10
Application Deadline	April 1

The University

The University of Louisville is located in Louisville, Kentucky, a metropolitan area 15 minutes from a major airport and accessible via many major interstate highways. The School of Dentistry, founded in 1887, is located on the University of Louisville Health Sciences campus, close to downtown Louisville, sharing a 12-block area with many health facilities.

Admissions

The committee on admissions selects students using a numerical admissions index, 60 percent of which is based on academic factors such as undergraduate GPA and DAT scores, and 40 percent of which is based on personal factors such as recommendations and other factors determined by a personal interview. Applicants are considered on their own merits without prejudice regarding race, religion, sex, age, handicap, color, or national origin. Nontraditional students with experiences outside the usual predental experiences are evaluated on an individual basis.

Undergraduate Preparation

Although most students enter the School of Dentistry with a baccalaureate degree, students who have earned 60 or more credits of undergraduate study will be considered. Prospective dental students should complete at least one year each of biology, inorganic chemistry, organic chemistry, and physics. Courses in business, mathematics, and communication skills are also considered advantageous.

Costs

Annual tuition totals $4,110 for Kentucky residents and $15,798 for nonresidents. Four-year lab and classroom expenses, including books and instruments, total about $6,865.

Financial Aid

The School of Dentistry participates in the Stafford, HPL SLS, LEAL, NHSC, EFN, and FADHPS loan programs. The school also offers work-study programs, summer research assistantships, minority scholarships, and scholarships through the university and alumni. Funds are limited and based on the principle that the primary responsibility for meeting educational cost rests with the student and family.

Minority Programs

The American Fund for Dental Health Scholarships for Minority Students offers aid to needy minority students.

Student Organizations

The School of Dentistry offers chapters of the American Association of Dental Schools and the American Student Dental Association. Other student organizations include the Christian Medical and Dental Society, International Association for Dental Research, Student Senate, and three professional fraternities.

Faculty

The School of Dentistry staffs 104 full-time and 50 part-time faculty and lecturers.

Curriculum

Basic science and pre-clinical courses comprise most of the first two years of study; the final two years focus on patient treatment. Requirements also include practice management courses and an externship in a private practice setting. Fourth-year students may enroll in the Senior General Practice Clinical Program.

Facilities

The School of Dentistry occupies almost 200,000 square feet of space at the Health Sciences campus. Clinical areas are divided into individual cubicles; laboratories are "multidisciplinary units" with high and low benches. The campus is also situated amongst a wide array of health facilities, including the Humana Hospital University, J. Graham Brown Cancer Center, Norton Hospital, Kosair Children's Hospital, Kentucky Lions Eye Research Institute, Louisville and Jefferson County Board of Health, and many other health institutions. The Kornhauser Health Sciences Library is shared by all components of the campus and houses 175,000 volumes.

Grading Procedures

All courses are letter graded, except for some preclinical and clinical courses at the course directors' discretion.

Special Programs

The School of Dentistry offers a summer research program for 20 to 30 dental students annually; these students may present their research at state, regional and national meetings, and summer research often leads to rewarding post-graduate training opportunities. The Accelerated Studies program offers exceptionally-qualified students the opportunity to complete their studies in less than four years, while the Decelerated Studies program allows part-time students to complete the first two years of study in three years. Exceptionally-qualified students may also take part in the Senior Honors program, departmental honors, or Senior Selectives Series. The School of Dentistry also offers a joint B.S./D.M.D. and an early acceptance program for high school seniors (Inside Track).

Application Procedures

Students must apply through AADSAS. The deadline for applications is April 1. Notification begins on December 1, and applicants are strongly urged to take the DAT in October of the year preceding entry into dental school. The committee on admissions requires letters of recommendation and a personal interview.

Contact

School of Dentistry
Health Sciences Center
University of Louisville
Louisville, Kentucky 40292
(502) 588-5081
(800) 334-8635

LOYOLA UNIVERSITY OF CHICAGO SCHOOL OF DENTISTRY

820 North Michigan Avenue
Maywood, Illinois 60153
(708) 216-3500

Accreditation	CDA
Degrees Offered	D.D.S.
# Students Applied	841
Enrollment	94 / class
Mean GPA	2.7
% Men / % Women	63% / 28%
% Minorities	32%
Tuition	$14,100
Application Fee	$30
Application Deadline	March 31

The University

The Loyola University School of Dentistry was founded on February 20, 1883, as the Chicago Dental Infirmary. In 1923, it was incorporated as part of Loyola University, a Catholic University in the Jesuit tradition. Under the leadership of Drs. Brophy, Logan, and Johnson, a Class A rating was attained for the dental school from the Dental Education Council of America. They established the Foundation for Dental Research in 1935, which today is the Brophy-Johnson-Logan Research Fund. The school was located at Wood and Harrison Streets in Chicago until 1969, when it moved to its present location in Maywood.

Admissions

The DAT is required for admission. Preference is given to applicants who have completed the Bachelor's degree. The admissions committee of the dental school admits students on the basis of previous academic records, the results of the ADA Dental Admissions Test, personal character, work experience, extracurricular activities, and knowledge of the dental profession. Transfer applications are not encouraged, as the difference between schools may make direct transfers difficult. However, individual requests for transfer are judged on their own merits.

Undergraduate Preparation

A minimum of three years of credit (90 semester hours) at a recognized college of liberal arts and sciences is required for admission. Preference is given to students who have a Bachelor's degree. The following coursework (including necessary laboratory work) is required: English, six semester hours; inorganic chemistry, eight semester hours; organic chemistry, four semester hours; biology or zoology, 16 semester hours; physics, eight semester hours.

Strong consideration is given to applicants who have a year of credit in organic chemistry.

It is recommended that students receive extra instruction in the biological sciences as well as advanced courses in the humanities and social and political sciences.

Student Body

More than half of the students enrolled in the dental school are residents of Illinois. More than a quarter are female.

Costs

Tuition is $14,100 per year and may be paid in three trimester installments. Student fees are $200. Books, instruments, and dental supplies (per year) amount to the following: freshman, $5,135; sophomore, $3,225; junior, $335; and senior, $10.

Financial Aid

Several financial aid programs are available through the university, including the Loyola Dental Alumni Centennial Fund, the Robert Wood Johnson Foundation Dental Student Aid Program (which provides loan awards to students from groups underrepresented in the health professions), The Loyola University of Chicago Parent/Student Loan, and need-based grants. Part-time jobs and a college work-study program are available. Financial aid is also available from other federal, state, and private offices. For information, contact the Medical Center Financial Aid Office (Building 124-W).

Minority Programs

Minority need-based grants are available. For further information, contact the office of admissions.

Student Organizations

Student organizations of special interest to dental students include the American Dental Association, American Student Dental Association, the American Association of Dental Schools, and the Student Congress, which is composed of representatives elected by each class in the School of Dentistry and a faculty moderator.

Faculty

Faculty members combine their practice and research with their work in teaching.

Curriculum

The dental school curriculum is based on the trimester system. Each 14-week trimester consists of six instructional weeks, followed by one week of exams, then six more instructional weeks followed by one week of final exams. The curriculum is continually reviewed by the curriculum committee, and suggestions from the Student Congress are given consideration.

The first year consists of the basic sciences and pre-clinical training. The second year includes basic sciences, a review of pre-clinical dentistry and clinic orientation. The third year includes clinical courses and lecture on jurisprudence and ethics. The senior year includes a review of clinical dentistry, a northeast regional board review, departmental clinical conferences, grand clinical conferences, and electives. During the last few years, the dental school has started a program of student research. Qualified students are encouraged to pursue original research under faculty direction.

Certain well-qualified students are selected for an honors program.

Facilities

In the School of Dentistry, there are 270 patient positions. Clinical areas are modular in concept and open in design. Each student operatory is a cubicle simulating a modern private office. In the freshman-sophomore teaching laboratories, necessary equipment and a separate work area are provided for thorough instruction.

The University Hospital supports a fully-equipped Department of Dentistry. All hospital dental staff are faculty of the dental school. The operating rooms are equipped for general dentistry and dental surgical specialties. The hospital also supports a dental clinic.

The Medical Center Library contains over 119,000 bound volumes of books and periodicals and maintains 1,909 subscriptions.

Grading Procedures

Letter grades are given. Students progressing satisfactorily are recommended for promotion to the next trimester by the promotion committee. In order to be eligible to take either Part I or Part II of the National Board Examination, a student must have passing grades in all subjects included in the exam.

Application Procedures

The school participates in the American Association of Dental Schools Application Service (AADSAS). Applications may be filed on or after June 1 of the year before entering. Applications must be received by March 31 of each year. An application fee of $20 is charged to each applicant after the preliminary review of the formal application.

Contact

Office of Admissions—School of Dentistry
Loyola University Medical Center
2160 South First Avenue
Maywood, Illinois 60153
(708) 216-3500

MARQUETTE UNIVERSITY SCHOOL OF DENTISTRY

604 North 16th Street
Milwaukee, Wisconsin 53233
(414) 228-3532

Accreditation	CDA
Degrees Offered	D.D.S., M.S., B.S./D.D.S., D.D.S./M.S., M.S.
# Students Applied	753
Enrollment	64 / class
Mean GPA	2.74
% Men / % Women	72% / 28%
% Minorities	50%
Tuition	$19,310
Application Fee	$25
Application Deadline	April 1

The University

The School of Dentistry, an independent, coeducational dental college, was established in 1907. It was created when Milwaukee Medical College and Marquette College joined to form Marquette University. Located in Milwaukee, Wisconsin (population 640,000), Marquette University School of Dentistry is not far from commerce and culture. The School of Dentistry is among the largest U.S. dental colleges.

Admissions

Applicants must have at least three years of college prior to entrance into the D.D.S. program. Students are selected on the basis of grades and DAT scores. The admissions committee also considers trend in academic performance, desire to succeed, honesty, and potential for the field of dentistry. Of the 753 students who applied for admission to the 1989-90 entering class, 64 are enrolled. These students had a mean academic DAT score of 14.71. Their mean PAT score was 15.78. Their mean total GPA was 2.74, while their mean science GPA was 2.56.

Undergraduate Preparation

Students are required to take eight semester hours each in inorganic chemistry, organic chemistry, biology (zoology and a course in comparative anatomy are preferred)—all with lab— and six semester hours of English. A course in quantitative and qualitative analysis may be accepted for one course in general inorganic chemistry. Students should also consider taking courses in biological sciences, mathematics, English composition and literature, speech, history, philosophy, sociology, political science, economics, accounting, personal finance, and psychology.

Student Body

Of the 64 students enrolled during the 1989-90 school year, there were 18 women, two American Indians, two Blacks, six Asians or Pacific Islanders, and 24 Hispanics. Ages ranged from 21 to 39, with a mean age of 24. Half had earned bachelor's degrees. Thirty-nine came from out of state.

Costs

Tuition for the year totals $19,310. During the first year instruments cost $4,400, books $575, and lab gowns $50. Other first year expenses total approximately $5,025. In all, freshmen can expect to pay about $24,335; $87,110 over the four-year period.

Financial Aid

Grants and scholarships are available. Students may apply for loans such as the Guaranteed Student Loan/Federally Insured Student Loan, the Health Professions Loan, and the Federal Health Education Assistance Loan. Ten $5,000 and 43 $3,000 scholarships and grants are awarded each year by the college. Comparable amounts are distributed to sophomores and juniors who demonstrate academic excellence and ability to motivate others through the Schweiger Fund. The student employment service is responsible for placing students in the work/study program.

Minority Programs

The minority affairs office coordinates recruitment, addresses minority concerns, and offers a pre-enrollment summer program and academic and support services. An American Indian office handles programs and services specifically for this group of students. The Robert Wood Johnson loan fund allows minority students to borrow up to $2,000 per year. Marquette's Multi-Cultural Center provides a social and educational base for minority interaction.

Student Organizations

Student organizations include the ASDA, two honor societies, and three professional fraternities, in addition to the student council. Project Outreach offers oral hygiene counseling to area children.

Faculty

The School of Dentistry staffs 64 full-time and 224 adjunct faculty members.

Curriculum

The D.D.S. program takes four years, including two seven-week summer sessions, to complete. The freshman and sophomore years focus on basic sciences. Students begin participating in the clinical part of the program as freshmen and may choose to participate in a number of hospital and community experiences as seniors.

Facilities

The learning resource center has eight carrels with videocassettes and slide-tape sets along with other audiovisual materials. The science library holds more than 170,000 volumes.

Grading Procedures

Students receive grades based on classroom performance and examinations. Courses are graded A, AB, B, BC, C, CD, and F; some are graded S (satisfactory) or U (unsatisfactory).

Special Programs

Students may earn a bachelor's degree while in dental school as part of a program sponsored by Marquette University College of Liberal Arts and Mount Mary College. A D.D.S./M.S. program is also available. A five-year preclinical program is offered to special students by the admissions committee and the dean.

Application Procedures

Students should apply through AADSAS by April 1. After that date, application should be made directly to Marquette College. A $25 application fee is to be sent with the application. Acceptance notification may be expected between December 1 and August 1. Interviews are not required and are conducted only at the request of the admissions committee.

Contact

Director of Admissions
School of Dentistry
Marquette University
604 North 16th Street
Milwaukee, Wisconsin 53233
(414) 228-3532 or (800) 445-5385

UNIVERSITY OF MARYLAND AT BALTIMORE DENTAL SCHOOL BALTIMORE COLLEGE OF DENTAL SURGERY

666 W. Baltimore Street
Baltimore, Maryland 21201-1586
(301) 328-7460

Accreditation	CDA
Degrees Offered	D.D.S., Ph.D., D.D.S./Ph.D., B.S., M.S., B.S./D.D.S.
# Students Applied	677
Enrollment	95 / class
Mean GPA	3.05
% Men / % Women	62% / 38%
% Minorities	26%
Tuition	$6,778 In-State
	$15,550 Out-of-State
Application Fee	$25
Application Deadline	March 1

The University

The Baltimore College of Dental Surgery, Dental School at the University of Maryland at Baltimore was founded in 1840 as the first dental college in the world. The school is located on a 32-acre campus in downtown Baltimore, along with five professional schools, an interprofessional graduate school, and a major medical center. Since 1983, the Dental School has boasted the Center for the Study of Human Performance in Dentistry, which studies such subjects as the positioning of dentist and patient relative to each other for most efficient care. The complex is unique in the Western Hemisphere and is a World Health Organization (WHO) Collaborating Center. Baltimore residents find the Dental School a convenient source of dental care. The Maryland Science Center, National Aquarium, and many other cultural and recreational facilities are available to students.

Admissions

Admission to the Dental School is based on academic performance, the quality of previous academic programs, letters of recommendation, extracurricular activities, and a personal interview. Applicants must also score 15 or higher in the Academic Average and Perceptual Ability sections of the Dental Admissions Test (DAT), which is regarded as a complement to the application rather than a separate criteria. Science and cumulative GPAs should be at least 2.5 for Maryland residents and at least 2.8 for nonresidents.

Undergraduate Preparation

Applicants must have completed at least 90 semester hours of credit, including a year of general biology with lab and inorganic chemistry with lab. A maximum of 60 semester hours will be accepted from a junior college.

Student Body

Three hundred sixty-nine students were enrolled in the dental program in 1989-90, which was comprised of 26 percent minority and 38 percent female students. Their mean science GPA was 2.91 and mean cumulative GPA was 3.05.

Placement Records

About 80 percent of dentists practicing in the state were trained at the Baltimore Dental School.

Costs

Annual tuition is $6,778 for Maryland residents and $15,550 for nonresidents. Additional costs for fees, food, lodging, and personal expenses bring the yearly total to $13,000 for state residents and $21,500 for nonresidents.

Financial Aid

Students desiring financial aid should apply annually in January for the following year. Aid comes in the form of loans, grants, scholarships, and work-study programs. University grants are available to Maryland residents who demonstrate financial need. Awards include Dean's scholarships, desegregation grants, other race grants, and tuition waivers.

Student Organizations

Honor societies include The Gamma Pi Delta Prosthodontic Honorary Society, The Gorgas Odontological Honorary Society, and The Phi Chapter of Omicron Kappa Upsilon. Dental fraternity chapters include Alpha Omega and Psi Omega.

Faculty

Over 250 faculty members teach at the Dental School, including practitioners who teach part-time.

Curriculum

The first three years of study consist of both lecture courses and clinical instruction. The fourth year concentrates on clinical work. The course Conjoint Sciences runs through all four years and presents certain subjects in a multidisciplinary manner. Students learn clinical skills by participating in one of eight available practice group clinics, each consisting of two dozen students, including sophomores, juniors, seniors and dental hygiene students. Courses include biochemistry, anatomy, microbiology, physiology, oral and maxillofacial surgery, dental anatomy/occlusion, operative dentistry, oral health care delivery, periodontics, biomedicine, pediatric dentistry, pharmacology, endodontics, fixed prosthodontics, orthodontics, removable prosthodontics, and oral medicine and diagnostic sciences. A candidate graduates upon satisfying all departmental requirements, passing all fourth-year courses, and achieving a minimum GPA of 2.0 during the fourth year.

Facilities

In 1990 all clinical facilities were renovated to provide the most up-to-date health care environment possible. The Health Sciences Library, ranked in size among the top 15 libraries of its kind in the U.S., serves as the regional medical library for 10 states and the District of Columbia. The library is part of the biomedical information network of the National Library of Medicine and houses 290,000 volumes, including 3,100 current journals. A wide range of automated databases are also available. Microcomputers and an IBM 4341 mainframe are available for faculty, staff, and student use through Computing/Health Informatics (CHI).

Grading Procedures

Courses are graded on an A through F letter scale.

Special Programs

Those interested in careers in academic dentistry may pursue a combined D.D.S./Ph.D. in physiology. The dental school offers baccalaureate and master's degree programs in dental hygiene as well as master's and doctoral degree programs in anatomy, biochemistry, microbiology, oral pathology, and physiology. Advanced dental education programs include the specialties of endodontics, oral and maxillofacial surgery, orthodontics, pediatric dentistry, periodontics, and prosthodontics. School- and hospital-based residency programs are also available. Graduates of the Honors Program offered by the University of Maryland Eastern Shore will be admitted to the corresponding professional school on the Baltimore campus. The University of Maryland College Park, University of Maryland Baltimore County, Bowie State College, Coppin State College, Morgan State University, and Salisbury State College offer a combined B.S./D.D.S. curriculum in which undergraduate requirements are met in three years before dental school studies are begun. Preprofessional, biology, or chemistry majors are eligible during January of any college year to experience a two-week minimester internship. Participants take the one-credit course Introduction to Fundamentals in Microbiology and observe delivery of dental care. A similar program geared towards exposing undergraduates to a dental career is Operation Dental Career held during the first week in June.

Application Procedures

Applications are processed through the American Association of Dental Schools Application Service (AADSAS) and must be filed by March 1. Applicants are urged to file early and take the DAT no later than October of the year preceding matriculation. Letters of recommendation must be written by either a preprofessional or predental committee, or, in the absence of such a committee, by one biology professor and one chemistry professor. Only applicants who are seriously being considered will be interviewed. Upon accepting an offer of admission, an applicant must pay a $200 fee. Intent to matriculate is confirmed by a $100 fee before June 1.

Contact

Baltimore College of Dental Surgery, Dental School
University of Maryland at Baltimore
Office of Admissions and Recruitment
666 W. Baltimore Street
Baltimore, Maryland 21201-1586
(301) 328-7472

MEDICAL COLLEGE OF GEORGIA SCHOOL OF DENTISTRY

Augusta, Georgia 30912-7300
(404) 721-2117

Accreditation	ADA
Degrees Offered	D.M.D., M.S./D.M.D.
# Students Applied	176
Enrollment	53 / class
Mean GPA	3.25
% Men / % Women	65% / 35%
% Minorities	9%
Tuition	$3,942 In-State
	$7,884 Out-of-State
Application Fee	None
Application Deadline	November 1

The University

The Medical College of Georgia was created in 1828. A state institution, it is among the oldest colleges in the nation. The School of Dentistry was founded in 1965. The school is strongly committed to excellence in education and has made substantial contributions to the field of dental research. The school offers a four-year D.M.D. program and has extensive, modern facilities for study.

The college is located in Augusta, Georgia, a main regional center hosting industry, banking, the arts, and other cultural and recreational attractions. Beaches and mountains are both nearby.

Admissions

High grades and DAT scores give an indication of how well the student will perform in the rigorous dental curriculum. The pattern of grades and proficiency in science courses are important factors in the admissions decision. A range of other factors are considered as well. These include letters of recommendation, results of interviews, motivation, and perceived ability to successfully deal with patients. The school admits 50 students per year and gives preference to residents of Georgia. Only applicants to the freshman class are considered.

In the past, the average accepted student had a 16.1 score on the academic portion of the DAT and a 16.5 on the PAT portion of the DAT. The average student's GPA is 3.25.

Undergraduate Preparation

Candidates must have at least 90 quarter hours (60 semester hours) of undergraduate coursework at an accredited institution. The required preprofessional courses include a minimum of ten quarter hours (or two semesters) of each of the following: inorganic chemistry (with lab); organic chemistry (with lab); biology (with lab); physics (with lab); and English. The undergraduate science course sequences should be those intended for science majors. A minimum grade of C must be attained in all required courses; most successful applicants will have grades of A or B in the required courses. All candidates for admission must take the DAT.

Student Body

The majority of students entering the school possess the baccalaureate degree. In recent years, the entering classes at the school have averaged over 35 percent women. The student body comprises about nine percent minorities.

Placement Records

Since the founding of the school, 96 percent of all enrolled students have graduated. Most dentists eventually establish a private practice, and it is estimated that there will be a great need for dentists in Georgia in the coming years. Currently, the ratio of dentists to the general population of Georgia is 45.8 dentists per 100,000 citizens.

Costs

Georgia residents pay $3,942 for tuition in the first and fourth years. The second and third years cost approximately $4,500 each. Nonresident tuition is $2,628 per quarter ($7,884 per year) plus the matriculation fee of $3,942 for a three-quarter year. Student health and activity fees are approximately $200 to $300 per year. Books and supplies cost $650 the first year, but these expenses decrease over the remaining years. Instruments and equipment cost $5,000 the first year.

Financial Aid

About 75 percent of the School of Dentistry students receive some form of financial aid, from scholarships and grants to loans and employment opportunities. Numerous institutional loan funds have been established by individuals and associations. Federal loan funds are also available. Most financial aid is need based, although some institutional awards are based on academic merit.

To apply, students must submit the FAF in addition to a supplemental form from the Medical College of Georgia. The supplemental form must be submitted to the college by February 15.

Faculty

The school has 85 full-time faculty. All members of the basic sciences faculty are dentists. The student/faculty ratio is 1:2.35.

Curriculum

The four-year curriculum is divided into 14 quarters. Classroom, laboratory, and clinical experiences are included in the program, with the bulk of patient care experience in the fourth year. The school stresses the relationship of the basic sciences to the clinical practice of dentistry.

While basic sciences and clinical sciences make up most of the first year, students also have their first exposure to clinical practice in this year. Throughout the curriculum, students are taught to examine the health needs of the society and are exposed to courses on public health dentistry, epidemiology of caries and periodontal disease, dental ethics, behavioral aspects of patient care, and other pertinent issues. Students have field experience in the community and are exposed to working with a health team—assistants, technicians, hygienists, and others.

Electives are available each year for the student to pursue an area of special interest. Students are encouraged to participate in research.

Facilities

The school's facilities were completed in 1972 and have since been modernized. The school building has 110,000 square feet of space and houses classrooms, labs, clinics, and offices. There are 240 patient care areas. Students also participate in patient care activities at ambulatory dental facilities in remote areas. On-campus housing is available.

Special Programs

The school offers a joint master of science in oral biology/ D.M.D. degree. To be eligible for the program, students must be enrolled in the School of Dentistry and must be in good academic standing. Candidates fulfill the requirements of both degrees and have the opportunity to conduct research in oral biology.

Application Procedures

Application is made directly to the school. The deadline for submission of applications is November 1 of the year preceding the year of enrollment. The school asks applicants to submit letters of recommendation and to attach a photo to their application. There is no application fee. Applicants may be invited for interviews.

Contact

Office of Student Affairs
Medical College of Georgia
Augusta, Georgia 30912-7300
(404) 721-3186

MEDICAL UNIVERSITY OF SOUTH CAROLINA COLLEGE OF DENTAL MEDICINE

171 Ashley Avenue
Charleston, South Carolina 29425
(803) 792-3811

Accreditation	CDE, ADA
Degrees Offered	D.M.D.
# Students Applied	310
Enrollment	46 / class
Mean GPA	2.91
% Men / % Women	65% / 35%
% Minorities	27%
Tuition	$3,500 In-State
	$9,800 Out-of-State
Application Fee	$25
Application Deadline	December 30

The University

The Medical University of South Carolina, founded in 1824 by the Medical Society of South Carolina, is the oldest medical institution in the southern United States. MUSC has informal agreements with all accredited institutions of higher learning in South Carolina on undergraduate preparation for health careers.

The College of Dental Medicine admitted its first students in 1967. In 1970, the college opened the Basic Sciences/

College of Dental Medicine building, with one-half of the building devoted to teaching facilities for dental medicine.

Admissions

Preference is given to residents of South Carolina, although out-of-state applicants with superior credentials will be considered. Applicants not presently living in South Carolina, but who believe they have adequate reason to claim South Carolina residency should write to the university registrar and director of admissions. The admissions committee evaluates an applicant's GPA and DAT scores to judge an applicant's intellectual abilities, and uses letters of recommendation and personal interviews to evaluate an applicant's personal characteristics. Selection is based on the applicant's total attributes.

Undergraduate Preparation

A minimum of three years of college work (90 semester hours) are required for admission. Preference is given to applicants who have completed a bachelor's degree. At least eight semester hours (including two semester hours of laboratory work) each of organic chemistry, inorganic chemistry, physics, biology (or zoology), and science electives (microbiology, biochemistry, comparative anatomy, genetics, etc.) are required. The biology/zoology requirement may be satisfied by taking four semester hours each of zoology and botany, but not by botany alone. At least six semester hours of English composition and mathematics are required. Suggested electives include three to six hours of advanced zoology, psychology, advanced mathematics, and advanced chemistry. The college also encourages students to study six additional semester hours of both English and history.

Student Body

Among the 46 dental students who entered MUSC-CDM in 1989, 16 were women, all but 16 were state residents, and 32 had bachelor's degrees. The mean DAT scores (both academic and PAT) were 15; the mean overall GPA was 2.91 and the mean science GPA was 2.82.

Costs

Tuition charges are subject to change. Tuition costs, per year, including Maymester and two summer sessions, amount to $3,500 for residents and $9,800 for nonresidents. Additional fees amount to approximately $520. All books, instruments, and supplies must be obtained through the university's student stores. All items must be purchased new, and no substitutions are allowed. The cost for instruments, supplies, and lab fees for the first year is estimated to be $3,179; for the second year, $3,397. The cost of books for the first year is estimated to be $650; for the second year, $680; and for the third year, $60.

Financial Aid

All applications for financial aid should be filed no later than May for the following academic year. The medical university uses the American College Testing Service (ACT) to determine the financial need of each student. These forms can be obtained through the office of student financial management and placement services, other university financial aid offices, or high school guidance counselors. Foreign students who do not have a permanent visa or have not been awarded political asylum are not eligible for financial aid. Financial aid is available from a variety of federal, state, and private offices.

Minority Programs

The minority affairs office at the medical university offers an active program to recruit minority students and faculty to all colleges of the medical university. It also offers academic and social support to minority and international students enrolled at the university. The office works closely with accredited, historically black South Carolina colleges. The area health education centers offer summer health education programs designed to recruit minority students into the health professions.

Student Organizations

Student representatives are elected to the honor council and to the inter-school council. Other organizations of interest to dental students include the Student American Dental Association, the Student National Dental Association, Omicron Kappa Upsilon, Psi Omega, Delta Sigma Delta, and the dental student's wives association.

Curriculum

The four-year curriculum is designed to allow students a balanced work load as well as extra time for weaker students to review material, a broadening of the student's clinical experience, and an opportunity for the honor student to gain additional experience in areas of special interest.

The first two years include preclinical dental sciences courses, as well as clinical observations and experiences. The final two years concentrate on clinical practice. During the fourth year, students are assigned rotations at various facilities.

Facilities

The Basic Sciences/College of Dental Medicine building contains teaching facilities for all six colleges, laboratories, and office space for the basic sciences departments, and the division of laboratory animal resources. The dental clinics resemble modern dental operating rooms.

The Medical University of South Carolina library develops collections to support the curriculum, research, and patient care goals of the university. The library's automated integrated management system offers on-line access to a collection of over 190,000 volumes. The library also subscribes to 2,900 current serial subscriptions. MiniMEDLINE provides access to some medical journal articles.

The Macaulay Museum of Dental History contains a large

collection of antique dental instruments, books, and memorabilia.

Grading Procedures

A numerical grade-point system is used, ranging from 1 to 4 points and zero. Each college curriculum committee may approve a grade reporting system of honors/pass/fail for specific courses.

Special Programs

The dental medicine scientist training program provides an opportunity for well-qualified students to earn the D.M.D. and the Ph.D. degrees. Applicants must apply simultaneously to the College of Dental Medicine and to the College of Graduate Studies. In addition, the candidate must write to the DMST committee requesting admission to the combined program and must describe how this program will fit into his or her career goals. The program takes at least six years to complete.

Application Procedures

The college participates in the American Association of Dental Schools Application Service (AADSAS). Applications must be received between June 1 and December 31 of the year prior to enrollment. After the AADSAS application has been received, the college will mail a supplementary application packet, which contains applicant appraisal forms and a supplementary application to qualified students. This form should be returned with an application fee of $25. Personal interviews are arranged with selected students and are required for admission. The DAT is required, and should be taken no later than the fall of the year preceding planned enrollment.

Contact

Office of the University Registrar
and Director of Admissions
Medical University of South Carolina
171 Ashley Avenue
Charleston, South Carolina 29425
(803) 792-8617

UNIVERSITY OF MEDICINE AND DENTISTRY OF NEW JERSEY, NEW JERSEY DENTAL SCHOOL

110 Bergen Street
Newark, New Jersey 07103-2400
(201) 456-4633

Accreditation	CDA
Degrees Offered	D.M.D.
# Students Applied	470
Enrollment	90 / class
Mean GPA	2.95
% Men / % Women	56% / 44%
% Minorities	22%
Tuition	$10,457 In-State
	$13,723 Out-of-State
Application Fee	$25
Application Deadline	March 1

The University

The University of Medicine and Dentistry of New Jersey (UMDNJ) is the state's primary provider of medical and dental education. The school has campuses across the state, and offers programs leading to the M.D., D.O., D.M.D., and Ph.D. degrees, in addition to various postgraduate programs. The entering class of 1956 was the first that could pursue the D.D.S. degree; the first class for the D.M.D. degree was admitted in 1965.

Admissions

Because UMDNJ-New Jersey Dental School is state supported, state residents are given preference. Currently, about 80 percent of the students are New Jersey residents. Applicants must be U.S. citizens or have a green card. Academic ability takes presidence over professional motivation in deciding among applicants. Mean DAT scores of a recent class was 4.55 (academic) and 4.27 (PAT). The average overall GPA was 3.35.

Undergraduate Preparation

Students should have a strong background in natural sciences. Courses in government, economics, and social and behavioral sciences are recommended. The minimum predental requirements include eight semester hours of biology including zoology, six semester hours of English, eight semester hours of inorganic chemistry including analytical chemistry, eight semester hours of organic chemistry, eight semester hours of physics, and enough electives to complete two full years of study. All science classes should include a lecture and a lab.

Student Body

A majority of dental school students have earned a bachelor's degree or a minimum of three years of study towards an undergraduate degree prior to matriculation. About 10 percent of the students have earned graduate degrees. Thirty-two of the 90 members of the graduating class of 1993 are women; 20 are various minorities.

Costs

Tuition is $10,457 for residents and $13,723 for nonresidents. Fees include a $25 nonrefundable application fee, a $500 acceptance fee (applied toward tuition), $496 per year for student health insurance for a single student, a $100 loan equipment use fee, about $50 for clinic coats, approximately $2,600 for instruments during the first year and $600 for the second year, a $125 student activity fee, and a $50 gold deposit fee.

Financial Aid

Financial aid in the form of grants, scholarships, loans, or paid employment is awarded on the basis of need or merit by federal and state agencies, the university, foundations, and corporations. Financial need is determined by deducting the student's and family's contribution from the cost of attending dental school. Students who apply for financial aid should complete a GAPSFAS form. Most financial aid is given as student loans. The financial aid office assesses a student's need and awards loans based upon this assessment. Funds are available from Perkins/NDLS, Health Professions Student Loan, Stafford Student Loan, Supplemental Loan to Students, and Health Education Assistance Loan. The Alternative Loan Program is recommended for students who have not demonstrated need, but require more financial aid.

Minority Programs

Minority students may be eligible for funds from the Minority/Disadvantaged Fund or Martin Luther King Scholarship. A need-based program has been established for minority students with an average grant award of at least $7,000.

Curriculum

The first two years of the professional dental program comprise an integrated, interdepartmental course of study focusing on the basic medical sciences. Clinical science is introduced in the second year, and students get a foundation in diagnosis, public health, preventive medicine, and psychiatry. In the third year, closely supervised students rotate through clinical departments, evaluating patients and receiving instruction via personal tutors and small group discussions. Fourth-

year students complete advanced program requirements and take electives.

Grading Procedures

The school uses grades of honors, high pass, pass, and fail. Students must take Parts I and II of the National Board exams.

Application Procedures

Applications to the UMDNJ-New Jersey Dental School should be filed with AADSAS before March 1. An application request card for AADSAS can be obtained from the office of student affairs-D.M.D. admissions. The DAT should be taken the April before applying to the dental school. The admissions committee selects candidates for interviews. Only students who have been interviewed are accepted.

Contact

Office of Student Affairs-D.M.D. Admissions
Room B-829
New Jersey Dental School
110 Bergen Street
Newark, New Jersey 07103-2400
(201) 456-4633

MEHARRY MEDICAL COLLEGE SCHOOL OF DENTISTRY

Nashville, Tennessee 37208
(615) 327-6669

Accreditation	CDA
Degrees Offered	D.D.S.
# Students Applied	353
Enrollment	46 / class
Mean GPA	2.59
% Men / % Women	60% / 40%
% Minorities	95%
Tuition	$12,000
Application Fee	$25
Application Deadline	March 15

The University

Meharry Medical College is a private, nonprofit institution. Its primary goal is to educate health professionals from disadvantaged backgrounds, who will then provide health care to members of the population who are traditionally underserved. The college was established in 1876 and, 10 years later, the dental school was added. Other schools comprising the college are the schools of medicine, graduate studies and research, and allied health. The School of Dentistry is a contract participant in the Southern Regional Education Board (SREB).

The college enrolls 751 students, of whom 179 are in the dental school. The campus is located near the center of Nashville, a city of about 500,000.

Admissions

The college has a philosophy of concern for the disadvantaged, the importance of community-based health care, and excellence in health care education and studies. The college admits students with this mission in consideration, looking at academic record, intelligence, overall character, and aptitude for medical studies.

Preference is given to those who come from underserved regions, who are economically disadvantaged, and who have been involved in community activities. In addition, Meharry gives preference to students from SREB states that have contracts with the college, and from specific schools that have contracts with the college.

Undergraduate Preparation

Students must have a minimum of three years of preprofessional coursework at a college or university. Required predental courses are eight semester hours of general chemistry, four semester hours of organic chemistry, eight semester hours of general physics, eight semester hours of general biology, zoology, or botany, and six semester hours of English composition.

The school also recommends courses in a variety of other areas, including psychology, physical sciences, and languages. Strong reading and study skills are also important. All students must take the DAT. The cumulative GPA must be at least a C and the minimum average in all required courses must be a C.

Student Body

Of the 1989-90 entering class of 35, 14 were women and 33 were black. Sixteen of the students held the bachelor's degree. Five were residents of Tennessee and 30 were from out of state.

The mean GPA was 2.59 and the mean science GPA was 2.44. The mean DAT (academic) score was 2.34 and the mean DAT (PAT) score was 2.60.

The school's 1991-92 entering class is comprised of 46 students.

Costs

Tuition for the 1991-92 academic year is $12,000 per year. The purchase of instruments is $1,165 the first year and $5,686 the second year. The purchase of books for the total program is expected to cost about $1,370. There is a student health fee of $150 per year. Microscope rental for the first year is $150.

Financial Aid

The school awards certified students from SREB participant states a $900 grant toward tuition. The school has limited loans and scholarships, and qualified students may be eligible to participate in the college work-study program. Students may wish to apply to their local bank for state or other guaranteed loans.

Curriculum

The dental curriculum consists of four years of 36 weeks each. Methods of instruction include lectures and labs, with some audiovisual and computer support.

The first year concentrates on the basic sciences, with a few preclinical courses. The second year shifts to a focus on the preclinical aspect of dentistry. In the third year, students take oral pathology and some preclinical/didactic courses, but the primary focus is on clinical experience (about 860 hours of clinical work). The fourth year consists of clinical work and seminars.

The school has a team approach (using committees) to integrate the basic and clinical sciences. Research opportunities may be available. Individual academic counseling, group study, and computer assistance are also provided.

Facilities

The college campus is comprised of 14 acres. There have been major renovations to the facilities in the last decade, and the new dental school was completed in 1978. Fully equipped laboratories, library facilities, and computer facilities are available.

Special Programs

Students may earn a bachelor's degree concurrently with the D.D.S. by arrangement with an undergraduate institution.

Application Procedures

The School of Dentistry participates in AADSAS. Applications must be filed between April 1 and March 15 of the year preceding the year of desired enrollment. The school has a $25 application fee. The school does not participate in an early decision plan.

Applicants are notified of acceptance between December 1 and July 15. A $100 deposit is required to hold the student's place in class; this nonrefundable deposit is applied toward tuition.

Contact

Meharry Medical College
Director of Admissions and Records
Nashville, Tennessee 37208
(615) 327-6669

THE UNIVERSITY OF MICHIGAN SCHOOL OF DENTISTRY

Ann Arbor, Michigan 48109-1078
(313) 763-3311

Accreditation	ADA
Degrees Offered	D.D.S., M.S., Ph.D., B.S., D.D.S./B.S., D.D.S./B.A., D.D.S./B.G.S.
# Students Applied	545
Enrollment	96 / class
Mean GPA	3.11
% Men / % Women	67% / 33%
% Minorities	24%
Tuition	$9,086 In-State
	$16,814 Out-of-State
Application Fee	$30
Application Deadline	April 1

The University

The University of Michigan has three campuses; the School of Dentistry is located on the Ann Arbor campus. The School of Dentistry was founded in 1875, and now enrolls 492 of the university's 36,000 students.

Admissions

The School of Dentistry received 545 applications for 96 spots in its 1990 entering class. Students must have an undergraduate GPA above 2.7 and DAT scores above 15/15 to receive serious consideration. Averages of each are 3.1 and 17/17, respectively.

Undergraduate Preparation

Dental students must have completed one year each of biology, inorganic chemistry, organic chemistry, physics (all with labs), and English. It is preferred that the biological science credits be taken in zoology and that four hours of an advanced course (animal physiology, comparative anatomy, or developmental biology) be included. Also, students are urged to take introductory courses in psychology and biochemistry, and either an additional course in psychology or a course in sociology or anthropology. Grades lower than C will not be accepted.

Student Body

About three-quarters of the School of Dentistry's students are residents of Michigan. The 1990 entering class is comprised of 24 percent minority students and 33 percent women. The average age of entering students is 23; three percent have master's degrees; 60 percent have bachelor's degrees; and three percent have two years of undergraduate study.

Costs

Annual tuition and fees total $9,086 for Michigan residents and $16,814 for nonresidents. The School of Dentistry estimates that lab expenses total $9,375 for four years of study.

Financial Aid

The School of Dentistry participates in the Perkins, Stafford, HPL, LSL, and HEAL loan programs, and sponsors its own self-named loan fund, largely to help students with unexpected financial problems. Financial aid also comes in the forms of grants, scholarships, and research stipends.

Minority Programs

The International Center, Michigan League, and the Center for the Education of Women all serve the interests of minorities and women. The comprehensive studies program (CSP) is a support unit of the University of Michigan that provides comprehensive academic counseling and intensive courses for minority students.

Student Organizations

Student organizations include the student council, Taft honorary dental society, Black Dental Student Association, and Michigan Association of Women Dental Students.

Faculty

The School of Dentistry has a full-time faculty of 144 (including 45 professors emeriti) and 82 adjunct faculty and lecturers.

Curriculum

D.D.S. candidates must complete four years of residency. The School of Dentistry is implementing a new program of study for D.D.S. students; currently, students are trained in clinical work beginning in the fall term of their first year. The first three years contain 40 weeks of instruction; the fourth year is 34 weeks. An eight-week break is scheduled during the program; students may use this time for vacation, research projects, internships, fellowships, or other enrichment activities. Students may take electives occasionally.

Facilities

The School of Dentistry contains lecture rooms, technical laboratories, general and specialty clinics, and a library that holds 47,000 volumes. The W.K. Kellogg Foundation Institute also provides facilities for the study of dentistry. The University Hospital (one of seven hospitals in Michigan's Medical Center complex) houses modern dental facilities including nine operatories, a recovery room, and an area for dental radiography. The C.S. Mott Children's Hospital has a new facility for pediatric dentistry.

Special Programs

The School of Dentistry offers many specialized and advanced degrees, including 10 master of science degrees and joint D.D.S./B.S., D.D.S./B.A., and D.D.S./B.G.S. degrees. Dental students may also undertake graduate study in oral biology leading to a Ph.D.

Application Procedures

Deadline for applications through AASDAS is April 1. The application must include two letters of recommendation from faculty members in different sciences and one letter of recommendation from a faculty member in a nonscience area. The School of Dentistry may also require interviews of some students. The nonrefundable application fee is $30.

Contact

Assistant Dean of the School of Dentistry
University of Michigan
School of Dentistry
Ann Arbor, Michigan 48109-1078
(313) 763-3316

UNIVERSITY OF MINNESOTA SCHOOL OF DENTISTRY

Minneapolis, Minnesota 55455
(612) 625-9982

Accreditation	CDA
Degrees Offered	D.D.S., B.S., M.S., Ph.D. in Oral Biology
# Students Applied	349
Enrollment	76 / class
Mean GPA	3.02
% Men / % Women	71% / 29%
% Minorities	14%
Tuition	$6,278 In-State
	$9,416 Out-of-State
Application Fee	$30
Application Deadline	April 1

The University

The Minnesota College Hospital was taken over by the University of Minnesota in 1888 to establish its own Department of Medicine. The dentistry school of the new Department of Medicine became a separate unit in 1892, and its name was changed in 1932 to the School of Dentistry. The Twin Cities campus serves as the largest and oldest in the university. The major cities of Minneapolis and St. Paul provide flourishing centers for the campuses along the banks of the Mississippi River. Filled with attractive, historic buildings, Minneapolis offers various cultural centers including the Guthrie Theater, Orchestra Hall, Science Museum and Omnitheater, the Institute of Arts, and the Dudley Rigg's Brave New Workshop. Outdoor activities are abundant with 150 nearby parks and 200 lakes. The university Rec Sports program is the largest of its kind on any campus nationwide. Stores tailor-made for students are located in the nearby Stadium Village, Dinkytown, and Cedar-Riverside neighborhoods.

Admissions

All applicants are required to have a minimum GPA of 2.0. In addition, all students must take the dental admissions test (DAT) prepared by the American Dental Association. Students are urged to take the DAT by October of the academic year preceding enrollment.

Undergraduate Preparation

Required undergraduate courses for students hoping to gain

entry into the professional dental program are: eight semester hours in English, eight semester hours of general chemistry (including a course in quantitative or qualitative analysis), six semester hours of organic chemistry (including the aliphatic and aromatic series), seven semester hours of biology or zoology, seven semester hours of physics, and three semester hours of applied human psychology. At least one course in college algebra, or precalculus by college credit or college validation, computer science, or statistics is also required.

Student Body

The 1989 entering class of 76 students includes 22 women and 10 students of minority background. Ages ranged from 21 to 42, with the mean age being 24. Thirty had bachelor's degrees, and 40 were residents of Minnesota.

Costs

Annual tuition for residents is $6,278; nonresidents pay $9,416. Student services fees and instrument usage fees run about $335 and $975 per year, respectively. Typodonts for the first year cost $300. Books run about $830 for the first year, $710 for the second, $400 for the third, and $77 for the last year. In the second year, students must buy precious metals at a cost of about $750.

Financial Aid

Qualified students in the School of Dentistry are eligible for special loans, scholarships, fellowships, awards, and honors sponsored by various individuals, foundations, commercial firms, etc. Several research fellowships are offered during the summer for dental students.

Student Organizations

The campus hosts four active dental societies: Alpha Omega, Delta Sigma Delta, Psi Omega, and Xi Psi Phi. The faculty elects several superior fourth-year dental students to the national honor society, Omicron Kappa Upsilon, each year.

Curriculum

The School of Dentistry's professional program is a four-year curriculum. The year is divided into three quarters: a 14-week fall quarter, a 10-week winter quarter, and a 10-week spring quarter. Students are required to participate in clinical activity in the summer following the third year of study. First year students can expect to take gross human anatomy, histology, oral biology, biochemistry, system physiology, operative dentistry, and oral radiology. Second year begins the study of prosthodontics and periodontology. During the third year students will be exposed to pharmacology, oral surgery, and

initial examination. The fourth year consists of physical evaluation, hospital dentistry, and emergency clinic. Each quarter averages about 23 credits of study.

Facilities

All of the basic science teaching laboratories are located in the Malcolm Moos Health Sciences Tower. The anatomy laboratories are adjacent to the tower. An extensive selection of reference materials is located in the biomedical library in Diehl Hall, one block south of the tower. The Wilson Library on the West Bank is headquarters of the large Twin Cities campus library system.

Grading Procedures

The university uses a grading system of A, B, C, D, F, S, and N. Students are evaluated every quarter and are expected to maintain a minimum GPA of 2.0 to be promoted to the next year's class.

Special Programs

The UM Graduate School offers accredited programs leading to the M.S. degree in seven dental specialties. A Ph.D. can be earned in oral biology and in the basic medical sciences. Two post-D.D.S. residency and training programs in general dentistry are available, as well. Important research work is available in areas such as oral microbiology, fluoride chemistry, bone substitutes, viruses, and microcirculation. Special services and teaching clinics are in operation to assist in cleft palate and maxillofacial work, and complicated pain problems. Dental students can participate in exchange programs with Denmark, Norway, Germany, and Peru.

Application Procedures

The University of Minnesota School of Dentistry participates in the American Association of Dental Schools Application Service (AADSAS). Students must send applications to the AADSAS by April 1. Students must send one official college transcript along with three written letters of recommendation. There is a $30 application fee. Personal interviews are not required but highly recommended for all applicants.

Contact

Office of Admissions
School of Dentistry
University of Minnesota
240 Williamson Hall
231 Pillsbury Drive SE
Minneapolis, Minnesota 55455
(612) 625-2006

UNIVERSITY OF MISSISSIPPI SCHOOL OF DENTISTRY

2500 North State Street
Jackson, Mississippi 39216-4505
(601) 984-6000

Accreditation	ADA
Degrees Offered	D.M.D.
# Students Applied	68
Enrollment	30 / class
Mean GPA	3.3
% Men / % Women	83% / 17%
% Minorities	10%
Tuition	$4,050 In-State
	$10,038 Out-of-State
Application Fee	$25 In-State; $50 Out-of-State
Application Deadline	March 1

The University

The University of Mississippi Medical Center houses the Schools of Dentistry, Medicine, Nursing and Health-Related Professions, Graduate Studies in the Medical Sciences, and the University Hospital. The School of Dentistry was founded in 1973, and has been accredited by the American Dental Association Council on Dental Education.

Admissions

When considering an applicant for admission, the admissions committee evaluates his/her college record, DAT scores, letters of recommendation from the preprofessional advisor, and personal interview. The committee also attempts to identify the "properly motivated person with scientific curiosity, intelligence, ambition, and social consciousness" who has the potential to provide excellent patient care and to benefit the profession. Strong preference is given to residents of Mississippi.

Undergraduate Requirements

Applicants must have completed at least three years of college work (90 semester hours) to be considered for admission. Completion of the Bachelor's degree is recommended. Courses in military science, physical education, certain professional courses and correspondence courses are not applied to the 90 semester hours requirement. A maximum of 65 semester hours of junior college credit may be applied toward admission. Completion of the following courses is required: En-

glish, six semester hours in composition (three semester hours may be in communications); behavioral sciences, six semester hours; mathematics, six semester hours (including college algebra, trigonometry, or calculus); inorganic chemistry, eight semester hours; organic chemistry, eight semester hours; biology or zoology, eight semester hours; advanced biology or chemistry, four semester hours (suggested courses include bacteriology, biochemistry, cell biology or cell physiology, comparative anatomy, embryology, histology, immunology, microbiology, physical chemistry, and quantitative analysis). Recommended electives are genetics, calculus, foreign language, and courses in the humanities.

Costs

Tuition for Mississippi residents is $4,050 annually, including registration, laboratory, activities and library fees. Tuition for nonresidents is $10,038 per year. Instrument usage and microscope fee is currently $190 each quarter, used; books and supplies, $1,000 per year in the first two years, $400 the third, and $300 the fourth year; the refundable instrument deposit fee is $100. Various additional expenses (not including living expenses) are estimated to be about $6,000 for the four years.

Financial Aid

Information about financial aid and student housing is available through the Medical Center Division of Student Services and Records, 2500 North State Street, Jackson, Mississippi 39216-4505. Additional financial aid is available through the School of Dentistry, Office of the Assistant Dean for Student Programs.

Facilities

The School of Dentistry is located in the University of Mississippi Medical Center, which also houses the 531-bed University Hospital. A five-story dental education building was completed in 1977.

Application Procedures

Candidates for admission must contact the Division of Student Services and Records by mail or by phone to receive an application form. Applications should be received between July 1 of the year preceding planned enrollment and March 1 of the year of planned enrollment. The DAT is required. The school recommends that the DAT be taken in the spring, but not later than the fall, of the year preceding the desired date of admission. DAT scores must not be more than three years old. The DAT must be taken within three years of the entering fall registration date.

All transcripts and correspondence concerning applications must be addressed to the Division of Student Services and Records. Before an application can be reviewed by the admissions committee, the following items must be received: an application fee of $25 for residents, $50 for nonresidents; a recent photograph (optional); an official transcript from each college attended; a list of courses the applicant plans to take; a brief autobiography; a current predental advisor's appraisal; ACT scores; and DAT scores.

Contact

Division of Student Services and Records
University of Mississippi Medical Center
2500 North State Street
Jackson, Mississippi 39216-4505
(601) 984-1080

UNIVERSITY OF MISSOURI-KANSAS CITY
SCHOOL OF DENTISTRY

650 East 25th Street
Kansas City, Missouri 64108-2795
(816) 276-2010

Accreditation	ADA
Degrees Offered	D.D.S., B.S., M.S., B.A./ D.D.S.
# Students Applied	444
Enrollment	69 / class
Mean GPA	3.23
% Men / % Women	68% / 32%
% Minorities	16%
Tuition	$6,378 In-State
	$10,119 Out-of-State
Application Fee	None
Application Deadline	April 1

The University

The University of Missouri-Kansas City School of Dentistry began as the Kansas City Dental College in 1881. In 1919, the Kansas City Dental College merged with Western Dental College to form the Kansas City Western Dental College, which became the School of Dentistry of the University of Kansas City in 1941. In 1963, the school became an official part of the University of Missouri system. The UMKC School of Dentistry is fully accredited by the ADA. Located on the Missouri side of the twin ports of the two Kansas Cities,

UMKC lies in the midst of one of the most important industrial and commercial centers of the American West. The area was the starting place for many western expeditions. Points of interest include the Nelson Art Gallery, the Atkins Museum, and several theaters. Across the river in Kansas students may visit an agricultural museum and a Shawnee mission. Professional football and baseball prosper and have an enthusiastic following.

Admissions

Priority is given to Missouri residents. Applicants must have a minimum of 30 semester hours of college credit. Factors taken into consideration include academic credentials, DAT scores, letter of evaluation, motivation, and all other information the applicant might submit. The DAT scores are required, and UMKC strongly recommends applicants take the DAT no later than October of the year before intended entry. A minimum of 60 semester hours must have been completed before an accepted candidate may begin school. With 30 to 60 hours of credit, the GPA mean should be 3.60, with 60 to 90 hours, 3.20, and with 90 to 120 hours, 2.80.

Undergraduate Preparation

No specific college major is required. Students must have graduated from an accredited high school with a 75 percent GPA ranking or higher. By the end of the winter semester of the year of application, students must have completed (with lab) eight to ten hours each of college biology, general and organic chemistry, and physics. Six hours of college English are also required.

Student Body

More than 400 students applied for the 69 spots in the 1989 class. Successful applicants included 22 women, 11 minorities, 31 Missouri residents, and 36 students who had baccalaureate degrees.

Placement Records

Alumni practice dentistry in every state of the union. More than 90 percent of the practicing dentists in Kansas graduated from UMKC School of Dentistry.

Costs

Estimated tuition for residents is $6,378 for the first two two-semester years, $7,374 for the third year (two semesters plus a four-week summer term), and $8,769 for the fourth year (two semesters plus a ten-week summer term). Nonresidents (those from states other than Missouri, Kansas, Arkansas, and New Mexico) pay an additional $3,741 per year, plus $1,581 in the third year and $3,794 in the fourth year for the summer terms. Books, equipment, and supplies run $5,300 the first year, $4,110 the second year, $1,490 the third year, and $680 the final year.

Financial Aid

About 85 percent of dental students need aid, but UMKC funds are limited. Applications are processed on a first-come, first-served basis. UMKC, however, ranks among the top 10 dental schools in the country in dollar amount of financial aid awarded. Students may apply for loans, part-time employment, grants, and scholarships. UMKC School of Dentistry offers six federal loan programs, 15 institutional grants and scholarships, 19 loan funds, and seven other assistance programs to help support students in their career study.

Student Organizations

UMKC has a variety of student organizations on campus for students to join. Most are affiliated with national dental offices. Non-dentistry organizations also offer further educational and recreational opportunities for interested students.

Faculty

The school's faculty consists of scholars, scientists, and specialists in all areas of oral health care. Instructors are both experienced teachers and dentists.

Curriculum

The D.D.S. course of study lasts four years. First-year students cover courses in basic sciences and dentistry and begin preliminary patient care. Second-year students continue class and laboratories and increase clinical practice. Third-year students spend less time in lectures and labs and begin to concentrate on clinic work. Fourth-year students are full-time practitioners, taking part in an occasional seminar or conference.

Facilities

The facilities include 305 fully-equipped dental operatories, with about 110,000 patient visits each year. Three dental-technique laboratories with fully-equipped working stations are available. The dental library has 15,000 volumes and more than 375 periodicals to choose from and operates in association with the university-wide library system. The School of Dentistry is affiliated with five local hospitals and medical centers for additional research and clinical facilities.

Grading Procedures

The school uses a letter and grade point system as follows: A (outstanding work) = 4; B (work of distinction) = 3; C (average) = 2; and D (passing but unsatisfactory) = 1. The F grade is for failure without credit. Students must maintain at least a 2.5 GPA each semester and get a passing grade on Parts I and II of the National Board Dental Examinations in order to graduate.

Special Programs

UMKC School of Dentistry offers the dental specialty certificate and the B.S. in dental hygiene. The M.S. degree is offered in oral biology or in dental hygiene education. The six-year B.A./D.D.S. combined degree program is unique to U.S. dental schools.

Application Procedures

Students must apply through the AADSAS by April 1 of the year of intended entry. Three letters of recommendation, one of which must be from the applicant's predental adviser or predental committee, must be submitted. UMKC School of Dentistry also recommends letters from college faculty, employers, dentists, or clergy. Applicants who meet the minimum GPA requirements are invited for a personal interview. Notices of acceptance begin after December 1. To preserve their class place, accepted students must submit a $200 nonrefundable deposit within 30 days of notice.

Contact

Office of Student Affairs
University of Missouri-Kansas City
School of Dentistry
650 East 25th Street
Kansas City, Missouri 64108
(816) 276-2080

UNIVERSITY OF NEBRASKA MEDICAL CENTER–LINCOLN COLLEGE OF DENTISTRY

40th and Holdrege Streets
Lincoln, Nebraska 68583-0740
(402) 472-1334

Accreditation	ADA
Degrees Offered	D.D.S., Ph.D., M.S.
# Students Applied	192
Enrollment	42 / class
Mean GPA	3.19
% Men / % Women	75% / 25%
% Minorities	9%
Tuition	$6,231 In-State
	$14,418 Out-of-State
Application Fee	$25
Application Deadline	March 1

The University

The University of Nebraska Medical Center College of Dentistry opened in 1899, as the Lincoln Dental College. The total enrollment was 24. In 1918, the dental college became a unit within the university and was recognized as a college by the state in 1919. The college is now located on Lincoln's UNL east campus. The college is fully accredited by the ADA. Located 55 miles from the major part of the medical center, the college has its own full-time faculty and an independent operating style. Lincoln has been listed near the top of almost every list of desirable cities to live, the most crime-free of 28 comparably sized cities studied by the FBI. Lincoln has a population of about 200,000 residents and enjoys an excellent public school system, public transportation, and many cultural, athletic, and social activities.

Admissions

Applicants must take the DAT, but the college has no specific minimum requirements for the scores. The college recommends taking the DAT in April, 15 months before enrollment. The DAT scores average about 16; the national mean is 15 on the new scale of 1 to 30. Nebraska residents get the highest consideration. A recent entering class had an average GPA of 3.24, the fourth highest of 57 dental schools in the U.S. Over the last four years, UNMC's dental students ranked among the top 20 percent on the National Board Examinations.

Undergraduate Preparation

UNMC College of Dentistry requires at least three years of college preparation (90 semester hours). Predental work may be completed at any accredited college, junior college, or community college in the United States. Required courses include eight hours each of physics, inorganic and organic chemistry, and biology or zoology. Six hours of English are also required.

Student Body

The college receives over 200 applications each year for its dental program. About 40 students are admitted each year. Twenty dental hygiene students and up to 25 students for advanced educational programs are also admitted. The total college enrollment is 185 dental students, 37 dental hygiene students and 36 graduate students. The average age of the entering class is 24.

Placement Records

The college has the highest passing percentage of any school in the central regional board area (10 states). In 1989, the graduating class was completely placed, and the college still had 90 practice opportunities available.

Costs

Resident tuition for 1990-91 was $6,231; nonresident tuition was $14,418. Fees for activities, books, and instruments total about $3,134. Living expenses are about $675 per month, or $8,100 a year. The total cost for four years amounts to about $35,000 for residents and $65,000 for nonresidents.

Financial Aid

Nearly 90 percent of students receive some form of financial assistance—either grants, scholarships, or loans. Awards vary from $200 to full tuition. The top 10 percent of each class receives scholarship awards; of these, about 80 are academic-based scholarships. In 1988-89, over $208,000 in grants and scholarships were given to students and over $1.6 million in loan aid. Foreign students on F-1 visas are not eligible for federal financial aid. Some college work-study programs are available.

Student Organizations

Student clubs at the college help promote social and recreational life. Social events are regularly held both informally and as all-college parties, such as the annual pig roast.

Faculty

UNMC College of Dentistry has 138 faculty members, 63 full time and 75 part time. The student/faculty ratio is about 4:1. All 10 of the basic science faculty members have a Ph.D. and each has an average of over 10 years teaching. Many of the clinical faculty are board certified. All of the dental hygiene faculty are registered dental hygienists and have an M.S. UNMC faculty now publish over 100 articles a year and bring in over $400,000 each year in external grants for teaching and research.

Curriculum

Students learn the basic sciences during the first two years in school. Also in the first year, students experience clinical observation. The second year brings on clinical work and the opportunity to work with patients. The third and fourth years are clinical in nature, as students perfect their dental skills and learn dental techniques.

Facilities

The college contains its own library and basic sciences and clinical areas. Support laboratories are available to help students complete clinical requirements, particularly in fixed and removable prosthodontics. The college has 11 separate clinical areas including some 155 individual clinical cubicles in specialty areas and 20 operating units in the dental hygiene clinic. About 50,000 patients have dental work done at the college each year.

Special Programs

The college offers the only baccalaureate dental hygiene program in Nebraska and it offers the Ph.D. Nine specialty educational programs lead to a certificate or M.S. degree. Most require two years beyond the D.D.S. degree. The oral surgery program takes five years, and the general practice programs take one year. The specialty programs include pediatric dentistry, prosthodontics, geriatrics, orthodontics, periodontics, oral surgery, endodontics, general practice residency, and advanced education in general dentistry. About 12 students a year take a hospital-based residency program.

Application Procedures

Dental students enroll in the college each August. You must apply through AADSAS. Apply as soon as possible after June 1 of the year before intended entry. The deadline for the application cycle is March 1 of the year before matriculation. The nonrefundable AADSAS application fee is $85 for the first school, and $10 for each additional school. In addition, there is an application fee of $25 to the University of Nebraska. Applicants under serious consideration may be invited for an interview. After December 1, the college will call applicants with an acceptance notice. The College of Dentistry does not require letters of recommendation, but evaluations of a student's progress by a predental advisor or committee are appreciated.

Contact

Admissions—University of Nebraska Medical Center
College of Dentistry
40th and Holdrege Streets
Lincoln, Nebraska 68583-0740
(402) 472-1363

NEW YORK UNIVERSITY, COLLEGE OF DENTISTRY, DAVID B. KRISER DENTAL CENTER

345 East 24th Street
New York, New York 10010
(212) 998-9900

Accreditation	MSACS
Degrees Offered	D.D.S., B.A./D.D.S.
# Students Applied	716
Enrollment	158 / class
Mean GPA	2.87
% Men / % Women	61% / 39%
% Minorities	41%
Tuition	$22,282
Application Fee	$35
Application Deadline	June 1

The University

New York University (NYU) is a private, urban university that enrolls over 45,000 students. The university is accredited by the Middle States Association of Colleges and Schools. Classes began at the university in 1831. The College of Dentistry (NYUCD) was founded in 1865 and received its present name in 1925. NYUCD is on First Avenue, between East 24th and 25th Streets, in the center of a renowned health sciences complex. The College of Dentistry students have access to the "Big Apple's" vast cultural opportunities, including historic Greenwich Village, Lincoln Center, theaters, and museums, all within easy reach through public transportation systems.

Admissions

NYUCD considers applicants based on a variety of criteria, including social, academic, and personal character. NYUCD candidates have a GPA of at least 3.0 and above-average DAT scores.

Undergraduate Preparation

Students must take the DAT and have a minimum of three years at an accredited college or university. NYUCD recommends students achieve their baccalaureate degree. Minimum course requirements include six to eight semester hours each (with lab) of biology, physics, and organic chemistry. Students also should have eight to 12 hours in inorganic chemistry (with lab) and six semester hours in English (two years are recommended). Recommended courses include comparative anatomy, embryology, and histology.

Student Body

More than 900 predoctoral and 70 graduate students study at the college. The 1990 entering class consisted of 158 students, of whom 61 (38.6 percent) were women. The students come from 74 colleges and universities across the United States and from five foreign countries.

Placement Records

Over 9,000 dentists nationwide are graduates of NYUCD. Two-thirds of the dentists practicing in New York City and more than half of those practicing in New York State graduated from NYUCD. Many NYUCD graduates serve as presidents of the major specialty associations and professional societies throughout the country.

Costs

Tuition is $22,282, plus $6,564 for first-year students for all books and required instruments. NYUCD estimates the four-year cost for books and instruments to total $11,275. Student housing is provided by NYU and is located nearby on East 25th Street. Room and board for students residing in NYU apartments is $354 per month, including utilities.

Financial Aid

About 80 percent of NYU's students receive financial aid. NYU offers 12 full four-year Dean's Merit Scholarships annually, and a comprehensive aid package is offered to all qualified students. Students must file the financial aid form (FAF) at the college scholarship service (CSS). In the Robert T. Stafford Loan Program, students may borrow up to $7,500 per year with a limit of $54,750. Similar terms exist for other loan programs. NYUCD offers a number of federal programs, some 23 other loan programs, the NYS Tuition Assistance Program, and 47 awards and prizes for academic excellence.

Student Organizations

The Omicron Kappa Upsilon society has a chapter on campus. Other organizations include the American Student Dental Association, the American Association of Dental Schools, the Student National Dental Association, the Dental Health Organization, the American Association for Dental Research, the International Association of Dental Students, the American Association of Women Dentists, the American Society of Dentistry for Children, and student fraternities.

Curriculum

The course of study lasts four years. During the first and second years, students cover the basic sciences and begin clinical practice. Courses include gross anatomy, inheritance and development, neuroscience, histology, physiology and pharmacology, biochemistry, microbiology, pathology, and materials science. Second-year students begin treating patients in prosthodontics, periodontic, and restorative clinics, and continue in all the dental specialities through the third year. The third year of study expands and intensifies the clinical areas begun earlier. The whole fourth year is given to the comprehensive care and applied practice administration (CCAPA) program. Students in this program take their patients through a complete treatment cycle, including diagnosis, treatment planning, and completion of all dental needs.

Facilities

Three centers comprise NYUCD: the David B. Kriser Dental Center, the Arnold and Marie Schwartz Hall of Dental Sciences, and the K.B. Weissman Clinical Science Building. The Hall of Dental Sciences has 292 modern operatories on five floors and houses a library of 33,000 bound volumes and 311 professional journals. Rare books and other memorabilia are stored here as well. NYU dental students may use one of the largest dental research libraries in the country (over 2 million books and journals, plus microfilms, video- and audiotapes in open stacks) and the 24 hours-a-day computer access to the NYU Bobst Library. NYU is also part of a national network of affiliated libraries.

Special Programs

Postdoctoral work is available in all specialties, and special programs lead to the combined B.A./D.D.S. degree. Programs are possible for graduates of foreign dental schools. The advanced professional certificate (APC) program is offered through the Stern School of Business.

Application Procedures

The deadline for applications is June 1 of the year in which the student seeks admission. Students may get applications from the college admissions office but must apply through AADSAS. The fee is $35 and is nonrefundable. Students must submit DAT scores and must complete all prerequisites before enrollment in September. In addition to the application form, students should submit three letters of recommendation, an official college transcript, a signed photograph, and take part in a personal interview.

Contact

Office of Admissions
Director of Admissions
New York University College of Dentistry
345 East 24th Street
New York, New York 10010
(212) 998-9818

UNIVERSITY OF NORTH CAROLINA SCHOOL OF DENTISTRY

105 Brauer Hall
Chapel Hill, North Carolina 27599-7450
(919) 966-2731

Accreditation	CDA
Degrees Offered	D.D.S., B.S., D.D.S./Ph.D., D.D.S./M.P.H.
# Students Applied	380
Enrollment	66 / class
Mean GPA	3.1
% Men / % Women	65% / 35%
% Minorities	5%
Tuition	$3,011 In-State
	$17,034 Out-of-State
Application Fee	$35
Application Deadline	December 1

The University

The University of North Carolina at Chapel Hill has the distinction of being the first state university founded in the nation. Both its chartering and George Washington's first inauguration occurred in 1789. The college town of Chapel Hill, near the center of North Carolina, is graced with a mild climate and located within a few hours drive of the Carolina beaches and the Blue Ridge Mountains. The university now consists of 190 permanent buildings in which 1,900 full-time faculty members instruct 22,000 students. The School of Dentistry was formed in 1949. The Division of Health Affairs includes the schools of medicine, pharmacy, public health, dentistry, and nursing.

Admissions

All applicants must take the Dental Admission Test in April or October of the year preceding matriculation. Selected applicants are invited to attend a series of interviews with faculty and student members of the admissions committee. Applicants who are not invited may contact the office of admissions regarding interviews.

Undergraduate Preparation

Applicants should preferably complete a BA or BS degree, or must at least complete three years or 96 semester hours at an accredited college or university. A maximum of 64 semes-

ter hours may be completed at a two-year community college, but required science courses must be taken at an accredited four-year institution. Academic requirements include eight semester hours of general chemistry with lab, two lecture courses with a minimum of four semester hours of organic chemistry, eight semester hours of general biology or zoology with lab, two college level courses in physics, and two semesters of English. Courses in drawing and sculpture that develop psychomotor skills are suggested.

Placement Records

The Career Counseling Service sponsors seminars designed to help students prepare for practice or apply for postgraduate programs. A practice placement service helps to locate available associateships and practices in the state.

Costs

Tuition and fees (library, student activities, student union, instructional supplies, and dental equipment usage) for North Carolina residents is $3,011 for the first two years, $3,057 for the third year, and $2,155 for the fourth year. For nonresidents, tuition and fees are approximately $17,034. Instruments and lab supplies are estimated to cost $3,315, $2,513, and $92 for the first three years, respectively. Textbooks currently cost about $978 for freshmen, $630 for sophomores, and $130 for juniors. Other fees are incidental and vary by year. Additionally, students must have use of an approved microscope, which currently sells for $465 and up. They can be rented for $50 per year.

Financial Aid

North Carolina residents may borrow up to $7,500 per year under the North Carolina Loan Program for Health Science and Mathematics. Students may borrow up to $7,500 per year under the Guaranteed Student Loan Program. The Health Professions Student Loan (HPSL) Program offers maximum awards of $2,500 per year plus tuition. Other loans include the Carl Perkins Loan Program, Supplemental Loans for Students (SLS), and loans from the UNC student aid office. The priority filing date for the HPSL, Perkins Loan, and UNC loans is March 1. The UNC Board of Governors Dental Scholarship Program provides funds for tuition, fees, instruments, and supplies, as well as a $5,000 stipend. Minority and disadvantaged North Carolina residents are eligible, with a view towards aiding those who will provide needed dental care in North Carolina. The Outland Scholarship is awarded by merit to North Carolina residents for their first year of dental study. The G. Randolph and Ann Babcock Fellowship is awarded to a candidate interested in academic dentistry and research after training has been completed in a dental specialty or advanced education program.

Minority Programs

The minority presence grant program for doctoral study provides stipends of up to $6,000 per year for Black North

Carolina residents. North Carolina School of Dentistry minority scholarships are available to first-year minority students. American Indians, Blacks, Mexican-Americans, and Puerto Ricans are eligible to receive $2,000 for their first year from the American Fund for Dental Health minority scholarship program. The scholarship may be renewed the second year. American Indians are eligible to apply for grants through the Indian Health Service Scholarship Programs administered by the Department of Education. Service obligation, rather than financial need, is a major condition for the award. All direct educational costs are covered and a monthly stipend of $623. The Indian Fellowship Program awards vary in amount and are based on financial need. The application deadline is February 1. Entering Black students who demonstrate financial need are eligible for minority presence grants for dentistry. Priority filing date is March 1. Women in their final year who show promise of distinction in their field and demonstrate financial need are eligible for the American Association of University Women fellowship. Awards average $3,500 for the year and applications must be filed by January 2 of the junior year. Women who are over 21 years old, are residents of the southern U.S., and who have been forced by marriage or other reasons to defer their career goals are eligible for the Diuguid fellowships. The stipend is for one year and the maximum amount is $8,000. Applicants must demonstrate financial need and apply by January 1.

Curriculum

The first year of the dental curriculum includes the basic sciences, introductory dental sciences, oral biology, and introduction to patient care, which includes delivery of preventive care. The basic sciences consist of gross anatomy, microscopic anatomy, biochemistry, physiology, microbiology, and general pathology. The introductory dental sciences include dental anatomy, materials science, conservative dentistry, periodontics, oral diagnosis and radiology, growth and development, and occlusion. Second-year studies include pharmacology, oral pathology, growth and development, life cycle courses, preclinical endodontics, orthodontics, removable and fixed prosthodontics, and a physical diagnosis course. In the spring semester students assume full patient care privileges and deliver comprehensive care. Third-year studies involve caring for patients in the comprehensive care and specialty services. Students may participate in research projects and externships during the summer. During the fourth year, students administer advanced dental care, take elective courses, do research, and participate in required extramural rotations. Students spend six weeks at off-campus sites, including three at a community dentistry health service and three at a hospital dental service. Students may learn about a specialty through patient care, research, and coursework.

Facilities

North Carolina's library system, containing more than three million volumes, is ranked among the top research libraries in the U.S. and Canada by the Association of Research Libraries. Included in the system are the Davis Library, Wilson Library, House Undergraduate Library, Health Sciences Library, and 12 school and departmental libraries. The Health Sciences Library of UNC contains over 233,700 volumes and 4,500 current serial titles. It has a large audiovisuals center and a microcomputer learning lab, as well as the on-line databases of MEDLINE and TOXLINE. The library also houses a learning laboratory that includes a computer center. The North Carolina Memorial Hospital, opened on campus in 1952, serves as the major teaching hospital and is accredited for residency programs in dentistry. The dental research center provides inclusive dental research facilities and operates one of the largest oral biomedicine research programs in the country. The university provides housing for about 6,900 students, both graduate and undergraduate. Apartments are available for student family housing. Dining facilities are located near the residence halls. Three privately-owned residence towers, which have their own cafeterias, are located close to campus.

Grading Procedures

Letter grades are given for core courses, and pass/fail grades are given for elective courses.

Special Programs

A certificate or B.S. degree may be earned in dental hygiene. Undergraduates may earn a B.S. in dentistry in three years; the last year of predental study must be completed at UNC at Chapel Hill. Both a combined D.D.S./M.P.H. degree and a combined D.D.S./Ph.D. degree are offered. The Ph.D. may be earned in the basic or behavioral sciences. Three-year advanced education programs are available in endodontics, orthodontics, pediatric dentistry, periodontology, prosthodontics, oral biology, oral epidemiology, oral radiology, and geriatric dentistry. The dental auxiliary teacher education program requires two years of study. The dentist scientist program provides stipends and support for those with the D.D.S. or D.M.D. degree to pursue clinical specialty training and the Ph.D. in a research discipline. The 12-month advanced education in general dentistry program is a postdoctoral certificate program with an emphasis on clinical dentistry. A similar 24-month general practice in dentistry emphasizes medical management and consists of a clinical program and a residency program. Residency rotations include physical diagnosis and internal medicine, anesthesiology, and oral surgery.

Application Procedures

Applications must be filed with the American Association of Dental Schools Application Service (AADSAS) by December 1. Applicants who wish to be notified by December 1 must send the required material several months prior to this date. Both AADSAS and School of Dentistry supplemental applications are required. Candidates must send a nonrefundable application fee, letters of recommendation, DAT scores, and official transcripts to the university. Foreign applicants must submit acceptable scores in the Test of English as a Foreign Language (TOEFL) and satisfactory scores on the DAT or Part 1 of the National Board Dental Examination. A nonrefundable application fee of $35 is charged.

Contact

Office of Admissions
School of Dentistry
University of North Carolina—Chapel Hill
105 Brauer Hall
Chapel Hill, North Carolina 27599-7450
(919) 966-4565

NORTHWESTERN UNIVERSITY DENTAL SCHOOL

Chicago, Illinois 60208
(312) 908-5932

Accreditation	ADA
Degrees Offered	D.D.S., B.A./D.D.S., M.S.
# Students Applied	646
Enrollment	64 / class
Mean GPA	2.99
% Men / % Women	65% / 35%
% Minorities	11%
Tuition	$20,283
Application Fee	$35
Application Deadline	March 1

The University

The Dental School of Northwestern University began in 1887 as a private school located in Chicago. In 1891, a group of prominent dentists reorganized the school to become an integral part of Northwestern. Dr. Greene Vardiman Black, the "father" of modern dentistry, was a founder of Northwestern University Dental School and served as dean for 18 years. The Dental School is on the Chicago campus. The various schools there enroll more than 5,000 students, about half of whom are full-time graduate students. The Dental School is fully accredited by the ADA.

Located in an attractive neighborhood, the Chicago campus is near Lake Michigan and all the recreational opportunities of the lakefront. Just outside the lakefront residence halls are beaches and miles of bicycle and jogging paths. Blocks away is North Michigan Avenue's "magnificent mile" of shopping and dining establishments. Theater, sports, and other cultural opportunities abound in the Windy City.

Admissions

Students must have at least two years of study at an accredited college or university. Although 60 semester (or 90 quarter) hours are acceptable, Northwestern recommends three or four years of undergraduate study. Applicants must submit DAT scores. An above-average science and cumulative GPA is expected. Entering freshmen must show proof of hepatitis vaccine.

Undergraduate Preparation

One year of study in English is required. In addition, one year each (with lab) is required in zoology or biology, organic and inorganic chemistry, and physics. Especially appropriate electives include business and accounting, computer science, economics, comparative anatomy, ethics, genetics, history, mathematics, psychology, sociology, speech, and statistics.

Student Body

Of the 64 members of the graduating class of 1993, 22 are women and seven are minorities. Almost half are Illinois residents. Fifty-three had earned bachelor's degrees before enrolling. The mean overall GPA was 2.99; the mean science GPA was 2.85.

Placement Records

The Dental School has graduated over 7,000 dentists who practice in each of the 50 states and in 44 countries.

Costs

Tuition is $20,283. Northwestern estimates room and board to be $7,332 per year. Instruments, books, and supplies cost about $3,576, and personal expenses and transportation amount to $2,931 and $1,212, respectively. Housing is guaranteed on campus for all four years of enrollment. Housing assignments begin after April 1.

Financial Aid

Students who show demonstrated financial need through GAPSFAS are eligible for assistance. Students awarded financial aid must, nonetheless, pay a minimum of $1,200 each year toward their education. Students are typically enrolled for three terms and receive one-third of their financial aid in each of those terms. Students must apply for aid annually.

Student Organizations

Three professional dental fraternities have chapters on campus: Alpha Omega, Delta Sigma Delta, and Xi Psi Phi. In addition, Omicron Kappa Upsilon has a chapter here. Student chapters of AADS, ADA, and the Apollonian Society also are very active at Northwestern. These and other student government and social groups make for a full student life on campus.

Curriculum

The program of study lasts four years. The first year covers the basic sciences. However, students may pursue electives throughout the four years. Juniors and seniors have the most elective time. Northwestern operates on the trimester system. First-year courses include gross anatomy, biochemistry, neuroanatomy, microbiology, physiology, operative dentistry, and pharmacology. Clinical courses begin in the sophomore year and increase in number through senior year, as do electives. Students may choose from some 60 elective courses.

Facilities

Programs are offered with the five hospitals that make up the McGraw Medical Center. Three member hospitals are on the Chicago campus. The Health Science Building contains 283 operatories, each of which is designed to accommodate both left- and right-handed students. The Ward and Searle buildings, shared with the medical school, house the multidisciplinary laboratories, preclinical laboratory, medical school library, and main dental school library (60,000 volumes and over 23,000 pamphlets, monographs, and periodicals). The dental library also has a 1,390-volume rare books collection of early masterpieces of dental literature.

Grading Procedures

Required courses are graded as follows: A (superior), B (good), C (satisfactory), D (poor but passing), E (conditional failure), and F (failure). Elective courses are graded on an honor, pass, or fail basis. Progress report grades are given for clinical practice courses, and departments award final grades at the end of the junior and senior years. A student may be placed on probation for incurring one or more E or F grades, or if the GPA falls below 2.0.

Special Programs

The college offers a special five track curriculum that allows students to graduate with a D.D.S. and an area of additional expertise. The Colorado Program allows students to work for one summer in two clinics outside Boulder with migrant workers and their families. The M.S., postgraduate courses in clinical subjects, and certificate and degree programs for dental hygienists are also available. A B.A./D.D.S. degree is offered.

Application Procedures

Applicants must apply through AADSAS, and the deadline is March 1 of the year before the year of intended entry. Applicants may begin applying to the school by July 1 for the class entering in August of the following year. In addition to the AADSAS fee, a $10 nonrefundable processing fee is required. Submit all transcripts from all colleges and universities attended, as well as a pre-health professions committee recommendation. Applicants may then be invited to submit a formal application to the school ($35 application fee). Supplemental information (such as letters of recommendation and personal essays) is welcome. Northwestern recommends students arrange for an interview early in the process. Provisional acceptances are issued beginning after December 1. Deposits of $500 and $300 applied to tuition are required before final notice of acceptance after August 1.

Contact

Office of Admissions and Student Affairs
Northwestern University Dental School
Ward Building 10-142
311 East Chicago Avenue
Chicago, Illinois 60611-3008
(312) 908-8334

THE OHIO STATE UNIVERSITY COLLEGE OF DENTISTRY

1800 Cannon Drive
Columbus, Ohio 43210-1200
(614) 292-9755

Accreditation	CDA
Degrees Offered	D.D.S., Ph.D., M.S.
# Students Applied	536
Enrollment	101 / class
Mean GPA	2.93
% Men / % Women	71% / 29%
% Minorities	12%
Tuition	$4,849 In-State
	$14,497 Out-of-State
Application Fee	$20
Application Deadline	March 1

The University

The Ohio State University College of Dentistry began as a department of Ohio Medical University in 1890, merged with Starling Medical College in 1906, and became part of Ohio State in 1914. Since 1925 the College of Dentistry has been located in Columbus, Ohio. In 1944 the dental hygiene program was established. Besides the preprofessional programs, the college offers graduate education and continuing education programs.

Admissions

Admission requirements include the completion of at least 60 semester hours in predental study, above-average achievement in required courses, satisfactory completion of the Dental Admissions Test, a personal interview at the college, two letters of recommendation, official transcripts, and college entrance scores. DAT scores are highly rated, and although there is no minimum GPA requirement, science grades are given the most consideration. The mean DAT scores for the students who matriculated in 1989 were 4.93 (academic) and 5.09 (PAT). The same class had mean GPAs of 2.93 (total) and 2.77 (science). Emphasis is also placed on marked scholastic improvement, personal characteristics, and knowledge of dentistry through observation. Interviews are by invitation only.

Undergraduate Preparation

Applicants must have completed two semesters of English composition and literature, one year of biology or zoology with lab, one year of general chemistry with lab, two semesters of organic chemistry with lab, and two semesters of physics with lab.

Student Body

Of the 101 students enrolled in the entering class of 1989, 29 percent were women and 12 percent were minorities. Seventy-five percent had undergraduate degrees, and 81 percent were state residents.

Costs

Tuition for 1990-91 was $4,849 for residents and $14,497 for nonresidents. Books and instruments cost $3,232 for the first year, $2,180 for the second year, and about $860 for the third year. There are no such costs during the final year. On-campus room and board costs $3,500 annually. Miscellaneous fees, including health insurance, amount to about $400. There is a $20 application fee and a $25 acceptance fee. Within 30 days after notification of admission, students wishing to reserve a place in the class must return a signed statement of acceptance with a $100 deposit.

Financial Aid

Available financial aid includes Ohio State Scholarships, the Health Profession Student Loan (HPSL), the Perkins Loan, University Loan Funds, the Guaranteed Student Loan (GSL), Supplemental Loans for Students and/or Parents, the Health Education Assistance Loan (HEAL), a federal college work-study program, and a student employment program.

Minority Programs

The office of student life provides various programs and services for Black and Hispanic students, including orientation, counseling, tutoring, and financial aid. Over 100 excellence scholarships are awarded annually to minority high school seniors who have achieved a GPA of 3.0 or better in college prep programs; these and other scholarships may pay for full tuition for Ohio residents

Student Organizations

Students may join the student council, American Dental Association, Student National Dental Association, and the chapters of dental fraternities Alpha Omega, Delta Sigma Delta, Psi Omega, and Xi Psi Phi.

Curriculum

The freshman and sophomore years consist of three academic quarters each; the junior and senior years consist of four quarters each. Each quarter lasts 11 weeks. The first six quarters concentrate on the major basic sciences. Courses include human anatomy for dental students, oral anatomy, community dentistry, restorative dentistry, periodontology, behavioral factors, orientation and history of dentistry, dental biochemistry, removable complete prosthodontics, orthodontics, microbiology, pharmacology, advanced physiology, oral radiology, physical evaluation, oral and physical evaluation, endodontics, local anesthesiology, oral microbiology, and orthodontic technique. The third and fourth years concentrate on the clinical facets of these courses. Clinical experience is gained in college, hospital, and remote-site clinics. Ten credit hours in approved elective courses must be completed for graduation certification.

Facilities

Graduate and professional housing is available, and family housing is available at Buckeye Village. The office of dental career opportunities assists students and graduates in finding practice locations. The learning resources center has material to supplement the dentistry curriculum. The main library has a mechanized information center that provides computer-based literature searches. The Health Sciences Library contains more than 169,000 volumes and 1,908 scientific journals and indexes. About 2,000 books and 200 journals pertain to dentistry in particular.

Grading Procedures

The College of Dentistry uses a letter grading system of evaluation (A = 4, B = 3, C = 2, D = 1, E = 0). Students must earn a minimum GPA of 2.0 during the professional program to be eligible for graduation.

Special Programs

Postgraduate studies include a two-year program in dental anesthesiology, a 24-month program in endodontics, a three-year program in oral pathology, a four-year program in oral and maxillofacial surgery, a 36-month program in orthodontics, a 24-month program in pediatric dentistry, a 36-month program in periodontics, and a 24-month program in prosthodontics. Study with a view towards an advanced academic degree is optional in these programs, with the exception of orthodontics and periodontics.

Application Procedures

Applications must be filed first with the American Association of Dental Schools Application Service (AADSAS). Those candidates who qualify will be sent a university application. Applications may be accepted until the first day of classes, but most admissions decisions are made by spring quarter of the preceding school year. The DAT must be taken within two years of the application filing period. One letter of recommendation must be from a college faculty member whose class the student has taken or from a college professional committee, whose report includes anecdotal comments from faculty members who have taught the student.

Contact

Admissions Office
Ohio State University College of Dentistry
Third Floor Lincoln Tower
1800 Cannon Drive
Columbus, Ohio 43210-1200
(614) 292-3980

UNIVERSITY OF OKLAHOMA COLLEGE OF DENTISTRY

Oklahoma City, Oklahoma 73190
(405) 271-5444

Accreditation	ADA, CDA
Degrees Offered	D.D.S.
# Students Applied	203
Enrollment	50 / class
Mean GPA	3.18
% Men / % Women	64% / 36%
% Minorities	20%
Tuition	$4,860 In-State
	$12,060 Out-of-State
Application Fee	$10 In-State, $15 Out-of-State
Application Deadline	March 1

The University

The University of Oklahoma was founded in 1890, 17 years before Oklahoma became a state. The main campus, which includes the colleges of arts and sciences, education, law, and business administration, is located in Norman. The Health Sciences Center is the state's main educational resource for training physicians, dentists, nurses, pharmacists, public health specialists, and a wide range of allied health professionals. Approximately 3,000 students are enrolled at the center. The Graduate College serves the Oklahoma City campus and the Tulsa campus.

Admissions

Preference is given to residents of Oklahoma. A minimum GPA of 2.0 is required, although most applicants for admission have earned a considerably higher GPA. Mean GPAs of a recent class are 3.18 (total) and 3.08 (science). Mean DAT scores are 15.5 (academic) and 16.4 (PAT).

Undergraduate Preparation

A minimum of 60 semester hours of coursework from an accredited college or university is required for admission. Many applicants have completed a bachelor's degree. At least eight semester hours each (including laboratory work) of biology, inorganic chemistry, organic chemistry, and physics are required for admission. Six semester hours of English are also required. Recommended electives include scientific writing, psychology, sociology, business management, and public speaking. Advanced studies in the biological sciences are also encouraged. A minimum grade of C is required for each prerequisite course.

Some colleges will award a bachelor of science degree following the completion of the first year in the College of Dentistry to students who have completed at least 90 semester hours in their predental programs. Interested students should request information from the appropriate officials at their predental college or university.

Student Body

Of the 50 members of a recent entering class, 18 were women and 10 were minorities. All but six were Oklahoma residents, and 30 had attained at least an undergraduate degree.

Costs

Basic annual tuition for a resident of Oklahoma amounts to $4,860. For a nonresident, tuition amounts to $12,060. Costs for laboratory instruments during the first year are estimated to be $3,700. Second-year expenses are estimated to be between $2,200 and $2,500. During the third year, these expenses are approximately $350. Fourth-year students should have no expenses for laboratory instruments. The first- and second-year costs for textbooks and uniforms are estimated at about $1,000 and $800, respectively. During the final two years, these costs average about $400 per year. Tuition costs and fees are subject to change.

Financial Aid

Financial aid is available from federal, state, and private sources. Some scholarships and grants are administered by the university. During the 1989-90 academic year, 95.5 percent of the dental students received some form of financial aid.

Student Organizations

Elected members of the student representation committees serve with voting rights on the admissions committee appeals board, the clinic policies committee, the curriculum committee, the instrument committee, the student clinic governance committee, and the academic misconduct board. Organizations available to dental students include the Staples Society (a community service organization), the Dental Student Council, the Student American Dental Association, and the Council of Students of the American Association of Dental Schools.

Curriculum

The dental studies program demands a large commitment of time. In addition to the traditional two semesters of each academic year, students participate in four additional weeks of instruction during the first and second year and also provide patient care in a 10-week summer session following the third year. Instruction is provided in the basic biological sciences, behavioral sciences, and clinical dental sciences.

The first year includes the basic biological sciences, em-

phasizing the basic structure and function of the human body. The first in a series of human behavior courses is introduced. Students begin patient care in the first year. Second-year students study the processes of disease and infection, and more advanced instruction is given in the clinical disciplines. The student assumes more responsibilities for patient care. In the third year, more than half of the student's time is spent providing dental care to patients. The student also receives instruction in the basic, clinical, behavioral, and social sciences. Students work in collaborative groups. The fourth year consists mostly of patient care, and the correlation of the basic, behavioral, and social sciences as well as the effective and efficient management of dental services. A five-week rotation or special preceptorship in private offices and/or institutions is required. Some students are given the opportunity to pursue elective study to concentrate on further development of knowledge and skills in selective clinical specialties, or to engage in research.

Facilities

The basic sciences education building is equipped with multidisciplinary laboratories which are designed for small group instruction in the basic sciences. Preclinical technique instruction takes place in a laboratory which is designed to simulate working at chairside.

Dental clinical instruction takes place in the dental clinical sciences building, which provides 180 general practice operatories for student use as well as additional operatories for oral diagnosis, radiography, oral surgery, pedodontics, periodontics, and graduate programs.

Grading Procedures

A letter grading system is used.

Application Procedures

The University of Oklahoma College of Dentistry participates in the American Association of Dental Schools Application Service (AADSAS). Applications may be submitted while the candidate is working toward completion of one or more of the required courses. Candidates are urged to apply early. Applications should be submitted between July 1 of the year preceding planned enrollment and March 1 of the year of planned enrollment. Selected applicants will be invited for a personal interview. Travel expenses are the responsibility of the applicant. The DAT is required and should be taken during the spring of the year preceding planned enrollment.

Applications should include an application fee of $15, letters of recommendation from a preprofessional advisory committee or two science instructors, a DAT transcript, official transcripts from each postsecondary institution attended, and a recent wallet-sized photo. These items should be mailed directly to the office of admissions.

Contact

Office of Admissions
College of Dentistry
University of Oklahoma
PO Box 26901
Oklahoma City, Oklahoma 73190
(405) 271-3530

OREGON HEALTH SCIENCES UNIVERSITY SCHOOL OF DENTISTRY

611 South West Campus Drive
Portland, Oregon 97201-3097
(503) 279-8801

Accreditation	CDA
Degrees Offered	D.M.D.
# Students Applied	325
Enrollment	67 / class
Mean GPA	3.3
% Men / % Women	82% / 18%
% Minorities	13%
Tuition	$3,510 In-State
	$8,610 Out-of-State
Application Fee	$40
Application Deadline	November 15

The University

The Oregon Health Sciences University School of Dentistry was founded in 1945 through an act of the Oregon legislature, which incorporated the facilities of the North Pacific College of Oregon into the Oregon State System of Higher Education. In 1974, the University of Oregon schools of dentistry, medicine, and nursing were unified as the Oregon Health Sciences University.

The Portland metropolitan area has a population of 1.3 million, and offers a wide variety of cultural and recreational activities. An annual jazz festival and world-class zoo add additional attraction. Ocean beaches and the coastal range are about 90 minutes away.

Admissions

Priority is given to Oregon residents first, followed by residents of the Western states participating in the WICHE program second, residents of the United States and Canada third, and foreign residents fourth. When evaluating the applicant, the admissions committee considers performance on the DAT compared with the science GPA, letters of recommendation, and interest and knowledge about the profession of dentistry. Of the students accepted to the 1989-90 entering class, the mean DAT score (academic) was 17, the mean PAT was 18. Both the mean total GPA and the mean science GPA were 3.3. Transfer students will be considered on an individual basis depending upon available space. Foreign-trained transfer students will be considered if they qualify as residents of the state of Oregon.

Undergraduate Preparation

Applicants must have completed at least 60 semester hours (90 quarter hours) of college-level coursework. At least 45 credit hours must have been earned at an accredited four-year institution. A one-year sequence of each of the following courses is required (including necessary laboratory work): general chemistry, general biology/zoology, and general physics. Six semester hours of organic chemistry are also required. The minimum amount of English composition required by the student's predental college will fulfill the English composition requirement. Electives should include additional biological science courses, such as anatomy and physiology, cell biology, and biochemistry, as well as courses in the social sciences and the humanities.

Student Body

Of the 67 members of the 1989-90 entering class, 34 were residents of Oregon, six were students funded by WICHE, 26 were from out of state, and one was from a foreign country. Sixteen had completed three years of college, and 44 had completed a bachelor's degree. Two had completed a master's degree. Twelve were women and nine were minority students.

Costs

Tuition and fees are subject to change. Tuition (per year) for a resident student (or a student from one of the states that participate in the WICHE program) amounts to $3,510. For a nonresident student, tuition amounts to $8,610. General fees, including instruments and books, are estimated to cost $5,767.

Financial Aid

Financial aid is available from a variety of federal, state, and private offices. Limited work opportunities are also available. All students accepted to the School of Dentistry will be mailed an application for an OHSU scholarship, to be completed before March 1. Applicants who plan to apply for financial aid should complete a financial aid form (available at any college or university financial aid office) and send it to the College Scholarship Service. These forms should be completed between January 1 and March 1 of the year of planned enrollment. The financial aid form should be completed before an offer of acceptance from the School of Dentistry is received. Applicants selected as alternates should also complete a financial aid form before March 1.

Minority Programs

The Disadvantaged Student Recruitment Program considers motivated and qualified applicants from underrepresented minority groups for admission. For further information, contact the assistant dean for admissions and student affairs at (503) 494-5274.

Student Organizations

Organizations of special interest to dental students include: the All-Hill Council and the Associated Students of the School of Dentistry (the student government association), the American Student Dental Association, the American Society of Dentistry for Children, and the American Association of Women Dentists. Nationally recognized dental fraternities with branches on campus include Omicron Kappa Upsilon, Delta Sigma Delta, Psi Omega, and Xi Psi Phi.

Faculty

There are 929 full-time and 583 part-time faculty members. An additional 1,614 community health professionals volunteer their time and skills to university programs. Most faculty members are involved in research and patient care in addition to their teaching responsibilities.

Curriculum

The curriculum is designed to help students prepare for careers in general dentistry. The sequence in which subject matter is taught is coordinated by the various biological science and preclinical technique departments. Some subjects are organized into conjoint courses, which are taught cooperatively by several departments.

The first two years consist of the basic sciences and preclinical techniques. During a first-year course dealing with the prevention of dental disease, students see their first patient. Behavioral science and public health aspects of dentistry are studied during the second year. The third and fourth years consist mostly of clinical practice, and include courses in practice planning and management. Students gain experience by treating patients in the dental clinics. Development of ethical standards of practice, opportunities for community service,

and elective courses are also presented during the last two years.

Facilities

The School of Dentistry houses the dental clinics, classrooms, microcomputers available for student use, and student laboratories. The building includes a modern clinic where about 12,000 outpatients are seen yearly by undergraduate and advanced education students. The main clinic areas contain 200 dental work stations, and individual X-ray rooms are available. The campus libraries contain 198,560 volumes of books, bound and unbound periodicals, and subscribe to 2,187 current periodicals. The library participates in an active interlibrary loan service.

Student housing is available.

Grading Procedures

A letter grading system is used. To be promoted from one year to the next, a student must have achieved a GPA (in most classes) of at least 2.0. Students take Part I of the National Board Examinations of the ADA in July after the sophomore year, and Part II in December of the senior year.

Special Programs

An optional fifth-year fellow program is available. Selected students will have an opportunity to practice for one year after graduation in successful general dental offices in Oregon to gain additional business and clinical expertise.

Students entering without a bachelor's degree may earn their degree if it is granted by the predental school or university. Students who intend to use School of Dentistry courses to complete their baccalaureate degree should consult with their faculty advisors.

Application Procedures

The School of Dentistry participates in AADSAS. Application materials must be received between June 1 and November 15 of the year preceding anticipated enrollment. An application fee of $40 is due upon request for additional materials. The DAT must be taken by October of the application year. There is no minimum score requirement. Interviews are arranged by invitation of the admissions committee.

Contact

Director of Admissions
School of Dentistry
611 South West Campus Drive
Portland, Oregon 97201-3097
(503) 494-5274

UNIVERSITY OF THE PACIFIC SCHOOL OF DENTISTRY

San Francisco, California 94115
(415) 929-6464

Accreditation	CDA
Degrees Offered	D.D.S.
# Students Applied	549
Enrollment	120 / class
Mean GPA	2.77
% Men / % Women	70% / 30%
% Minorities	30%
Tuition	$29,100
Application Fee	$35
Application Deadline	March 1

The University

The School of Dentistry of the University of the Pacific was incorporated in 1896 as the College of Physicians and Surgeons. In 1962, the College of Physicians and Surgeons joined with the University of the Pacific, and a nine-story building was completed in 1967 for the teaching of clinical dentistry and conducting of dental research. The alumni association provided a 12-operatory dental clinic in 1973.

The university is located in the heart of San Francisco, a picturesque yet cosmopolitan city. Many cultural and recreational activities are available.

Admissions

Admission to the School of Dentistry is competitive. First consideration is given to applicants with an overall GPA of at least 2.8. Transfer students are admitted only under special circumstances. No student will be admitted to advanced standing beyond the second year. Mean DAT scores for a recent entering class are 4.32 (academic) and 4.82 (PAT). Mean GPAs are 2.77 (overall) and 2.61 (science).

Undergraduate Preparation

Applicants must have completed at least 90 semester units (135 quarter units) at an accredited university or college. Thirty semester units (45 quarter units) must be completed at an accredited four-year institution. Completion of the following courses, including necessary laboratory work, is required: eight semester hours each of biology (or zoology), general physics, inorganic chemistry, and organic chemistry. The school also requires the completion of six semester hours of English composition; three semester hours of another English course may be substituted for composition.

Preference is given to candidates who will have completed a bachelor's degree at the time of matriculation. For those with a B.S. degree, a minor in English, philosophy, political science, or humanities is recommended. Pass/fail grades in required courses are unacceptable.

Student Body

Among the 120 members of the 1989 entering class there were 40 women and 47 minorities (mostly Asian Pacific Islanders). Fifty-eight percent had undergraduate degrees, and 81 percent were state residents.

Costs

Tuition amounts to $29,100 for the first year, $30,300 for the second year, and $31,500 for the third year. Tuition for the international dental studies D.D.S. degree program amounts to $27,894 for the first year and $29,200 for the second year. General fees (including instruments) amount to approximately $9,355 for the first year, $1,835 for the second year, and $1,163 for the third year. Tuition and fees are subject to change.

Financial Aid

Financial aid is awarded on the basis of need and/or ability. It is available from a variety of federal, state, and private sources. Applicants needing financial aid of any kind must contact the financial aid office at the School of Dentistry for applications by December of the year preceding admission. Students from Alaska, Hawaii, Idaho, Montana, Nevada, New Mexico, North Dakota, and Wyoming may be eligible for funds offered by the Western Interstate Commission for Higher Education (WICHE), and should contact their state's WICHE representative by September of the year preceding admission.

Student Organizations

Organizations of special interest to dental students include the American Student Dental Association, the California Dental Association, and the American Association of Dental Schools, as well as chapters of Omicron Kappa Upsilon and Tau Kappa Omega.

Curriculum

The academic year begins in July and is divided into 13-week quarters consisting of 10 weeks of instruction, an examination week, and two weeks of vacation. The program combines three major areas of instruction: basic sciences, preventive and community services, and preclinical/clinical sciences. The first year consists of the basic sciences and the teaching of preclinical skills, which are used with clinical patients in each major discipline, including dental radiology, endodontics, fixed prosthodontics, operative dentistry, oral diagnosis, and treatment planning. Preventive dentistry is taught in all four years of study. During the second and third years, students learn to provide comprehensive dental care to assigned patients. In the third year, students learn to provide dental care in community clinics, and are involved in community screenings and rotations at Laguna Honda Hospital and various senior citizens centers throughout the city. They also participate in health fair activities.

Facilities

A nine-story building on campus provides space for teaching clinical dentistry and conducting dental research. The university purchased and renovated a building within seven blocks of the school to help meet student needs for housing at a reasonable cost. The facility houses 252 residents in 66 apartments, and provides a contemporary dental technique laboratory and a physical fitness center for residents. Through the extramural clinic program, students provide dental care (under faculty supervision) in selected northern California community clinics, which resemble private practice settings.

Limited student housing is available for single and married students.

Grading Procedures

A letter grading system is used. Students who are in academic good standing are automatically recommended for promotion by the student academic performance and promotions committee.

Special Programs

The international dental studies curriculum offers qualified graduates of foreign dental programs the opportunity to earn the doctor of dental surgery degree. This 24-month program provides training in dental techniques as practiced in the United States.

The school also offers a five-year honors program leading to the D.D.S. degree and a six-year program leading to baccalaureate/D.D.S. degrees.

Application Procedures

The university participates in the American Association of Dental Schools Application Service (AADSAS). The completed AADSAS application material must be received by AADSAS no later than March 1. Applicants must have taken the DAT no later than April to qualify for the class entering in July. The School of Dentistry requires a $35 application fee, which is in addition to and separate from the AADSAS fee. Interviews are required and are arranged by invitation of the admissions committee.

Contact

Office of Admissions
School of Dentistry
The University of the Pacific
2155 Webster Street
San Francisco, California 94115
(415) 929-6400

UNIVERSITY OF PENNSYLVANIA SCHOOL OF DENTAL MEDICINE

4001 Spruce Street
Philadelphia, Pennsylvania 19104-6003
(215) 898-5000

Accreditation	CDA
Degrees Offered	D.M.D., D.M.D./M.B.A., D.M.D./M.D., D.M.D./Ph.D.
# Students Applied	495
Enrollment	80 / class
Mean GPA	3.07
% Men / % Women	65% / 35%
% Minorities	25%
Tuition	$21,210
Application Fee	$35
Application Deadline	February 1

The University

The University of Pennsylvania's School of Dental Medicine is one of the oldest university-affiliated dental institutions in the country. Since 1878 it has served as the teaching stage for scientist, diagnostician, clinician, artist, engineer, teacher, business manager, and all of the many roles that the profession of dentistry demands. The university dental school was funded in 1897 by the estate of Thomas W. Evans, a brilliant dentist to the courts of Europe during France's Second Empire. The name was officially changed from the Thomas W. Evans Museum and Dental Institute to the School of Dental Medicine in 1964. Located in the heart of Philadelphia, the school is surrounded by a metropolis of entertaining and educational resources. Along the banks of the Schuylkill River students can enjoy the famed South Street marketplace, the U.S. Mint, and Independence Park. The city also offers performances in theater, opera, the Philadelphia Orchestra, professional sports, and museums.

Admissions

The admissions committee evaluates applicants on their level of performance in academic courses, participation in worthy extracurricular activities, and community involvement. Students are required to take the DAT test preferably in the spring of the junior year. In addition, applicants must submit their scores from the American Dental Association admission test.

Undergraduate Preparation

Students are encouraged to have a broad educational background. Applicants with a four-year college degree are most desirable, however, thoughtful consideration will be given to applicants who are strongly motivated. Minimum course requirements for admission are: three semesters of chemistry, including inorganic chemistry and a complete course in organic chemistry with lab; two semesters of biology or zoology with lab that includes mammalian dissection; a two-semester course in physics covering introductory atomic theory, radioactivity, and electronics; one year of English; one semester of college mathematics (students should be comfortable with advanced quantitative data; calculus is preferred). Recommended courses include elementary biochemistry, additional organic chemistry and physical chemistry, anatomy, physiology, and genetics. A well-rounded academic background that includes coursework in the humanities, social sciences, the arts, and physical education is favored. The dental school will accept placement credits that were accepted by the undergraduate college toward fulfillment of degree requirements, if these credits are clearly indicated on the college transcripts.

Student Body

Geographically, the vast majority of students come from the Pennsylvania-New York-New Jersey region. The remaining enrollees are primarily California, Connecticut, and Massachusetts residents. As many as 30 may come from foreign countries. The current total enrollment of 368 consists of 251 male and 117 female students.

Costs

For the 1989-90 school year, first-year students paid a tuition of $20,210. Second-, third-, and fourth-year students paid $19,590. Additional D.M.D. general fees (which include the student health service) ran $664 each year. Four-objective microscopes are available to all students taking certain courses for a rental fee of $25. Instruments required for the first year of study cost $5,800; for the second year, $2,800. Books cost $840 the first two years and $760 the last two years.

Financial Aid

Federally-funded, campus-based loan programs and grants from the School of Dental Medicine are the two forms of financial assistance available to D.M.D. students. Students must submit financial aid applications every year to be considered for the aid awards that are granted. The student's need is determined by the information on the Graduate and Professional School Financial Aid Service (GAPSFAS) application. Inquiries should be sent to the School of Dental Medicine, office of student affairs or the student financial information center. Some of the available loans include the National Direct Student Loans and the Health Professions Loans.

Student Organizations

Single and married graduates who are able to make positive contributions to undergraduate life are recruited by the residential life staff, which organizes a counseling and older brother/sister group for new students.

Faculty

There are close to 260 professional staff members on the School of Dental Medicine faculty. This makes a student/faculty ratio of less than 2:1.

Curriculum

The first and second years of study are oriented toward developing competence in the fundamental sciences governing human biology and the normal structure and function of the oral cavity. Competencies basic to general practice include biochemistry, histology/embryology, orthodontics, and microbiology. The third and fourth years emphasize the continued development in therapeutics and general patient care. The approach to master clinician includes the continued study of orthodontics, endodontics, and over 500 hours of restorative dentistry, in addition to a hospital extramural assignment.

Facilities

The School of Dental Medicine has affiliations with several clinical facilities and learning centers. The general dentistry clinic has been completely rehabilitated since 1984. Additional facilities include the microbiological testing laboratory, microcomputer program, implant dentistry treatment center, periodontal diseases research center, center for research in oral biology, the clinical research center, and the Melvin Page Oral Medicine Diagnostic Clinic and Laboratory. One of the world's most complete collections of dental literature is housed in the Leon Levy Library, which contains approximately 42,000 volumes of periodicals and monographs on dental medicine.

Special Programs

A special bio-dental consortial program leads to a combined bachelor/dental degree through the College of Arts and Sciences of the University of Pennsylvania, Rennselaer Polytechnic Institute, Muhlenberg College, Villanova University, and Lehigh University. The program normally requires seven years to complete. Additional combined degree programs include the D.M.D./M.B.A., M.D./D.M.D. (oral and maxillofacial surgery), and the D.M.D./Ph.D. degrees.

Application Procedures

The School of Dental Medicine participates in the American Association of Dental Schools Application Service (AADSAS). Students should apply no later than February 1 preceding the calendar year in which admission is desired. There is a nonrefundable application fee of $35. One letter of recommendation from the applicant's undergraduate predental advisory committee, or, if the school has no such committee, one letter each from a biological science professor and a chemistry or physics instructor. High school transcripts, SAT scores, and scores from the dental aptitude test must be forwarded by March 1. The admissions committee reserves the right to request interviews with selected applicants.

Contact

Office of Admissions
School of Dental Medicine
University of Pennsylvania
4001 Spruce Street
Philadelphia, Pennsylvania 19104-6003
(215) 898-5570

UNIVERSITY OF PITTSBURGH SCHOOL OF DENTAL MEDICINE

Pittsburgh, Pennsylvania 15260
(412) 648-8900

Accreditation	AADS, CDE, CDA
Degrees Offered	D.D.S.
# Students Applied	335
Enrollment	75 / class
Mean GPA	2.96
% Men / % Women	73% / 27%
% Minorities	Not Available.
Tuition	$13,940 In-State
	$19,700 Out-of-State
Application Fee	$25
Application Deadline	March 1

The University

Founded in 1787, the University of Pittsburgh is a private, nonsectarian educational institution located on 125 acres in the city's Oakland district. The School of Dental Medicine was founded in 1896 by four dentists, a physician, and a pharmacist. It was moved to its present location in 1912.

The Oakland community offers a wide variety of cultural activities, including a museum of natural history and the Carnegie Music Hall. Many recreational activities are available at Schenley Park, with 500 acres of wooded land and facilities for ice skating, tennis, golf, ball games, riding, and picnicking. Downtown Pittsburgh is five minutes away by bus or auto.

Admissions

All candidates are seriously considered for admission. Nontraditional candidates are encourage to send resumes, certificates, letters from employers, and/or publications to support their applications. Applications for advanced standing from students who are in good academic and disciplinary standing from another accredited dental program will be considered. Transfer students may be required to take written and/or practical examinations to determine where they will be placed in the curriculum.

Undergraduate Preparation

Applicants should have completed at least 90 semester hours at an accredited college with an overall and science GPA above 2.0. Preference is given to applicants who have completed a bachelor's degree. The following courses are required: English (six semester hours), biology (eight semester hours, including laboratories), physics (eight semester hours), general chemistry (six semester hours), and organic chemistry (six semester hours). The School of Dental Medicine requires laboratories in biology, but strongly recommends laboratories in the other sciences as well. Most required coursework should have been completed at a four-year college. Proficiency in written and spoken English is required.

Student Body

Nineteen of the 72 members of the graduating class of 1993 are women, 10 are from out of state, and 40 had earned baccalaureate degrees prior to matriculation. The mean DAT score (academic) was 4.39; the mean DAT (PAT) was 4.15. The mean GPA was 2.96 (overall) and 2.88 (science).

Costs

Tuition and fees are subject to change. The tuition (per year) for a resident student amounts to $13,940. A nonresident pays $19,700 in tuition. Living expenses amount to approximately $9,000 for one year. The costs of various fees, books, and supplies for the first year are approximately $7,860; for the second year, $3,880; for the third year, $1,230; and for the fourth year, $1,710.

Financial Aid

Financial aid is available from a variety of federal, state, and private offices. Loans and scholarships are awarded on the basis of need and/or ability. The Graduate and Professional Student Financial Aid Service (GAPSFAS) form is used to determine need.

Minority Programs

Information about minority programs is available from the Office of Affirmative Action, 901 William Pitt Union, University of Pittsburgh, Pittsburgh, PA 15260; Telephone: (412) 648-7860.

Student Organizations

Organizations of interest to dental students include the American Student Dental Association, the Student National Dental Association, the American Association of Women Dental Students, the Student American Society of Dentistry for Children, and chapters of Psi Omega and Delta Sigma Delta.

Curriculum

The importance of integrating basic scientific knowledge with clinical skills is stressed. Conditions of dental practice are simulated in clinical instruction. Clinical skills are taught in a developmental sequence (child, young adult, etc.). Students learn about interprofessional relations through work with oral hygienists and dental technicians.

The first year consists of basic sciences and clinical experience. First-year students examine, record findings, and perform some techniques for one another. The second year includes basic sciences, and the assignment of their first clinical patients in the winter term. Many elective clinical programs are offered in the third and fourth years. Students are encouraged to generate projects for elective study. A series of hospital externships and extramural assignments are available.

Facilities

Salk Hall, home of the School of Dental Medicine, contains clinical operatories, offices, lecture halls, and the Edward J. Forrest Continuing Education Auditorium. The Maurice and Lena Falk Library of the Health Professions contains approximately 200,000 volumes and receives more than 3,000 periodicals. The combined university libraries contain more than one million volumes. Reference material on almost any technical subject may be obtained by interlibrary loan.

Student housing is available.

Application Procedures

The school participates in the American Association of Dental Schools Application Service. Candidates are encouraged to complete AADSAS paperwork before November 1 of the year before planned enrollment. After the AADSAS packet is received, further data and a $25 application fee are requested. Three letters of recommendation (or a compilation from the preprofessional advisory committee) and transcripts of high school and college activity may be sent to the school before the AADSAS packet is received. The DAT should be taken in the spring or fall of the year before planned matriculation. Interviews are not always required for admission, although a visit to the School of Dental Medicine is strongly recommended.

Contact

Office of Admissions
School of Dental Medicine
345 Salk Hall
University of Pittsburgh
Pittsburgh, Pennsylvania 15261
(412) 648-8424 or (800) 833-3204

UNIVERSITY OF PUERTO RICO SCHOOL OF DENTISTRY

San Juan, Puerto Rico 00936
(809) 758-2525, ext. 1800

Accreditation	ADA
Degrees Offered	D.M.D, M.S.D.
# Students Applied	97
Enrollment	250
Mean GPA	3.25
% Men / % Women	50% / 50%
% Minorities	Not Available
Tuition	$2,500
Application Fee	$15
Application Deadline	December 15

The University

The University of Puerto Rico is a state-supported university system. The University of Puerto Rico Medical Sciences Campus has its roots in the establishment of the School of Tropical Medicine in 1926. In the late 1940s, the School of Medicine was created, and, in 1956, the School of Dentistry was established. Today, the campus comprises programs not only in medicine and dentistry but in pharmacy, public health, and health-related professions.

Admissions

The minimum GPA for admission is 2.0, both in general coursework and required science coursework. The admissions committee also considers changes in the undergraduate GPA, breadth of educational experience, letters of recommendation, and DAT scores. The entering class of 1990 had average DAT scores (both the academic average and PAT average) of 16 and a general mean GPA of 3.25. The school gives preference to residents of Puerto Rico.

Undergraduate Preparation

Candidates for admission must have completed at least 90 semester hours (or 135 quarter hours) of undergraduate coursework. Undergraduate courses must include 12 semester hours of Spanish, leading to fluency; 12 semester hours of English; eight semester hours each of zoology, biology, physics, inorganic chemistry, and organic chemistry, all with lab. Six semester hours of social and behavioral sciences are also required. These courses must be completed before the end of the second semester of the year of enrollment.

Student Body

The School of Dentistry enrolls about 250 students. Of the 39 students enrolled in the entering class of 1990, 20 were women. Twenty-six members of the class held college degrees. The average age of the class was 22. All students were residents of Puerto Rico.

Costs

Tuition for Puerto Rican residents is $2,500 per year. Books, instruments, and supplies are estimated to cost about $4,000 for the first year. Housing is estimated to cost about $2,500 per year.

Financial Aid

Legislative scholarships can be obtained by dental students who agree by contract to provide one year of professional service to the Commonwealth Government of Puerto Rico, its municipalities or instrumentalities. There is also a Legislative Loan program, which can be repaid by professional service. Other financial aid programs include Health Professions Loan Program, National Direct Student Loan Program, Bank Loan with Federal Guarantee Program, Health Education Assistance Loan Program, and college work-study program.

Student Organizations

The campus has a chapter of the Student American Dental Association. In 1961, the Beta Gamma Chapter of the honorary dental professional fraternity Omicron Kappa Upsilon was established at the school.

Faculty

There are about 100 faculty members of various ranks at the School of Dentistry.

Curriculum

The curriculum is geared toward educating practitioners fully qualified to serve the oral health needs of the Puerto Rican community, and is organized into four areas: basic biological sciences, basic dental sciences, the clinical program, and a program of electives.

The basic biological sciences include human anatomy, biochemistry and nutrition, physiology, dental anatomy, and general pathology. The basic dental sciences include courses related to restorative, ecological (behavioral and social), and surgical sciences. Clinical experience is obtained at the school and at affiliated hospitals. The elective part of the program consists of at least 12 credit hours taken in the junior and senior years. Elective courses include: advanced oral surgery, periodontics occlusion seminar, implant dentistry, and geriatric dentistry.

Facilities

The School of Dentistry occupies about 81,600 square feet of space in the main building of the Medical Sciences Campus. There are 123 dental units and chairs for individual clinical skills training. The freshman and sophomore multidisciplinary laboratories are designed to accommodate 66 students. Facilities also include specialty clinics in various areas such as orthodontics, oral surgery, and pediatric dentistry. The library collection totals over 110,000 volumes, including medical periodicals, monographs, and textbooks. A range of nonprint materials are also available. Library services include interlibrary loans and computer literature search capabilities.

Grading Procedures

The school uses a letter grading system: A, B, C, D, and F.

Special Programs

The school offers a Master of Science in Dentistry (M.S.D.) in oral and maxillofacial surgery (36 months) and in pediatric dentistry (24 months). The school also offers a certificate program in these fields.

Application Procedures

The University of Puerto Rico School of Dentistry participates in AADSAS. AADSAS applications must be filed by December 15 of the year prior to the year of intended enrollment. The DAT must have been taken by this date. Candidates must submit the official undergraduate transcript, a photograph, and evaluation forms from undergraduate institutions directly to the school. There is a $15 application fee.

Contact

University of Puerto Rico
Medical Sciences Campus
School of Dentistry
Office of Admissions
GPO Box 5067
San Juan, Puerto Rico 00936
(809) 758-2525, ext. 5212

UNIVERSITY OF SOUTHERN CALIFORNIA SCHOOL OF DENTISTRY

Los Angeles, California 90089-0641
(213) 743-2811

Accreditation	ADA, CDA
Degrees Offered	D.D.S., B.S., M.S., Ph.D.
# Students Applied	792
Enrollment	109 / class
Mean GPA	3.07
% Men / % Women	57% / 43%
% Minorities	41%
Tuition	$22,380
Application Fee	$40
Application Deadline	April 1

The University

Founded in 1897, the School of Dentistry of the University of Southern California today is held in high esteem for its teaching programs. For more than half a century, it was the only dental school south of San Francisco and west of the Rocky Mountains.

The school is a private institution that has produced many recognized leaders in the art and science of dental practice. Its affiliated hospitals include the Los Angeles County/USC Medical Center and Rancho Los Amigos Hospital.

Admissions

The school seeks a student body that is culturally and geographically diverse. As such, USC uses the same criteria for out-of-state applicants as for California residents. A strong science background is considered favorably. Students in the 1989 entering class had a mean overall GPA of 3.07 and a mean science GPA of 3.02. Mean PAT and academic DAT scores were both 16.

Undergraduate Preparation

At the time of application, candidates should have taken a minimum of 60 semester units of coursework at an accredited college or university in the U.S. or Canada. One year of each of the following courses is required for admission: general biology (with lab), inorganic chemistry (with lab), organic chemistry (with lab), general physics (with lab), English composition, and philosophy, history, or fine arts. The school strongly advises students to take additional upper-level courses

in areas such as biochemistry, human anatomy, histology, and physiology.

The DAT must be taken no later than April of the year for which application is made.

Student Body

Forty-eight of the 109 enrollees in 1989 were women; 45 comprised various minorities. About 67 percent had undergraduate degrees. All but 19 were state residents.

Costs

Annual tuition for 1990-91 is $22,380. Instruments cost $5,500 the first year and $3,500 the second year. Precious metals must be purchased the first year, which cost $1,700. Books cost about $600 the first and second years, and $50 the third year. Total financial output for the first year is approximately $30,780; for the second year, $27,116; for the third year, $23,030; and for the last year, $16,046.

Financial Aid

A large percentage of USC dental students receive some form of financial aid. Aid programs are based both on need and merit, and include state and federal financial aid assistance plans.

Curriculum

The D.D.S. program consists of 11 consecutive 14-week trimesters. The emphasis is on patient treatment throughout the curriculum, and students begin their clinical education as early as the first trimester of study. Biomedical and dental sciences are also emphasized. With its emphasis on clinical skills, the USC School of Dentistry has earned a reputation for excellence in preparing students to enter private practice.

Students gain experience in the lab and in the school's clinical facilities. Each student is supervised on a one-to-one basis and individually evaluated. Students are encouraged to participate in basic and clinical science research.

Application Procedures

USC School of Dentistry participates in AADSAS. Completed applications should be submitted to AADSAS by April 1 of the year of anticipated enrollment. Candidates must also submit the following directly to the school while applying to AADSAS: a $40 application fee, two letters of recommendation (from science professors or one preprofessional committee letter), official transcripts of all undergraduate and graduate coursework, and a passport-style photograph. DAT test scores that are more than two years old may not be acceptable.

Contact

Admissions and Student Affairs
University of Southern California
School of Dentistry, Room 124
University Park-MC0641

Los Angeles, California 90089-0641
(213) 743-2841

SOUTHERN ILLINOIS UNIVERSITY SCHOOL OF DENTAL MEDICINE

2800 College Avenue
Alton, Illinois 62002-9918
(618) 463-3920

Accreditation	ADA
Degrees Offered	D.M.D., B.S./D.M.D.
# Students Applied	206
Enrollment	49 / class
Mean GPA	2.93
% Men / % Women	70% / 30%
% Minorities	25%
Tuition	$3,100 In-State
	$9,300 Out-of-State
Application Fee	$20
Application Deadline	April 1

The University

Southern Illinois University has two campuses, the main campus at Edwardsville and one in Carbondale. The School of Dental Medicine itself is located in Alton, 15 miles northwest of Edwardsville and 30 minutes from St. Louis. Transportation to the Edwardsville campus is available; there, dental students have access to all university facilities. The School of Dental Medicine was founded in 1969 and now enrolls 200 of the university's 35,000 students. The city of St. Louis boasts many activities, such as riverboat drama, Six Flags Over Mid America amusement park, a zoo, art museum, botanical gardens, opera, theater, the city symphony, and much more.

Admissions

The first-year class at the School of Dental Medicine generally numbers about 50 students. Scores from the October 1987 DAT test are the earliest the school will accept. Of the 1989 entering class, the mean DAT scores were 3.90 for the academic portion and 4.45 for the PAT portion. Mean GPA scores were 2.82 for science and 2.93 overall.

Undergraduate Preparation

School of Dental Medicine students must have completed at least two academic years of undergraduate coursework. These courses must include six semester hours each of inorganic chemistry, biology or zoology, and physics; four semester hours of organic chemistry (although six semester hours are preferred); and six semester hours of coursework in English. All science courses must include lab work.

Student Body

Of the 49 students enrolled in the 1989 entering class, 29 percent were women and about 25 percent were minorities. Students ranged in age from 20 to 37, with 25 being the mean age. Forty-one percent had an undergraduate degree, and 71 percent were residents of Illinois.

Placement Records

An active professional placement service assists students in choosing and pursing post-graduate interests. Traditionally, about half of the dental school's new graduates enter private practice. Another one-fourth continue education in graduate residency and specialty programs; others pursue options including military or public health service, dental research, dental education, and government service.

Costs

Annual tuition totals $3,100 for Illinois residents and $9,300 for nonresidents. Fees vary from year to year. Other first-year fees, including books and instruments, total about $5,325; second-year fees, when the cost of books and instruments are reduced, total about $3,060, and third- and fourth-year fees total about $486.

Financial Aid

The School of Dental Medicine participates in the Stafford, Perkins, SLS, HEAL, and HPL loan programs. Scholarships include the Illinois General Assembly Scholarship, the Illinois Veteran's Scholarship, and awards for first-year students in "exceptional" financial need.

Student Organizations

The university's Edwardsville campus (SIUE) hosts more than 90 student organizations, clubs, and special interest groups.

Faculty

The School of Dental Medicine staffs 42 full-time faculty and 49 part-time faculty. They are active in dental research, professional dental organizations, and private practice.

Curriculum

D.M.D. candidates must complete four years of study. Students begin in the first year with basics of biomedical and clinical science, and begin direct patient care in the second year. Graduated students may also do a one-year general practice residency.

Facilities

Facilities include a recently expanded dental clinic with 72 patient care stations, a comprehensive biomedical library, and biomedical and clinical research laboratories.

Special Programs

Summer research programs are available to interested students. SIU-Edwardsville students may study for a joint B.S./ D.M.D. degree, studying preprofessionally for three years at Edwardsville and then doing professional studies at Alton.

Application Procedures

Students must apply through the AADSAS between June 1 of the year preceding entry into dental school and April 1 of the following year. The nonrefundable application fee is $20. Interviews are not required but may be granted by the school.

Contact

Office of Admissions and Records
Southern Illinois University
School of Dental Medicine
2800 College Avenue
Alton, Illinois 62002-9918
(618) 463-3864

STATE UNIVERSITY OF NEW YORK AT BUFFALO, SCHOOL OF DENTRSTRY

Buffalo, New York 14214
(716) 831-2836

Accreditation	ADA
Degrees Offered	D.D.S., M.S., Ph.D., B.S./ D.D.S., D.D.S./Ph.D., M.S./ Ph.D.
# Students Applied	451
Enrollment	80 / class
Mean GPA	3.01
% Men / % Women	80% / 20%
% Minorities	Not Available
Tuition	$5,670 In-State
	$13,070 Out-of-State
Application Fee	$50
Application Deadline	March 1

The University

The State University of New York at Buffalo is recognized as one of the nation's top public research universities. The campus became part of the State University of New York (SUNY) system in 1962. In 1989, SUNY-Buffalo was admitted to the Association of American Universities. The SUNY School of Dental Medicine was established in 1892. Its facilities for oral health education are recognized as being among the best of their kind in the nation.

Admissions

The school considers undergraduate transcripts and DAT scores as well as letters of recommendation. The school also encourages students to gain some experience in dentistry before applying for admission. High school transcripts and records of SAT scores must also be submitted. Selected candidates are asked to participate in a personal interview. The first-year class of 1989-90 had a mean GPA of 3.01 and an average academic DAT score of 16.8. In 1989-90, the school processed 451 applications. Most students admitted are residents of New York State.

Undergraduate Preparation

Applicants must have completed at least 90 credit hours of undergraduate study to be considered for admission. Baccalaureate degrees are preferred. Undergraduate coursework must include two semesters of English, two semesters each of general chemistry, general biology, organic chemistry, and general physics, all with lab.

Student Body

Of the 80 entering students for the 1989-90 school year, 26 were women and four were minorities. Sixty-seven were in-state residents.

Placement Records

In 1990, 62 percent of the graduating class went into residency training, while 67 percent went into general practice residencies. About 21 percent entered private practice, and the remaining graduates went into specialties and graduate programs or joined the armed services.

Costs

Residents of the State of New York pay an annual tuition of $5,670. Nonresidents pay $13,070. Instrument rental is estimated to cost $770 per year. The cost of supplies varies from year to year; the highest cost is about $1,500 in the second year. Affordable off-campus housing is available.

Financial Aid

The school considers students for financial aid based on financial aid transcripts from undergraduate colleges attended and on the FAF, both of which must be filed with the financial aid office.

The university and state government offer the Perkins Loan Program, college work-study program, and Tuition Assistance Program. Benefits administered by the federal government include Stafford Loans and Supplemental Loans to Students. Dental students may also qualify for Health Professions Student Loans, New York State Regents Scholarships for Professional Education (for minorities), and other programs.

Minority Programs

The university's Special Programs division handles minority affairs and is charged with making the learning environment more supportive of minority students. The university makes special efforts to financially, socially, and academically support its students from underrepresented minority groups. Enrollment for 1988-89 represented the highest-ever percentage of minorities among the SUNY at Buffalo student body.

Student Organizations

Student organizations include the American Student Dental Association and the American Association of Women Dentists. The school also has chapters of Alpha Omega and Delta Sigma Delta fraternities.

Faculty

The school's faculty comprises 92 full-time members and 86 part-time members, who hold expertise in clinical and research areas of dentistry, including many board-certified specialty areas.

Curriculum

The curriculum comprises four "core areas"—biomedical sciences, dental sciences (oral biology, oral medicine, stomatology, and interdisciplinary sciences), dental clinical disciplines, and effective practice management.

The biomedical science core courses focus on the health of the oral cavity and its interrelationships to the health and disease of other body systems. The dental science courses include those areas concerned with the masticatory system and diseases, including oral biology and oral medicine.

The focus of the dental clinical disciplines is to develop excellence in clinical application. This core area includes studies in oral radiology, operative dentistry, prosthodontics, and oral and maxillofacial surgery.

The practice management core area focuses on the efficient delivery of care and issues surrounding patient communication. Throughout the program, students are encouraged to participate in research experience as well as clerkships and summer externships. The third- and fourth-year clinical experience includes rotations at any of the school's affiliated hospitals.

Facilities

Facilities include six clinics with modern equipment created especially for the school. The Patient Evaluation and Management/Emergency Service Clinic has 15 operating positions and laboratory space.

The Basic Technique Laboratory is available to first-year students; there is also a Junior/Senior Laboratory.

State-of-the-art facilities include the Zonarc (for visualization of very thin sections of bony structure in the head and neck), laser technology, prosethetic labs, and a pain control center.

The Health Sciences Library houses more than 270,000 volumes and 2,700 series for the programs in medicine, dentistry, pharmacy, nursing, and health-related professions. The university libraries system is among the leading research libraries in North America.

Special Programs

The school has a seven-year B.S./D.D.S. combined degree program. The school offers M.S. degrees in Biomaterials, Oral Sciences, and Orthodontics, and has a multidisciplinary Ph.D. program in oral Biology.

Selected students are chosed for the joint D.D.S./Ph.D. program either as first-year students or as sophomores. This is normally a seven-year program. The school also offers certificates of proficiency in a number of specialty fields.

Application Procedures

The School of Dental Medicine participates in AADSAS. The application deadline is March 1. In addition to the

AADSAS application, students must submit directly to the school the following materials: an application fee of $50, DAT scores, high school and college transcripts, and a letter of recommendation from the undergraduate preprofessional committee.

Selected applicants are invited to visit the school and meet with faculty and students. The school also participates in an early decision plan.

Contact

State University of New York at Buffalo
Admissions Office—School of Dental Medicine
327 Squire Hall
Buffalo, New York 14214
(716) 831-2839

STATE UNIVERSITY OF NEW YORK AT STONY BROOK, SCHOOL OF DENTAL MEDICINE

Stony Brook, New York 11794
(516) 632-8950

Accreditation	ADA
Degrees Offered	D.D.S., M.S., Ph.D.
# Students Applied	302
Enrollment	28 / class
Mean GPA	3.24
% Men / % Women	57% / 43%
% Minorities	18%
Tuition	$5,550 In-State
	$12,950 Out-of-State
Application Fee	$50
Application Deadline	March 31

The University

The University at Stony Brook was founded in 1957 as a small college whose mission was to educate math and science teachers. As one of four university centers in the state university system, SUNY-Stony Brook is today recognized as one of the nation's outstanding institutions of higher learning. The university's world-class faculty attracts a high volume of feder-

ally sponsored research. SUNY is a comprehensive research university producing a high percentage of Ph.D.s.

Established in 1973, the School of Dental Medicine is one of five professional schools comprising the university's Health Sciences Center. The five schools enroll a total of 1,900 students and conduct programs of research, service, and continuing professional education.

The 1,100-acre SUNY campus is located 60 miles east of Manhattan on Long Island's wooded north shore.

Admissions

The school seeks a diverse, highly qualified student body. Selection is based on an overall appraisal of the applicant's suitability for dentistry. Factors considered in the admission process include academic achievement with competence in the sciences, letters of recommendation, manual skill, and personal qualities. Preference is given to residents of New York State. Mean DAT scores were 17.9 and 17.5 (academic and PAT, respectively); GPA means were 3.24 (overall) and 3.17 (science).

Undergraduate Preparation

Undergraduate coursework must include one year of introductory courses in inorganic chemistry, organic chemistry, physics, and general biology or zoology—all with labs; one year of mathematics (calculus or statistics); and one year of behavioral or social sciences. It is recommended that candidates for admission take the DAT no later than October of the year before the intended matriculation date.

Student Body

In the fall of 1989, student enrollment in the Health Sciences Center included about 560 undergraduates, 830 graduates, and 500 graduate professional students. Of the 28 students who matriculated in the dental school in 1989, all were state residents, and 24 had undergraduate degrees. Twelve were women and five were minority students.

Costs

New York State residents pay an annual tuition of $5,550, for a four-year total of $22,200. Nonresidents pay $12,950 per year, for a total of $51,800. Expenses, including fees, insurance, microscope rental, instrument purchase, and books, total approximately $3,000 for the first year. These costs decrease in subsequent years.

The total cost for New York State residents to attend the school of dentistry is currently estimated to be $32,500; for nonresident, $62,104.

Financial Aid

Financial aid is awarded on the basis of demonstrated need. Types of assistance include programs administered by off-campus agencies to which the student applies directly; special funds administered by the Health Sciences Center; and campus-based programs administered by the office of student services and the university office of financial aid.

These programs include Health Professions Loans, Health Education Assistance Loans, the state-funded Tuition Assistance Program, Pell Grants, New York State Health Service Corps Scholarships, and Veterans Educational Benefits. Campus-based programs include the Aid Program for part-time study, college work-study program, Educational Opportunity Program, and Perkins Loans.

Student Organizations

The school has a Sigma Tau chapter of Omicron Kappa Upsilon on campus, an honors society for high-achieving students.

Faculty

Over 2,000 professionals from the Long Island area have faculty appointments and participate in the schools of the Health Sciences Center.

Curriculum

The goal of the curriculum is to allow graduates to readily enter into general practice, advanced training for specialty practice, public health, teaching, and/or research. Dental students take about 900 hours of instruction in the basic sciences, including anatomy, biochemistry, pathology, and physiology. Dental students receive comprehensive training in the recognition of normal form and function of oral tissues and the recognition of pathologic conditions of the mouth and related structures. The student is given an education in the social and behavioral sciences as related to the practice of dentistry.

Clinical training begins in the latter part of the first year, with the major portion being taken in the third and fourth years. Students are responsible for complete care of the patients assigned to them. Students learn to obtain histories and to develop a treatment plan for the patient. Each student is introduced to patient care in a carefully controlled environment according to one's individual ability. Third- and fourth-year required courses include children's dentistry, radiology, oral facial genetics, practice development, and physiologic emergencies. During the fourth year, students take 112 hours of selective courses at the school or at one of its affiliated institutions.

Facilities

Students have access to more than 130 dental operatories similar to those used in the general practice of dentistry. The operatories allow students to work alone or together with dental auxiliary personnel as a team.

The Health Sciences Library houses approximately 237,700 volumes. The library subscribes to over 4,300 periodical and serial titles covering the fields of allied health, medicine, basic sciences, dental medicine, nursing, and social welfare.

Grading Procedures

Student performance in didactic and technique courses is evaluated using the letter grades A, B, C, D, and F. Patient care courses and seminars are graded with the letters H (honors), S (satisfactory), and U (unsatisfactory).

Special Programs

The school has postgraduate programs in orthodontics (24 months), general dentistry (one year), and dental care for the developmentally disabled (a fellowship program).

Application Procedures

The school participates in AADSAS. The deadline for submission of AADSAS applications is March 31. Students are encouraged to apply early, since acceptances are made on a rolling basis.

Applicants must arrange to have DAT scores forwarded to the school directly. A $50 application fee must be received at the school before AADSAS applications will be considered.

A required part of the application process is a letter of recommendation from the applicant's preprofessional advisory committee (or, in lieu of this letter, two letters from science faculty members may be substituted). All applicants under serious consideration will be asked to participate in a personal interview.

Contact

Office of Academic Affairs and Admission
School of Dental Medicine
SUNY at Stony Brook
Rockland Hall, South Campus
Stony Brook, New York 11794-8709
(516) 632-8980

TEMPLE UNIVERSITY SCHOOL OF DENTISTRY

3223 North Broad Street
Philadelphia, Pennsylvania 19140
(215) 787-7000

Accreditation	CDA
Degrees Offered	D.D.S., D.M.D., D.M.D./ M.B.A.
# Students Applied	800
Enrollment	100 / class
Mean GPA	Not Available
% Men / % Women	65% / 35%
% Minorities	17%
Tuition	$12,482 In-State
	$18,950 Out-of-State
Application Fee	$30
Application Deadline	March 1

The University

Founded in 1884, Temple University is today one of the nation's major higher education and research institutions. The university enrolls over 30,000 students, and its health sciences campus comprises the schools of dentistry, medicine, pharmacy, and allied health professions. Temple has campuses in the urban and suburban areas of Philadelphia and Montgomery County, Pennsylvania, as well as campuses in Italy and Japan that carry out the university's specialized foreign programs of study.

The School of Dentistry began in 1863 as the Philadelphia Dental College. Its Hospital for Oral Surgery, opened in 1878, was the first hospital in the country devoted exclusively to oral and maxillofacial surgery. The college became affiliated with Temple University in 1907.

The school is the second oldest dental school in continuous operation in the country. A multimillion-dollar, state-of-the-art clinical facility, opened in 1990, houses the most modern preclinical and clinical facilities in the nation.

Historic Philadelphia is a major northeastern city rich in recreational and cultural attractions, including the Philadelphia Zoo, the Philadelphia Museum of Art, the Opera Company of Philadelphia, and an array of major league sports teams. Philadelphia is 90 miles from New York City, 100 miles from the nation's capital, and a short drive to both the Pennsylvania Dutch country and the ocean beaches of New Jersey.

Admissions

Factors considered in the admission process include undergraduate academic record, the college or university attended, DAT scores, letters of recommendation, results of the personal interview, essay, and work experience. The admissions committee evaluates candidates also on the basis of personal characteristics and skills, including motivation, approach to problems, and human relations capability.

Undergraduate Preparation

Completion of a minimum of 60 semester hours from an accredited college or university is required for admission; however, most students have completed over 90 semester hours and preference is given to those who complete the baccalaureate degree. A minimum of six semester hours is required in each of the following subjects: biology, inorganic chemistry, organic chemistry, physics (all with laboratory), and English. A broad undergraduate education is desirable, with aptitude in the sciences. Nonscience majors are considered as well as science majors.

The DAT should be taken in the fall of the year before application, or sooner if possible. The mean PAT and academic DAT scores for the 1989 entering class were both 16.

Student Body

The student body at the School of Dentistry is extremely diverse. Approximately 40 percent of first-year students are from out of state. More than 30 states are represented. About 10 to 12 percent come from a wide range of foreign countries. In recent years, about 35 percent of the student body have been women, and 17 to 26 percent have been underrepresented minorities.

Costs

Tuition in 1990-91 for state residents is $12,482. Nonresidents pay $18,950. Books are estimated to cost about $300 annually. Instruments cost about $5,200 for the first year, with the cost decreasing significantly in subsequent years. Nearby off-campus apartments, utilities, and food are estimated to total between $350 and $500 per month.

Financial Aid

Most students are eligible for federally funded loans. Determination of need is based on analysis of the information provided by the applicant and his or her family. Applications can be obtained by contracting the financial aid office.

A limited number of scholarships are available to students with an outstanding undergraduate record (science GPA of 3.5 or better) and who have demonstrated a longstanding interest in a dental career. Special scholarships are also available for underrepresented minorities and financially disadvantaged students.

Minority Programs

The School of Dentistry actively identifies and encourages qualified minority candidates for admission. Year-round support services are available to enrolled minority and disadvantaged students.

Student Organizations

The school has chapters of the American Student Dental Association, the Student National Dental Association, and the Latin American Dental Students. Fraternities on campus include Alpha Omega and Delta Sigma Delta. Students also have the opportunity to participate in student council.

Curriculum

The curriculum is designed to provide significant experience in all phases of dental practice, and to impart the basic science knowledge and patient management skills necessary to the dental practitioner. The emphasis is on general practice, but the program also provides a foundation for careers in specialties of dentistry, dental education, and research.

The first and second years concentrate on the basic sciences and on skill development for dental practice. First- and second-year courses include biochemistry, gross anatomy, oral radiology, preventive dentistry, microbiology, periodontology, operative dentistry lecture and lab, and oral pediatrics. Patient care experience begins at the end of the second year. The last two years concentrate on providing clinical services for patients. Temple dental students have the opportunity to provide dental care for more than 20,000 patients annually, and gain exposure to many complicated procedures, such as reconstructive surgery and maxillofacial prosthetic replacement. Electives are taken over the course of the dental education.

In addition to providing routine dental care, students gain experience in providing comprehensive oral health care to patients with a wide range of disabilities. Students are assigned clinical rotations in the head and neck tumor clinic at Temple University Hospital.

Facilities

The school is equipped with laboratories, lecture halls, seminar rooms, treatment planning and audiovisual rooms, and more than 325 fully-equipped dental operatories. The university opened a new $41 million state-of-the-art clinical facility in 1990.

The dental library, located less than a block from the school of dentistry, houses a vast collection of volumes related to dentistry and regularly receives more than 200 journals. Students have access to standard dental and medical indexes and computerized databases for literature review and search. The medical school library is also conveniently located for dental students.

Special Programs

The school has graduate programs in a range of specialties, including endodontics, prosthodontics, and oral and maxillofacial surgery. A five-year D.M.D./M.B.A. program awards the joint degree from the dental school and Temple's School of Business and Management.

Application Procedures

Temple University School of Dentistry participates in AADSAS. Completed applications should be returned to AADSAS by March 1 of the year for which the application is made. About 400 students are invited to the school for personal interviews (some interviewing is routinely conducted out of state for those applicants who cannot travel to Philadelphia). About 100 students are ultimately selected for admission. Notification of acceptance is normally made by June 1 of the year in which application is made.

Contact

Office of Admissions and Student Affairs
Temple University School of Dentistry
3223 North Broad Street
Philadelphia, Pennsylvania 19140
(215) 221-2801 or 221-7663

UNIVERSITY OF TENNESSEE COLLEGE OF DENTISTRY

875 Union Avenue
Memphis, Tennessee 38163
(901) 528-6200

Accreditation	CDA
Degrees Offered	D.D.S., M.S.
# Students Applied	187
Enrollment	90 / class
Mean GPA	2.99
% Men / % Women	81% / 19%
% Minorities	10%
Tuition	$4,264 In-State
	$8,230 Out-of-State
Application Fee	$25
Application Deadline	February 28

The University

The Memphis campus of the University of Tennessee was founded in 1911. The health science center is the only comprehensive health science university in Tennessee. It provides both graduate and undergraduate education, and operates clinical and educational programs at the UT medical centers in Knoxville, Chattanooga, Nashville, and Jackson.

Memphis is a large city with a rich cultural history. Modern Memphis is a center for health science education and research, agriculture, a growing tourist industry, and an internationally renowned music and recording center. The area offers a wide variety of cultural and recreational activities.

Admissions

The university admits one class per year in August. State residents are given preference. However, 23 Arkansas students are accepted each year under formal agreement with that state. Other highly qualified nonresidents will also be considered, with preference given to children of alumni. A minimum GPA of 2.5 is required, although most students enrolled in the college have higher averages. Applicants should strive to maintain a GPA of 3.0 or higher. All applicants are required to take the DAT. A score of 15 or above is desired in each category. Very few incoming transfers are possible.

Undergraduate Preparation

A minimum of 90 semester hours (or 135 quarter hours) is required for admission. Preference is given to applicants who have earned a bachelor's degree, or who have completed the coursework required by their college to enable them to receive a bachelor's degree upon completion of the first year of dental school. The following coursework is required (including necessary laboratory work): English composition, six semester hours; general biology, eight semester hours; general chemistry, eight semester hours; organic chemistry, eight semester hours; physics, eight semester hours; and electives, 52 semester hours.

Upper-level biology courses, such as cell biology, comparative anatomy, embryology, genetics, histology, microbiology, and physiology are recommended elective courses. CLEP and other advanced placement credit will be accepted for required courses provided additional coursework (beyond the general requirements) in the same area has been completed.

Student Body

Of the 90 students who were admitted in 1989, 17 were women and nine were of minority backgrounds. Twenty-two were from states other than Tennessee or Arkansas; 41 had earned baccalaureate degrees. The age range was 20 to 39 years, with the mean age being 23.

Costs

Annual tuition for residents (from Tennessee or Arkansas) is $4,264; nonresidents pay $8,230. Fees, instruments, books, and supplies for the first year are estimated to cost $5,643; for the second year, $5,199; for the third year, $1,085; and for the fourth year, $475. All students are required to purchase a kit of instruments from the university bookstore semiannually.

Financial Aid

Financial aid is awarded based solely on need. Work-study programs are available.

Minority Programs

The office of minority affairs operates the Tennessee minority health careers program, which provides learning experiences, career awareness activities, workshops, and related opportunities to high school and college-level students from groups underrepresented in the health professions.

Student Organizations

The student government organization consists of elected officers from each of the colleges, who serve as the official liaison between the chancellor and UT Memphis students. There are also several religious organizations on campus.

Faculty

There are more than 900 full-time and part-time faculty members, as well as an additional 1,200 or so volunteer faculty.

Curriculum

Students learn clinical skills in the first year and start working with patients the second year. A standard four-year program, including coursework and clinical work, is observed.

Facilities

Most basic science courses are taught in the Cecil C. Humphreys general education building, which houses lecture and conference rooms, teaching laboratories, a microcomputer laboratory, and audiovisual facilities. Gross anatomy teaching laboratories are located in the Wittenborg building.

The C.P.J. Mooney Memorial Library holds just over 155,000 bound volumes, including more than 37,000 books and more than 2,100 periodical titles. The library also provides services including interlibrary loans, photocopying, and reference and bibliographic searches.

Grading Procedures

A letter grading system is used.

Application Procedures

The earliest date for submitting an application is July 1 of the year preceding enrollment. The application deadline is February 28 (although applications after this date may be considered). A nonrefundable application fee of $25 must accompany the application. Interviews are required, and are arranged by invitation from the committee on admissions after a review of the applicants' records. An evaluation must be obtained from the official prehealth sciences advisory committee, or, where such a committee does not exist, the academic dean of the undergraduate college. This must be obtained from a college the applicant has attended for at least one academic year. Letters of recommendation are also considered. Transfer students must present a statement of withdrawal in good standing from the dean or other responsible officer of the institution previously attended.

Contact

Admissions Office
College of Dentistry
University of Tennessee, Memphis
875 Union Avenue
Memphis, Tennessee 38163
(901) 528-6201
(800) 821-6165, ext. 6201 (In-State)
(800) 821-6682, ext. 6201 (Out-of-State)

UNIVERSITY OF TEXAS HEALTH SCIENCE CENTER AT HOUSTON DENTAL BRANCH

Houston, Texas 77225
(713) 792-4021

Accreditation	ADA
Degrees Offered	D.D.S., M.S.
# Students Applied	332
Enrollment	95 / class
Mean GPA	2.94
% Men / % Women	61% / 39%
% Minorities	48%
Tuition	$4,511 In-State
	$18,044 Out-of-State
Application Fee	$35 In-State; $70 Out-of-State
Application Deadline	November 1

The University

The University of Texas formally opened in 1883. Today, the university has numerous colleges, divisions, schools, and branches throughout the state.

The Health Science Center at Houston was established in 1972 to administer and provide for the operation of the several biomedical and health-related units located in the city. Eight professional schools are part of the Health Science Center, including the Dental Branch (founded in 1905 as the Texas Dental College). The center also comprises the Graduate School of Biomedical Sciences, the Medical School, the School of Nursing, and several other health-related schools.

Houston is the nation's fourth most populous city. Houston and surrounding Harris County have a population of 2.75 million residents with a median age of 27.5. There are approximately 121,000 students enrolled in the city's 28 colleges and universities. The city is known for its cultural attractions and is home to the Johnson Space Center, a focal point for the U.S.-manned spaceflight program. Houston is an hour away from Gulf beaches.

Admissions

The committee on admissions reviews academic performance, the evaluation of the health professions advisory committee, DAT scores, and personal qualities including maturity, motivation, integrity, and social awareness. Preference in admission is given to Texas residents. Recent mean GPAs were 2.94 (overall) and 2.84 (science); DAT mean scores were 15.3 (academic) and 16.4 (PAT).

Undergraduate Preparation

Students are advised to choose a course of study that leads to the bachelor's degree. Students should strive for an overall GPA of 3.0 or better and at least a 2.0 in the preprofessional required courses, which are as follows: one year of English, two years of biology, one year of physics, one year of general chemistry, and one year of organic chemistry. The science classes must include labs and must be classes required of science majors.

All applicants must take the DAT, preferably at least eight months before expected enrollment. Candidates are advised to take the test after they have completed at least one year of predental college work.

Student Body

The Health Science Center at Houston enrolls nearly 3,000 students in the various health and biomedical disciplines at its component schools. Of the 95 students enrolled in the Dental Branch in 1989, 37 were women, 45 were of various minority backgrounds, 55 had earned a baccalaureate degree, and all but four were state residents.

Costs

In 1989-90, annual resident tuition was set at $4,511; nonresident tuition was set at $18,044. Tuition is prorated for students enrolled at less than full-time status. Tuition and fees are subject to change. Fees include a laboratory fee of $43 for the first year and a professional liability insurance fee of $92 per year. Books for the first year are estimated to cost $800 to $900; instruments and supplies, $3,800. Costs for books and supplies decrease substantially in subsequent years.

Financial Aid

The Dental Branch of the University of Texas Health Science Center at Houston has limited loan and scholarship funds. These funds may be available on the basis of demonstrated financial need and/or academic excellence.

Student Organizations

Student organizations include the American Dental Association, the American Student Dental Association, the Zeb Ferdinand Poindexter Chapter of the Student National Dental Association, and the Texas Association of Women Dentists Chapter of the American Association of Women Dentists.

Honor societies include the Mu Mu Chapter of Omicron Kappa Upsilon, established in 1940 to recognize outstanding dental students.

Faculty

The Health Science Center at Houston employs a faculty and staff totalling more than 3,200.

Curriculum

The curriculum consists of "clusters" as opposed to traditional lock-step courses, allowing flexibility in the academic program. The curriculum is presented in a student-centered environment, allowing motivated students to progress at faster rates.

Subjects studied in the first two years include gross anatomy, cell and tissue biology, dental anatomy, operative dentistry, dental pharmacology, and pediatric dentistry.

Subjects studied in the third and fourth years include oral pathology and radiology, practice administration, removable prosthodontics, and occlusion. Although some electives are offered in the first two years, most electives are taken in the third and fourth years. Among the types of electives are table clinics, lecture courses, research projects, and seminars.

Facilities

The Dental Branch (includes the school of dentistry as well as programs in dental hygiene and dental assisting) is housed in the Texas Medical Center. Comprehensive facilities include laboratories, fully equipped clinical cubicles, lecture rooms, and the auditorium and library.

Students learn clinical skills and obtain patient contact in affiliated health care sites; there are also outreach clinics for teaching in Laredo, Brownsville, and Houston.

The library houses 24,000 volumes on medicine and dentistry. Students also have access to the Houston Academy of Medicine-Texas Medical Center Library.

Grading Procedures

The school uses a pass/fail system of student evaluation. A grade of 70 or above is considered passing; however, an overall average of 76 must be maintained for promotion and graduation. A grade of 69 or below is considered failing.

Special Programs

In the M.S. program (dental graduate program), students can pursue advanced study in a number of areas, including endodontics, oral and maxillofacial surgery, pediatric dentistry, and general dentistry. The dental branch also offers a certificate program in dental postgraduate work, and carries out the programs in dental hygiene and dental assisting.

Application Procedures

All applications are processed by the medical and dental application center of the University of Texas system. Applications are accepted between April 15 and November 1 of the year preceding the year of anticipated enrollment.

In addition to the completed application, candidates must submit official transcripts from all academic institutions attended, an evaluation from the health professions advisor or advisory committee, DAT scores, a nonrefundable filing fee ($35 for Texas residents and $70 for nonresidents), and a photograph. The committee on admissions may ask candidates to participate in an on-campus interview.

Contact

Director of Student Affairs
Dental Branch
University of Texas
Health Science Center at Houston
P.O. Box 20068
Houston, Texas 77225
(214) 828-8230

UNIVERSITY OF TEXAS HEALTH SCIENCE CENTER AT SAN ANTONIO, DENTAL SCHOOL

San Antonio, Texas 78284
(512) 567-3161

Accreditation	CDA
Degrees Offered	D.D.S., D.D.S./M.S., D.D.S./Ph.D.
# Students Applied	435
Enrollment	96 / class
Mean GPA	3.05
% Men / % Women	62% / 38%
% Minorities	38%
Tuition	$4,511 In-State
	$18,044 Out-of-State
Application Fee	$35 In-State, $70 Out-of-State
Application Deadline	November 1

The University

The University of Texas Health Science Center at San Antonio (UTHSCSA) is one of 14 components of the University of Texas system. Approximately 2,200 students are enrolled in the Health Center's five schools—the Dental School, the Medical School, the School of Nursing, the School of Allied Health Sciences, and the Graduate School of Biomedical Sciences.

San Antonio is a large city, known for its mild climate and bicultural population. There are many cultural centers, including museums, galleries, historical sites, a symphony orchestra, and theaters. Nearby lakes and rivers provide areas for fishing, boating, and swimming.

Admissions

The DAT is required. The average science GPA of the 1990 entering class was 3.09. Of 90 applicants that were accepted, 49 had received the baccalaureate degree. When evaluating applicants, the admissions committee considers the undergraduate GPA, DAT scores, evaluations by professional advisors or professors, extramural achievements, and an applicant's conduct during the interview. Preference is given to Texas residents, although highly qualified nonresidents will be considered. Applications for admission with advanced standing are accepted from students who can provide certification of good standing and rank at an accredited dental school.

Through the Dual Degree/Early Acceptance Option, students can obtain both a bachelor's degree and a dental degree in seven years. Through an affiliation between the Dental School and a number of undergraduate schools, students accepted for the dual degree option gain early acceptance to the Dental School, some as early as the freshman year in college.

Undergraduate Requirements

Applicants must have completed a minimum of 60 semester hours of credit from an accredited college or university. At least one year of English, physics, general chemistry, and organic chemistry are required (including lab). At least two years of biology are required, including one year of lab. A minimum grade of C must be earned for all required courses.

Student Body

Eighty-five of the 90 members of the 1990 entering class were Texas residents. Of these, 72 came from areas with populations of more than 50,001. Thirty-four members of the entering class were women, and 35 were minorities.

Costs

Tuition costs are subject to change. Tuition (per year) for a resident student is $4,511, for a nonresident student, $18,044. Required fees amount to $250 for the first year. Costs for instrument rental, supplies, and required manuals amount to $1,625 for the first year.

Financial Aid

Over 90 percent of students who apply for financial assistance receive aid. Students may apply for financial aid after they have been accepted for admission. After financial aid forms have been submitted, the financial aid office considers an applicant for every loan grant or scholarship program that he/she is eligible for. Applicants who qualify for assistance on the basis of need receive funds based on a maximum expense budget for the program they are about to enter. Nonresidents are eligible for all forms of financial aid. Foreign students are not eligible for traditional forms of financial aid.

Minority Programs

The Office of Special Programs supports minority students through a support network, which provides tutoring, study groups, mentors, resource materials, and referrals. Several minority student organizations and group functions are also supported by the Office of Special Programs.

Curriculum

The first and second years include the basic sciences, with some clinical experience beginning in the first year and increasing each year, until it predominates in the junior and senior years. The third and fourth years consist of a continuation of basic and dental sciences with clinical experiences.

Facilities

The Dental School's Outpatient Clinic and the Medical Center Hospital (the Medical School's primary teaching facility) offer opportunities for students to observe and ultimately treat patients under the supervision of faculty. The Dolph Briscoe, Jr. Library, the fifth-largest medical library in the nation, contains over 191,000 books and journals. Additional scientific information is available through computer access to a variety of national and international networks.

Special Programs

The University offers a double degree option, allowing students an opportunity to earn an M.S. or Ph.D. degree in addition to the D.D.S. Students must satisfy the entrance requirements of both the Dental School and the Graduate School of Biomedical Sciences. Five years are usually required to earn the D.D.S./M.S. degree, and seven years are usually required for the D.D.S./Ph.D.

Application Procedures

The DAT must be taken by the fall of the year preceding enrollment. DAT scores more than three years old are not acceptable. The central application center at Austin processes applications to all medical and dental schools of the University of Texas system. Applicants must notify the Division of Educational Measurements of the ADA that DAT results must be sent directly to the University of Texas Medical and Dental Application Center at Austin. Applications are accepted between April 15 and November 1 of the year preceding matriculation. Applicants for admission with advanced standing must request an application for admission with advanced standing from the office of the registrar. Interviews are arranged through a written invitation from the admissions committee.

Contact

Dental Admissions
Office of the Registrar
UTHSCSA
7703 Floyd Curl Drive
San Antonio, Texas 78284-7702
(512) 567-2660

TUFTS UNIVERSITY SCHOOL OF DENTAL MEDICINE

One Kneeland Street
Boston, Massachusetts 02111
(617) 956-6512

Accreditation	ADA
Degrees Offered	D.M.D., M.S., B.S./D.M.D.
# Students Applied	749
Enrollment	129
Mean GPA	2.86
% Men / % Women	57% / 43%
% Minorities	23%
Tuition	$19,285
Application Fee	$35
Application Deadline	April 1

The University

Tufts University was founded in 1850 as the Tufts Institute of Learning. The Tufts University School of Medicine began as Boston Dental School in 1868. The first graduation took place in 1869. Today, one in three dentists practicing in New England is an alumnus or alumna of Tufts. The school is located in downtown Boston. The school shares its space with Boston's Chinese community and the theater district. Historic Boston, with all of its cultural and historic appeal, is within easy reach of the interested student. The school is fully accredited by the ADA.

Admissions

The admissions committee seriously considers applicants with averages of 2.5 or above, and with at least the national average on the academic and PAT sections of the DAT. Admission to advanced standing is possible.

Undergraduate Preparation

Applicants must have completed not less than three years of study at an accredited college or university. Required are one full year of English, physics, biology, and inorganic chemistry and a half year of organic chemistry. Tufts also recommends that applicants study physiology, biochemistry, general psychology, histology, mathematics, economics, statistics, anthropology, genetics, comparative anatomy, and take an English course to develop writing technique.

Student Body

Of the more than 500 applicants interviewed each year, Tufts admits 125 students in the first year program, and 35 in the full-time postdoctoral program. For the class of 1990, 21 percent were from Massachusetts, seven percent were from other New England states, and 72 percent were from the rest of the country and abroad. About 43 percent were female and 57 percent male. Some 63 percent are from five states: Massachusetts, New York, California, Florida, and New Jersey.

Costs

Tuition for the 1990-91 entering class was $19,285. Other fees and supplies came to an additional $5,653. Living costs are estimated at $1,050 per month.

Financial Aid

Financial aid is based solely on need. During 1988-89, 65 percent of Tufts financial aid applicants received an award, the average award totalling $7,500. Students must apply prior to May 1 of the spring before the fall matriculation. The school encourages students to apply annually. The Tufts Aid Program offers federal and other loans through the Health Professions Student Loan Program. Students must file a GAPSFAS form and a family income tax return. About 19 student scholarship funds are available along with some 51 student loan funds. A special liaison with Maine, Rhode Island, and New Mexico offers tuition funds to exceptional students from those states.

Student Organizations

The Xi Xi chapter of the Omicron Kappa Upsilon, National Dental Society has a chapter on campus. The George A. Bates Society adds to the cultural, social and scientific knowledge of students, and the Robert R. Andrews Society promotes research in honor of its namesake.

Curriculum

The D.M.D. program takes four years to complete. The first year consists of basic science and preclinical technique courses. Normal human anatomy and physiology is the main theme, and courses include biochemistry, histology, gross anatomy, physiology, embryology, nutrition, and microbiology. The second year students begin their clinical experience. Second year courses deal with the pathology of the bodily systems. Dental didactic and technique courses continue into the third year. The third and fourth year programs are primarily clinical. During the fourth year electives are possible, and students take part in a special five-week externship program in a clinical facility.

Facilities

The school has a total of 160 operatories. The library, located in the M. Sackler Center for Health Communications, has a state-of-the-art communications network and is linked with the National Library of Medicine and other regional libraries. Library facilities include 95,000 volumes and 1,550 periodical subscriptions.

Special Programs

In association with Adelphi University, Tufts has a seven-year combined program for the B.S. and D.M.D. degrees in its Tufts-Adelphi Combined Degree Program. A two-year M.S. degree is available with a major in dental science. Tufts maintains an International Student Program. Graduate and postgraduate programs in dental specialties and dental postgraduate certificate courses are also available.

Application Procedures

Students must apply through AADSAS as soon as possible after June 1 (15 months prior to matriculation). The last acceptance date for applications is April 1. At the same time the $35 application fee should be sent, as well as a 2" x 2" photograph, DAT scores, and committee recommendations. Applicants will not be notified before December 1 of the year prior to their admission. Tufts requires a $500 deposit, credited toward tuition, within 45 days of notification.

Contact

Office of Admissions
Tufts University School of Medicine
One Kneeland Street
Boston, Massachusetts 02111

VIRGINIA COMMONWEALTH UNIVERSITY, MEDICAL COLLEGE OF VIRGINIA, SCHOOL OF DENTISTRY

Richmond, Virginia 23284
(804) 786-9183

Accreditation	CDA
Degrees Offered	D.D.S., D.D.S./M.S., D.D.S./Ph.D.
# Students Applied	531
Enrollment	35 / class
Mean GPA	3.02
% Men / % Women	78% / 22%
% Minorities	23%
Tuition	$5,770 In-State
	$10,800 Out-of-State
Application Fee	$35
Application Deadline	April 1

The University

In 1893, the University College of Medicine opened with a dental department division. In 1913, the dental department was merged with the dental education program founded by the Medical College of Virginia to form the Medical College of Virginia (MCV) School of Dentistry. Today, it is the only school of dentistry in Virginia.

Virginia Commonwealth University is composed of two campuses. The Academic Campus is located in the Fan District, a restored residential area of turn-of-the-century townhouses. The MCV Campus is located two miles east in the financial, governmental, and shopping areas of downtown Richmond. Richmond is a large city with a population of approximately 700,000. A wide variety of cultural and recreational activities are available.

Admissions

The DAT is required. Preference is given to candidates who have completed 120 credit hours and have received a bachelor's degree. Preference is given to residents, although nonresidents are considered. The university encourages qualified international students, both immigrant and non-immigrant, to seek admission. Transfer students from other accredited U.S. and Canadian dental schools will be accepted for the sophomore and junior years.

Undergraduate Preparation

Applicants must have a minimum of 90 semester hours (or the equivalent) at an accredited college or university. The following required coursework (including necessary laboratory work) should be completed by July of the year of matriculation: general biology, emphasizing zoology, general chemistry, organic chemistry, physics, and English.

Courses in biochemistry, general microbiology, the behavioral sciences and courses involving psychomotor skills are strongly recommended. Generally, no more than two years at the community college level are accepted for credit.

Student Body

Approximately half of the students accepted for the 1989-90 academic year were residents of Virginia. Twenty-nine were from out of state and two were from foreign countries. The average DAT score was 18.0 (academic) and 17.8 (PAT). The mean science GPA score was 2.98. Out of 81 applicants who were accepted, 10 had not received their bachelor's degree.

Costs

Tuition and fees are subject to change.

Tuition (per year) is $5,770 for residents and $10,800 for nonresidents. Other expenses (including fees, instruments and books) totaled $3,555 for the first year.

Financial Aid

The School of Dentistry makes an effort to provide financial aid to all qualified students. Rural Virginia Dental Scholarships and local college funds are designed to give financial aid to dental students. Other financial aid is available from federal, state and private offices.

Minority Programs

Applicants from minority groups underrepresented in the health sciences are encouraged to contact the Office of the Health Careers Opportunity Program, Virginia Commonwealth University, Richmond, VA 23298-0549.

Student Organizations

The School of Dentistry has a chapter of Omicron Kappa Upsilon, the national honorary dental society.

Curriculum

The four-year program leading to the D.D.S. degree emphasizes study in three broad areas: basic sciences, clinical sciences, and social sciences. The social sciences cover such topics as dental health needs, the system of health care delivery, dental practice management, professional ethics, and behavioral matters. Classes are taught in conjunction with laboratory and clinical experiences throughout the four years. The first year consists of the basic sciences. The second year includes study of the basic and clinical sciences, including preclinical lectures, laboratory preparation, and comprehensive patient care. The third year consists of rotations in radiology, diagnosis, and DAU. Elective courses are offered during the senior year to allow students to gain additional experience in a particular area. Electives also allow students who have not defined their goals to participate in varied courses. A Special Studies Program is also available, which allows a qualified fourth-year student to focus his/her time and energy in a defined area of study, service, and/or research.

Facilities

The School of Dentistry is housed in the Wood Memorial and the Lyons Buildings, which contain clinical facilities, classrooms, student laboratories, a media library, and a closed circuit color television studio with receiver units in laboratories and classrooms.

Grading Procedures

A letter grading system is used.

Special Programs

An Early Acceptance Honor Program has been established between the professional schools on the MCV campus and the academic campus of the University. Interested candidates should contact the dental school admissions office or the College of Humanities and Sciences. Combined D.D.S./M.S. or D.D.S./Ph.D. degrees are offered in conjunction with the School of Basic Sciences. Each program is individually developed by the two schools.

Application Procedures

The School of Dentistry participates in AADSAS. Applications will be accepted on or after June 1 of the year preceding admission. Application materials must be received by April 1. An application fee of $35 is due upon request to submit supplemental application materials to the School of Dentistry. The DAT should be taken by October of the year before a student enrolls. Interviews are standardized and are arranged by the admissions committee. The school does not participate in the early decision plan.

Contact

Office of Admissions and Student Affairs
School of Dentistry
Medical College of Virginia Commonwealth University
Richmond, Virginia 23298-0566
(804) 786-9196

UNIVERSITY OF WASHINGTON SCHOOL OF DENTISTRY

Seattle, Washington 98195
(206) 543-5982

Accreditation	CDA
Degrees Offered	D.D.S.
# Students Applied	450
Enrollment	200
Mean GPA	3.19
% Men / % Women	75% / 25%
% Minorities	25%
Tuition	$4,926 In-State
	$12,513 Out-of-State
Application Fee	$35
Application Deadline	December 1

The University

The dental school was established in 1945 as one of six professional schools that are part of the university. The University of Washington is located on 700 acres in the Puget Sound area of Seattle, Washington. The campus location offers opportunities for a variety of cultural and recreational activities. The Seattle climate is moderate year round.

Admissions

The entering class size is about 50. The majority of students accepted hold bachelor's degrees. Two percent of the 1990-91 entering class were admitted with three years of college. The mean DAT (academic) for entering first-year students is 18.2. The mean DAT (PAT) is 19.2.

Student Body

Of the entering class of 1990-91, 40 were men and 13 were women. Fourteen were from minority groups and 26 were from out of state. The class represented a diversity of undergraduate majors.

Costs

For 1990-91, tuition for residents was $4,926 and $12,501 for nonresidents. Other costs for the first year were estimated to total $4,467.

Financial Aid

All federally subsidized loan programs and state-sponsored

grants and scholarships are available through the university's office of student financial aid. Students anticipating a financial need must complete the FAF by the university's filing deadline of March 1.

Minority Programs

Special admissions consideration is given to applicants from ethnically underrepresented groups and economically disadvantaged backgrounds through the Dental Upward Bound Program, which provides the opportunity for extension of curriculum beyond the four years of enrollment. Comprehensive support systems are made available to Dental Upward Bound students.

Curriculum

The four-year curriculum includes required summer study after the second and third years. The first year consists of lecture, lab, and preclinical studies in the basic sciences, dental anatomy, and dental material. The second year teaches methods in which basic science principles apply to clinical work. Actual clinical work begins in the second year, and continues in the third and fourth years along with lectures which refine the student's diagnostic and technical skills. Students participate in the clinical portion of the program at sites such as hospitals and community clinics.

Special Programs

Students may enroll in either M.S. or Ph.D. programs concurrently with the dental degree program.

Application Procedures

The School of Dentistry participates in AADSAS. A supplemental application is required in addition to the AADSAS application. Competitive applicants are invited for an interview with members of the admissions committee. Applications are accepted from June to December 1.

Contact

University of Washington School of Dentistry
Office of Student Services
Warren G. Magnuson Health Sciences Center
Suite D323, SC-62
Seattle, Washington 98195-9950
(206) 543-5840

WEST VIRGINIA UNIVERSITY SCHOOL OF DENTISTRY

Morgantown, West Virginia 26506
(304) 293-2521

Accreditation	CDA
Degrees Offered	D.D.S., M.S., B.S., Ph.D.
# Students Applied	217
Enrollment	250
Mean GPA	Not Available
% Men / % Women	70% / 30%
% Minorities	Not Available
Tuition	$3,839 In-State
	$8,413 Out-of-State
Application Fee	$30
Application Deadline	November 1

The University

An integral part of the West Virginia University Medical Center, the School of Dentistry was founded in 1951 and enrolled its first class in 1957. The school offers the D.D.S. degree as well as a variety of advanced degrees and residencies. The school is situated in Morgantown, West Virginia, a town with a population of about 30,000.

Admissions

The school examines the applicant's academic record and seeks those with a broad cultural background. The school also evaluates personal qualities that relate to the candidate's suitability to practice dentistry. Other important factors include recommendations from the student's preprofessional committee and DAT scores. Residents of West Virginia are given preference in the admissions process. Nonresident candidates should have a GPA of at least 3.0 and average scores on the academic and PAT sections of the DAT of at least 4.4.

Undergraduate Preparation

Applicants must have completed a minimum of two years of college; however, three years is more acceptable. The required science courses are: eight semester hours each of inorganic chemistry, organic chemistry, physics, and zoology or biology, all with lab. There is also a requirement of six semester hours of English composition or an equivalent subject.

Student Body

The 1989-90 entering class was comprised of 35 students.

Ten were women. Twelve members of the class held the bachelor's degree at time of entry. Twenty-four were from West Virginia. The mean DAT score (academic section) was 17. The mean DAT score (PAT section) was 17.

Costs

For 1990-91, tuition for residents was $3,839 per year. Tuition for nonresidents was $8,413 for the first three years and $6,872 for the fourth year. Other major expenses run about $7,100 the first year and decrease over the following years.

Financial Aid

A variety of scholarships are available through the Board of Regents of West Virginia University. The school also administers several loan funds.

Curriculum

The four-year program leading to the D.D.S. consists of eight semesters, each 15 weeks in length, plus three required summer sessions. The core required courses are taught within the first seven semesters and during two summer sessions. During the third year, students have the opportunity to choose a specialization form three areas: general practice, biological sciences, or clinical specialty. Each student designs an individualized curriculum that must be approved by the faculty advisor. Electives are available in the fourth year. All students must also complete mock board examinations in the fourth year and three weeks of remote-site training.

Special Programs

The school offers the M.S. and the Ph.D. in basic sciences, and has two oral surgery residency programs and seven general practice residencies. There is an M.S. degree program for those wishing to specialize in endodontics or orthodontics, and a B.S. in dental hygiene is offered. The school also offers two combined degree programs—D.D.S./M.S. and D.D.S./Ph.D.

Application Procedures

The school participates in AADSAS. The application period is June 1 to November 1 of the year preceding the year of desired enrollment. There is a $30 nonrefundable application fee. The school does not have an early decision plan. Applicants are notified of acceptance no earlier than December 1. Nonresidents must submit a $100 deposit to hold their place in class; the required deposit for residents is $50.

Contact

West Virginia University
Office of Student Admissions and Records
1170 HSN
Health Science Center
Morgantown, West Virginia 26506
(304) 293-3521

CANADIAN DENTAL SCHOOLS AT A GLANCE

School	Accreditation	Degrees Offered	# Students Applied	Enrollment
University of Alberta, Faculty of Dentistry	CEA of CDA	D.D.S., M.Sc., Ph.D.	366	51 / class
University of British Columbia Faculty of Dentistry	CEA of CDA	D.M.D., M.Sc., Ph.D.	210	40 / class
Dalhousie University Faculty of Dentistry	CEA of CDA	D.D.S., M.S.	192	34 / class
Université Laval, école de Médecine Dentaire	CEA of CDA	D.M.D.	403	46 / class
University of Manitoba Faculty of Dentistry	CEA of CDA	M.S., Ph.D., D.M.D.	108	20 / class
McGill University Faculty of Dentistry	CEA of CDA	D.D.S., B.Sc., M.S.	236	31 / class
Université de Montréal Faculté de Médecine Dentaire	CEA of CDA	D.M.D.	489	178 / class
University of Saskatchewan College of Dentistry	CEA of CDA	D.M.D.	70	21 / class
University of Toronto Faculty of Dentistry	CEA of CDA	D.D.S., D.D.S./Ph.D.	621	64 / class
University of Western Ontario Faculty of Dentistry	CEA of CDA	D.D.S., M.S.	500	40 / class

* Not Available   ** Not Applicable   C/S – Contact School   The CEA of CDA stands for the Committee on Education of the Canadian Dental Association

Mean GPA	% Male / % Female	% Minorities	In-State Tuition	Out-of-State Tuition	Application Fee	Application Deadline
*	72% / 28%	*	$2,000	**	C/S	February 1
3.32	94% / 6%	*	$2,913	**	$25	December 15
80.8%	65% / 35%	*	$2,341	**	$20	December 1
4.16	61% / 39%	*	C/S	C/S	$15	March 1
3.54	75% / 25%	*	$2,346	**	$100	January 2
3.2	64% / 36%	*	$1,848	$4,350	$25	December 1 February 1
3.6	44% / 39%	*	$1,078	$3,480	$15	March 1
*	67% / 33%	*	$2,250	**	None	February 28
2.7	58% / 42%	*	$2,084	**	$50	February 1
*	75% / 25%	*	$1,929	**	C/S	December 3

* Not Available   ** Not Applicable   C/S – Contact School   The CEA of CDA stands for the Committee on Education of the Canadian Dental Association

UNIVERSITY OF ALBERTA FACULTY OF DENTISTRY

Edmonton, Alberta
Canada T6G 2N8
(403) 492-2945

Accreditation	CDA, ADA
Degrees Offered	D.D.S., M.Sc., Ph.D.
# Students Applied	366
Enrollment	51 / class
Mean GPA	Not Available
% Men / % Women	72% / 28%
% Minorities	Not Available
Tuition	$2,000
Application Fee	Contact School
Application Deadline	February 1

The University

The Faculty of Dentistry of the University of Alberta is approved by the Canadian Dental Association and the American Dental Association. The school is located in Edmonton, the capital city of Alberta province. Edmonton, situated on the No. Saskatchewan River, has a population of about 521,000. Founded as a major fur-trading center in 1795, Edmonton is one of Canada's fastest growing cities. Edmonton serves as the gateway to the developing Peace River and Athabasca frontier country. The rugged outdoor sports activist will find abundant opportunity for boating, fishing, and other such activities.

Admissions

Five percent foreign students and 10 percent non-Alberta Canadians may be accepted as part of the class. The university may reserve the remaining 85 percent for Canadian citizens who are residents of Alberta or of the Northwest Territories or Yukon. Students must successfully complete the Canadian DAT, have an average GPA between 7.0 and 7.5, have an acceptable average in the applicable science courses, and complete a successful interview. Alberta will not consider students with a GPA below 6.5. The GPA mean for the 1990 class was 7.6; scores in the science range averaged 7.5.

Undergraduate Preparation

The Faculty of Dentistry requires the satisfactory completion of two full years (10 full courses) of university work (five full courses must be taken during one winter session).

Preprofessional studies may be completed either at the University of Alberta or at any comparable post-secondary institution. These studies must include organic chemistry, inorganic chemistry, physics, and biology. Proficiency in English, the language of instruction at Alberta, is required. Scores at 80 percent or better in the Alberta English 30 course are required. Also acceptable is a grade of 6 or 7 on the International Baccalaureate Higher Level English course, a score of at least 580 on the TOEFL test, or a score of at least 90 on the MELAB. Students must also receive a score of 200 or better on the TSE.

Student Body

Of 366 applicants for 1990, 116 were qualified for acceptance, and 50 were accepted for the first year class. In 1990, 45 out of the 50 accepted students in the entering class were Canadian citizens or landed immigrants and Alberta residents. The other five were Canadians from other provinces. Of the entering class, 36 were male and 14 female.

Costs

Tuition is $2,000. Books cost about $100 for the first year; dental instruments cost about $5,900. While tuition remains the same over the next three years, costs for books and instruments decrease significantly. Tuition, books, and dental instruments for each of the four years total $1,795.

Financial Aid

Some faculty assistantships and fellowships are available.

Faculty

The faculty at Alberta consists of about 200 academic professors, clinical professors, and instructors from all the related disciplines, suggesting a student/faculty ratio of 1:1.

Curriculum

The course of study lasts four years. The first two years emphasize studies in the basic biological sciences (biochemistry, anatomy, physiology, pharmacology, and bacteriology) with an introduction to the dental sciences. The final two years shift emphasis from classroom and laboratory learning to the clinical programs, including the actual treatment of patients in the dental clinics. Each year includes coursework in operative dentistry.

Facilities

The Medical Sciences reading room of the John W. Scott Health Science Library contains a comprehensive selection of reference materials and textbooks on dentistry. It also contains the most current dental journals in English and other languages, and the Index to Dental Periodical Literature, going back to 1839. Senior students are assigned to the Dental Department and the Department of General Anesthesia at the University Hospital. An experience in the General Practice Clinic, the

Satellite Dental Clinic, and the Geriatric Youville Hospital is a requirement for the final year.

Grading Procedures

Students must pass both the practical and the theoretical examinations of any course having these components. An overall GPA of 5.5 is considered excellent work. A grade of 5 is also good. A grade of 4 is a conditional pass and will permit the student to be promoted or graduate. Course grades of 3, 2, and 1 are failing. Re-examinations are possible at the discretion of the faculty and with certain specific requirements of the university in place.

Special Programs

Besides the D.D.S. degree, Alberta offers the M.Sc. and Ph.D. degrees. Dental graduates may take graduate programs in either oral biology or clinical science. In addition, students may pursue a Dental Hygiene Diploma and an M.Sc. degree and Certificate in Orthodontics. Courses in continuing education are also available.

Application Procedures

Applicants should apply through the University of Alberta. The earliest date for filing applications is September 30 of the year before admission. The deadline for the D.D.S. program is February 1. For postgraduate clinical programs, the deadline is October 15. Upon notification of acceptance, a $50 deposit is required to reserve the applicant's place in class. Alberta requires a dental examination of all accepted students.

Contact

Office of Admissions
Faculty of Dentistry
3039 Dentistry/Pharmacy Building
University of Alberta
Edmonton, Alberta, Canada T6G 2N862
(403) 492-2945

UNIVERSITY OF BRITISH COLUMBIA FACULTY OF DENTISTRY

345-2194 Health Sciences Mall
Vancouver, British Columbia
Canada V6T 1W5
(604) 228-5323

Accreditation	CDA
Degrees Offered	D.M.D., M.Sc., Ph.D.
# Students Applied	210
Enrollment	40 / class
Mean GPA	3.32
% Men / % Women	94% / 6%
% Minorities	Not Available
Tuition	$2,913
Application Fee	$25 (for college work completed outside British Columbia)
Application Deadline	December 15

The University

As the result of two surveys conducted in 1955 and 1961 regarding the need for dental education facilities in the Province of British Columbia, the Faculty of Dentistry was established in 1962. A small class of undergraduate dental students was first admitted in September 1964.

Admissions

The admissions committee requires that all applicants have an overall undergraduate grade point average of at least 2.5 on a 4.0 grading scale. Students must also take the MCAT.

Undergraduate Preparation

Students must have completed at least three academic years in the Faculty of Arts or the Faculty of Science at The University of British Columbia, or the equivalent. The following courses are required: English, mathematics, chemistry (general), organic chemistry, physics, biology, and biochemistry.

Student Body

Of the 40 students in the 1989-90 entering class, 15 were women, 36 were residents of British Columbia, and 30 had earned bachelor's degrees.

Costs

Tuition as of September 1989 was $2,913. There is a $20

fee for a cardiopulmonary resuscitation course in the second year and a NDEB Certificate fee in the fourth year of $400. Instruments, supplies, and lab attire are expected to cost around $1,765 in the first year, $2,305 in the second year, $1,561 in the third year, and $907 in the fourth year. Textbooks and supplies cost a minimum of $800 per year.

Financial Aid

Scholarships, prizes, bursaries, and loans are available to all students. Information on financial assistance can be obtained through the Awards and Financial Aid Office, 101-2075 Wesbrook Mall, The University of British Columbia, Vancouver, B.C. V6T 1W5, telephone (604) 228-5111.

Curriculum

During the first year, medical and dental students study side by side, except in the dental aspects of basic science and in the dental sciences. Clinical instruction begins during the second half of the second year.

Facilities

The teaching, research, and clinical facilities are contained in the John Barfoot Macdonald Building. The Woodward Biomedical Library provides library facilities.

Special Programs

Graduate programs in dental science at the master's and Ph.D. levels are available, as well as a postgraduate diploma course in periodontics.

Application Procedures

Application materials may be obtained from Undergraduate Admissions, Office of the Dean, Faculty of Dentistry, 350-2194 Health Sciences Mall, The University of British Columbia, B.C. V6T 1W5. The application, which is due by December 15, must include official transcripts of all college and university work completed. If any of the college work has been completed outside the Province of British Columbia, a $25 fee should be included with the application.

Contact

Faculty of Dentistry
345-2194 Health Sciences Mall
The University of British Columbia
Vancouver, BC Canada V6T 1W5
Admissions: (604) 228-3416
Information: (604) 228-5323

DALHOUSIE UNIVERSITY FACULTY OF DENTISTRY

Halifax, Nova Scotia
Canada B3H 3J5
(902) 494-2275

Accreditation	CDA
Degrees Offered	D.D.S., M.S.
# Students Applied	192
Enrollment	34 / class
Mean GPA	80.8%
% Men / % Women	65% / 35%
% Minorities	Not Available
Tuition	$2,341
Application Fee	$20
Application Deadline	December 1

The University

Dalhousie University, founded in 1818, is located on a 60-acre campus in Halifax, Nova Scotia. The university is within easy walking distance of natural parkland and the ocean. The small city of Halifax features historical buildings, a wide variety of entertainment, and various leisure facilities. It is also near many of the Atlantic region's major research centers and teaching hospitals.

The Faculty of Dentistry was opened in 1958 and was extensively enlarged and renovated in 1980. The school is proud to have the most modern dental clinic and laboratory facilities for student instruction in Canada.

Admissions

Although qualified students from all provinces will be considered, preference is given to residents of the Atlantic provinces. In order to be competitive, students should have received a score of 15 or better on the manual dexterity portion of the DAT. Applicants should have a minimum overall GPA of 3.0. A broad academic background and good written and verbal English skills are a decided asset. Besides academic factors, an applicant's letter of recommendation and interview(s) are also important considerations.

Undergraduate Preparation

Students must have completed a minimum of 10 full-year academic classes, although students are encouraged to finish their bachelor's degree before applying to the Faculty of Dentistry. Among the predental curriculum required are full-year courses in biology, general chemistry, organic chemistry, and physics, and three full-year academic classes in the humanities and/or social sciences, one of which must involve a significant writing component. The science classes must include laboratory instruction or seminar periods.

Student Body

Of the 32 students who enrolled in the dental school in 1989, 14 were women. All were from the Atlantic provinces, and 24 had earned bachelor's degrees. The students ranged in age from 20 to 35; the mean age was 24.2 years.

Costs

In 1989-90, tuition and fees for the Faculty of Dentistry were $2,341. Instruments were estimated to cost about $2,440 in the first year, $2,279 in the second year, and $81 in the third year. There is a $500 user fee applied in each of the four years. Textbooks, manuals, and handouts were estimated at $1,186 for the first year, $1,078 for the second year, $280 for the third year, and $150 for the fourth year.

Financial Aid

Financial aid consists of various scholarships, prizes and medals, and bursaries. Among these is an entrance scholarship for $1,000; plus in-course scholarships, Dalhousie University Dental Scholarships of $1,000, and a Dr. I.K. Lubetsky Scholarship of $500.

Student Organizations

Over 70 clubs and societies are registered with the student union at Dalhousie University representing academic, political, recreational, and special interest organizations. Students in the Faculty of Dentistry are also members of the Dalhousie Dental Students' Society or the Dalhousie Dental Hygiene Students' Society.

Curriculum

During the first year, dentistry students take foundation sciences, such as human anatomy and physiology, neuro-anatomy, pathology, biochemistry, and microbiology/immunology. In the second year, dental science is integrated with these foundation sciences. More emphasis is placed on dental laboratory sciences and beginning clinical patient treatment. In the third year, students engage in extensive patient treatment with a few lecture and seminar courses. During the fourth year, the emphasis is on restorative dentistry and comprehensive and integrated patient care.

Facilities

The facilities at the Dalhousie Faculty of Dentistry are some of the most modern in North America. The university library system includes five libraries, which contain a total of approximately 1.3 million volumes and over 300,000 microforms and nonprint items. The dental library is adjacent to the dentistry building in the Sir Charles Tupper Medical Building. Second-, third-, and fourth-year students are assigned a fully-equipped clinic office space in which to provide individual patient treatment. The faculty operates a complete dental laboratory, and full-time dental assistants are available to assist students in clinic activities. Students also have access to PCs in the computer workroom.

Special Programs

The Faculty of Dentistry at Dalhousie University offers a two-year diploma in dental hygiene program, a two-year postgraduate program in periodontics, and a four-year post-graduate program in oral and maxillofacial surgery.

Application Procedures

Applications, sent directly to the school, are due by December 1 and must be accompanied by a $20 fee. With the application form, applicants must submit Canadian Dental Association Dental Aptitude Test results, official transcripts, three confidential evaluations, an assessment by a college advisory committee from the institution the applicant is attending, and a medical and dental certificate ensuring physical, mental, and dental fitness. An interview may be required.

Contact

Faculty of Dentistry
Dalhousie University
Halifax, Nova Scotia, Canada B3H 3J5
(902) 494-2275

UNIVERSITÉ LAVAL, ECOLE DE MÉDECINE DENTAIRE

Quebec
Canada G1K 7P4
(418) 656-5293

Accreditation	CDA
Degrees Offered	D.M.D.
# Students Applied	403
Enrollment	46 / class
Mean GPA	4.16
% Men / % Women	61% / 39%
% Minorities	Not Available
Tuition	Contact School
Application Fee	$15
Application Deadline	March 1

The University

The School of Dental Medicine was established in 1969. All of the instruction is performed in French. Sponsorship is offered by the province of Quebec where most of the expenses are covered by funds from the government.

Admissions

The Canadian DAT is required. Students may take the exam in French. The American Dental Association DAT may be substituted. Applicants must have a GPA in the upper third. Residents of Quebec have priority in admissions; at least 90 percent of the students must come from this province.

Undergraduate Preparation

Students must have completed 11 years of high school in addition to two years of junior college (CECEP) work. Non-residents must attend a university. All applicants must complete eight semester hours of inorganic chemistry, biology, and mathematics. Four credit hours are required of organic chemistry and 12 of physics. Predental students should maintain an undergraduate program that emphasizes the health sciences

and human biology. It is recommended that the applicant have a GPA in the upper third of the undergraduate class.

Student Body

Of the 46 enrolled students in the 1989-90 entering class, 29 were women. The average age was 21.5. Most students have at least two years of predental education. Only three students came from outside Quebec.

Financial Aid

Students should contact campus credit unions, banking establishments, or the university Service des bourses et de l'aide financiére. Supply houses offer student loans to sophomores and juniors. Several loans and scholarships are available through the federal, city, and provincial governments.

Curriculum

The basic and preclinical sciences are covered during the first two years. Nearly all of the work of the last two years consists of clinical material. Electives of any discipline are open to fourth-year students. Students can choose from electives in hospital dentistry, public health, or applied research.

Grading Procedures

Students are evaluated on written and oral examinations.

Special Programs

There is a certificate program in oral and maxillofacial surgery.

Application Procedures

The application period runs from January 1 to March 1. There is a $15 application fee. The School of Dental Medicine does not participate in the AADSAS. Students may be required to have an interview as part of the screening process. Those accepted applicants must submit a certificate of fine health. Students should receive word of acceptance by August 15. At this time candidates have 15 days to respond to the university.

Contact

Comité d'admission
Université Laval
Ecole de Médecine Dentaire
Quebec, Canada G1K 7P4
(418) 656-5293

UNIVERSITY OF MANITOBA FACULTY OF DENTISTRY

Winnipeg, Manitoba
Canada R3T 2N2

Accreditation	CDA
Degrees Offered	M.S., Ph.D., D.M.D.
# Students Applied	108
Enrollment	20
Mean GPA	3.54
% Men / % Women	75% / 25%
% Minorities	Not Available
Tuition	$2,346
Application Fee	$100
Application Deadline	January 2

The University

The University of Manitoba Faculty of Dentistry, established in 1957, is funded by the province of Manitoba. The Health Science campus in the city of Winnipeg is home to the Faculty of Dentistry. Winnipeg has a population of 600,000.

Admissions

Students must achieve a minimum carving dexterity score of 14 and a PMAT average of 14 on the Canadian DAT. A GPA requirement is not specified. Applicants must be citizens of Canada or have permanent residency status. Residents of Manitoba and science majors are preferred. Academic achievement and an upward trend in scholastic performance are considered. For the 1989-90 entering class, the mean DAT was 18.90 and the mean PAT was 6.20. The mean DAT for chalk carving was 16.45. The mean GPA was 3.54.

Undergraduate Preparation

An applicant should have at least two years of undergraduate schooling. Candidates are required to take three years of chemistry, two years of physics, one year of biology, and one year of biochemistry, each with a lab. Students should also have one year of mathematics, two years of English, and four electives, including one class in the social sciences.

Student Body

There are 100 full-time undergraduate students in the dental program, 50 dental hygiene students, and 15 graduate students. Of the 108 students who applied for the 1989-90 school year, 20 students were enrolled. Five of these students were women. Ages ranged from 19 to 27, the mean age being 21.75. Most had bachelor's degrees. Seventeen were residents of the province, two came from another province in Canada, and one came from another country.

Costs

Students can expect to pay $2,346 for tuition each year. Other costs over the four-year period include $220 for laboratory fees, $16,229 for instruments, $3,285 for other supplies and materials, $2,480 for books, $64 for lab coats, and $22,278 for other expenses including living expenses. In all, costs total $53,940 for four years.

Faculty

There are 45 full-time faculty, 40 part-time faculty, and 70 support staff members.

Curriculum

The four-year program stresses the basic sciences. Students study biochemistry, physiology, microbiology, and pathology through the Department of Oral Biology. The Faculty of Medicine teaches the anatomy and pharmacology classes. Sophomore year includes the first clinical experience in scaling technique. Seniors may choose electives. Two weeks each are spent in a teaching hospital and a rural externship.

Facilities

The Health Sciences Centre is composed of four hospitals where dental skills and services are taught. The Medical College's Department of Anatomy offers laboratories. The main clinic includes 60 units, with an additional 40 units in other parts of the building. The Health Sciences Centre also has units. Cassette tapes and audiovisual equipment is available at the Dental Faculty library.

Grading Procedures

Letter grades are awarded for didactic and clinical performance.

Special Programs

Eligible students may receive a Bachelor of Science in Dentistry at the Faculty of Dentistry.

Application Procedures

Students should apply for admissions by January 2. The application fee is $100. The Faculty of Dentistry notifies students of acceptance between June 26 and August 30. Students must complete a personal interest inventory in lieu of an interview.

Contact

Admissions Officer
University of Manitoba
Winnipeg, Manitoba, Canada R3T 2N2

McGILL UNIVERSITY FACULTY OF DENTISTRY

3640 University Street
Montreal, Quebec
Canada H3A 2B2

Accreditation	CDA
Degrees Offered	D.D.S., B.Sc., M.S.
# Students Applied	236
Enrollment	31 / class
Mean GPA	3.2
% Men / % Women	64% / 36%
% Minorities	Not Available
Tuition	$1,848 In-Province
	$4,350 Out-of-Province
Application Fee	$25
Application Deadline	December 1, Non-Quebec; February 1, Quebec

The University

McGill University is located in Montreal, Québec. The school was founded in 1821 at the bequest of the Hon. James McGill, who died in 1813 and bequeathed a 46-acre estate and a large sum of money for the purpose of building a college bearing his name. The college, now called McGill University, comprises 12 faculties and 10 schools.

Admissions

The Faculty of Dentistry accepts 30 students yearly into its four-year program. Candidates for the Faculty of Dentistry must have a minimum undergraduate GPA of 3.2 and must score a minimum of 17 on all three sections of the DAT. Students applying to the five-year program should have better qualifications. Students who do not gain admittance after four applications are discouraged from applying again.

Undergraduate Preparation

Dental students must have completed one year each of general biology, inorganic chemistry, organic chemistry, physics, mathematics, and human or mammalian physiology. Dental students must also have completed one semester each in microbiology, immunology, cell biology, and molecular biology. One year of biochemistry may be substituted for the courses in cell and molecular biology.

Student Body

Of the 31 students admitted in 1989, 11 are women. Fifteen had undergraduate degrees, and all were Canadian.

Placement Records

The Canada Employment Centre assists Canadian students in finding part-time, summer, and permanent employment. The Employment Centre also maintains a resource library and holds seminars.

Costs

Annual tuition and fees for 1989-90 totalled $1,848 for residents and $4,350 for nonresidents. The Faculty of Dentistry estimates that lab expenses will total $5,225 for all four years of schooling.

Financial Aid

The school of dental medicine offers a number of entrance scholarships to students of high academic achievement; these awards are open to Canadian citizens or permanent residents and to students entering dental school for the first time. The university makes loans to students of good academic standing. L'Ordre des Dentistes du Quebec has created a loan fund to assist students; other available funds include the W.K. Kellogg Loan Fund, Dental Students' Society Dean D.P. Mowry Memorial Fund, and Dr. Stan Smaill bursary.

Student Organizations

McGill sponsors over 250 extracurricular activities for its students, including international clubs, religious groups, political clubs, fraternities, intramural athletics, and communications groups.

Faculty

The Faculty of Dentistry staffs 63 full-time faculty and 72 lecturers.

Curriculum

D.D.S. candidates must complete the standard four-year curriculum, achieving at least a C+ in each course and maintaining a minimum GPA of 2.9 to advance. Students must also participate annually with elementary schools, present at least one table clinic, and do a project at the summer clinic between junior and senior years. The five-year dental program is available to students in the Quebec Colleges of General and Professional Education; these students must register for a full year of courses at the Faculty of Science. All classes are taught in English, but students may write examinations and term papers in French, and, in any case, all dental students must demonstrate proficiency in writing and speaking French.

Facilities

McGill University has five university teaching hospitals and is affiliated with six others. The Montreal General Hospital houses the McGill University Dental Clinic. The Health Sciences Library holds 200,000 volumes in all aspects of medicine and houses all materials relating to dentistry.

Grading Procedures

Final grades are based on oral, written, and practical assessments; most subjects have final examinations. Letter grades are A, A-, B+, B, B-, C+, and F.

Special Programs

McGill awards the B.S. degree to McGill Faculty of Science students who enter the Faculty of Dentistry upon completion of 60 credits out of a 90-credit science program. The Faculty of Dentistry awards the M.S. degree in oral and maxillofacial surgery to students who, upon completion of the D.D.S. or D.M.D. degree, complete four years of residency at the Montreal General Hospital and a master's thesis.

Application Procedures

Applicants outside of Quebec must apply by December 1; Quebec residents applying to the four-year program must apply by February 1; and Quebec residents applying to the five-year program must apply by March 1. The nonrefundable application fee is $25 but is waived for McGill undergraduates.

Contact

Administrative Assistant for Student Affairs
McGill University
Faculty of Dentistry
3640 University Street
Montreal, Quebec, Canada H3A 2B2

UNIVERSITÉ DE MONTRÉAL, FACULTÉ DE MÉDECINE DENTAIRE

Montreal, Quebec
Canada H3C 3T5
(514) 343-6305

Accreditation	CDA
Degrees Offered	D.M.D.
# Students Applied	489
Enrollment	178 / class
Mean GPA	3.6
% Men / % Women	44% / 39%
% Minorities	Not Available
Tuition	$1,078 In-Province
	$3,480 Out-of-Province
Application Fee	$15
Application Deadline	March 1

The University

The Université de Montréal established its Faculté de Médecine Dentaire in 1904. Provisions are made by the state to support this private institution. The Faculté de Médecine Dentaire has the distinction of being one of two schools where instruction in a North American school is given in French. At the head of the St. Lawrence Seaway in Quebec, Montreal offers countless facilities and resources with libraries, museums, and recreational attractions. Montreal is the largest city in Canada.

Admissions

All applicants are required to take the Canadian Dental Admission Test (DAT). A score of 15 is the minimum requirement for the carving dexterity test. Students should score a 17 on the perception aptitude test. The ADA DAT is not permitted as a substitute for the Canadian DAT.

Undergraduate Preparation

A minimum of two predental college years are required of all applicants. In addition, students should have six semester credits of inorganic chemistry, organic chemistry, and biology. Nine credits are expected in physics and mathematics. Twelve semester hours are required in French and philosophy. Factors that influence the selection process include the reputation of the predental college, official transcripts, class rank, and scores on the Canadian DAT.

Student Body

Of the 83 enrolled students, 39 are women. The average age is 21.5. Most students possess a bachelor's degree. Only five students come from outside the province of Montreal. There are no foreign students. Applicants must be Canadian residents.

Costs

Each year's class will pay a tuition of $1,078 whether residency is established in Montreal or not. Instruments and books will cost close to $4,100. In addition, there is a $40 microscope rental fee. Students should allow $5,298 for the first year's expenses and at least $16,134 for the four-year program.

Financial Aid

Students wishing to serve in the Canadian military can be eligible to earn support through the Canadian Armed Forces. Scholarships are also available from the province of Quebec and the federal government. Special loan funds are offered to sophomores and juniors by the Faculté under certain restrictions.

Curriculum

With no summer sessions, the curriculum consists of eight 15-week semesters. The first two years are devoted to the study of basic sciences, while clinical training is reserved for the final two years. Students of the senior class rotate through hospitals to become familiar with dental surgery procedures and pedodontics. Faculty funds for research are of limited proportions for seniors.

Facilities

There is a computerized system which calculates student performance by measuring clinical performance with actual student ability. In addition, audiovisual facilities and the computer center are available for student and faculty use.

Grading Procedures

Quantitative and qualitative factors are considered. Clinical performance is determined by a number/point system.

Application Procedures

The application period runs from January 1 to March 1. There is a $15 application fee. Students should receive word of acceptance by July. The Faculté does not participate in the AADSAS.

Contact

Université de Montreal
C.P. 6205 Succ. A.
Montreal, Quebec, Canada H3C 3T5
(514) 343-2221

UNIVERSITY OF SASKATCHEWAN COLLEGE OF DENTISTRY

Saskatoon, Saskatchewan
Canada S7N 0W0
(306) 966-5117

Accreditation	CDA
Degrees Offered	D.M.D.
# Students Applied	70
Enrollment	21 / class
Mean GPA	Not Available
% Men / % Women	67% / 33%
% Minorities	Not Available
Tuition	$2,250
Application Fee	None
Application Deadline	February 28

The University

The University of Saskatchewan College of Dentistry was established in 1965 in Saskatoon. It became Canada's ninth school of dentistry. Research and continuing education programs have been established at the college, and a graduate studies program is in the developmental stages.

Admissions

One year of undergraduate work is required for admission. Students must take the Canadian DAT and be citizens of Canada or have landed immigrant status. Grades, trend in scholastic achievement, personality, physical fitness, Saskatchewan residency status, and letters of recommendation or references are considered in the selection of students. There are no set requirements in terms of DAT scores or GPA.

Undergraduate Preparation

Eligible students must study for one year at the University of Saskatchewan College of Arts and Science where they must complete the following courses: English 110, Literature 110 or a language course numbered 120, Biology 110, Chemistry 110, Physics 111, and either Psychology 110, Sociology 110, Philosophy 110, or Anthropology 110.

Student Body

Of the 70 students that applied in 1989-90, 21 were enrolled. Seven of these students were women. The ages of the students ranged from 19 to 23 with a mean age of 20. Most students had either four years of undergraduate work with no degree or a Bachelor of Science degree. All of the students came from Saskatchewan.

Costs

Tuition is $2,250 each year or $11,250 over the course of the five-year program. Other expenses include a $60 student activity fee and $1,000 for rental of a microscope per year. Students can expect to pay a total of $8,600 for instruments and $3,250 for books for all five years.

Financial Aid

Students may apply for scholarships, loans, and bursaries directly from the university.

Curriculum

The D.M.D. program covers five years of study. Basic sciences comprise the majority of courses during the first years with a few courses in dental sciences. By the third year, most of the courses focus on the dental sciences. First year students study biochemistry, cell biology, oral biology, organic chemistry, gross anatomy, embryology, physiology, histology, introduction to clinical dentistry, restorative dentistry, and occlusion. During the second year, courses include microbiology, neuroanatomy, oral biology including oral biochemistry and physiology, general pathology, pharmacology, social and preventative dentistry, periodontics, prosthodontics, diagnosis and oral radiology and restorative dentistry including operative and fixed prosthodontics. Third year courses encompass microbiology, general pathology, oral biology including oral pathology, oral medicine, oral surgery and anesthesiology, orthodontics, endodontics and social and preventative dentistry in private practice. Oral biology, clinical techniques, oral medicine and practice management are part of the fourth-year curriculum. The last year concentrates on oral biology, diagnosis and oral radiology, oral surgery and anesthesiology, pediatric dentistry including pediodontics and orthodontics, periodontics, prosthodontics, restorative dentistry including operative, fixed prosthodontics and endodontics, and social and preventative dentistry with seminars in dentistry and office and practice management.

Facilities

The Dental College Clinical Building is located adjacent to the Health Science Building. Students participate in clinical experiences in the Hospital Dental Department of the University Hospital.

Special Programs

During the fifth year, students who have completed all other requirements may participate in an option program where they choose classes from other departments in the college or at another university as approved by the curriculum committee.

Application Procedures

Applications must be filed by February 28. Applicants will learn of their acceptance between June and July.

Contact

Office of the Dean
College of Dentistry
University of Saskatchewan
Saskatoon, Sask., Canada S7N 0W0
(306) 966-5117

UNIVERSITY OF TORONTO FACULTY OF DENTISTRY

124 Edward Street
Toronto, Ontario
Canada M5G 1G6
(416) 979-4373

Accreditation	CDA
Degrees Offered	D.D.S., D.D.S./Ph.D.
# Students Applied	621
Enrollment	64 / class
Mean GPA	2.7
% Men / % Women	58% / 42%
% Minorities	Not Available
Tuition	$2,084
Application Fee	$50
Application Deadline	February 1

Admissions

Students applying for admission must have completed at least two years at a university in order to enter the D.D.S. program. The undergraduate minimum GPA should be at least 2.7. Although the Canadian Dental Association Aptitude Test is a requirement, scores are not taken into consideration as part of the criteria for admission. Students whose first language is not English are required to take a test of English proficiency. Applicants must be Canadian citizens, permanent residents, or hold student visas and be sponsored by an international agency. Selection is based upon scholarship, the applicant statement, and letters of reference.

Undergraduate Preparation

Applicants should have completed the following courses: a full course in first year biology, chemistry, physics, and organic chemistry, all with lab. Courses in English, the humanities, social sciences, and advanced biology are strongly suggested.

Placement Records

Among the career opportunities available to graduates are general practice, hospital internships, postgraduate diplomas, M.Sc. and Ph.D. graduate degrees, and research and university teaching.

Costs

Tuition during the 1990-91 academic year was $2,084. Campus services and student societies cost $255 and costs for dental instruments totaled $3,899. Other costs include $3,500 for housing, $2,800 for food and meals, $480 for clothing, and $800 for books and supplies.

Financial Aid

Specific information regarding financial aid is available from the Faculty of Dentistry. Students may request Ontario Student Assistance Program applications from the financial aid office. Outstanding first-year students are invited to apply for the Tom Lykos Memorial Scholarship by sending a letter of application by February 1.

Curriculum

During the first year, coursework focuses on an introduction to dental materials, restorative dentistry, and the development of digital skills through classes in biochemistry, biomaterials science, community dentistry, gross anatomy, histology, clinical and preventative dentistry, nutrition, oral anatomy and occlusion, oral biochemistry, oral biology, physiology, and restorative dentistry. Second-year classes emphasize basic sciences and the treatment and prevention of oral disease. Clinical study begins during the third year as an addition to coursework. During the fourth year, clinical practice continues along with courses dealing with more advanced treatment, electives, clinical conferences, and hospital visits.

Special Programs

The University of Toronto Faculty of Dentistry and School of Graduate Studies offers a joint Doctor of Dental Surgery/ Doctor of Philosophy program in preparation for academic or biomedical research in dentistry. Eligible candidates will already have been admitted to the D.D.S. program and be able to fulfill the requirements of the School of Graduate Studies and the Graduate Department. Applicants should apply to the Faculty of Dentistry for admission to the D.D.S. program and send a letter to the Chairman of the Graduate Department of Dentistry informing the Chairman of application to the D.D.S. program along with a curriculum vitae and two letters of reference to be sent separately.

Application Procedures

Applications are available from the admission office of the Faculty of Dentistry as of August 1. A signed and completed application form, a $50 application service fee, a photocopy of proof of Canadian citizenship, proof of English facility, if applicable, and the applicant statement are due in the Admission Office by February 1. Transcripts and certificates should be sent directly to the admission office by February 1. Current-year transcripts are due by June 28.

Contact

Admission Office
Faculty of Dentistry
124 Edward Street
Toronto, Ontario, Canada M5G 1G6
(416) 979-4373

UNIVERSITY OF WESTERN ONTARIO FACULTY OF DENTISTRY

London, Ontario
Canada N6A 5C1
(519) 679-2111

Accreditation	CDA
Degrees Offered	D.D.S., M.S.
# Students Applied	500
Enrollment	40 / class
Mean GPA	Not Available
% Men / % Women	75% / 25%
% Minorities	Not Available
Tuition	$1,929
Application Fee	Contact School
Application Deadline	December 3

The University

The University of Western Ontario Faculty of Dentistry has a longstanding reputation of achievement in dental education and research. The faculty offers the D.D.S. degree in a comprehensive program of study.

Admissions

Admission is competitive. Out of about 500 applications, the faculty accepts 40 students per year. A range of factors is considered in the admissions process. Academic criteria as well as DAT scores are examined. The Canadian DAT is required. Competitive candidates have an "A" (80 percent) average in two of the preprofessional years. Personal qualities and personal references are also important factors in the admissions decision.

Undergraduate Preparation

Full-year laboratory courses in biology, chemistry, and physics are required. In addition, a full-year lab course in organic chemistry is also required. Students must have several courses at the honors level, including organic chemistry. Because curricula vary among universities, students are encouraged to contact the Faculty of Dentistry for assistance in adequately meeting the course requirements.

Student Body

Twenty-five percent of the 40 students admitted in 1989 are women. More than half the class had undergraduate degrees; 50 percent were between 20 and 22 years of age. All but two students were from the Ontario region.

Placement Records

Graduates are extremely successful in the profession, and most become associates in dental practice in the province of Ontario upon graduation. Those from other provinces usually return to their home province to practice. A few open their own practices upon graduation.

Costs

Tuition (1990-91) for Canadian citizens (or permanent residents) was $1,929. The instrument fee (including the purchase or rental of instruments, equipment, materials, lab costs, and books) is $4,235 for the first year. These costs decrease in subsequent years. Foreign students should contact the Faculty of Dentistry for information on tuition.

Financial Aid

Most financial assistance will come from the Ontario Student Assistance Program, which is government funded. This helps students who are residents of Ontario and who show financial need.

Curriculum

The curriculum presents the basics in the first two years and the primary clinical experience—patient care—in the last two years. It is a challenging program, designed to prepare graduates for the demands of health care into the 21st century.

The first two years consist of the basic medical and dental sciences, clinical sciences, and clinical methods that make up the foundation of practice. Students are exposed to topics such as biomaterials, community dentistry, and operative dentistry, and have their first clinical experience in an introductory course.

Second-year courses emphasize clinical aspects of practice and are meant to prepare students for the third and fourth years of clinical experience and hospital-based elective study. Second-year topics include anesthesia, oral medicine and radiology, endodontics, and fixed and removable prosthodontics.

The third and fourth years consist of increasing amounts of time caring for patients and attending specialty clinics. Students will participate in clinical rotations and hospital-based electives. In these years, students are also trained in the management aspects of private practice.

Facilities

Students practice and study in both dental clinics and affiliated hospitals in London, Ontario. Facilities for dental students are considered state-of-the-art.

Special Programs

The faculty offers postgraduate specialty training in orthodontics and oral pathology. For more in-depth study, including graduate research, students can pursue the M.S. or clinical dentistry degrees.

Application Procedures

Application is made directly to Western's Faculty of Dentistry. Applications are usually available in early October. The application deadline is December 3 of the year preceding the year of intended enrollment. The admissions committee generally notifies candidates of acceptance by late June.

Contact

Admissions Secretary
Faculty of Dentistry
University of Western Ontario
Dental Sciences Centre
London, Ontario
Canada N6A 5C1
(519) 679-2111, ext. 6137

REA's Problem Solvers

The "PROBLEM SOLVERS" are comprehensive supplemental text-books designed to save time in finding solutions to problems. Each "PROBLEM SOLVER" is the first of its kind ever produced in its field. It is the product of a massive effort to illustrate almost any imaginable problem in exceptional depth, detail, and clarity. Each problem is worked out in detail with a step-by-step solution, and the problems are arranged in order of complexity from elementary to advanced. Each book is fully indexed for locating problems rapidly.

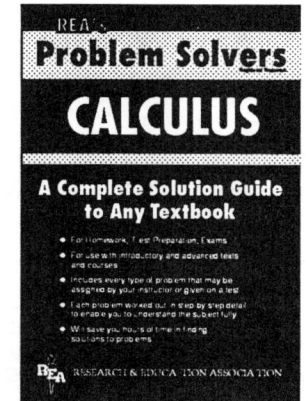

ADVANCED CALCULUS
ALGEBRA & TRIGONOMETRY
AUTOMATIC CONTROL
   SYSTEMS/ROBOTICS
BIOLOGY
BUSINESS, MANAGEMENT, & FINANCE
CALCULUS
CHEMISTRY
COMPLEX VARIABLES
COMPUTER SCIENCE
DIFFERENTIAL EQUATIONS
ECONOMICS
ELECTRICAL MACHINES
ELECTRIC CIRCUITS
ELECTROMAGNETICS
ELECTRONIC COMMUNICATIONS
ELECTRONICS
FINITE & DISCRETE MATH
FLUID MECHANICS/DYNAMICS
GENETICS
GEOMETRY

HEAT TRANSFER
LINEAR ALGEBRA
MACHINE DESIGN
MATHEMATICS for ENGINEERS
MECHANICS
NUMERICAL ANALYSIS
OPERATIONS RESEARCH
OPTICS
ORGANIC CHEMISTRY
PHYSICAL CHEMISTRY
PHYSICS
PRE-CALCULUS
PSYCHOLOGY
STATISTICS
STRENGTH OF MATERIALS &
   MECHANICS OF SOLIDS
TECHNICAL DESIGN GRAPHICS
THERMODYNAMICS
TOPOLOGY
TRANSPORT PHENOMENA
VECTOR ANALYSIS

If you would like more information about any of these books,
complete the coupon below and return it to us or go to your local bookstore.

RESEARCH & EDUCATION ASSOCIATION
61 Ethel Road W. • Piscataway, New Jersey 08854
Phone: (908) 819-8880

Please send me more information about your Problem Solver Books

Name _____

Address _____

City _____ State _____ Zip _____

REA's Test Preps
The Best in Test Preparations

The REA "Test Preps" are far more comprehensive than any other test series. They contain more tests with much more extensive explanations than others on the market. Each book provides several complete practice exams, based on the most recent tests given in the particular field. Every type of question likely to be given on the exams is included. Each individual test is followed by a complete answer key. **The answers are accompanied by full and detailed explanations.** By studying each test and the pertinent explanations, students will become well-prepared for the actual exam.

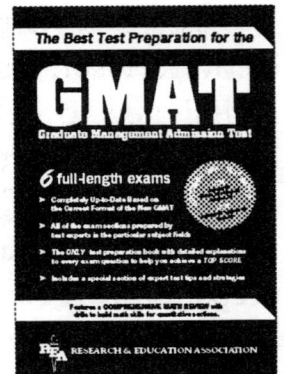

REA has published 20 Test Preparation volumes in several series. They include:

Advanced Placement Exams
Biology
Calculus AB & Calculus BC
Chemistry
English Literature & Composition
European History
United States History

College Board Achievement Tests
American History
Biology
Chemistry
English Composition
French
German
Spanish
Literature
Mathematics Level I & II

Graduate Record Exams
Biology
Chemistry
Computer Science
Economics
Engineering
General
Literature in English
Mathematics
Physics
Psychology

FE - Fundamentals of Engineering Exam
GMAT - Graduate Management Admission Test
MCAT - Medical College Admission Test
NTE - National Teachers Exam
SAT - Scholastic Aptitude Test
LSAT - Law School Admission Test
TOEFL - Test of English as a Foreign Language

RESEARCH & EDUCATION ASSOCIATION
61 Ethel Road W. • Piscataway, New Jersey 08854
Phone: (908) 819-8880

Please send me more information about your Test Prep Books

Name _____

Address _____

City _____ State _____ Zip _____

"The ESSENTIALS" of Math & Science

Each book in the ESSENTIALS series offers all essential information of the field it covers. It summarizes what every textbook in the particular field must include, and is designed to help students in preparing for exams and doing homework. The ESSENTIALS are excellent supplements to any class text.

The ESSENTIALS are complete, concise, with quick access to needed information, and provide a handy reference source at all times. The ESSENTIALS are prepared with REA's customary concern for high professional quality and student needs.

Available in the following titles:

Advanced Calculus I & II
Algebra & Trigonometry I & II
Anthropology
Automatic Control Systems /
    Robotics I & II
Biology I & II
Boolean Algebra
Calculus I, II & III
Chemistry
Complex Variables I & II
Differential Equations I & II
Electric Circuits I & II
Electromagnetics I & II
Electronic Communications I & II

Electronics I & II
Finite & Discrete Math
Fluid Mechanics /
    Dynamics I & II
Fourier Analysis
Geology
Geometry I & II
Group Theory I & II
Heat Transfer I & II
LaPlace Transforms
Linear Algebra
Mechanics I, II & III
Modern Algebra

Numerical Analysis I & II
Organic Chemistry I & II
Physical Chemistry I & II
Physics I & II
Real Variables
Set Theory
Statistics I & II
Strength of Materials &
    Mechanics of Solids I & II
Thermodynamics I & II
Topology
Transport Phenomena I & II
Vector Analysis

*If you would like more information about any of these books,
complete the coupon below and return it to us or go to your local bookstore.*

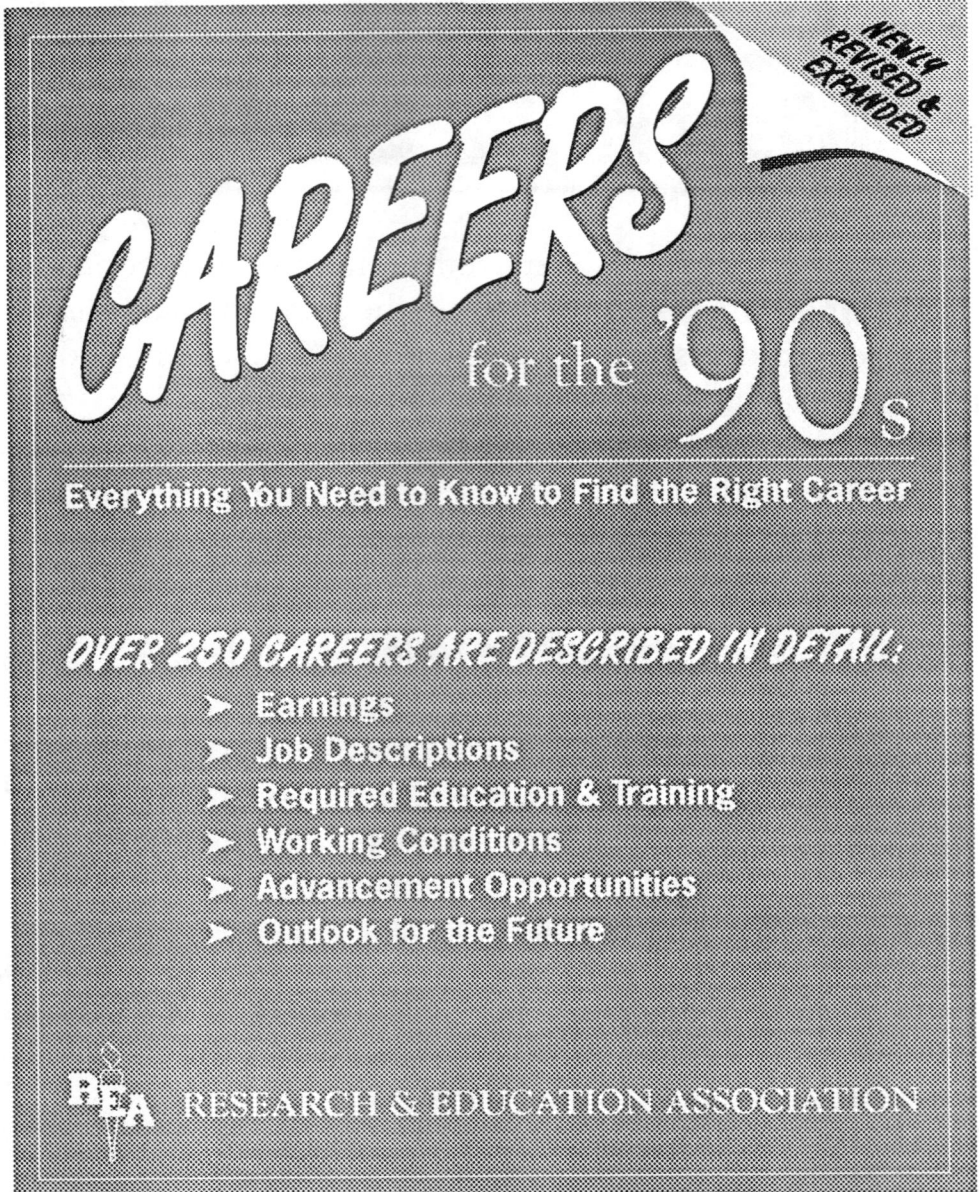

Available at your local bookstore or order directly from us by sending in coupon below.

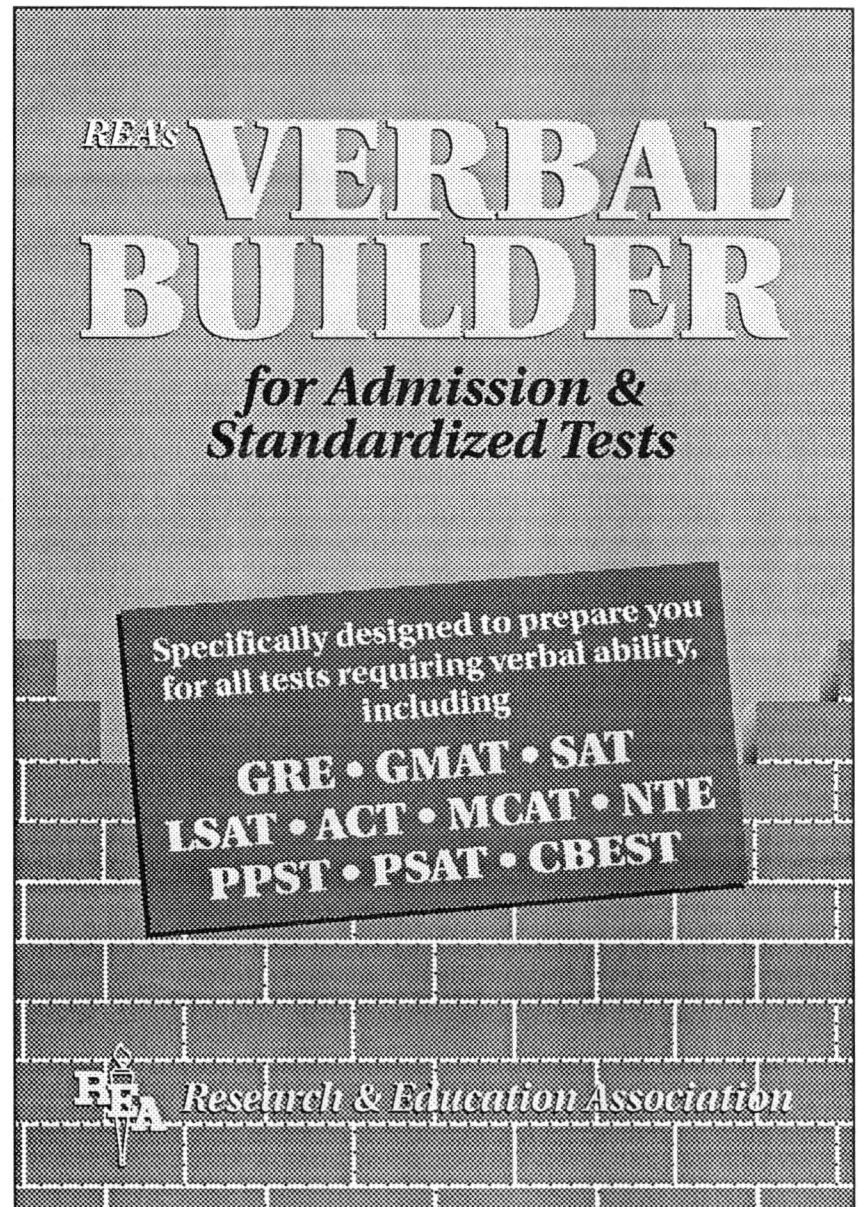

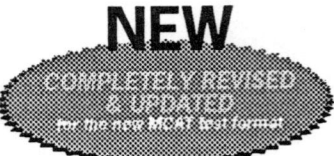
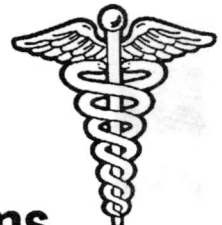